SYNTHETIC REPERTORY

Karl F. Haug Verlag GmbH & Co.

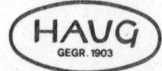

(HAUG) GEGR. 1903

Fritz-Frey-Straße 21
Postfach 10 28 40
Tel. ✆ 0 62 21 / 4 99 74
Telex 4 61 683 hvvfm d

6900 Heidelberg 1

Karl F. Haug Verlag GmbH & Co., Postfach 10 28 40, 6900 Heidelberg 1

Geschäftsleitung

Ihr Zeichen	Ihre Nachricht	Unser Zeichen	Datum
			April 24, 1987

Dear reader:

This is the only legal edition of the SYNTHETIC REPERTORY in English language published by B. Jain Publishers (P) Ltd. and no other publisher is authorized to print and distribute the English edition of the book.

If he does so, this is illegal and the publisher can take legal action.

Dr. E. Fischer

- Publisher -

SYNTHETIC REPERTORY

Psychic and General Symptoms
of the Homoeopathic Materia Medica

Published by
Dr. med. Horst Barthel, Wilhelmsfeld

Volume II: General Symptoms

Dr. med. Horst Barthel, Wilhelmsfeld

4th improved edition

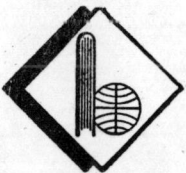

B. Jain Publishers (P) Ltd.

CIP-Kurztitelaufnahme der Deutschen Bibliothek

Synthetic repertory: psychic and general symptoms of the homoeopathic materia medica = Répertoire synthétique = Synthetisches Repertorium / publ. by Horst Barthel. – Heidelberg : Haug
  ISBN 3-7760-0925-X
NE: Barthel, Horst [Hrsg.]; 1. PT; 2. PT
Vol. 1. Psychic symptoms / Horst Barthel. Trad. en français P. Schmidt ; J. Baur. – 3. impr. ed. – 1987.
  ISBN 3-7760-0892-X

Published in India by :

B. Jain Publishers (P) Ltd.

1921, Street 10, Chuna Mandi,
Paharganj, New Delhi-110055
Post Box : 5775
Gram : BOOKCENTRE. Phones : 7770430, 7770572
Fax : 91-11-7510471

Reprint 1993

Price : **Rs. 500** (Indian Edition)

© 1973 Karl F. Haug Verlag Heidelberg

2. Auflage 1982
3. Auflage 1987

Printed at :
J. J. Offset Printers
Kishan Kunj, Delhi - 110 092

ISBN 81-7021-183-2
ISBN 81-7021-185-9
BOOK CODE B-2045

To the master and teacher of Hahnemannian Homoeopathy

Dr. med. Jost Künzli von Fimelsberg
St. Gallen

PREFACE

Over the years the plan to supplement and continue Kent's repertory was influenced by various intermediate concepts and resulted in the present Synthetic Repertory. The resumption of the original title was the result of a threefold synthesis: the supplement from the oldest to the latest homeopathic literature, the register of equivalents and related symptoms, and the composition of individual subjects, as for example, complaints due to psychic trauma.

Progress in homeopathy comes about on the one hand by collecting materia medica and composing it practically for the repertory, and on the other hand by adding symptoms of newly proven drugs. Therefore colleagues are kindly requested by the authors to cooperate with them in increasing the verification of drugs. Furthermore, help is requested in eliminating mistakes carried over from other sources, and others which the authors have overlooked.

The trilinguality brought about problems of translation for the German speaking authors. In most cases the English titles could be used as originally stated. Dr. Pierre Schmidt of Geneva undertook with great competence the very difficult task of translating the mental symptoms. He also translated the preface and the introduction for this volume. In addition the French versions of the third volume were improved by his critical revision. The authors extend to him their warmest thanks for his work in the translation, and are grateful for all the advice and understanding with which Dr. P. Schmidt assisted them in the creation of this work. Dr. Roger Schmidt and Mr. Alain Naude of San Francisco revised the English version of the preface and the introduction for this volume. The authors feel very obliged to them.

Mr. Dr. med. Jacques Baur, Lyon, was not only the french translater of all the titles in Vol. II, he also translated the new additional symptoms in this volume. We give our special gratitude for his valuable help!

The publishers thank Mr. Dr. med. Jost Künzli von Fimmelsberg, St. Gallen, for the permission of printing his supplements in the new edition which he took out of the classic homoeopathic literature into his own Repertory. In that way his long and unprecedented struggle about the sources, especially about Hahnemann's Arzneimittellehren is now made publicly known and available for everyone.

We give our gratitute to Mr. Dr. med. Artur Braun, to Dr. med. Klaus-Henning Gypser and Dr. A. Rehman, Lahore (Vol I–III), for some corrections of Vol. III and we also like to give our thanks to Mr. Martin Weber, Genf, for his help in translating the new french rubrics in Vol. III.

To Dr. Herbert Schindler of Karlsruhe, who contributed significantly to the international nomenclature of homeopathic drugs, the authors are indebted for much information, as well as for the corrections and the final verification of the drug index.

The editors wish to express their thanks to the authors of publications included in this work: to Dr. O. A. Julian† of Paris, Dr. J. Mezger† of Stuttgart, Dr. Pierre Schmidt of Geneva, and Dr. J. Stephenson of New York, for their kind permission to use their publications. We wish also to thank the publishers Peyronnet of Paris, Masson of Paris, Roy & Co. of Bombay, and Ternet-Martin of Vienne (Isere).

Dr. E. Fischer, publisher, and Mr. Sieber, production manager, have been responsible for making this book as practical as possible, by responding in the most cooperative manner to all our proposals concerning the book and its printing design. To them we wish to express our special thanks.

INTRODUCTION

The need for the repertory comes from the character of homeopathy itself. Homeopathy means medical action according to the law of similars of Hahnemann (1755–1843): similia similibus curentur. According to this law the drug picture and the characteristic symptoms of the patient have to agree to an optimum degree. Thus we seek the simillimum for the patient.

In the Homeomethodology the homeopathic materia medica is the means by which the results of drug provings and clinical observation of drugs are classified. In practice the choise of a drug needs the classification of drugs according to symptoms. The repertory serves that purpose. The materia medica contains the symptoms of drugs and the repertory relates the drugs to the symptoms. Through the repertory the doctrine of drugs and therapy according to symptoms complement each other.

In the beginning of homeopathy the drug symptoms had already increased to such a degree that it seemed impossible to bear them all in mind. Therefore in 1817 Hahnemann developed the first of his two "symptomdictionaries", which was the first repertory. Compared with the partial information of the materia medica remembered by chance, the repertory permits the choice of a drug through extensive homeopathic knowledge.

Until now almost 110 repertories have been published. The "Repertory of the Homeopathic Materia Medica" by J. T. Kent (1849–1916) is the most appropriate, most complete, and most reliable of all. Kent used older works of the materia medica and clinical observations, but refused numerous insufficiently confirmed symptoms and drugs. Until his death he added by hand into his own copies new symptoms and drugs, and classified them according to his own experience into various degrees.

To keep the repertory continually up to date requires the preservation of symptoms and drugs not listed in Kent's repertory, and also their confirmation by cures. It is also of great importance to make available the primary and repeated provings of younger authors.

Supplements to general and particular symptoms result in a multitude of material which requires a decision as to whether we should limit the number of authors and headings, or whether we should list only the general symptoms. Since the general symptoms will affect the choice of drugs for chronic patients, this Synthetic Repertory is limited to general symptoms. For particulars Kent s "Repertory" is still the best reference book.

According to the hierarchy of general symptoms the Synthetic Repertory is separated into the following three volumes: Vol. I contains the mental symptoms, Vol. II contains the general symptoms in a more selective way. The symptoms for food and drink which in Kent's repertory are separated into different chapters and headings according to aggravation, improvement, aversion and desire, are now summed up in one single heading. Vol. III contains the chapters of sleep symptoms and dreams, as well as the male and female sexual symptoms.

Sources of the Synthetic Repertory

1. KENT, J. T.: Kent's repertory is a climax in the evolution of the repertory because of its extensive contents and logical structure, its moderation between the generalizations and differentiations of tendencies found in other authors, and

finally its reliability and practicability. For more than 70 years it has proven true all over the world; the English version is available in the 6th American and the 3rd Indian edition. There exists a French translation in extracts; a German translation appeared in 1971, in its 2nd edition. The chapters and headings of the above mentioned general symptoms are totally included. Mistakes detected during the last revision were corrected. As further sources Kent's "Lectures on Homeopathic Materia Medica" and "New Remedies" were used.

2. KNERR, C. B.: With his "Guiding Symptoms" C. Hering wrote a classic materia medica of 10 volumes supported by clinical experience. Hering's student Knerr transformed this work into a repertory of two volumes. These detailed empirical data concerning modalities and clinical symptoms are difficult to understand for lack of clarity in the way they are set out; this disadvantage is eliminated in the Synthetic Repertory.

3. VON BOENNINGHAUSEN, C.; BOGER, C. M.: The repertory written by v. Boenninghausen on the advice of Hahnemann was the first repertory to be published, and is still in use. The Synthetic Repertory has used C. M. Boger's English translation and supplement. We have taken into consideration a certain tendency to generalize in this work: the inclusion of modalities into main headings and local symptoms into general symptoms, for instance.

In the 2nd. edition we added symptoms and remedies from C. M. Boger's "Additions to Kent's Repertory" and from his Repertory in "A Synoptic Key of the Materia Medica". By technical reasons we gave all these additions the index number 3.

4. JAHR, G. H. G.: His "Systematic-alphabetic repertory of homeopathic remedy doctrine" which appeared in 1848–49 and is no longer available is noted for its comprehensive listing of symptoms. But because it is split up into synonyms and because of its arrangement it is not practical.

5. GALLAVARDIN, J. P.: In his experience of mental diseases Gallavardin tested and extended the drugs which treat psychiatric patients, which Dulac took from the works of Jahr. The repertory and the materia medica from "Psychisme et Homeopathie", published after the author's death, have been used as sources.

6. STAUFFER, K.: The "Symptom-index" represents Stauffer's vast and critically controlled practical experiences. Apart from verifying drug symptoms it also conveys new additions to the materia medica.

7. SCHMIDT, P.: The supplements by 35 authors to his four repertories of Kent have been integrally included. Further material from the courses of the "Groupement Hahnemannien de Lyon", which have been published in the reports of those meetings, have been included. P. Schmidt obtained his homeopathic knowledge in direct line from Kent, and was instructed by Kent's collaborators in the technical details of establishing the repertory. This, and his 50 years of practical experience, have given him the authority to classify higher grades, and to introduce the fourth grade of drugs in the case of several symptoms. This fourth grade of drugs has been especially useful to him whenever there have been no differentiating symptoms allowing him to consider other drugs under the same heading.

8. BOERICKE, O. E.: The materia medica of W. Boericke, which has been widely used in the English-speaking world, was transcribed into a repertory by O. E. Boericke. It has the advantage of presenting a great many new drugs in English. However, it does not contain a list of drug abbreviations, and there are mistakes

in the nomenclature of the drugs and the symptom complex. Its classification is not always consistent.

9. STEPHENSON, J.: This work, which is laid out as clearly as Kent's repertory, contains drug provings of the years 1924–59, which originate especially from the English and German-speaking countries.

10. MEZGER, J.: The symptoms of 35 reproven or new drugs have been taken from his critical work "Gesichtete Homeopathische Arzneimittellehre" (Selected Homeopathic materia medica).

11. ALLEN, T. F.: The ten volumes of the "Encyclopedia of Pure Materia Medica", which only contain pure drug symptoms, have a two-volume index, "A General Symptom Register of the Homeopathic Materia Medica", of which pertinent parts were added to the Synthetic Repertory. They provide access to the older proven symptoms for future verification. They also contain numerous rare remedies.

12. CLARKE, J. H.: His "A Clinical Repertory to the Dictionary of Materia Medica" from his three-volume materia medica, remaining to this day one of the best, reports mainly clinical indications and rare drugs.

13. The most recent drug provings published in various journals.

14. JULIAN, O. A.: His "Matière Médicale d'Homéothérapie" of 1971 is up to the present day the most complete summary of drug provings in the international literature. We incorporated it even though we had completed the manuscript. The 2nd edition contains also the ca. 30 remedies, supplementary published by Dr. Julian in his new edition of this work, now titled "Dictionnaire de Matière Médicale de 130 Nouveaux Homéothérapeutiques" by Masson, Paris (1981).

15. KÜNZLI, J.: Supplements taken from the international homoeopathic literature.

16. HAHNEMANN, S.: "Pure Materia Medica" and "Chronic diseases". Symptoms and remedies which are missing in Kent's Repertory are added according to the supplements of Künzli.

The abbreviation of the tuberculinum not otherwise defined by the authors 2, 6, 7, and 8 is tub., as for the tuberculinum Kent.

The Synthetic Repertory mentions for the first time the exact sources of symptoms or drugs added to Kent's repertory, and uses a numbering system. Symptoms and drugs from Kent's original repertory have not been numbered. Additions made by Kent in his own hand are marked[1], supplements from his "Lectures" and "New Remedies" by[1'], the figures[2-14] coincide with the enumeration of the above mentioned sources. According to Pierre Schmidt, his and Gallavardin's experiences justify classifications of certain drugs of Kent into higher grades. These drugs are marked by both figures, as[1,5] or[1,7]. Since we mention the sources of this material the reader can decide for himself the importance of the authors quoted, and test their indications in the light of his own practical experience.

The corrections of Kent which he made personally in his own Repertory, owned later on by Mr. Dr. Pierre Schmidt were now published by Mr. Dr. D. H. Chand ("Kent's Final General Repertory", New Delhi, 1980). But we had already used them in the 1st edition of the "Synthetic Repertory", and therefore there was now no reason to take them into consideration anymore.

Different gradings of the drugs were found in the sources. These were adapted to the three grades of Kent with a certain amount of liberty. As the individual gradings could not be indicated for drugs added from various sources, the highest grade from among those sources has been indicated.

The grades of the drugs are clearly differentiated in print. Drugs of the first and second grades are printed in small letters, those of the second, third and fourth in bold type, those of the third and fourth in capitals, those of the fourth in underlined capitals.

The transformation of the drugs into the grading system of the Synthetic Repertory, and the transformation of varying arrangements of systems in the sources into the present system of headings, making the clearest possible differentiations, has demanded serious and difficult decisions.

The headings are indicated by printing-type, indentation and spacing. In the main heading the key word of the symptom title is printed in bold type capitals, in the sub-heading, in bold type only, whilst times of day, clock-times, and other sub-headings are printed in ordinary type. The main headings start at the beginning of a line, the first indentation indicates the first sub-heading, the second indentation indicates the next sub-heading, and so on. Each indented title refers to the key word of the main title. Under each symptom title the remedies are printed in normal spacing to show that they belong together.

The titles were partly clarified by supplements, whereas in Vol. I – delusions – and in Vol. III – dreams – they were simplified by using the indicative or the infinitive.

Headings and symptom titles are given in English, French, and German, with the exception of clock-times and Latin terms. The English titles were mostly taken from the English literature, without changing American expressions and spelling. Most of the French and German titles are translations from the English whenever they have been found in existing French and German sources.

The preference given to English titles comes from the importance of the English literature on Homeopathy, and the importance of English as a world language. French represents the languages of the Latin-American continent and South Europe.

The abbreviations agg. and am. have been used in all languages to mean the modalities of aggravation and amelioration respectively. They are to be understood as nouns or verbs, as the case may be.

For French- and German-speaking readers there is a complete and clearly arranged index at the end of each volume which uses the column numbering of the repertory to locate any required heading. Since the English listing of symptoms is already alphabetical, the English index is limited to synonyms and cross references (in vol. I, II). In addition the use of the repertory is facilitated by many references among the symptoms and in the index. The asterisk of the titles of symptoms refers to one of 138 new collected rubrics of the index of vol. I and II.

The remedy index of the Synthetic Repertory lists abbreviations of the drugs in alphabetical order, and, after each abbreviation, the remedy and its synonym. It contains 1594 drugs, whilst Kent's index contains 591. Obsolete drugs like Electricitas. Galvanism, Magnes Artificialis and the complex snake drug ophiotoxicum were not retained. Double entries, lack of clarity, and wrong nomenclature were corrected wherever possible. The traditional nomenclature of homeopathic drugs has been in use for the last 170 years, and this establishes its priority over the modern pharmacological, pharmaceutic terminology. Since homeopathic drugs have always been used in the same way, homeopathic literature remains valid regardless of its age, and can only be understood in the traditional nomenclature.

For practical reasons Kent's abbreviations have been kept, in spite of certain inconsistencies like arg-m. and nat-m. Only inconsistent abbreviations of small drugs were changed. The different abbreviations in the sources, including those of Clarke, were changed to conform to the more comprehensible, accentuated abbreviations of Kent. We tried to establish a uniform abbreviation throughout, e. g. ar. for the anion arsenicosum (compare with Kent's kali-ar. and nat-a.).

Whenever possible wrong spellings of drug abbreviations in the literature have been corrected.

In the field of general symptoms the Synthetic Repertory represents the synthesis of the homeopathic knowledge of the last 170 years. By internationalizing the nomenclature of the drugs, by using three languages for the symptoms and the indexes, we hope to have contributed to a closer understanding among homeopathic physicians in the world. The common language of homeopathic physicians can only come from commonly used terms for drugs and symptoms.

Dr. med. Horst Barthel   Dr. med. Will Klunker
Alte Römerstraße 70   Am Rosenberg 1375
D-6901 Wilhelmsfeld   CH-9410 Heiden

BIBLIOGRAPHY/BIBLIOGRAPHIE/BIBLIOGRAPHIE

1 KENT, J. T.: Repertory of the Homoepathic Materia Medica. 6th Edition, Ehrhart & Chicago (1957)

Kent's Repertorium der homöopathischen Arzneimittel. Herausgegeben von G. v. Keller und J. Künzli von Fimelsberg. 2., verb. Auflage, Karl F. Haug Verlag, Heidelberg (1971)

KENT, J. T.: Lectures on Homoeopathic Materia Medica. 1st ind. Edition, M. Bhattacharyya, Calcutta (1965)

KENT, J. T.: New Remedies. Ind. Edition, Sett Dey & Co., Calcutta (1963) pp. 1—151

2 KNERR, C. B.: A Repertory of Hering's Guiding Symptoms of our Materia Medica. M. Bhattacharyya, Calcutta (1951)

3 BOGER, C. M.: Boenninghausens's Characteristics and Repertory. 2nd Edition, Roy & Co., Bombay (1952)

BOGER, C. M.: Additions to Kent's Repertory. Jain Publishing Co., Chuna Mandi, Paharganj, New Delhi-55 (1972)

BOGER, C. M.: A Synoptic Key of the Materia Medica. Salzer & Co., Calcutta 6th Edition

4 JAHR, G. H. G.: Systematisch-alphabetisches Repertorium der Homöopathischen Arzneimittellehre. Herrmann Bethmann, Leipzig (1848)

5 GALLAVARDIN, J.-P.: Psychisme et Homoeopathie. Ed. Ternet-Martin, Vienne (Isère) (1960)

6 STAUFFER, K.: Symptomen-Verzeichnis nebst vergleichenden Zusätzen zur Homöopathischen Arzneimittellehre. Joh. Sonntag, Regensburg (1951)

7 SCHMIDT, P.: Annotations in Kent's Repertory/Annotations dans le Repertoire de Kent/Anmerkungen in Kents Repertorium

SCHMIDT, P.: passim in: Groupement Hahnemannien de Lyon, Comptes rendus des réunions

8 BOERICKE, O. E.: Repertory; in: W. Boericke, Pocket Manual of Homoeopathic Materia Medica. 9th Edition, Boericke & Runyon, New York (1927)

9 STEPHENSON, J.: A Materia Medica and Repertory, Hahnemannian Provings 1924—1959. Roy & Co., Bombay (1963)

10 MEZGER, J.: Gesichtete Homöopathische Arzneimittellehre. 3. Auflage, Karl F. Haug Verlag, Ulm (1964, 1966)

11 ALLEN, T. F.: Index ("A General Symptom Register of the Homoeopathic Materia Medica"); in: The Encyclopedia of Pure Materia Medica, vol. XI, Gregg Press Inc., Ridgewood N. J. (1964)

12 CLARKE, J. H.: A Clinical Repertory to the Dictionary of Materia Medica. The Homoeopathic Publishing Comp., London (1904)

13 KLUNKER, W.: Eine Arzneiprüfung von Espeletia grandiflora. Allg. homöop. Ztg. 217: 5—14 (1972)

KLUNKER, W.: Zu den Rubriken der Säuglings- und Stillbeschwerden im Kentschen Repertorium, Ztschrft. f. Klass. Homöop. Bd. 17/6, 269—272 (1973)

LODISPOTO, A.: Diät und Homöopathie, Ztschrft. f. Klass. Homöop. Bd IV/3, 95-141 (1960)

SÉROR, R.: Pathogénésies homeopathiques françaises. Cahiers de Biothér. (1966), 79—86

14 JULIAN, O. A.: Matière Médicale d'Homéotherapie. Peyronnet, Paris (1971). Dictionnaire de Matière Médicale de 130 Nouveaux Homéothérapeutiques. Masson, Paris (1981)

15 KUNZLI, J.: Nachträge aus der internationalen homöopathischen Literatur

16 HAHNEMANN, S.: Reine Arzneimittellehre. 3., vermehrte Auflage. Dresden und Leipzig (1830), Nachdruck Karl F. Haug Verlag, Heidelberg (1979)

HAHNEMANN, S.: Die chronischen Krankheiten. 2., vermehrte Auflage. Dresden und
Leipzig (1835), Nachdruck Karl F. Haug Verlag, Heidelberg (1979)

REMEDIES AND THEIR ABBREVIATIONS

abel.	abelmoschus	agar.	agaricus muscarius
abies-c.	abies (pinus) canadensis	agar-cit.	agaricus citrinus
abies-n.	abies nigra	agar-cpn.	agaricus campanulatus
abr.	abrus precatorius	agar-cps.	agaricus campestris
		agar-em.	agaricus emeticus
abrot.	abrotanum	agar-pa.	agaricus pantherinus
		agar-ph.	agaricus phalloides
absin.	absinthium		
		agar-pr.	agaricus procerus
acal.	acalypha indica	agar-se.	agaricus semiglobatus
	acanthia lectularia	agar-st.	agaricus stercorarius
		agar-v.	agaricus vernus
		agarin.	agaricinum
acet-ac.	aceticum acidum	agav-a.	agave americana
acetan.	acetanilidum	agav-t.	agave tequilana
		agn.	agnus castus
		agra.	agraphis nutans
achy.	achyranthes calea	agre.	agremone ochroleuca
		agri.	agrimonia eupatoria
acon.	aconitum napellus		
acon-a.	aconitum anthora	agro.	agrostema githago
acon-c.	aconitum cammarum	ail.	ailanthus glandulosa
acon-f.	aconitum ferox	alco.	alcoholus
acon-l.	aconitum lycoctonum	ald.	aldehydum
acon-s.	aconitum septentrionale	alet.	aletris farinosa
aconin.	aconitinum	alf.	alfalfa
act-sp.	actaea spicata	all-c.	allium cepa
adel.	Adelheid aqua	all-s.	allium sativum
adeps-s.	adeps suis	allox.	alloxanum
adlu.	adlumia fungosa	aln.	alnus rubra
adon.	adonis vernalis	aloe	aloe socotrina
adonin.	adonidinum	alst.	alstonia constricta
adox.	adoxa moschatellina	alst-s.	alstonia scholaris
adren.	adrenalinum	alth.	althaea officinalis
		alum.	alumina
		alum-p.	alumina phosphorica
aesc.	aesculus hippocastanum	alum-sil.	alumina silicata
aesc-g.	aesculus glabra		
		alumin.	aluminium metallicum
aeth.	aethusa cynapium	alumin-a.	aluminium aceticum
aether	aether	alumin-m.	aluminium muriaticum
aethi-a.	aethiops antimonialis	alumn.	alumen
aethi-m.	aethiops mineralis		alumen chromicum
aethyi-n.	aethylium nitricum		

am-a.	ammonium aceticum	anil-s.	anilinum sulphuricum
		anis.	anisum stellatum
am-be.	ammonium benzoicum		antifebrinum = acetan.
am-br.	ammonium bromatum	ant-ar.	antimonium arsenicosum
am-c.	ammonium carbonicum	ant-c.	
am-caust.	ammonium causticum		
am-i.	ammonium iodatum	ant-i.	antimonium iodatum
am-m.	ammonium muriaticum	ant-m.	antimonium muriaticum
am-n.	ammonium nitricum	ant-o.	antimonium oxydatum
am-p.	ammonium phosphoricum	ant-s-aur.	antimonium sulphuratum
am-pic.	ammonium picricum		auratum
am-t.	ammonium tartaricum		
am-val.	ammonium valerianicum		
am-van.	ammonium vanadinicum	ant-t.	antimonium tartaricum
ambr.	ambra grisea		
ambro.	ambrosia artemisiaefolia		
amgd-p.	amygdalus persica	anth.	anthemis nobilis
aml-ns.	amylenum nitrosum	antho.	anthoxanthum odoratum
ammc.	ammoniacum gummi	anthraci.	anthracinum
amn-l.	amnii liquor	anthraco.	anthracokali
amor-r.	amorphophallus rivieri	antip.	antipyrinum
ampe-qu.	ampelopsis quinquefolia	ap-g.	apium graveolens
ampe-tr.	ampelopsis trifoliata	ap-v	apium virus
amph.	amphisbaena vermicularis	aphis	aphis chenopodii glauci
amyg.	amygdalae amarae aqua		
amylam.	amylaminum	apiol.	apiolum
		apis	apis mellifica
anac.	anacardium orientale	apisin.	apisinum
anac-oc.	anacardium occidentale	apoc.	apocynum cannabinum
anag.	anagallis arvensis	apoc-a.	apocynum
anagy.	anagyris foetida		androsaemifolium
anan.	anantherum muricatum	apom.	apomorphinum
		aq-calc.	aqua calcarea
		aq-chl.	aqua chlorata
		aq-mar.	aqua marina
		aq-pet.	aqua petra
andr.	androsace lactea		
ane-n.	anemone nemorosa	aq-sil.	aqua silicata
		aqui.	aquilegia vulgaris
ane-r.	anemone ranunculoides	arag.	aragallus lamberti
anemps.	anemopsis californica	aral.	aralia racemosa
		aral-h.	aralia hispida
ang.	angustura vera		
		aran.	aranea diadema
ange.	angelica atropurpurea		
ange-s.	radix angelicae sinensis	aran-ix.	aranea ixobola
ango.	angophora lanceolata	aran-sc.	aranea scinencia
anh.	anhalonium lewinii	aranin.	araninum
		arb.	arbutus andrachne
anil.	anilinum	arbin.	arbutinum

arec.	areca catechu	asper.	asperula odorata
aren.	arenaria glabra		
arg-cy.	argentum cyanatum		
arg-i.	argentum iodatum		
arg-m.	argentum metallicum		
arg-mur.	argentum muriaticum		
arg-n.	argentum nitricum	astac.	astacus (cancer) fluviatilis
arg-o.	argentum oxydatum	aster.	asterias rubens
arg-p.	argentum phosphoricum	astra-e.	astragalus excapus
arge.	argemone mexicana	astra-m.	astragalus menziesii
		atha.	athamanta oreoselinum
arist-cl.	aristolochia clematitis	atra-r.	atrax robustus
arist-co.	aristolochia colombiana	atri.	atriplex hortensis
arist-m.	aristolochia milhomens		
		atro.	atropinum
		aur.	aurum foliatum
arn.	arnica montana		
ars.	arsenicum album		
ars-br.	arsenicum bromatum	aur-ar.	aurum arsenicicum
ars-h.	arsenicum hydrogenisatum	aur-br.	aurum bromatum
ars-i.	arsenicum iodatum	aur-fu.	aurum fulminans
ars-met.	arsenicum metallicum		
ars-n.	arsenicum nitricum	aur-i.	aurum iodatum
ars-s-f.	arsenicum sulphuratum flavum	aur-m.	aurum muriaticum
		aur-m-k.	aurum muriaticum kalinatum
ars-s-r.	arsenicum sulphuratum rubrum	aur-m-n.	aurum muriaticum natronatum
		aur-s.	aurum sulphuratum
		auran.	aurantii cortex
		aven.	avena sativa
		aza.	azadirachta indica
art-v.	artemisia vulgaris	bac.	bacillinum Burnett
arum-d.	arum dracontium	bac-t.	baccillinum testium
arum-dru.	arum dracunculus	bach	bacillus Bach-Paterson
arum-i.	arum italicum		
arum-m.	arum maculatum		
arum-t.	arum triphyllum	bad.	badiaga
arund.	arundo mauritanica	baj.	baja
arund-d.	arundo donax		
asaf.	asa foetida		
		bals-p.	balsamum peruvianum
		bals-t.	balsamum tolutanum
asar.	asarum europaeum	bapt.	baptisia tinctoria
asar-c.	asarum canadense	bapt-c.	baptisia confusa
asc-c.	asclepias cornuti	bar-a.	baryta acetica
asc-i.	asclepias incarnata	bar-c.	baryta carbonica
asc-t.	asclepias tuberosa	bar-i.	baryta iodata
		bar-m.	baryta muriatica
		bar-p.	baryta phosphorica
asim.	asimina triloba	bar-s.	baryta sulphurica
		barb.	barbae cyprini ova
ask.	askalabotes laevigatus	baros.	barosma crenulatum
aspar.	asparagus officinalis		

bart.	Bartfelder aqua	bry.	bryonia alba aut dioica
bell.	belladonna	bufo	bufo rana
		bufo-s.	bufo sahytiensis
bell-p.	bellis perennis	bung.	bungurus fasciatus
ben.	benzinum	buni-o.	bunias orientalis
ben-d.	benzinum dinitricum		
ben-n.	benzinum nitricum	but-ac.	butyricum acidum
benz-ac.	benzoicum acidum	buth-a.	buthus australis
benzo.	benzoinum oderiferum		
benzol.	benzolum	buth-af.	buthus afer
berb.	berberis vulgaris	buth-oc.	buthus occitanus
berb-a.	berberis aquifolium	bux.	buxus sempervirens
		cac.	cacao
berbin.	berberinum		
beryl.	beryllium metallicum	cact.	cactus
beta	beta vulgaris		
betin.	betainum muriaticum	cadm-br.	cadmium bromatum
beto.	betonica aquatica	cadm-i.	cadmium iodatum
betu.	betula alba	cadm-m.	cadmium muriaticum
bism.	bismuthum subnitricum	cadm-met.	cadmium metallicum
		cadm-o.	cadmium oxydatum
		cadm-s.	cadmium sulphuratum
bism-met.	bismuthum metallicum	cael.	caela zacatechichi
bism-o.	bismuthum oxydatum	caes.	caesium metallicum
bism-val.	bismuthum valerianicum		
bix.	bixa orellana	cain.	cainca
blatta	blatta orientalis		
blatta-a.	blatta americana	caj.	cajuputum
bol-la.	boletus laricis		
bol-lu.	boletus luridus		
bol-s.	boletus satanas	cal-ren.	calculus (lapis) renalis
bold.	boldo	calad.	caladium seguinum
		calag.	calaguala
bomb-chr.	bombyx chrysorrhea	calam.	calamus aromaticus
bomb-pr.	bombyx processionea	calc.	calcarea carbonica
bond.	Bondonneau aqua		
bor.	borax veneta		
bor-ac.	boricum acidum	calc-a.	calcarea acetica
both.	bothrops lanceolatus	calc-ar.	calcarea arsenicosa
		calc-br.	calcarea bromata
botul.	botulinum	calc-caust.	calcarea caustica
		calc-chln.	calcarea chlorinata
bov.	bovista lycoperdon	calc-f.	calcarea fluorica naturalis
brach.	brachyglottis repens	calc-hp.	calcarea hypophosphorosa
bran.	branca ursina	calc-i.	calcarea iodata
brass.	brassica napus	calc-lac.	calcarea lactica
		calc-m.	calcarea muriatica
brom.	bromium		
bruc.	brucea antidysenterica	calc-o-t.	calcarea ovi testae
brucel.	brucella melitensis	calc-ox.	calcarea oxalica
brucin.	brucinum	calc-p.	calcarea phosphorica
	brugmansia candida	calc-pic.	calcarea picrica
		calc-s.	calcarea sulphurica

calc-sil.	calcarea silicata	cast.	castoreum canadense
		cast-eq.	castor equi
calc-st-sula.	calcarea stibiato-	cast-v.	castanea vesca
	sulphurata	caste.	castella texana
		catal.	catalpa bignonoides
		catar.	cataria nepeta
calen.	**calendula officinalis**	caul.	caulophyllum
calli.	calliandra houstoni		
		caust.	causticum Hahnemanni
		cean.	ceanothus americanus
calo.	calotropis gigantea	cean-tr.	ceanothus thrysiflorus
		cecr.	cecropia mexicana
calth.	caltha palustris	cedr.	cedron
camph.	camphora		
		celt.	celtis occidentalis
camph-ac.	camphoricum acidum	cench.	cenchris contortrix
camph-br.	camphora bromata		
		cent.	centaurea tagana
canch.	canchalagua		
		ceph.	cephalanthus occidentalis
cann-i.	cannabis indica	cer-ox.	cerium oxalicum
cann-s.	cannabis sativa	cere-b.	cereus bonplandii
canna	canna angustifolia	cere-s.	cereus serpentinus
canth.	cantharis	cerv.	cervus brasilicus
canthin.	cantharidinum	ceto.	cetonia aurata
capp.	capparis coriaccea	cetr.	cetraria islandica
		cham.	chamomilla
caps.	capsicum annuum		
		chamae.	chamaedrys
car.	carissa		
		chap.	chaparro amargoso
carb-ac.	carbolicum acidum	chaul.	chaulmoogra
		cheir.	cheiranthus cheiri
carb-an.	carbo animalis	chel.	chelidonium majus
carb-v.	carbo vegetabilis	chel-g.	chelidonium glaucum
carbn.	carboneum	chelin.	chelidoninum
carbn-chl.	carboneum chloratum	chelo.	chelone glabra
carbn-h.	carboneum		
	hydrogenisatum	chen-a.	chenopodium
carbn-o.	carboneum oxygenisatum		anthelminticum
carbn-s.	carboneum sulphuratum	chen-v.	chenopodium vulvaria
carc.	carcinosinum Burnett	chim.	chimaphila umbellata
card-b.	carduus benedictus	chim-m.	chimaphila maculata
card-m.	carduus marianus	chin.	china officinalis
cardam.	cardamine pratensis		
carl	Carlsbad		
caru.	carum carvi	chin-ar.	chininum arsenicosum
cary.	carya alba	chin-b.	china (cinchona) boliviana
cas-s.	cascara sagrada	chin-m.	chininum muriaticum
		chin-s.	chininum sulphuricum
casc.	cascarilla	chin-val.	chininum valerianicum
cass.	cassada	chinid.	chinidinum

chion.	chionanthus virginica	cocc.	cocculus indicus
		cocc-s.	coccinella septempunctata
chlf.	chloroformium	coch.	cochlearia armoracia
chlol.	chloralum hydratum		
chlor.	chlorum	coch-o.	cochlearia officinalis
chloram.	chloramphenicolum	cod.	codeinum purum aut
chlorpr.	chlorpromazinum		
cho.	cholas terrapina		
chol.	cholesterinum	coff.	coffea cruda
cholin.	cholinum	coff-t.	coffea tosta
chr-met.	chromium metallicum	coffin.	coffeinum
chr-ac.	chromicum acidum	colch.	colchicum autumnale
chr-o.	chromium oxydatum	colchin.	colchicinum
chr-s.	chromium sulphuricum	coli.	colibacillinum
chrys-ac.	chrysophanicum acidum	coll.	collinsonia canadensis
chrysan.	chrysanthemum leucanthemum	coloc.	colocynthis
chrysar.	chrysarobinum		
cic.	cicuta virosa	colocin.	colocynthinum
cic-m.	cicuta maculata	colos.	colostrum
cice.	cicer arietinum	com.	comocladia dentata
cich.	cichorium intybus		
cimic.	cimicifuga racemosa		
		con.	conium maculatum
cimx.	cimex lectularius	conch.	conchiolinum
cina	cina maritima		
		conin.	coniinum
		conin-br.	coniinum bromatum
		conv.	convallaria majalis
		convo-a.	convolvulus arvensis
		convo-d.	convolvulus duartinus
		convo-s.	convolvulus stans
cinch.	cinchoninum sulphuricum		
cine.	cineria maritima	cop.	copaiva
cinnb.	cinnabaris		
		cor-r.	corallium rubrum
cinnm.	cinnamomum ceylanicum	corh.	corallorhiza odontorhiza
cist.	cistus canadensis	cori-m.	coriaria myrtifolia
cit-ac.	citricum acidum	cori-r.	coriaria ruscifolia
		corn.	cornus circinata
		corn-a.	cornus alternifolia
cit-d.	citrus decumana	corn-f.	cornus florida
cit-l.	citrus limonum	corn-s.	cornus sericea
cit-v.	citrus vulgaris	cortico.	corticotropinum
clem.	clematis erecta		
clem-vir.	clematis virginiana	cortiso.	cortisonum
clem-vit.	clematis vitalba	cory.	corydalis formosa
cloth.	clotho arictans		
cob.	cobaltum metallicum	cot.	cotyledon umbilicus
cob-n.	cobaltum nitricum	coto	coto
coc-c.	coccus cacti	crat.	crataegus oxyacantha et
coca	coca		
cocain.	cocainum hydrochloricum		

croc.	crocus sativus	del.	delphinus amazonicus
crot-c.	crotalus cascavella	delphin.	delphininum
crot-chlol.	croton chloralum		
crot-h.	crotalus horridus		
crot-t.	croton tiglium	dema.	dematium petraeum
cryp.	cryptopinum	der.	derris pinnata
cub.	cubeba officinalis		
cuc-c.	cucurbita citrullus		
cuc-p.	cucurbita pepo	des-ac.	desoxyribonucleinicum acidum
culx.	culex musca		
cumin.	cumarinum	dicha.	dichapetalum
cund.	cundurango	dict.	dictamnus albus
		dig.	digitalis purpurea
cuph.	cupnea viscosissima	digin.	digitalinum
cupr.	cuprum metallicum	digox.	digitoxinum
cupr-a.	cuprum aceticum	dios.	dioscorea villosa
cupr-am-s.	cuprum ammoniae	diosm.	diosma lincaris
	sulphuricum	dip.	dipodium punctatum
cupr-ar.	cuprum arsenicosum	diph.	diphtherinum
cupr-c.	cuprum carbonicum	diphtox.	diphtherotoxinum
cupr-cy.	cuprum cyanatum		
cupr-m.	cuprum muriaticum	dirc.	dirca palustris
cupr-n.	cuprum nitricum	ditin	ditainum
cupr-o.	cuprum oxydatum nigrum	dol.	dolichos (mucuna)
cupr-s.	cuprum sulphuricum	dor.	doryphora decemlineata
cupre-au.	cupressus australis		
cupre-l.	cupressus lawsoniana		
cur.	curare	dros.	drosera rotundifolia
curc.	curcuma javanensis	dub.	duboisinum
		dubo-h.	duboisia hopwoodi
cycl.	cyclamen europaeum	dubo-m.	duboisia myoporoides
cyd.	cydonia vulgaris	dulc.	dulcamara.
cymin.	cymarinum		
cyn-d.	cynodon dactyion	dys.	bacillus dysenteriae
cyna.	cynara scolymos	eaux	Eaux bonnes aqua
cyno.	cynoglossum officinale	eberth.	eberthinum
cypr.	cypripedium pubescens		
cyt-l.	cytisus laburnum	echi.	echinacea
		echi-p.	echinacea purpurea
cytin.	cytisinum		
		echit.	echites suberecta
		elae.	elaeis guineensis
dam.	damiana	elaps	elaps corallinus
		elat.	elaterium officinarum
daph.	daphne indica		
dat-a.	datura arborea	elem.	elemuy gauteria
		emetin.	emetinum
dat-f.	datura ferox	enteroc.	enterococcinum
dat-m.	datura metel	eos.	eosinum
dat-s.	datura sanguinea	ephe.	ephedra vulgaris
		epig.	epigaea repens
datin.	daturinum	epih.	epihysterinum
datis.	datisca cannabina	epil.	epilobium palustre

epiph.	epiphegus virginiana	eupi.	eupionum
equis.	equisetum hyemale	eys.	eysenhardtia polystachia
equis-a.	equisetum arvense		
eran.	eranthis hyemnalis	fab.	fabiana imbricata
erech.	erechthites hieracifolia		
ergot.	ergotinum	faec.	bacillus faecalis
erig.	erigeron canadensis	fago.	fagopyrum esculentum
		fagu.	fagus silvatica
erio.	eriodyction californicum		
		fel	fel tauri
		ferr.	ferrum metallicum
erod.	erodium cicutarium	ferr-a.	ferrum aceticum
ery-a.	eryngium aquaticum	ferr-ar.	ferrum arsenicosum
ery-m.	eryngium maritinum	ferr-br.	ferrum bromatum
		ferr-c.	ferrum carbonicum
		ferr-cit.	ferrum citricum
eryt-j.	erythrophlaeum judiciale	ferr-cy.	ferrum cyanatum
eryth.	erythrinus	ferr-i.	ferrum iodatum
		ferr-lac.	ferrum lacticum
esch.	eschscholtzia californica	ferr-m.	ferrum muriaticum
esin.	eserinum	ferr-ma.	ferrum magneticum
		ferr-o-r.	ferrum oxydatum rubrum
esp-g.	espeletia grandiflora	ferr-p.	ferrum phosphoricum
		ferr-pern.	ferrum pernitricum
eucal.	eucalyptus globulus	ferr-p-h.	ferrum phosphoricum
eucal-r.	eucalyptus rostrata		hydricum
eucal-t.	eucalyptus tereticortis	ferr-pic.	ferrum picricum
eucol.	eucalyptolum	ferr-prox.	ferrum protoxalatum
		ferr-py.	ferrum pyrophosphoricum
		ferr-r.	ferrum reductum
eug.	eugenia jambosa		
euon.	euonymus europaea	ferr-s.	ferrum sulphuricum
euon-a.	euonymus atropurpurea	ferr-t.	ferrum tartaricum
euonin.	euonyminum	ferul.	ferula glauca
eup-a.	eupatorium aromaticum		
eup-per.	eupatorium perfoliatum		
eup-pur.	eupatorium purpureum	fic.	ficus religiosa
euph.	euphorbium officinarum	fic-v.	ficus venosa
		fil.	filix-mas
euph-a.	euphorbia amygdaloides		
euph-c.	euphorbia corrolata	fl-ac.	fluoricum acidum
euph-cy.	euphorbia cyparissias	flav.	flavus
euph-he.	euphorbia heterodoxa	foll.	folliculinum
euph-hy.	euphorbia hypericifolia	flor-p.	flor de piedra
euph-ip.	euphorbia ipecacuanhae		
euph-l.	euphorbia lathyris	foen.	foeniculum sativum
euph-m.	euphorbia marginata	form.	formica rufa
euph-pe.	euphorbia peplus	form-ac.	formicicum acidum
euph-pi.	euphorbia pilulifera	formal.	formalinum
euph-po.	euphorbia polycarpa	frag.	fragaria vesca
		fram.	framboesinum
euph-pr.	euphorbia prostata	franc.	franciscaea uniflora
euph-re.	euphorbia resinifera		
euphr.	euphrasia officinalis	franz.	Franzensbad aqua

frax.	fraxinus americana		gunp.	gunpowder
fuc.	fucus vesiculosus		gymne.	gymnema silvestre
fuch.	fuchsinum		gymno.	gymnocladus canadensis
fuli.	fuligo ligni		haem.	haematoxylum
gad.	gadus morrhua			campechianum
gaert.	bacillus Gaertner		hall	Hall aqua
gal-ac.	gallicum acidum		halo.	haloperidolum
gala.	galanthus nivalis		ham.	hamamelis virginiana
galeg.	galega officinalis		harp.	harpagophytum
galeo.	galeopsis ochroleuca			procumbens
			hecla	Hecla (Hekla) lava
gali.	galium aparine			
galin.	galinsoga parviflora		hed.	hedera helix
galph.	galphimia glauca		hedeo.	hedeoma pulegioides
gamb.	gambogia		hedy.	hedysarum ildefonsianum
			helia.	helianthus annuus
			helin.	heloninum
gast.	Gastein aqua		helio.	heliotropinum
gaul.	gaultheria procumbens			peruvianum
gels.	gelsemium sempervirens		hell.	helleborus niger
genist.	genista tinctoria		hell-f.	helleborus foetidus
gent-c.	gentiana cruciata		hell-o.	helleborus orientalis
gent-l.	gentiana lutea		hell-v.	helleborus viridis
gent-q.	gentiana quinquefolia		helm.	helminthochortos
geo.	geoffrova vermifuga		helo.	heloderma suspectum
			helon.	helonias dioica
ger.	geranium maculatum		helx.	helix tosta
gerin.	geraninum		hep.	hepar sulphuris calcareum
get.	Gettysburg aqua			
geum	geum rivale			
gink-b.	ginkgo biloba			
gins.	ginseng			
			hepat.	hepatica triloba
			hera.	heracleum sphondylium
			heuch.	heuchera americana
glech.	glechoma hederacea			
glon.	glonoinum			
glyc.	glycerinum			
gnaph.	gnaphalium polycephalum		hip-ac.	hippuricum acidum
			hipp.	hippomanes
gonotox.	gonotoxinum		hippoz.	hippozaeninum
goss.	gossypium herbaceum			
gran.	granatum			
graph.	graphites naturalis		hir.	hirudo medicinalis
grat.	gratiola officinalis			
grin.	grindelia robusta		hist.	histaminum muriaticum
gua.	guaco		hoit.	hoitzia coccinea
quaj.	quajacum officinale			
guajol.	guajacolum			
guan.	guano australis		hom.	homarus
			home.	homeria collina
guar.	guarana		hume.	humea elegans
guare.	guarea trichiloides		hura	hura brasiliensis
guat.	guatteria gaumeri			
			hura-c.	hura crepitans

hydr.	hydrastis canadensis
hydr-ac.	hydrocyanicum acidum
hydrang.	hydrangea arborescens
hydrc.	hydrocotyle asiatica
hydrin-m.	hydrastinum muriaticum
hydrin-s.	hydrastinum sulphuricum
hydro-v.	hydrophyllum virginicum
hydrobr-ac.	hydrobromicum acidum
hydroph.	hydrophis cyanocinctus
hyos.	hyoscyamus niger
hyosin.	hyoscyaminum bromatum
hyper.	hypericum perforatum
hypo	hypophyllum sanguineum
hypoth.	hypothalamus
iber.	iberis amara
ichth.	ichthyolum
ictod.	ictodes foetida
ign.	ignatia amara
ille.	illecebrum verticillatum
ilx-a.	ilex aquifolium
ilx-c.	ilex casseine
imp.	imperatoria ostruthium
ind.	indium metallicum
indg.	indigo tinctoria
indol.	indolum
influ.	influenzinum
ins.	insulinum
inul.	inula helenium
iod.	iodium purum
iodof.	iodoformium
ip.	ipecacuanha
	ipomoea bona-nox
ipom.	ipomoea purpurea
irid.	iridium metallicum
irid-m.	iridium muriaticum
iris	iris versicolor
iris-fa.	iris factissima
iris-fl.	iris florentina
iris-foe.	iris foetidissima
iris-g.	iris germanica
iris-ps.	iris pseudacorus
iris-t.	iris tenax
itu	itu

jab.	jaborandi
jac.	jacaranda gualandai
jac-c.	jacaranda caroba
jal.	jalapa
jasm.	jasminum officinale
jatr.	jatropha curcas
jatr-u.	jatropha urens
joan.	joanesia asoca
jug-c.	juglans cinerea
jug-r.	juglans regia
junc-e.	juncus effusus
junc-p.	juncus pilosus
juni.	juniperus virginiana
juni-c.	juniperus communis
just.	justicia adhatoda
kali-a.	kali aceticum
kali-ar.	kali arsenicosum
kali-bi.	kali bichromicum
kali-biox.	kali bioxalicum
kali-bit.	kali bitartaricum
kali-br.	kali bromatum
kali-c.	kali carbonicum
kali-caust.	kali causticum
kali-chl.	kali chloricum
kali-chls.	kali chlorosum
kali-chr.	kali chromicum
kali-cit.	kali citricum
kali-cy.	kali cyanatum
kali-f.	kali fluoratum
kali-fcy.	kali ferrocyanatum
kali-hp.	kali hypophosphoricum
kali-i.	kali iodatum
kali-m.	kali muriaticum
kali-n.	kali nitricum
kali-ox.	kali oxalicum
kali-p.	kali phosphoricum
kali-perm.	kali permanganicum
kali-pic.	kali picricum
kali-s.	kali sulphuricum
kali-s-chr.	kali sulphuricum chromicum
kali-sal.	kali salicylicum
kali-sil.	kali silicicum
kali-sula.	kali sulphuratum

kali-sulo.	kali sulphurosum
kali-t.	kali tartaricum
kali-tel.	kali telluricum
kali-x.	kali xanthogenicum
kalm.	kalmia latifolia
kam.	kamala
kara.	karaka
karw-h.	karwinskia humboldtiana
kerose.	kerosenum
keroso.	kerosolenum
kino	kino australiensis
kiss.	Kissingen aqua
kola	kola
kou.	kousso (= brayera anthelmintica)
kreos.	kreosotum
kres.	kresolum
kurch.	kurchi
lac-ac.	lactis acidum
lac-c.	lac caninum
lac-d.	lac vaccinum defloratum
lac-f.	lac felinum
lac-v.	lac vaccinum
lac-v-c.	lac vaccinum coagulatum
lac-v-f.	lactis vaccini flos
lacer.	lacerta agilis
lach.	lachesis muta
lachn.	lachnanthes tinctoria
lact.	lactuca virosa
lact-s.	lactuca sativa
lactrm.	lactucarium thridace
lam.	lamium album
lap-a.	lapis albus
lapa.	lapathum acutum
lappa	lappa arctium
laps.	lapsana communis
lat-h.	latrodectus hasselti
lat-k.	latrodectus katipo
lat-m.	latrodectus mactans

lath.	lathyrus sativus aut
laur.	laurocerasus
lec.	lecithinum
led.	ledum palustre
lem-m.	lemna minor
leon.	leonurus cardiaca
lepi.	lepidium bonariense
lept.	leptandra virginica
lesp-c.	lespedeza capitata
lesp-s.	lespedeza sieboldii
lev.	Levico aqua
levist.	levisticum officinale
levo.	levomepromazinum
liat.	liatris spicata
lil-a.	lilium album
lil-s.	lilium superbum
lil-t.	lilium tigrinum
lim.	limulus cyclops
limx.	limex ater
lina.	linaria vulgaris
linu-c.	linum catharticum
linu-u.	linum usitatissimum
lip.	lippia mexicana
lipp.	Lippspringe aqua
lith-be.	lithium benzoicum
lith-br.	lithium bromatum
lith-c.	lithium carbonicum
lith-lac.	lithium lacticum
lith-m.	lithium muriaticum
lith-sal.	lithium salicylicum
loa.	loasa tricolor
lob.	lobelia inflata
lob-a.	lobelia acetum
lob-c.	lobelia cardinalis
lob-d.	lobelia dortmanna
lob-e.	lobelia erinus
lob-p.	lobelia purpurascens
lob-s.	lobelia syphilitica
lobin.	lobelinum
lol.	loleum temulentum
lon-c.	lonicera caprifolium
lon-p.	lonicera pericylmenum
lon-x.	lonicera xylosteum

luf-act.	luffa actangula	mati.	matico
luf-op.	luffa operculata		
		matth.	matthiola graeca
lup.	lupulus humulus	mec.	meconium
lupin.	lupulinum	med.	medorrhinum
lyc.	lycopodium clavatum	medus.	medusa
lycpr.	lycopersicum esculentum	melc.	melastama ackermanni
		melal.	melaleuca hypericifolia
lycps.	lycopus virginicus		
lycps-eu.	lycopus europaeus	meli.	melilotus officinalis
lysi.	lysimachia nummularia	meli-a.	melilotus alba
lyss.	lyssinum	melis.	melissa officinalis
		melit.	melitagrinum
m-arct.	magnetis polus arcticus	melo.	melolontha vulgaris
m-aust.	magnetis polus australis	meningoc.	meningococcinum
macro.	macrotinum	menis.	menispermum canadense
		menth.	mentha piperita
macroz.	macrozamia spiralis	menth-pu.	mentha pulegium
		menth-v.	mentha viridis
mag-c.	magnesia carbonica	mentho.	mentholum
mag-bcit.	magnesia borocitrica	meny.	menyanthes trifoliata
mag-f.	magnesia fluorata	meph.	mephitis putorius
mag-i.	magnesia iodata	merc.	mercurius solubilis
mag-m.	magnesia muriatica		
mag-p.	magnesia phosphorica		
mag-s.	magnesia sulphurica	merc-a.	mercurius aceticus
mag-u.	magnesia usta	merc-aur.	mercurius auratus
magn-gl.	magnolia glauca		
magn-gr.	magnolia grandiflora	merc-br.	mercurius bromatus
		merc-c.	mercurius corrosivus
maland.	malandrinum		
malar.	malaria officinalis	merc-cy.	mercurius cyanatus
malatox.	malariatoxinum	merc-d.	mercurius dulcis
		merc-i-f.	mercurius iodatus flavus
manc.	mancinella		
		merc-i-r.	mercurius iodatus ruber
mand.	mandragora officinarum		
mang.	manganum aceticum aut	merc-k-i.	mercurius biniodatus cum kali iodato
mang-coll.	manganum colloidale		
mang-m.	manganum muriaticum	merc-meth.	mercurius methylenus
mang-o.	manganum oxydatum	merc-ns.	mercurius nitrosus
mang-s.	manganum sulphuricum		
mangi.	mangifera indica		
manz.	manzanita		
marr.	marrubium album	merc-p.	mercurius phosphoricus
		merc-pr-a.	mercurius praecipitatus albus
mate	maté	merc-pr-f.	mercurius praecipitatus flavus

merc-pr-r.	mercurius praecipitatus ruber	muscin.	muscarinum
		mut.	bacillus mutabilis
		mygal.	mygale lasiodora
		myos-a.	myosotis arvensis
		myos-s.	myosotis symphytifolia
merc-s-cy.	mercurius sulphocyanatus	myric.	myrica cerifera
		myris.	myristica sebifera
		myrrha	myrrha
		myrt-c.	myrtus communis
merc-sul.	mercurius sulphuricus	myrt-ch.	myrtus cheken
merc-tn.	mercurius tannicus	myrt-p.	myrtus pimenta
		mytil.	mytilus edulis
merl.	mercurialis perennis	nabal.	nabalus serpentaria
mesp.	mespillus germanica	naja	naja tripudians
meth-ae-ae.	methylium aethylo-aethereum	napht.	naphta
		naphtin.	naphtalinum
meth-sal.	methylium salicylicum	narc-po.	narcissus poeticus
methyl.	methylenum coeruleum	narc-ps.	narcissus pseudonarcissus
methys.	methysergidum	narcin.	narceinum
mez.	mezereum	narcot.	narcotinum
		narz.	Narzan aqua
micr.	micromeria douglasii	nast.	nasturtium aquaticum
		nat-a.	natrum aceticum
		nat-ae-s.	natrum aethylosulphuricum
mill.	millefolium	nat-ar.	natrum arsenicosum
		nat-be.	natrum benzoicum
mim-h.	mimosa humilis	nat-br.	natrum bromatum
mim-p.	mimosa pudica	nat-bic.	natrum bicarbonicum
mit.	mitchella repens	nat-c.	natrum carbonicum
moly-met.	molybdaenum metallicum	nat-cac.	natrum cacodylicum
mom-b.	momordica balsamica	nat-ch.	natrum choleinicum
mom-ch.	momordica charantia	nat-f.	natrum fluoratum
		nat-hchls.	natrum hypochlorosum
		nat-hsulo.	natrum hyposulphurosum
monar.	monarda didyma	nat-i.	natrum iodatum
moni.	monilia albicans	nat-lac.	natrum lacticum
mono.	monotropa uniflora	nat-m.	natrum muriaticum
mons.	monsonia ovata	nat-n.	natrum nitricum
morb.	morbillinum	nat-ns.	natrum nitrosum
morg.	bacillus Morgan	nat-p.	natrum phosphoricum
morph.	morphinum aceticum	nat-s.	natrum sulphuricum
		nat-s-c.	natrum sulphocarbolicum
mosch.	moschus	nat-sal.	natrum salicylicum
muc-u.	mucuna urens	nat-sel.	natrum selenicum
mucor	mucor mucedo	nat-sil.	natrum silicicum
mucot.	mucotoxinum	nat-sil-f.	natrum silicofluoricum
		nat-suc.	natrum succinicum
mur-ac.	muriaticum acidum	nat-sula.	natrum sulphuratum
muru.	murure leite	nat-sulo.	natrum sulphurosum
murx.	murex purpureus	nat-taur.	natrum taurocholicum
musa	musa sapientum	nat-tel.	natrum telluricum

nect.	nectandra amare	onop.	onopordon acanthium
nectrin.	nectrianinum	onos.	onosmodium virginianum
neg.	negundium americanum		
		op.	opium
		oper.	operculina turpenthum
nep.	nepenthes distillatoria	opl.	oplia farinosa
nepet.	nepeta cataria	opop.	opopanax chironium
		opun-f.	opuntia ficus
neur.	neurinum		
nicc.	niccolum carbonicum aut	opun-v.	opuntia vulgaris
	metallicum	orch.	orchitinum
nicc-s.	niccolum sulphuricum	oreo.	oreodaphne californica
		orig.	origanum majorana
nicot.	nicotinum	orig-cr.	origanum creticum
nid.	nidus edulis	orig-v.	origanum vulgare
nig-d.	nigella damascena	orni.	ornithogalum umbellatum
nig-s.	nigella sativa		
nit-ac.	nitri acidum		
nit-m-ac.	nitromuriaticum acidum	oscilloc.	oscillococcinum
		osm.	osmium metallicum
nit-s-d.	nitri spiritus dulcis	ost.	ostrya virginica
		ouabin.	ouabainum
		ov.	ovininum (= oophorinum)
		ovi-p.	ovi gallinae pellicula
nitro-o.	nitrogenium oxygenatum		
		ox-ac.	oxalicum acidum
nuph.	nuphar luteum	oxal.	oxalis acetosella
		oxyd.	oxydendron arboreum
nux-a.	nux absurda		
		oxyg.	oxygenium
		oxyt.	oxytropis lamberti
nux-m.	nux moschata		
nux-v.	nux vomica	paeon.	paeonia officinalis
nyct.	nyctanthes arbor-tristis		
		pall.	palladium metallicum
nymph.	nymphaea odorata	palo.	paloondo
oci.	ocimum canum		
oci-s.	ocimum sanctum	pana.	panacea arvensis
oena.	oenanthe crocata		
oeno.	oenothera biennis	pann.	panna (= aspidium panna)
		papin.	papaverinum
oest.	oestrus cameli		
okou.	okoubaka aubrevillei	par.	paris quadrifolia
ol-an.	oleum animale aethereum	paraf.	paraffinum
	Dippeli	paraph.	paraphenylendiaminum
	oleum cajuputi = caj.		
ol-car.	oleum caryophyllatum		
ol-j.	oleum jecoris aselli	parat.	paratyphoidinum
ol-myr.	oleum myristicae	parathyr.	parathyreoidinum
ol-sant.	oleum santali		
ol-suc.	oleum succinum	pareir.	pareira brava
	oleum wittnebianum	pariet.	parietaria officinalis
	= caj.	paro-i.	paronychia illecebrum
olnd.	oleander (= nerium	parot.	parotidinum
	oleander)	parth.	parthenium hysterophorus
onis.	oniscus asellus		
	(= millipedes)	passi.	passiflora incarnata
onon.	ononis spinosa (arvensis)	past.	pastinaca sativa

paull.	paullinia pinnata	pime.	pimenta officinalis
		pimp.	pimpinella saxifraga (alba)
pect.	pecten jacobaeus		
ped.	pediculus capitis	pin-c.	pinus cupressus
pedclr.	pedicularis canadensis	pin-l.	pinus lambertiana
pelarg.	pelargonium reniforme	pin-s.	pinus silvestris
pellin.	pelletierinum		
pen.	penthorum sedoides	pip-m.	piper methysticum
penic.	penicillinum		
		pip-n.	piper nigrum
		pipe.	piperazinum
perh.	perhexilinum	pisc.	piscidia erythrina
peri.	periploca graeca	pitu.	pituitarium posterium
pers.	persea americana		
pert.	pertussinum	pitu-gl.	pituitaria glandula
pest.	pestinum	pituin.	pituitrinum
		pix	pix liquida
peti.	petiveria tetrandra		
petr.	petroleum	plan.	plantago major
petros.	petroselinum sativum	plan-mi.	plantago minor
		plat.	platinum metallicum
		plat-m.	platinum muriaticum
ph-ac.	phosphoricum acidum	plat-m-n.	platinum muriaticum
phal.	phallus impudicus		natronatum
phase.	phaseolus nanus	platan.	platanus occidentalis
phel.	phellandrium aquaticum	plb.	plumbum metallicum
phenac.	phenacetinum	plb-a.	plumbum aceticum
phenob.	phenobarbitalum	plb-c.	plumbum carbonicum
		plb-chr.	plumbum chromicum
		plb-i.	plumbum iodatum
phila.	philadelphus coronarius	plb-n.	plumbum nitricum
phle.	phleum pratense	plb-p.	plumbum phosphoricum
phlor.	phlorizinum	plect.	plectranthus fruticosus
phos.	phosphorus	plumbg.	plumbago litteralis
phos-h.	phosphorus hydrogenatus	plume.	plumeria celinus
phos-pchl.	phosphorus pentachloratus	pneu.	pneumococcinum
phys.	physostigma venenosum		
		podo.	podophyllum peltatum
		pole.	polemonium coeruleum
physal.	physalis alkekengi	poll.	pollen
		polyg-a.	polygonum aviculare
		polyg-h.	polygonum
physala-p.	physalia pelagica		hydropiperoides aut
phyt.	phytolacca decandra		
phyt-b.	phytolacca berry	polyg-m.	polygonum maritimum
		polyg-pe.	polygonum persicaria
pic ac.	picricum (picronitricum)	polyg-s.	polygonum sagittatum
	acidum	polym.	polymnia uvedalia
picro.	picrotoxinum		
pilo.	pilocarpinum	polyp-p.	polyporus pinicola
		polytr.	polytrichum juniperinum
		pop.	populus tremuloides
		pop-c.	populus candicans

pot-a.	potentilla anserina
pot-au.	potentilla aurea
pot-e.	potentilla erecta
pot-r.	potentilla reptans
pot-t.	potentilla tormentilla
pota.	potamogeton natans
prim-f.	primula farinosa
prim-o.	primula obconica
prim-v.	primula veris
prin.	prinos verticillatus
prop.	propylaminum
prot.	bacillus proteus
prun.	prunus spinosa
prun-d.	prunus domestica
prun-m.	prunus mahaleb
prun-p.	prunus padus
prun-v.	prunus virginiana
prune.	prunella vulgaris
psil.	psilocybe caerulescens
psor.	psorinum
psoral.	psoralea bituminosa
ptel.	ptelea trifoliata
pulm-a.	pulmo anaphylacticus
pulm-v.	pulmo vulpis
pulmon.	pulmonaria vulgaris
puls.	pulsatilla pratensis
puls-n.	pulsatilla nuttalliana
pulx.	pulex irritans
pyrar.	pyrarara
pyre-o.	pyrethrum officinarum
pyre-p.	pyrethrum parthenium
pyre-r.	pyrethrum roseum e floribus
pyro-ac.	pyrolignosum acidum
pyrog.	pyrogenium
pyrol.	pyrola rotundifolia
pyrus	pyrus americanus
quas.	quassia amara
queb.	quebracho
querc.	quercus e glandibus
quill.	quillaya saponaria
rad.	radium metallicum
rad-br.	radium bromatum
raja-s.	rajania subsamarata
ran-a.	ranunculus acris
ran-b.	ranunculus bulbosus

ran-fi.	ranunculus ficaria
ran-fl.	ranunculus flammula
ran-g.	ranunculus glacialis
ran-r.	ranunculus repens
ran-s.	ranunculus sceleratus
raph.	raphanus sativus
raphani.	raphanistrum arvense
rat.	ratanhia peruviana
rauw.	rauwolfia serpentina
rein.	Reinerz aqua
res.	resorcinum
reser.	reserpinum
rham-cal.	rhamnus californica
rham-cath.	rhamnus cathartica
rham-f.	rhamnus frangula
rheum	rheum palmatum
rhod.	rhododendron chrysan-thum
rhodi.	rhodium metallicum
rhodi-o-n.	rhodium oxydatum nitricum
rhus-a.	rhus aromatica
rhus-c.	rhus cotinus
rhus-d.	rhus diversiloba
rhus-g.	rhus glabra
rhus-l.	rhus laurina
rhus-r.	rhus radicans
rhus-t.	rhus toxicodendron
rhus-v.	rhus venenata
rhus-ver.	rhus vernix
rib-ac.	ribonucleinicum acidum
ric.	ricinus communis
rob.	robinia pseudacacia
ros-ca.	rosa canina
ros-ce.	rosa centifolia
ros-d.	rosa damascena
rosm.	rosmarinus officinalis
rub-t.	rubia tinctorum
rubu.	rubus villosus
rudb-h.	rudbeckia hirta
rumx.	rumex crispus
rumx-a.	rumex acetosa
russ.	russula foetens
ruta	ruta graveolens
sabad.	sabadilla
sabal	sabal serrulatum
sabin.	sabina

sacch.	saccharum officinale (album)	sed-t.	sedum telephium
		sedi.	sedinha
sacch-l.	saccharum lactis		
sacchin.	saccharinum		
sal-ac.	salicylicum acidum	sel.	selenium
sal-am.	salix americana	seli.	selinum carvifolium
sal-n.	salix nigra	sem-t.	semen tiglii
sal-p.	salix purpurea	semp.	sempervivum tectorum
salam.	salamandra maculata	senec.	senecio aureus
salin.	salicinum	senec-j.	senecio jacobaea
salol.	salolum	senecin.	senecinum
salv.	salvia officinalis	seneg.	senega
salv-sc.	salvia sclarea		
samb.	sambucus nigra	senn.	senna
samb-c.	sambucus canadensis	sep.	sepia succus
samb-e.	sambucus ebulus	septi.	septicaeminum
sang.	sanguinaria canadensis		
sang-n.	sanguinarinum nitricum	ser-ang.	serum anguillae
sang-t.	sanguinarinum tartaricum		
sanguiso.	sanguisorba officinalis	serp.	serpentaria aristolochia
sanic.	Sanicula aqua	sieg.	siegesbeckia orientalis
sanic-eu.	sanicula europaea	sil.	silicea terra
santa.	santalum album	sil-mar.	silica marina
santin.	santoninum	silpho.	silphion cyrenaicum
sapin.	saponinum	silphu.	silphium laciniatum
sapo.	saponaria officinalis	sima.	simaruba amara
sarcol-ac.	sarcolacticum acidum		
		sin-a.	sinapis alba
		sin-n.	sinapis nigra
saroth.	sarothamnus scoparius	sisy.	sisyrinchium galaxoides
		sium	sium latifolium
		skat.	skatolum
sarr.	sarracenia purpurea	skook.	Skookum chuck aqua
sars.	sarsaparilla	slag	slag
sass.	sassafras officinalis	sol-a.	solanum arrebenta
saur.	saururus cernuus	sol-c.	solanum carolinense
saxi.	saxifraga granulata		
scam.	scammonium		
scarl.	scarlatinum		
schin.	schinus molle		
scir.	scirrhinum	sol-m.	solanum mammosum
scol.	scolopendra morsitans	sol-n.	solanum nigrum
scolo-v.	scolopendrium vulgare	sol-o.	solanum oleraceum
scop.	scopolia carniolica	sol-ps.	solanum pseudocapsicum
scopin.	scopolaminum bromatum	sol-t.	solanum tuberosum
scor.	scorpio europaeus	sol-t-ae.	solanum tuberosum aegrotans
scroph-m.	scrophularia marylandica		
scroph-n.	scrophularia nodosa		
scut.	scutellaria laterifolia		
sec.	secale cornutum	solid.	solidago virgaurea
sed-ac.	sedum acre	solin.	solanium aceticum aut purum
sed-r.	sedum repens (alpestre)		

soph.	sophora japonica		sul-ac.	sulphuricum acidum
			sul-h.	sulphur hydrogenisatum
			sul-i.	sulphur iodatum
sphing.	sphingurus (spiggurus)			
spig.	spigelia anthelmia		sul-ter.	sulphur terebinthinatum
			sulfa.	sulfanilamidum
spig-m.	spigelia marylandica		sulfon.	sulfonalum
			sulfonam.	sulfonamidum
			sulo-ac.	sulphurosum acidum
spil.	spilanthes oleracea		sulph.	sulphur lotum (sublimatum)
			sumb.	sumbulus moschatus
spir-sula.	spiritus sulphuratus			
spira.	spiranthes autumnalis		syc.	bacillus sycoccus
spirae.	spiraea ulmaria		sym-r.	symphoricarpus racemosus
spong.	spongia tosta		symph.	symphytum officinale
squil.	squilla (scilla) maritima		syph.	syphilinum
stach.	stachys betonica		syr.	syringa vulgaris
stann.	stannum metallicum		syzyg.	syzygium jambolanum
stann-i.	stannum iodatum			
stann-m.	stannum muriaticum		tab.	tabacum
stann-pchl.	stannum perchloratum			
staph.	staphysagria		tam.	tamus communis
			tama.	tamarix germanica
			tanac.	tanacetum vulgare
staphycoc.	staphylococcinum		tang.	tanghinia venenifera
staphytox.	staphylotoxinum		tann-ac.	tannicum acidum
stel.	stellaria media			
stict.	sticta pulmonaria		tarax.	taraxacum officinale
stigm.	stigmata maydis		tarent.	tarentula (tarantula) hispanica
still.	stillingia silvatica		tarent-c.	tarentula (tarantula) cubensis
stram.	stramonium		tart-ac.	tartaricum acidum
strept-ent.	bacillus strepto-enterococcus			
streptoc.	streptococcinum			
stront.	strontium metallicum		tax.	taxus baccata
stront-br.	strontium bromatum		tela	tela araneae
stront-c.	strontium carbonicum			
stront-i.	strontium iodatum		tell.	tellurium metallicum
stront-n.	strontium nitricum		tell-ac.	telluricum acidum
stroph-h.	strophantus hispidus		tep.	Teplitz aqua
stroph-s.	strophantus sarmentosus		ter.	terebinthiniae oleum
stry.	strychninum purum		tere-ch.	terebinthina chios
stry-ar.	strychninum arsenicosum		terebe.	terebenum
stry-n.	strychninum nitricum			
stry-p.	strychninum phosphoricum			
stry-s.	strychninum sulphuricum		tet.	tetradymitum
stry-val.	strychninum valerianicum		tetox.	tetanotoxinum
strych-g.	strychnos gaultheriana			
			teucr.	teucrium marum verum (= marum verum)
stryph.	stryphnodendron barbatimam		teucr-s.	teucrium scorodonia
succ.	succinum		thal.	thallium metallicum aut aceticum
succ-ac.	succinicum acidum			

thal-s.	thallium sulphuricum		tub-d.	tuberculinum Denys
thala.	thalamus		tub-k.	tuberculinum Koch
			tub-m.	tuberculinum Marmoreck
thea	thea chinensis		tub-r.	tuberculinum residuum
thebin.	thebainum			
			tub-sp.	tuberculinum Spengler
ther.	theridion curassavicum			
thev.	thevetia nerifolia			
thiop.	thioproperazinum		tus-fa.	tussilago farfara
thiosin.	thiosinaminum			
			tus-fr.	tussilago fragans
thlas.	thlaspi bursa pastoris		tus-p.	tussilago petasites
			typh.	thypha latifolia
thuj.	thuja occidentalis		ulm.	ulmus campestris
thuj-l.	thuja lobii		upa.	upas tieuté
thym-gl.	thymi glandulae extractum			
thymol.	thymolum		upa-a.	upas antiaris
thymu.	thymus serpyllum		ur-ac.	uricum acidum
thyr.	thyreoidinum		uran.	uranium metallicum
			uran-n.	uranium nitricum
			uranoth.	uranothorium
thyreotr.	thyreotropinum		urea	urea pura
			urea-n.	urea nitrica
til.	tilia europaea			
tinas.	tinaspora cordifolia		urt-c.	urtica crenulata
titan.	titanium metallicum		urt-g.	urtica gigas
tol.	toluidinum		urt-u.	urtica urens
tong.	tongo		usn.	usnea barbata
			ust.	ustilago maydis
tor.	torula cerevisiae		uva	uva ursi
			uvar.	uvaria triloba
torm.	tormentilla erecta		uza.	uzara
tox-th.	toxicophloea thunbergi		v-a-b.	vaccin atténué bilié
toxi.	toxicophis pugnax			
trach.	trachinus draco			
trad.	tradescantia diuretica		vac.	vaccininum
trib.	tribulus terrestris			
			vacc-m.	vaccinium myrtillus
trich.	trichosanthes amara			
trif-p.	trifolium pratense		valer.	valeriana officinalis
trif-r.	trifolium repens		vanad.	vanadium metallicum
tril.	trillium pendulum		vanil.	vanilla aromatica
tril-c.	trillium cernuum			
			vario.	variolinum
			ven-m.	venus mercenaria
trinit.	trinitrotoluenum		verat.	veratrum album
trios.	triosteum perfoliatum		verat-n.	veratrum nigrum
tritic.	triticum		verat-v.	veratrum viride
			verb.	verbascum thapsus aut
trito	trito			
trom.	trombidium muscae		verb-n.	verbascum nigrum
	domesticae (= acarus)		verbe-h.	verbena hastata
trop.	tropaeolum majus		verbe-u.	verbena urticaefolia
tub.	tuberculinum bovinum Kent		verin.	veratrinum
tub-a.	tuberculinum avis		vero-b.	veronica beccabunga

vero-o.	veronica officinalis	wye.	wyethia helenoides
vesi.	vesicaria communis	x-ray	x-ray
vesp.	vespa crabro	xan.	xanthoxylum fraxineum
vib.	viburnum opulus		(americanum)
vib-od.	viburnum oderatissinum	xanrhi.	xanthorrhiza apifolia
vib-p.	viburnum prunifolium	xanrhoe.	xanthorrhoea arborea
vib-t.	viburnum tinus	xanth.	xanthium spinosum
vichy-g.	Vichy aqua, grande grille	xero.	xerophyllum
vichy-h.	Vichy aqua, hôpital	xiph.	xiphosura americana
vinc.	vinca minor		
vince.	vincetoxicum officinale		
		yohim.	yohimbinum
viol-o.	viola odorata	yuc.	yucca filamentosa
viol-t.	viola tricolor	zea-i.	zea italica
vip.	vipera berus		
		zinc.	zincum metallicum
vip-a.	vipera aspis	zinc-a.	zincum aceticum
vip-l-f.	vipera lachesis fel	zinc-ar.	zincum arsenicosum
vip-r.	vipera redi	zinc-br.	zincum bromatum
		zinc-c.	zincum carbonicum
visc.	viscum album	zinc-cy.	zincum cyanatum
visc-q.	viscum quercinum	zinc-fcy.	zincum ferrocyanatum
vit.	vitex trifolia	zinc-i.	zincum iodatum
vitr.	vitrum antimonii	zinc-m.	zincum muriaticum
voes.	Voeslau aqua	zinc-o.	zincum oxydatum
		zinc-p.	zincum phosphoricum
		zinc-pic.	zincum picricum
wies.	Wiesbaden aqua	zinc-s.	zincum sulphuricum
wildb.	Wildbad aqua	zinc-val.	zincum valerianicum
wildu.	Wildungen aqua	zing.	zingiber officinale
		ziz.	zizia aurea

DAYTIME

agar.³, **alum.**, am-c.³, am-m.,
arg-m.³, arg-n.³, calc.³, caust.³,
cimic., **euphr.³, ferr.**, guaj., lac-d.¹',
lach.³, **med., nat-ar.**, nat-c., **nat-m.**,
nit-ac., nux-v.⁶, phos.³, **puls.**,
rhust-t., sang., SEP., STANN.,
SULPH.

sunrise till sunset⁷

med.

am.³, ⁶
acon.⁶, **agar.**, arn., bry., cham.,
cob-n.⁹, **cycl.**, helon., **jal.**, kali-c.⁸,
mag-p., merc.¹', nat-p.¹', nat-s.¹',
petr., sep., syph.⁸

MORNING (5–9 h)

abies-n., abrot., absin., **acal.⁸,**
acon., aesc., **AGAR.**, agn., all-c.³,
aloe, alum., ALUM-P.¹', alumn.²,
am-c., **AM-M.**, ambr., **anac.,**
ang.², ³, ⁶, **ant-c., ant-t.**², ³, apis,
aran.³, aran-ix.¹⁰, **ARG-M.**, arg-n.,
arist-cl.¹⁰, **arn., ars., ARS-I.,**
ars-s-f.¹', asaf., asar., **AUR.,**
aur-ar.¹', aur-i.¹', **AUR-S.**¹', **bapt.,**
bar-c., bar-i.¹', **bar-m., bar-s.**¹', **bell.,**
benz-ac., **berb.**, bism., **bor., bov.,**
BRY., bufo, cadm-met.⁹, ¹⁴, calad.,
CALC., calc-i.¹', **CALC-P., calc-sil.**¹',
cann-i.⁸, cann-s., **canth., caps.,**
CARB-AN., CARB-V., CARBN-S.,
cast.³, ⁶, **caust., CHAM., CHEL.,**
chin., **chr-ac.**, cic., cimic., **CINA,**
cinnb., cist., clem., cob.³,
cob-n.⁹, ¹⁰, ¹⁴, coc-c., **coca, cocc.,**
cod., **coff.**, colch., coloc., **con.,**
convo-s.⁹, ¹⁴, corn., cortico.⁹, ¹⁴,
cortiso.⁹, ¹⁴, **CROC.**, crot-h., crot-t.,
cupr., cycl., **dig., dios.**, dros., dulc.,
echi.³, elaps³, erig.¹⁰, **eup-per.,**

euph., **euphr., ferr., ferr-ar.**, ferr-i.,
ferr-p., fl-ac.³, ⁸, form., **gamb., gels.,**
gran., **graph.**, grat., **guaj.**, harp.¹⁴,
hed.⁹, ¹⁰, ¹⁴, hell., **hep., hydr.,**
hydroph.¹⁴, hyos., **ign.**, iod., ip.,
iris³, **kali-ar., KALI-BI., kali-c.,**
kali-i., kali-m.¹', **KALI-N., kali-p.,**
kali-sil.¹', **kalm., kreos.**, lac-c.⁸,
LACH., laur., led., lept.³, lil-t.³, ⁸,
lith-c.⁸, lob.³, lyc., **mag-c.,**
mag-f.¹⁰, ¹⁴, **mag-m.**, mag-s.⁹, ¹⁰, ¹⁴,
magn-gr.⁸, mang., med.⁷, ⁸, meny.,
meph.⁴, **merc.**, merc-c., **merc-i-f.,**
mez., mosch., mur-ac., **naja**⁸, ⁶,
NAT-AR., nat-c., **NAT-M.,**
nat-n.³, ⁶, nat-p., **NAT-S.**, nat-sil.¹',
nicc., **NIT-AC.**, nuph.⁸, **nux-m.,**
NUX-V., oci-s.⁹, ¹⁴, olnd.², ³, **ONOS.,**
op., ox-ac., par., pareir., perh.¹⁴,
PETR., PH-AC., PHOS., phyt.,
pic-ac., **plan., plat.**, plb., **PODO.,**
psor., ptel., **PULS., ran-b.**, ran-s.,
rheum, RHOD., RHUS-T., RUMX.,
ruta, sabad., **sabin., sal-ac.**, samb.,
sang., sars., sec., **sel., senec.,**
seneg., SEP., sil., **SPIG.**, spong.,
SQUIL., stann., staph., stell.⁸,
stram., stront-c., stry.⁸, **SUL-AC.**¹,
sul-i.¹', **SULPH.**, tab., **tarax.**, tell.¹⁴,
teucr., **thuj., TUB.**⁷, **VALER.,**
ven-m.¹⁴., **verat.**, verat-v., verb.,
viol-o., viol-t., visc.⁹, ¹⁴, **zinc.,**
zinc-p.¹'

5 h
aloe³, apis³, ⁶, bov., **chin.**³, cob.,
dros.³, helon., **kali-c.**¹', ³, kali-i.,
nat-m.³, nat-p.³, ph-ac.³, **podo.,**
rumx.³, sep.³, sil.³, **sulph.**³

6 h
aloe, **alum.**³, arn.³, bov.³, calc-p.,
ferr.³, **hep.**³, lyc.³, nux-v.³, ox-ac.,
sep., sil., sulph., verat.

7 h
eup-per., **hep.**³, nat-c.³, **nux-v.**³,
podo., sep.³

8 h³
eup-per., nux-v.

breakfast.

and afternoon[3]

sars.

and evening[3]

alum., bov., **calc.**, caust., coc-c., **graph.**, guaj., **kali-c.**, lach., **lyc.**, phos., psor., **rhus-t.**, sang., **SEP.**, **stram.**, **stront-c.**, **thuj.**, verat., zinc.

and night[3]

iod., nat-c.

morning of one day and the afternoon of the next[3]

lac-c.

am.[3, 6]
acon., am-m., ambr.[4], apis[8], cench.[1'], jugl-c.[8], merc.[3, 4, 6], phos.[2, 3, 6], sang., still.[8], xero.[8], zinc.[4]

bed, in[3]

aloe, **am-m.**, ambr., bry., con., **kali-c.**, **lyc.**, **nux-v.**, phos., sep., **sulph.**

daybreak am.[3]

colch., syph.

sunrise, agg. before[3]

lyc.

sunrise, after

cham., **nux-v.**, puls., syph.[7]

waking see sleep–after–morning

FORENOON (9–12 h.)

aloe, alum., alum-p.[1'], **alumn.[2]**, am-c., am-m., ambr., anac.[3], ang.[2, 3], ant-c., ant-t., aran., **arg-m.**, arg-n.[3, 6], ars., ars-s-f.[1'], asaf., aur., aur-ar.[1'], aur-s.[1'], bar-c., bar-m., **bar-s.[1']**, bell., bor., bov., **bry.**, cact., calc., calc-sil.[1'], **CANN-I.[2]**, **CANN-S.**, canth., carb-an., **carb-v.**, carbn-s., caust., cedr., cham., chel., chin., cocc., coloc., con.[2, 3], cupr., cycl., dros., dulc., euph., euphr., ferr., **fl-ac.[3]**, graph.[2, 3], **guaj.**, halo.[14], hell., **hep.[2, 3]**, ign., ip., kali-ar., kali-c., kali-m.[1'], kali-n., kali-p., kali-sil.[1'], kreos., lach., **laur.**, lyc.[2, 3], mag-c., mag-m., **mang.**, merc., mez., mosch., mur-ac., **nat-ar.**, **NAT-C.**, **NAT-M.**, nat-p., **nat-sil.[1']**, nit-ac., **nux-m.**, nux-v., par., **pareir.[2]**, petr., ph-ac., phos., plat.[2, 3], plb., **PODO.**, puls., **ran-b.**, rhod., **rhus-t.**, rumx., SABAD., sars., sec., sel.[2], sil., seneg., **SEP.**, **sil.**, spig., spong.[2, 3], **STANN.**, staph.[2, 3], **stram.[3]**, stront-c., **SUL-AC.**, **SULPH.**, tarax., **teucr.**, valer., verat.[2, 3], verb., **viol-t.**, zinc., zinc-p.[1']

9 h
bry.[3], **cham.**, **eup-per.[3]**, kali-bi.[3], kali-c., lac-c.[3], nat-m.[3], nux-v.[3], podo., sep.[3] sumb., **verb.[3]**

9–11 h[6]
stann.

9–14 h[6]
nat-m.

10 h
ars.[3], bor.[3], chin.[3], chin-s.[3], cimic.,
eup-per.[3], gels., **iod.**[3], meli.[3],
NAT-M., nux-v., petr.[3], **phos.**[3],
rhus-t.[3], sep.[3], sil.[3], **stann.**[3], **sulph.**[3],
thuj.[3]

10–11 h agg.[8]
gels., **nat-m.**[6, 8], **sep.**, sulph.

10–15 h agg.[7]
tub.

11 h
arg-m., arg-n.[6, 7], ars., arum-t.,
asaf.[3], asar., bapt.[3], berb., cact.,
chin-s.[3], cimic., cob., cocc.[3], **gels.**[3],
hydr., hyos., ind.[6], ip., lach.[3, 6],
mag-p.[3], nat-c.[3], **NAT-M.**[3], nat-p.[3],
nux-v.[3], **phos.**[3], phyt., puls.[3],
rhus-t.[3], sep.[3], **stann.**[3], **SULPH.**,
zinc.[3]

am.
alum., lil-t.[8], **LYC.**, nat-sil.[1']

NOON (12 h)

alum., ant-c.[3], apis, **ARG-M.**,
arg-n.[3], ars., bol-la.[3], bruc.[4], carb-v.,
cham.[3], chel.[3], chin.[3], cic., coloc.[3],
elaps[3], **eup-per.**[3], gels.[3], kali-bi.,
kali-c.[3], lach.[3], mag-c.[3], **nat-m.**[3],
nux-m., nux-v.[3], paeon., phos.,
sang.[3], **sel.**[3], sep., **sil.**[3], spig.[3],
stram., sulph., **valer.**, verb.[3], **zinc.**

12–24 h[6]
lach.

eating, after[6]

grat.[3], halo.[14], **mag-m.**, **nat-c.**,
nux-m., valer.

am.
CHEL., nat-s.[6]

symptoms increasing till noon,
then decreasing[3, 6]

acon.[3], **arg-n.**, bry.[3], echi., gels.,
glon., kali-bi.[3], **kalm.**[1', 3, 6], nat-m.[3],
nux-v.[3], **sang.**[3, 7], sanic.[7], spig.[7],
stann., stram.[3], stront-c., sulph.[3]

AFTERNOON (13–18 h)

acon., aesc.[8], aeth., **agar.**, all-c.,
aloe, alum., ALUM-P.[1'], alum-sil.[1'],
am-c., am-m., ambr., anac., **ang.**[2, 3],
ant-c., ant-t., **apis, arg-m., arg-n.**,
arn., **ars.**, ars-i., **ars-s-f.**[1'], **asaf.**,
asar., aur., aur-ar.[1'], aur-i.[1'], aur-s.[1'],
aur-sil.[1'], aza.[14], bar-c., bar-i.[1'],
bar-m., bar-s.[1'], **BELL., bism.**, bor.,
bov., bry., buth-a.[9, 14], cact., calad.,
calc., calc-i.[1'], **calc-p.**, calc-sil.[1'],
camph., cann-s., **canth.**, caps.,
carb-an., carb-v., carbn-s., caust.,
cedr., **cench.**[7, 8], cham., **chel.**, chin.,
cic., cimic., cina, coc-c., cocc., coff.,
colch., **coloc.**, con., croc., **cycl.**,
cyn-d.[14], cyt-l.[10, 14], **dig.**, dios., dros.,
dulc., euphr., eys.[9], fago.[8], ferr.,
ferr-ar., ferr-i., ferr-m.[2], ferr-p.,
fl-ac.[3], gels., graph.[2, 3], grat.[4],
guaj.[3], hell., hep.[2, 3], hip-ac.[9, 14],
hyos., **ign.**, iod., ip., kali-ar.,
kali-bi., kali-c., kali-cy.[8], kali-m.[1'],
KALI-N., kali-p., kali-sil.[1'], kreos.,
lach., **laur., led.**, lil-t.[8], lob.[8], **LYC.**,
mag-c., mag-m., **mang.**, meli.,
meny., **merc.**, mez., **mosch.**,
mur-ac., naja[14], nat-ar., **nat-c.**[2, 3, 6],
nat-m., nicc., **nit-ac.**, nux-m.,
nux-v., ol-an., op., par., petr.,
ph-ac., phos., phyt., plan., plat.[2, 3],
plb., **ptel., PULS.**, ran-b., ran-s.,
rheum, rhod., **RHUS-T., rumx.**,
ruta, sabad., sabin., sal-ac., **sang.**,
sars., sel., seneg., SEP., SIL.,
SIN-N., spig., **spong.**[2, 3], squil.,
stann., **staph.**[2, 3], **still.**, sul-ac.,

sul-i.[1'], **sulph.**, tarax., **teucr.**,
thiop.[14], **THUJ., valer., ven-m.**[14],
verat.[2, 3], verb., **viol-t.**, wye.[1'],
x-ray[8], xero.[8], **ZINC., ZINC-P.**[1']

13 h
arg-m., **ars.**[3], cact.[3], chel.[3], cina[3],
grat.[3], kali-c.[3], **lach.**[3], mag-c., phos.[3],
puls.[3]

13–14 h[1']
ars.

13–21 h[6]
chel.

14 h
ars.[3], calc., chel.[3], cur.[7], **eup-per.**[3],
ferr.[3], gels.[3], lach., lob., mag-p.[3],
nit-ac., ol-an., puls., sang.

14, 15, 16 h till towards morning[6]

syph.

14.30 h
hell.

15 h
ang.[3], ant-t.[3], **apis,** ars., asaf.[3], asar.,
BELL., bry.[1', 7], cedr.[3], cench., chel.[3],
chin-s.[3], clem., con.[3], nat-m.[3],
samb.[3], sang.[3], sil., staph., sulph.,
thuj.

15–17 h
sep.

15–18 h[6]
apis

15–3 h[1']
bell.

16 h
aesc.[3], alum., anac., **apis**[3], ars.[3],
arum-t., cact.[3], calc-p., carb-v.,
caust., cedr.[3], chel., **chin-s.**[3], cob.,
coloc., gels., **hell.,** hep.[3], ip.[3],
kali-c., lachn., **LYC.,** mag-m.,
mang.[3], mur-ac., nat-m.[3], nat-s.,
nit-ac.[3], **nux-v.**[3], puls., rhus-t.[3],
stront-c., sulph.[3], verb.[3]

16–17 h[14]
allox.

16–18 h
alum.[16], eys.[9, 14], gels.[6], **sep.**[1]

16–19 h[6]
coloc., **lyc.**

16–20 h
alum., bov., buth-a.[9, 10], coloc.[3],
hell., LYC., mag-m., nux-m.,
sabad.[3, 8], sulph., zinc.[3]

16–22 h
alum., chel., plat.

16–4 h[6]
thuj.

17 h
alum.[3], bov.[3], caust.[3], cedr.[3], **chin.**[3],
cimic., **coloc.,** con., gels.[3], **hep.,**
hyper.[3], kali-c., **lyc.**[3], nat-m.[3],
nux-v.[3], **PULS.**[1, 7], **rhus-t.**[3], sulph.[3],
THUJ.[3], tub.[3], valer.[3]

17–18 h[14]
ange-s., methys.

17–20 h
lil-t.

and evening[3]

kali-c.

am.
cinnb., cob-n.[14], cortico.[9, 14], hecla[14],
hed.[14], kali-c.[14], **nat-s.**[3], phyt.[3],
rhus-t.[3], **sep.**[3, 6]

EVENING (18–21 h)

abrot., **acon.,** agar., agn., alf.[8],
all-c., aloe, **ALUM.,** alum-sil.[1'],
alumn.[2], am-br.[8], **AM-C., am-m.,**
AMBR., anac., ang.[2, 3], **ANT-C.,**

ANT-T., apis, **arg-m., arg-n., ARN.,
ars., ars-i.,** ars-s-f.[1]', **asaf., asar.,**
aur., aur-ar.[1]', aur-i.[1]', **aur-s.**[1]',
bapt., bar-c., bar-i.[1]', bar-m., bar-s.[1]',
BELL., berb., berb-a.[14], bism., **bor.,
bov., brom., BRY.,** bufo[3], buth-a.[9],
caj.[8], **calad., CALC.,** calc-ar.[1]',
calc-i.[1]', calc-p., **calc-s., CALC-SIL.**[1]',
camph., cann-s., canth., **CAPS.,
CARB-AN., CARB-V., CARBN-S.,**
carc.[9], **CAUST.,** cedr., **cench.**[1]', [7],
CHAM., chel., chin., chlorpr.[14], cic.,
cimic., cina, clem., **cocc.,** coff.,
COLCH., coloc., com., **con., croc.,**
crot-h., cupr., **cupr-s.**[2], **CYCL.,**
cyn-d.[14], cyt-l.[9, 10, 14], dig., dios.[8],
dirc., dros., **dulc.,** euon-a.[8],
EUPHR., eys.[9, 14], **ferr., ferr-ar.,
ferr-i., ferr-p., fl-ac.,** flor-p.[14],
form.[6], **gamb., graph., guaj.,** hecla[14],
HELL., hep., HYOS., ign., iod., **ip.,**
jatr., **kali-ar., kali-bi., kali-c.,
kali-i.,** kali-m.[1]', **KALI-N., kali-p.,
kali-s.,** kali-sil.[1]', **kalm.,** kreos.,
**LACH., laur., led., lil-t., LYC.,
MAG-C., mag-m., mang., MENY.,**
meph.[4], **MERC.,** merc-c.[8], **merc-i-r.,
MEZ.,** mosch., mur-ac., **nat-ar.,
nat-c., nat-m., NAT-P.,** nat-sil.[1]',
nep.[10, 13, 14], nicc., **NIT-AC., nux-m.,
nux-v.,** olnd.[2, 3], op., osm., **ox-ac.,**
palo.[14], **par.**[2, 3], penic.[13], **petr.,
PHOS-AC., PHOS.,** phyt., pic-ac.,
pitu.[14], plan., **PLAT., PLB., psor.,
ptel., PULS., ran-b., RAN-S.,** rheum,
rhod., rhus-t., RUMX., RUTA,
sabad., **sabin.,** sal-ac., **samb., sang.,
sars.,** sel., **seneg., SEP., SIL.,
SIN-N.,** spig., **spong.,** squil.,
STANN., staph., stict., **STRONT-C.,
SUL-AC., sul-i.**[1]', **SULPH., sumb.,**
syph.[3, 8], **tab.,** tarax., tarent.[2], teucr.,
thiop.[14], **thuj.,** trios.[14], v-a-b.[14],
VALER., verat., verb., vib., viol-o.,
viol-t., x-ray[9], **ZINC., ZINC-P.**[1]'

18 h
ant-t.[3], bapt., calc.[7], calc-p., caust.,
cedr.[3], dig., hep., hyper., **kali-c.**[3],
kali-i., lachn., nat-m.[3], **NUX-V.**[3],
penic.[13], petr.[3], **puls.**[3], **rhus-t.**[3],
sep.[3], **sil.**[3], **sumb.**

18–19 h
carc.[9], culx.[1]', **hep.**

18–20 h[14]
rauw.

18–22 h[14]
kali-c.

18–4 h[7]
guaj.

18–6 h
kreos., lil-t.[6], **syph.**

19 h
alum.[3], ant-c., bov., cedr.[3], chin-s.[3],
culx.[1]', ferr.[3], gamb.[3], gels.[3], **hep.**[3],
ip.[3], **lyc.,** nat-m.[3], **nat-s.**[3], **nux-v.**[3],
petr., puls.[3], pyrog.[3], rhus-t., **sep.**[3],
sulph.[3], tarent.[3]

20 h
alum.[3], **bov.**[3], caust.[3], coff.[3], elaps[3],
hep.[3], mag-c.[3], merc.[3], merc-i-r.,
phos.[3], **rhus-t.**[3], **SULPH.**[3], tarax.

20–3 h[8]
syph.

21 h
ars.[3], **bov.**[3], **BRY.,** calc.[7], **gels.**[3],
merc.[3], mur-ac., sulph.

and night

cenchr.[1]', lil-t.[6], mag-c.[3]

air agg., in open

am-c., carb-an., carb-v., **merc.,**
nit-ac., sulph.

am.
agar.[6], **alum.**, aran-ix.[10], arn.,
arg-m., asaf., **AUR.**, bor.[8], bruc.[4],
cast.[6], chel., cob-n.[9], cortiso.[14],
halo.[14], hed.[10, 14], kali-n.[4],
lob.[8], lyc., mag-c.[10], **med.**, nat-m.[6],
nicc.[8], nux-v.[8], podo.[6], **puls.**[3, 4, 6],
sep., stel.[8], thyr.[14], visc.[9, 14]

16 h till going to bed am.

alum.

eating, after

indg.

am.
sep.

every other evening

puls.

lying down agg., after

ars., graph.[6], hep.[6], **ign., led.,**
merc.[6], **phos.**, puls.[6], sel.[6],
stront-c., **sulph.**, thuj.

am.
kali-n.

sleep, before going to

plat.

sunset, after

ang.[3], bry., ign., lycps.[3], merc.[3],
phyt.[3], **puls.**, rhus-t., syph.[3]

am.[3]
coca, lil-t., med., sel.

till sunrise

aur., cimic., colch., **merc.**[3, 8],
phyt.[8], **SYPH.**[1, 7]

twilight agg.

am-m., ang.[3], arg-n.[3], **ars.,**
ars-s-f.[1'], berb.[3], **calc., caust.,**
cham.[3], dig., graph.[3], mang.[3],
nat-m., nat-s.[3], **phos.**, plat.[3], plb.,
PULS., rhus-t., staph., sul-ac.,
valer.

am.
alum., bry., meny.[3], **phos.**, tab.[3]

NIGHT (21–5 h)

abel.[14], abrot., acet-ac., **ACON.,**
agar., agn., agre.[14], aloe, alum.,
ALUM-P.[1'], alum-sil.[1'], alumn.[2],
am-br., am-c., **am-m.**, ambr., **ammc.,**
anac., **ang.**[2, 3], **ant-c., ant-t.,**
apis[3, 6, 8], apoc., **aral.**, aran.[3],
arg-m., **ARG-N.**, arist-cl.[9], **ARN.,**
ARS., ARS-I., ARS-S-F.[1'], asaf.,
asar., aster.[8], **aur.**, aur-ar.[1'], aur-i.[1'],
aur-m.[1'], **AUR-S.**[1'], bac.[8], **bar-c.,**
bar-i.[1'], **bar-m., bar-s.**[1'], **bell.,**
benz-ac., berb-a.[14], bism., bor.,
bov., brom., bry., bufo[3], buni-o.[14],
but-ac.[8], cact., caj.[8], calad., **CALC.,**
calc-ar.[1'], **CALC-I., CALC-P.,**
CALC-S., CALC-SIL.[1'], camph.,
cann-i., cann-s., canth., caps.,
carb-ac., **CARB-AN., carb-v.,**
CARBN-S., caust., cedr., **cench.**[1',7,8],
CHAM., chel.[1], **CHIN.**, chin-ar.,
chion.[8], cic., cimic.[3], **cina**[1], **CINNB.,**
clem., coc-c., **cocc., cod., COFF.,**
COLCH., coloc., com.[8], **CON.,**
convo-s.[14], **croc.**, crot-c.[8], **crot-h.,**
crot-t.[4], **cupr., CYCL.**, cyt-l.[9], **dig.,**
dios., dol., **dros., DULC.**, elaps,
erig.[10], eucal., **euphr., equis.,**
FERR., FERR-AR., FERR-I., ferr-p.,

fl-ac., flaw.[14], gamb., GRAPH.,
grat.[4], guaj., hed.[9], hell., HEP.,
hip-ac.[14], HYOS., ign., IOD., IP.,
iris[8], jal.[3, 6], KALI-AR., KALI-BI.,
kali-br., KALI-C., KALI-I., kali-m.,
kali-n., kali-p., kali-sil.[1'] kalm.[1'],
kreos., LACH., laur., led., LIL-T.,
lob.[3], lyc., MAG-C., MAG-M.,
mag-p.[3, 8], mand.[9], MANG., meny.,
meph.[3, 14], MERC., merc-c.,
merc-i-f., mez., moly-met.[14], mosch.,
mur-ac., nat-ar., nat-c., nat-m.,
nat-p., nat-s., nat-sil.[1'], nep.[10, 13, 14],
NIT-AC., nux-m., nux-v., olnd.,
op., ox-ac., par., pareir.[2], petr.,
ph-ac., phenob.[13], PHOS., phyt.,
pic-ac., plat., PLB., PSOR., PULS.,
pyrog.[3], ran-b., ran-s., rat.[3], rheum,
rhod., RHUS-T., RUMX., ruta[3, 6],
sabad., sabin., sal-ac., samb., sang.,
sarcol-ac.[14], sars., sec., sel., senec.,
seneg., SEP., sieg.[10], SIL., sin-n.,
spig., spong., squil., stann., staph.,
stict., still.[3], stram., STRONT-C.,
sul-ac., SUL-I.[1'], SULPH.,
SYPH.[1'-3, 6-8], tarax., tarent.,
TELL., ter.[3], teucr., thal.[14], thea[8],
thuj., trios.[14], valer., verat., vib.[8],
viol-t., vip.[3], visc.[14], x-ray[8], ZINC.,
ZINC-P.[1']

22 h
ars.[3], bov.[3], cham., CHIN-S.[3],
graph.[3], ign.[3], lach.[3], petr.[3], podo.,
puls.

23 h
aral.[3], ars.[3], bell., cact., calc.[3],
carb-an.[3], lach., rumx., sil., sulph.[3]

night-air agg.[3]

am-c., carb-v., merc., nat-s., nit-ac.,
sulph.

am.[3, 6]
alum.[3, 4], ang., arg-m.[3], caust.,
cupr-a.[8], laur.[3, 4], mand.[9], med.[7],
petr.[3]

every other night

    puls.

midnight[3]

ACON.[3, 7], aran.[8], arg-n.[3, 6],
ars.[3, 7, 8], ars-i.[6], brom.[6], calc.,
calad., canth., caust., chin.[1', 3],
dig., dros., ferr., hed.[14], kali-ar.[1'],
kali-c., lach.[3, 4], lyc., mag-m.,
mez.[8], mur-ac., nat-m., nux-m.,
nux-v.[3, 6], op.[3, 6], phos., puls.[3, 6],
rhus-t., samb., spong., stram.,
sulph.[3, 7], verat., zinc.[5]

before
alum., alum-p.[1'], am-m., ambr.,
anac., ang.[2, 3], ant-t., apis,
ARG-N., arn., ARS., ars-s-f.[1'],
asar., bell., brom., bry.,
calad.[2, 3], cann-s., caps.[3],
CARB-V., carbn-s., caust.,
CHAM., chel., chin., COFF.,
colch., cupr., cycl., dulc., ferr.,
ferr-ar., fl-ac.[3], graph., hep.,
ign., KALI-AR., kali-c.,
kali-m.[1'], lach., LED., LYC.,
mag-c.[3], mang., merc., mez.,
mosch., mur-ac., nat-m.,
nat-p.[1'], nat-s.[1'], nit-ac., nux-v.,
osm., petr., PHOS., phyt., plat.,
psor., PULS., ran-b., RAN-S.,
rhod., rhus-t., RUMX., ruta,
SABAD., samb., sep., spig.,
spong., STANN., staph.,
stront-c., sulph., teucr., thuj.,
valer., verat.[3], viol-t.

after,
acon., alum., alum-p.[1'],
alum-sil.[1'], am-m., ambr.,
ang.[2, 9], ant-c., apis[9], arist-cl.[9],
ARS., ars-i., asaf., aur.,
aur-ar.[1'], bar-c., bar-i.[1'], bar-m.,
bar-s.[1'], bell., bor., bry.,
calad.[2, 3], calc., calc-i.[1'],
calc-sil.[1'], cann-s., canth.,
caps., carb-an.[2, 3, 8], carb-v.,

caust., cham., **chel.**, chin.,
coc-c., cocc., coff., con., croc.,
cupr., DROS., dulc., euph.[2],
euphr., **ferr., ferr-ar.,** ferr-i.,
ferr-p., **gels.,** graph., hed.[9],
hell., hep., **ign.,** iod., **KALI-C.,**
kali-m.[1'], **KALI-N.,** kali-p.,
kali-sil.[1'], lyc.[2, 3], **mag-c.,**
mand.[9, 10], **mang., merc., mez.,**
mur-ac., **NAT-AR.,** nat-c.,
nat-m., nat-p., nat-s., nat-sil.[1'],
nit-ac., **NUX-V.,** par., **ph-ac.,**
PHOS., phyt., plat., **PODO.,**
puls., ran-b., **ran-s.,** rhod.,
RHUS-T., rumx., sabad., sabin.,
samb., sars., seneg., sep., **SIL.,**
spig., **spong.,** squil., staph.,
stram., sul-ac., sul-i.[3], **sulph.,**
tarax., **THUJ.,** viol-o.

0–4 h[6]: thuj.

1 h
    ARS., carb-v.[3], caul., cocc.,
    lachn., mag-m., mur-ac., psor.,
    puls.[3]

1–2 h[1']
    ars.

1–3 h
    kali-ar.

2 h
    all-c. (non[1]: ars.), aur-m.,
    benz-ac., **caust.**[3], com.[3], cur.[7],
    dros., ferr., graph.[3], **hep.,** iris[3],
    (non[1]: kali-ar.), **kali-bi., kali-br.,**
    KALI-C., kali-p.[3], lach.[3], lachn.,
    lyc.[3], mag-c., mez.[3], nat-m.[3],
    nat-s.[3], **nit-ac.**[3], ptel.[3], **puls.**[3],
    rumx., sars.[3], **sil.**[3], spig.[3], sulph.[3]

2–3 h
    gink-b.[14], kali-bi.[6]

2–4 h
    arist-cl.[9, 10], **KALI-C.**

2–5 h[8]
    aesc., aeth., **aloe,** am-c., bac.,
    bell., bell-p.[10], chel., cina, coc-c.,
    cur., hed.[10], **kali-bi., kali-c.,**
    kali-cy., kali-p., nat-s., **nux-v.,**
    ox-ac., **podo.,** ptel., rhod.,
    rumx., sulph., thuj., tub.

3 h
    adlu.[14], **am-c., am-m.**[3], ant-c.,
    ant-t., **ars.**[1], bapt., bor., **bry.**[3],
    calc., canth.[3], **cedr.**[3], chin., con.,
    euphr., dulc., ferr.[3], hed.[9, 10, 14],
    iris, **kali-ar.**[1], kali-bi.[1'], **KALI-C.,**
    kali-n., kali-p.[7], **mag-c.**[3, 10],
    mag-f.[10, 14], mag-m., **nat-m.**[3],
    nux-v., podo., **rhus-t.**[3], sec., **sel.**[3],
    sep., sil.[3], staph., **sulph.**[3], thuj.,
    zinc.

3–4 h[6]
    am-m., arist-cl.[10], caust., kali-bi.,
    kali-c., med.[7], nux-v.[6]

3–5 h[10]
    bor.[6], calc-f., mag-c., mand.,
    syph.[6]

4 h
    alum.[3], alumn., **am-m.**[3], anac.[3],
    apis[3], **arn.**[3], **bor.**[3], **caust.**[3],
    CEDR.[3], chel., coloc.[3], **con.**[3],
    cycl.[6], ferr.[3], **ign.**[3], kali-c.[3], **lyc.**[3],
    mag-c.[10], **mur-ac.**[3], **nat-s.**[3],
    nit-ac.[3], **NUX-V.**[3], penic.[13, 14],
    podo., **puls.**[3], rad-br.[3], sep.[3], sil.[3],
    stann.[3], **sulph.**[3], verat.[3]

4–16 h
    kali-cy.[7], **MED.**[7], nux-v.

am.
    LYC., mand.[9], nat-p.[1'], nat-s.[1']

until noon[8]

    puls.

until noon

    ars., cist.

ABSCESSES, suppurations

acon.[8, 11], all-c.[2], **anan.**, ant-c.,
ant-t., **ANTHRACI.**[1, 7], **apis**[2, 8, 12],
ARN.[2, 3, 6, 8, 12], ars., **ars-i.**, ars-s-f.[1'],
asaf., **bar-c.**, bar-m.[11], **bell.**[2, 6, 8, 12],
bell-p.[7], both.[11], **bry.**, bufo[3, 12],
calc., calc-f.[1', 10], **calc-hp.**[3, 6, 8],
CALC-I., **CALC-S.**, calc-sil.[1'],
CALEN.[2, 3, 7, 8, 12], **canth.**[2], caps.,
carb-ac.[8], carb-an.[6], **carb-v.**,
caust.[2], **cench.**[1'], **cham.**[2, 4], **chin.**[8, 12],
chin-ar.[10], chin-s.[8, 11], cic., **cist.**[2, 6],
cocc., con., conch.[11], **croc.**, crot-h.,
cupr.[6], digox.[12], **dulc.**, **echi.**[3, 6, 7],
elat.[12], **fl-ac.**[2, 6-8, 12], **guaj.**, **gunp.**[7],
HEP., **hippoz.**[2, 8, 12], kali-c., kali-chl.,
kali-s.[3], **kreos.**[2, 6], **LACH.**, **lap-a.**[2, 8],
led.[2, 8], **lyc.**[1'-3, 6, 8], mag-c., **mang.**[1', 2],
matth.[12], **MERC.**, merc-d.[3], methyl.[12],
mez., **myris.**[6-8, 10, 12], nat-c., nat-m.,
nat-sal.[12], nat-sil.[1'], **nit-ac.**, nux-v.,
ol-j.[1] (non: olnd.), paeon., petr.,
ph-ac.[1', 6, 8], **PHOS.**[1'-4, 6, 8],
phyt.[2, 6], plb.[11], psor.[6], ptel.[11], puls.,
pyrog., raja-s.[14],
rhus-t.[1'-3, 4, 6, 8], **sec.**, sep., sieg.[7, 10],
SIL., sil-mar.[8], staph., **stram.**,
sul-ac.[2], sul-i.[3, 6], **sulph.**, symph.[12],
syph.[1', 7, 8, 12], tarent.[2, 3], **tarent-c.**,
thyr.[12], tub.[6], vesp.[8, 11, 12], **vip.**[4],
wies.[11]

fistulae
reaction, lack

⌐ *wounds—suppurating*

abort, remedies to[8]

apis, arn.[7], bell., bry., calc.[1'],
calc-s.[2], hep., merc.

absorption of pus[3]

iod., **LACH.**, phos., **sil.**

bones, of[6]

ang., arg-m., arg-n., aur., calc-f.,
calc-hp., merc-aur., phos., puls.[3],
sil., staph., sulph.[3]

burning

ANTHRACI., **ARS.**, merc.[1'], **pyrog.**,
TARENT-C.

chronic[2, 8]

arg-m.[14], arn.[8], **asaf.**[2], aur.[2], calc.,
calc-f.[8], calc-i.[8], calc-p.[8], calc-s.[6],
carb-v., cham.[8], chin.[8], con.[2],
fl-ac.[6, 8], graph.[8], **hep.**, **iod.**, iodof.[8],
kali-i.[8], laur.[2], lyc.[2], mag-f.[14],
mang.[2], **merc.**, merc-c.[2], merc-i-r.[8],
nit-ac.[2], ol-j.[8, 12], phos.[2, 6, 8], sars.[2],
sep.[2], **SIL.**[2, 7, 8], **sulph.**

effects from[6]

abrot., **chin.**, chin-ar., ferr., kali-c.,
nat-m., ph-ac., **phos.**

fever, continued[7]

ph-ac.

foreign bodies, elimination of

arn.[7], **hep.**[1', 2], **lob.**[7, 12], **SIL.**[2, 7, 12]

gangrenous[2]

ars., asaf., carb-v., chin., chin-s.,
hep., kreos., **LACH.**, merc., **nit-ac.**,
phos., sil., sul-ac.

glands, of

aur.[4], aur-m-n.[2], bad.[3, 6], **bar-c.**[2, 3, 6], bar-m., **bell.,** brom., **CALC.,** calc-f.[10], **calc-hp.**[3, 6, 10], calc-i.[8], calc-p.[10], **CALC-S.,** canth., carb-an.[3, 6, 10], carb-v., cinnb.[1'], cist., clem.[3, 6], coloc., crot-h., **dulc.,** echi.[6], fl-ac.[3, 6, 10], **form.**[3, 6], **guaj.,** guare.[2], **HEP.,** hyos., ign., jug-r.[12], **KALI-I.,** kreos., **lach.,** lap-a.[8], **lyc., MERC.,** myris.[10], **nit-ac.,** petr., **phos., phyt.**[3], **pyrog., rhus-t., sars.,** sec.[12], **sep., SIL.,** sil-mar.[12], spig.[3], squil., sul-ac.[3], **SULPH., stram., syph.,** teucr-s.[6, 10], **tub.,** zinc.[3]

hasten suppuration remedies to[1'-3, 8]

ars.[3], bell.[3], guaj.[8], **hep.,** lach.[3, 8], **merc.,** nat-sil.[1'], oper.[8], phos.[8], phyt.[8], puls.[3], **sil.**[1-3, 7, 8], sulph.[1']

incipient[6]

apis, **arn.**[2, 6], ars., **bar-c.**[2], **bell., carb-an.,** euph., guaj., **hep., lach., merc.**[2, 6], rhus-t.

internal organs, of[2]

canth., LACH.

joints, of[6]

ang.:[2], ars-i., bac., calc., calc-f., **calc-hp.**[6, 8], **calc-p.**[2, 3], calc-s., conch.[11], fl-ac., guaj.[1'], kali-c., kali-i., **merc.**[1'-3, 6], myris.[12], nit-ac., ol-j.[12], ph-ac., **phos.**[3, 6], **psor.**[3, 6], puls., **sil.**[2, 3, 6, 8], ter., **teucr.,** thuj., tub.

muscles, of [1', 8]

calc.

pus, acrid[4]

ail.[3], **ARS.**[3, 4], asaf.[6], bell-p.[3], brom.[3], **carb-v., CAUST.**[2, 4, 6], **cham., clem.,** echi.[3], euphr.[3], fl-ac.[1'], gels.[3], **hep., kali-ox.**[3], lach., **lyc., merc.**[2, 4, 6], mez., **nat-c.,** nat-m., **NIT-AC.**[3, 4], nux-v., petr.[2], phos., plb., puls., **ran-b.**[3, 4], ran-s., **rhus-t.**[2, 4, 6], ruta, sabad.[3], sanic.[3], sars.[3], **sep., sil.**[2, 4, 6], spig., squil., **staph., sulph.**[2-4, 6], zinc.

excoriating[4]

am-c., anac., bell., calc., chel., con., cupr., graph., ign., iod., kreos.

black[4]

bry., chin., lyc., **sulph.**[2, 4]

bland[2]

bell., **calc., hep., lach.,** mang., **merc.,** phos., **PULS.,** rhus-t., **sil.,** staph., **sulph.**

bloody[4]

arg-n., arn., **ars.**[2, 4, 6], **ASAF.**[2, 4, 6], bell., calc-s.[1'], **carb-v.**[2, 4], **caust.**[2, 4], con., croc., dros., **HEP.**[2, 4, 6], iod., kali-c., kreos., lach., **lyc.**[2, 4], **MERC.**[2, 3, 4, 6], mez., nat-m., **nit-ac.**[2, 4, 6], ph-ac., phos., **phyt.**[2], **puls.**[2, 4], **rhus-t.**[2, 4], ruta, sabin., sec., **sep., sil.**[2, 4, 6], sul-ac., sulph., zinc.

brown[2, 4]

anac.[4], **ars.**, bry., calc.[4], **carb-v.**,
con.[4], puls.[4], **rhus-t., sil.**

fetid[4]

am-c., ant-t., **anthraci.**[2], arn.[7],
ars.[2-4, 6], **ASAF.**[2, 4, 6], aur., bapt.[3],
bar-m., **bell.**, bov., bry., **calc.**[2, 4, 6],
carb-an.[2], **CARB-V.**[2, 4, 6],
caust.[2, 4], chel., **chin.**[2, 4],
chin-s.[2, 4, 12], cic., clem., con.[2, 3, 4],
cycl., dros., fl-ac.[6], **graph.**[2, 4],
HEP.[2, 4, 6], kali-c., **kali-p.**[2],
KREOS.[2, 4], **lach.**[2, 4, 6], led.[3],
lyc.[2, 4], mang., **merc.**[2, 4], mez.,
mur-ac., nat-c., **nit-ac.**[2, 4, 6],
nux-m., **nux-v.**[2, 4], paeon.[6], petr.[6],
ph-ac.[2, 4, 6], phos.[2, 4, 6], **phyt.**[2],
plb., **psor.**[3, 6], **puls.**, pyrog.[3],
ran-b., **ran-s., rhus-t.**[2, 4], ruta,
sabin., sec., **sep.**[2-4], **SIL.**[2-4, 6],
squil., stann., **staph.**, sul-ac.[4, 6],
SULPH.[2-4, 6], syph.[3], thuj., vip.[4, 6],
vip-r.

gelatinous[2, 4]

arg-m.[4], arn.[4], bar-c.[4], cham.,
ferr.[4], merc., sep.[4], **sil.**

gray[2, 4]

ambr.[4], **ars.**, carb-an.[4], **caust.**,
chin.[4], lyc.[4], merc., sep.[4], **sil.**,
thuj.[4]

greenish[2, 4]

ars.[4], **asaf., aur.**, carb-v.[4], **caust.**,
kreos.[4], **MERC.**, nat-c.[4], nux-v.[4],
phos.[4], **puls.**, rhus-t.[4], sec.[1', 3],
sep., sil., staph.[4], syph.[3], tub.[3]

sour, smelling[2, 4]

calc., graph.[4], **hep.**, kalm., **merc.**,
nat-c.[4], sep.[4], sulph.

suppressed[3]

bry., calc.[2], cham.[2], dulc., **HEP.**[2],
lach.[2, 3], **merc.**[2], puls., **sil.**[2, 3],
stram., **sulph.**

tenacious[2, 4]

ars.[4], asaf., bor.[3], bov., cham.[4],
coc-c.[3], **con.**[2-4], hydr.[3], kali-bi.[3],
merc., mez.[4], ph-ac.[4], phos.[2],
sep., sil.[4], sulph.[4]

thick[3]

arg-n., **calc-sil.**[1'], euphr., hep.,
kali-bi., kali-s., **puls.**, sanic.

thin[3, 4]

ars.[3], **asaf.**[3, 4, 6], carb-v.[4],
caust.[3, 4, 6], dros.[4], fl-ac.[3], iod.[4],
kali-c.[4], **lyc.**[4], **merc.**[3, 4, 6], nit-ac.,
phos.[3], plb.[4], puls.[4], ran-b.[4],
ran-s.[4], rhus-t.[3, 4, 6], ruta[4],
sil.[3, 4, 6], staph.[4], **sulph.**[3, 4, 6],
thuj.[4]

watery[2, 4, 6]

agar-cps.[11], **ars., ASAF.**, calc.[2, 3, 4],
carb-v.[2, 4], **caust.**, cench.[1'],
cham.[2], clem.[4], con.[4], dros.[4],
fl-ac.[3], **graph.**[4], **iod.**[4], kali-c.[4],
lach.[4], **lyc.**[2, 4], **merc., nit-ac.**[2, 3, 4],
nux-v.[4], **phyt.**[2], plb.[4], puls.[4],
ran-b.[2, 4], **ran-s.**[4], rhus-t.[6], **sil.**[3, 6]

whitish[4]

am-c., ars., **calc.**[2, 4], carb-v., hell.,
lyc.[2, 4], nat-m., puls., sep., sil.,
sulph.

yellow[4]

acon., am-c., ambr., anac., ang.,
arg-m., ars.[2, 4], aur., bov., **bry.**,
calc.[2, 4, 6], calc-s.[1'], caps.,
carb-v.[2, 4, 6], **caust.**[2, 4, 6], cench.[1'],
cic., **clem.**, con., croc., dulc.,
euphr.[3], graph., **HEP.**[2, 4], iod.,
kali-n., kreos., lyc., mag-c., mang.,
merc.[2, 4, 6], **mez.**[3, 6], **nat-c.**[2, 4],
nat-m., **nit-ac.**[4, 6], **nux-v.**,
phos.[1', 2, 4], **PULS.**[2, 4, 6],
rhus-t.[2, 4], ruta, sec., sel.,
sep.[2, 4, 6], **sil.**[2, 4, 6], spig., **staph.**[2, 4],
sul-ac., **sulph.**[2], thuj., viol-t.

yellow-green[3]

ars-i., **calc-sil.**[1'], kali-bi., kali-s.,
merc.[1'], **puls.**[2, 3]

recurrent

pyrog., syph.

wounds–reopening

ACETONEMIA of the child[14]

phenob.

ACTIVITY am.[3]

cycl., helon., iod., kali-bi., lil-t.,
mur-ac., sep.

Vol. I: occupation
Vol. I: exertion

desire for[2]

acon., ars., aur., eucal.

increased[2]

acon., agar., ant-c., ant-t., camph.,
cic.[14], eucal., **hyos.**, lyss., nep.[13, 14],
op., ox-ac., plat., **stram.**

outer a. ceases[9]

anh.

physical[11]

ars., coca[7, 11], fl-ac.[7], lycps.,
nat-s., nep.[13, 14], **op.**, phos.

exertion

afternoon[11]

rhus-t.

evening[11]

lycps.

midnight, until[11]

COFF.

ADHESION of inner parts,
sensation of[3, 7]

arn., bry., coloc., **dig.**[7], euph., hep.,
kali-c.[3], kali-n., merc.[7], **mez.**, nux-v.,
par., petr., phos., **plb.**, puls., **ran-b.**[3],
RHUS-T., seneg., **sep., sulph.**, thuj.,
verb.

AGILITY[3]

apis, calc-p., coca[11], coff., form.[11, 12],
lach., mang., nux-v., op., rhus-t.,
stram., tarent., valer.

AGRANULOCYTOSIS[9]

cortico., lach.[10], sulfa.

AIR, draft agg.

acon., alum.[1'], anac., **ars.**, ars-s-f.[1'],
bapt.[2], **BELL.**, benz-ac., bov.,
brom.[1'], **bry.**[1, 7], cadm-s., **CALC.**,
calc-f.[1', 7, 10] **CALC-P.**, calc-s.,
calc-sil.[1'], camph., **canth.**[3], **caps.**
carb-an., **carbn-s.**[1, 7], **caust.**,
cench.[1'], **cham.**, chin., cist., cocc.,
colch.[3, 6], coloc., crot-h.[3], dulc.[1'],
ferr., gels., **graph.**, hep., **ign.**,
kali-ar., kali-bi.[3], **KALI-C.**, kali-m.[1'],
kali-n., kali-p., kali-s., kali-sil.[1'],
lac-c., **lach.**, led., **LYC.**[1, 7], **lyss.**,
mag-c.[1, 7], **mag-p.**, med., **merc.**,
mim-p.[14], mur-ac., nat-c., nat-m.[1, 7],
nat-p., nat-sil.[1'], **nit-ac.**, nux-m.,
nux-v., **ol-j.**, onop.[14], petr., **ph-ac.**,
phos., psil.[14], **psor.**, **PULS.**[1, 7],
ran-b., **RHUS-T.**, rumx., sang.[3, 6],
sanic., sars., **SEL.**, senec.[1'], **sep.**,
SIL., **spig.**[1, 7], stann.[1'], **stram.**[1, 7],
stront-c., **SULPH.**, **sumb.**, tep.[11],
tub.[1', 3, 7], valer., verb., vichy[11],
x-ray[9], **zinc.**, zinc-p.[1']

ailments from[12]

cadm-s., lach.

cold draft, when perspiring

dulc.[1'], merc-i-f.[12]

am.[3]
lycps.

sensation of, as if fanned

camph., canth., caust.[6], **chel.**,
coloc.[6], cor-r., croc., fl-ac., graph.,
lac-d., **laur.**, **mez.**[6], **mosch.**, **nux-v.**,
olnd., puls., rhus-t., sabin., samb.,
spig., squil., stram., **zinc.**

fanned
wind-sensation

indoor air agg.[2]

acon., **ALUMN.**, am-c., am-m.,
ambr., anac., ang., ant-c., arg-m.,
arn., ars., **asaf.**, **asar.**, aur., bar-c.,
bell., **bor.**, **bov.**, bry., calc., camph.,
cann-s., canth., caps., carb-an.,
carb-v., **caust.**, chel., **cic.**, cina,
coff., **colch.**, con., **CROC.**, dig.,
dulc., graph., **hell.**, hep., hyos., ign.,
iod., ip., kali-c., kali-n., **laur.**, **lyc.**,
MAG-C., mag-m., mang. **meny.**,
merc., **mez.**, mosch., mur-ac., nat-c.,
nat-m., nit-ac., nux-v., **op.**, **ph-ac.**,
phos., **plat.**, **plb.**, **PULS.**, **ran-b.**,
ran-s., **rhod.**, rhus-t., ruta, **SABIN.**,
sars., sel., **seneg.**, sep., spig.,
spong., **stann.**, staph., **stront-c.**,
sul-ac., **sulph.**, **tarax.**, thuj., **verat.**,
verb., viol-t., **zinc.**

am.[2]
agar., alumn., **am-c.**, **am-m.**,
ambr., anac., ang., **ant-c.**, arn.,
ars., bar-c., **bell.**, bor., bov., bry.,
calad., **calc.**, camph., **cann-s.**,
canth., caps., carb-an., carb-v.,
caust., **CHAM.**, **chel.**, **chin.**, cic.,
Cina, cit-v., **COCC.**, coff., **coloc.**,
con., dig., **dros.**, dulc., **euph.**,
ferr., graph., **GUAJ.**, hell., hep.,
hyos., **ign.**, iod., **ip.**, kali-c.,
kali-n., **kreos.**, lach., laur., **led.**,
lyc., mag-c., mag-m., mang.,
meny., **merc.**, mez., **mosch.**,

mur-ac., nat-c., nat-m., **nit-ac.,
NUX-M., NUX-V.,** oci-s.[9], **olnd.,**
op., **petr.,** ph-ac., phos., plat.,
plb., puls., ran-b., **rheum,** rhod.,
rhus-t., ruta, sabad., sabin., sars.,
sel., seneg., sep., **SIL., spig.,**
stann., **staph., stram.,** stront-c.,
sul-ac., sulph., tarent., **teucr.,
thuj., valer.,** verat., verb., **viol-t.,**
zinc.

night-air see night-air

open a. agg., in

acon., **agar.,** agn., agre.[14], alco.[11],
all-c.[3], alum., alumn.[2], **am-c.,**
am-m., ambr., anac., ang.[3], ant-c.,
ant-t., arg-m.[2], arn., **ars., ars-s-f.**[1'],
asar.[3], aur., aur-ar.[1'], aur-s.[1'],
aza.[14], **bar-c.,** bar-m., **bell.,**
benz-ac.[8], berb.[4], bor., bov.,
bruc.[4], **bry.,** bufo, cact., cadm-s.[8],
calad., **calc.,** calc-i.[1'], **calc-p.,**
camph.[3], cann-s.[3], canth., **caps.,**
carb-an., carb-v., carbn-o.[11],
carbn-s.[8], **caust.,** cedr., **cham.,**
chel., CHIN., chin-ar., cic.,
cimic.[3], cina, cist.[3], **clem., COCC.,**
coff., coff-t.[7], colch.[3], **coloc., con.,**
cor-r.[3, 8], crot-h.[8], crot-t., **cycl.**[8],
.dig., dros.[8], **dulc.,** epiph.[8], euph.,
euphr.[8], **ferr.,** ferr-ar., ferr-p.,
fl-ac.[3], form., **graph., GUAJ.,**
ham., hell., **helon., HEP.,** hyos.,
ign., iod., ip., **kali-ar., kali-bi.,**
KALI-C., kali-m.[1'], **kali-n.,**
kali-p., kali-sil.[1'], kalm., **kreos.,**
lach., laur., led.[3], lina.[8], **lyc.,**
lycpr.[8], **lyss.,** mag-c., mag-m.[2],
mag-p.[3], **mang.,** meny., **MERC.,**
merc-c., mez.[3, 11], mosch.[3, 8],
mur-ac., nat-ar., **nat-c.,** nat-m.,
nat-p., nat-sil.[1'], **NIT-AC.,**
NUX-M., NUX-V., olnd., op.,
par., **petr., ph-ac., phos.,** phyt.,
plat.[3], plb., **psor.,** puls., ran-b.,
rheum, rhod., **rhus-t., RUMX.,**
ruta, sabad.[3], sabin.[3], sang.[3],
sars.[3], **sel.,** senec., **seneg.**[1], **sep.,**
SIL., spig., spong.[3], **stann.,**

staph.[3], **stram., stront-c., sul-ac.,
SULPH.,** tarax.[3], **teucr.,** thea[8],
thuj., **valer.,** verat., verb., viol-t.,
voes.[11], x-ray[8], **zinc.**

am.

abrot., **acon.,** aesc.[3], agar., **agn.,
all-c.,** aloe, **ALUM.,** alum-p.[1'],
alum-sil.[1'], **ALUMN.**[2], am-c.[2, 3],
am-m., ambr., **aml-ns., anac.**[2, 3],
ang.[2, 3], ange-s.[14], **ant-c., apis,**
aran.[3], aran-ix.[10], **arg-m., ARG-N.,**
arist-cl.[10], arn., **ARS.,** ars-i.,
ars-s-f.[1'], **asaf.,** asar., **atro., aur.,**
aur-i.[1'], aur-m.[1'], **bapt.**[3],
bar-c.[2, 3, 16], bar-i.[1'], bar-s.[1'],
bell.[2, 3, 16], bism.[2], bor.[2, 3], **bov.,**
bry., buni-o.[14], **cact.,** caj., **calad.,**
calc.[2, 3], calc-i.[1'], **calc-s., camph.,**
CANN-I., cann-s., canth.,
caps.[2, 3], carb-ac., carb-an.,
carb-v., carbn-s., carc.[9], caust.[2, 3],
chel., chlor., cic., **cimic.,** cina[2, 3],
cinnb., coc-c., coca, **coff.,**
colch.[3], coloc., com., **con., CROC.,**
crot-c., culx.[1'], dicha.[14], dig.,
dios., dulc.[2, 3]. erig.[10], euphr.,
ferr-i., **fl-ac.,** flor-p.[14], **gamb.,**
gels., glon.[3], **graph.,** grat.[1'],
hed.[10], **hell.,** hep.[2, 3], hip-ac.[9, 14],
hydr-ac., hyos., iber.[3], ign.[2, 3],
ind., **IOD., ip.,** kali-bi.,
kali-c.[2, 3, 14, 16], **KALI-I., kali-n.,**
kali-s., lac-c.[7], **lach.,** lact.,
laur., **lil-t., lyc., MAG-C.,**
MAG-M., mag-p.[3], mag-s.,
mang., **med.**[7, 15], **meli.,** meny.,
merc.[2, 3], merc-i-f.[1'], merc-i-r.,
mez., mosch., mur-ac., myrt.,
naphtin., nat-c., **nat-m., NAT-S.,**
nep.[10], nicc., nit-ac.[2, 3], nux-v.[3],
op., **osm.,** ph-ac., phos., **phyt.,**
pic-ac., pip-n.[3], pitu.[14], **plat.,**
plb., pneu.[14], **PSOR.**[3, 7, 15],
ptel., PULS., ran-b., **ran-s.,** rat.,
rauw.[9, 14], **rhod.**[2, 3], **RHUS-T.,**
ruta[2, 3], **SABAD., SABIN.,** sal-ac.,
sang., sanic., saroth.[9], sars.[2, 3, 16],
sec., sel.[2, 3], **seneg., sep.,** spig.,
spong., stann.[2, 3], **staph.**[2, 3],
stront-c.[2, 3], sul-ac.[2, 3], **sul-i.**[1'],
sulph., tab., tarax., **tarent.**[1', 7],

tell., thiop.[14], thlas.[3], thuj., tril.,
TUB.[7, 15], valer.[3], verat.[2, 3], verb.[1],
vib., viol-t., visc.[9], zinc., zinc-p.[1']

aversion to

agar., alum., AM-C., am-m.,
ambr., anac., ang.[3], aran.[3], arn.[3],
ars.[3], ars-s-f.[1'], aur.[3], BAPT., bell.,
bry., CALC., calc-ar.[1'], CALC-P.,
calc-sil.[1'], camph., cann-s.[3],
canth., caps., carb-an., carb-v.,
caust., CHAM., chel., chin., cic.[3],
cina, cist., COCC., COFF., coloc.,
con., cycl., dig., dros.[3], ferr.,
ferr-ar., graph., guaj., helon.,
hep., IGN., ip., kali-ar., KALI-C.,
kali-m.[1'], kali-n., kali-p.,
kali-sil.[1'], kreos., lach., laur.,
led.[3], lyc., lyss., mag-m.[3, 11],
mang., meny., merc., merc-c.,
mosch., mur-ac.[3], NAT-C., nat-m.,
nat-p., NAT-SIL.[1'], nit-ac.,
nux-m., NUX-V., op., PETR.,
ph-ac., phos., plat.[3], plb., psor.,
puls.[3], rhod., rhust-t., RUMX.,
ruta[3], sabin.[3], sars.[3], sel., seneg.,
sep., SIL., spig., staph.[3], stram.[3],
stront-c., sul-ac., SULPH., teucr.,
thuj., tub.[3], valer., verb., viol-t.,
zinc.[3]

alternating with desire for [1']

ars-s-f.

desire for

acon., agn., aloe[3], alum.,
alum-p.[1'], alum-sil.[1'], am-c.[3],
am-m., ambr., aml-ns.[11], anac.,
ang.[3], ange-s.[14], ant-c., ant-t., apis,
aran-ix.[10], arg-m., ARG-N.[1, 7],
arn., ars., ars-i., asaf., asar.,
aster., AUR., aur-ar.[1'], aur-i.[1'],
AUR-M., AUR-S.[1'], bapt.[6], bar-c.,
bar-i.[1'], bar-m., bar-s.[1'], bell.[3],

bor., bov., brom., bry., bufo, calc.[3],
CALC-I., calc-s., cann-s.[3], caps.[3],
carb-an., CARB-V., carbn-h.,
carbn-s., caust., chel.[11], cic.[3],
cimic.[14], cina[3], cit-v.[11], coca[11],
CROC., dig., elaps, fl-ac., gels.,
graph., hell., hep.[3], hyos.[11], IOD.,
ip.[6], kali-bi.[3], kali-c., KALI-I.,
kali-n., KALI-S., lach., lact.[11],
laur., lil-t., LYC., mag-c., mag-m.,
mang., med.[1', 7], meny., mez.,
mosch.[3], mur-ac., nat-c., nat-m.,
nat-s., op., ph-ac., phos., plat.,
plb.[3], ptel., PULS., rhod.[3], rhus-t.,
ruta[3], sabin., sanic., sars., sec.,
sel.[3], seneg., sep., spig., spong.,
stann., staph.[3], stram., stront-c.[3],
sul-ac.[3], sul-i.[1'], SULPH., tab.,
tarax., tarent., tell., teucr., thuj.,
tub.[1', 3, 7], tub-r.[13], verat.[3], viol-t.,
zinc., zinc-p.[1']

cold air see cold–air–desire

but draft agg.[7]

acon., anac., ars., bor., bry.,
calc-s., carb-an., carbn-s., caust.,
graph., KALI-C., lach., LYC.,
mag-c., mur-ac., nat-c., nat-m.,
ph-ac., phos., PULS., RHUS-T.,
sars., sep., spig., stram., SULPH.,
zinc.

passing through glands, sensation of

spong.

through him[3]

calc., coloc.

seashore agg., air on the

aq-mar.[8], ars., brom.[3, 8, 10],
carc.[7, 9, 10], iod.[10], kali-i., mag-m.,
mag-s.[10], med.[3, 7], nat-m.[1, 7],
nat-s., rhus-t.[3], sep., tub.[7]

bathing–sea

ailments from[12]

aq-mar., brom.

am.
  brom.[1', 3, 7, 8], **carc.**[7, 9, 10], lyc.[3],
  med.[1, 7], **nat-m.**[7], **tub.**[7]

alcohol see food–alcohol agg.–
  brandy agg.

ALIVE sensation, internally[3]

anac., asar., bell., berb.[3, 6], calc.,
cann-s., chel., cocc., **CROC.**[3, 6], cycl.,
hyos., **ign.**, kali-i., lach., led., mag-m.,
meny., merc., nat-m., op., petr., phos.,
plb., puls., rhod., sabad., sabin., sang.,
sec., sil., spong., sulph., tarax.,
THUJ.[3, 6], viol-t.

ALTERNATING states[3] ✻

acon., **ars.**[1'], dulc., ign., **KALI-BI.**,
lyc., onop.[14], prot.[14], puls.

change–symptoms

contradictory

ıstasis

ALUMINIUM poisoning[2, 3]

alum.[10], **bry.**, cadm-o.[7], camph., cham.,
ip., puls.

ANAEMIA

abel.[14], **acet-ac.**, acon., agar., agn.[1']
alet.[6, 8, 12], aloe[6], alum., alum-p.[1'],
alum-sil.[1'], am-c.[6], ambr., anil.[11, 12],
ant-c., **ant-t.**[2, 3], apis[2], apoc.[1'],
aq-mar.[6], **arg-m.**, arg-n., **arg-o.**[8],
arn., **ARS.**, ars-i., **ARS-S-F.**[1'],
aur-ar.[8, 12], **bell.**, ben-d.[12], berb.[1'],
beryl.[9, 14], bism.[2, 8], bol-la.[2], **BOR.**,
bov., **bry.**, cadm-met.[9, 14], **CALC.**,
calc-ar.[8], calc-i.[1'], calc-lac.[8],
CALC-P., calen.[6], calo.[8], carb-an.[1'],
carb-v., **carbn-s.**[2, 12], casc.[2, 12],
caust., cedr., cham., **CHIN.**, chin-ar.,
chin-s.[8], chlol.[12], chloram.[14],
chlorpr.[14], cic.[8], cina, cob-n.[9, 14],
cocc., coff., colch.[11], coloc., **con.**,
cortico.[9], cortiso.[9], crat.[8], **crot-h.**,
cupr., cupr-ar.[8], cupr-s.[11], **cycl.**,
dig., eucal.[6], **FERR.**, **FERR-AR.**,
ferr-c.[8], ferr-cit.[8], **ferr-i.**, **ferr-m.**[8, 12],
ferr-o-r.[8], **ferr-p.**, ferr-pic.[6], **ferr-r.**[8],
goss.[8], **GRAPH.**, **ham.**[2], **HELL.**,
helon., hep.[3], **hydr.**[2, 6, 8], **ign.**, iod.,
ip.[6, 12], **irid.**[8, 12], **KALI-AR.**, **kali-bi.**,
kali-br.[2], **KALI-C.**, kali-n.[6],
KALI-P., kalm.[2], kres.[10, 13, 14],
lac-ac.[12], lac-d.[1', 3, 6, 12], **lach.**, lec.[8],
lyc., mag-c., mag-m., **MANG.**,
MED., **MERC.**, **merc-c.**, mez.,
MOSCH.[3], nat-ar., **nat-c.**, **NAT-M.**,
nat-n.[6, 12], **nat-p.**, **nat-s.**, **NIT-AC.**,
nux-m., **nux-v.**, ol-j., **olnd.**, oxyg.[12],
petr., **ph-ac.**, **PHOS.**, **phyt.**[8], **pic-ac.**,
PLAT.[3, 6, 8], **PLB.**, **plb-a.**[8], psor.,
PULS., rhod., **rhus-t.**, ric.[11],
rub-t.[6, 8, 12], ruta, sabin., sacch.[8],
sec., senec., **sep.**, sil., spig., **SQUIL.**,
stann., **STAPH.**, stroph-h.[12],
SUL-AC., sulfa.[9, 14], sulfonam.[14],
SULPH., tab.[11, 12], ther., **thyr.**[8, 12],
tub.[1'], urt-u.[12], valer., vanad.[7, 8],
verat., **x-ray**[9, 14], **zinc.**, zinc-ar.[8],
zinc-m.[8], zinc-s.[11]

🖐 *faintness–anaemia*

weakness

exhausting disease, from[8]

acet-ac., alst., **calc-p., chin.,** chin-s.,
ferr., helon., kali-c., **nat-m., ph-ac.,**
phos.[2, 8], sec.[2]

haemorrhage, after

arg-o.[8], **ars.**[8], **calc., carb-v., CHIN.,**
crot-h.[8], **FERR., helon.**[2], hydr.[2],
ign.[8], **lach.,** nat-br.[8], **nat-m., nux-v.,**
ph-ac., phos., sabin.[1'], staph.[2],
sulph.

menorrhagia, from[8]

arg-o., ars., **calc.,** calc-p., **cann-i.**[2],
crat., **cycl., ferr., graph., hydr.**[2],
kali-c., mang., **nat-m., puls.,** sep.[7, 8]

nutritional disturbance, from[9]

alet., alum., **calc-p.,** terr., helon.,
nux-v.

pernicious[8, 12]

ars.[8], calc.[1'], **crot-h.**[2], mang.[1'],
nat-m.[1'], **phos.,** pic-ac.[2, 8, 12], **thyr.,**
trinit.[8]

ANAESTHESIA

abrot., absin.[11], **acon.**[6, 11], alco.[11],
ambr.[4, 6], **anac.**[2, 6], ant-t.[4], arg-n.[6],
ars.[4, 6], ars-i.[1'], atro.[11], bar-m.[4, 6],
bell.[4, 11], berb.[6], cadm-s.[1'], **camph.**[8],
cann-i.[1', 2, 11], **caps.**[2], carb-ac.[6, 11],
carbn-chl.[11], carbn-h.[11], carbn-o.[11],
carbn-s.[1', 2, 11], caul.[2], **caust.**[6], cham.[6],
chlf.[2, 11], chlol.[2, 11], **cic.**[2], cocc.[6],
crot-chlol.[12], cupr-a.[4], cycl.[11],
eucal.[2], **HYDR-AC.**[4-6], hyos.[6]
nyper.[6], ign.[6], kali-br.[6, 12], **kali-i.**[2],

keroso.[11, 12], laur.[4], lyc.[4, 6], m-arct.[4],
mand.[10, 14], merc.[11], meth-ae-ae.[11],
methyl.[11], nitro-o.[11], **nux-m.**[6],
nux-v.[4], **olnd.**[2, 4, 6], **op.**[4, 6, 11],
ox-ac.[6], ph-ac.[6], **PLB.**[1', 2, 4, 6, 11, 12],
puls.[11], ran-a.[4], rhod.[4, 6], **sec.**[4, 6, 10],
spig.[6], stram.[6, 11], stront-c.[6], tab.[11],
ter.[2], verat.[4], **verat-v.**[2], vip.[4, 6],
zinc.[2, 4]

right side, of[11]

plb.

affected parts, of[11]

plb.

ANALGESIA

anh.[10], ant-c.[6], bell., chel., **cic.,**
COCC., con., hell., **hyos.,** ign.,
kali-br., laur., **LYC.,** mand.[10], merc.,
mosch., **OLND., OP., PH-AC.,**
phos., pic-ac., **PLB.**[1, 7], puls.,
rhus-t.[1], **sec., STRAM., sulph.**

irritability–lack

painlessness

inner parts

ars., bell., bov., hyos., **OP., PLAT.,**
spig.

parts affected

anac., asaf., **cocc.,** con., **lyc., olnd.,**
PLAT., puls., rhus-t.

ANXIETY, general physical

acon., agar., alum.[4], am-m., ambr.[4], aml-ns., ant-t., ARG-N., arn.[4], ARS., ars-i., ARS-S-F.[1'], bar-c., bar-m., bar-s.[1'], bell.[4], bor.[4], brom., bry., calc., calc-ar.[1'], calc-i.[1'], CAMPH., cann-s., canth., carb-v., caust.[4], cench.[1'], CHAM., chel., chin., chlor.[11], cic., cocc., coff., colch., con., cupr., DIG., euph., ferr., ferr-ar., ferr-i., ferr-p.[1], guaj., ign., iod., IP., kreos.[4], laur., lob., lyc., mag-c.[4], meph.[4], merc., mez., mosch., mur-ac., nat-c.[4], nat-m., nat-s.[1'], nux-m.[4], NUX-V., op.[4], petr.[4], PH-AC., PHOS., plat., plb., prun.[4], PULS., ran-b.[4], rhod.[4], rhus-t., ruta[4], sabad., sabin., sars.[4] sec., seneg., sep., sil.[4], spig.[4], squil.[4], stann., staph., stram., sul-ac., sul-i.[1'], SULPH., tarent.[1'], teucr., ther.[1'], thuj., verat., zinc., zinc-p.[1']

APOPLEXY *

ACON., agar.[10], alco.[11], ANAC.[2, 3, 12], ant-c.[3, 11, 16], ant-t.[3], apis[12], arn., ars.[2, 3], ars-s-f.[12], asar.[3, 6], aster.[2, 12], aur., bapt.[12], bar-c., BELL., brom.[12], BRY.[2, 3, 12], cact.[7, 12], cadm-br.[12], cadm-s.[2, 3, 11, 12], calc.[3, 6], camph., carb-v., carbn-h.[12], carbn-s.[12], caust.[12], chen-a.[10, 12], chin., chlol.[12], COCC., coff., con., croc.[3], crot-h., cupr., cupr-a.[12], dig.[3, 6, 11], erig.[10], ferr., fl-ac.[12], form.[2, 12], gast.[12], GELS., GLON.[2, 3, 6, 10, 12], guare.[12], hell.[12], hep.[3], hydr-ac.[3, 10, 11], hyos., ign.[3], iod.[2], IP., juni.[11, 12], kali-br.[12], kali-cy.[12], kali-m.[3], kali-n.[10], kreos.[3], LACH., laur., lim.[12], lith-br.[12], lol.[11], lyc., merc., mill.[1', 2, 11], morph.[11], nat-m., nat-n.[10], nat-ns.[12], nit-ac., nux-m., nux-v., oena.[2, 12], olnd.[3, 6, 10], OP., ox-ac.[11], ph-ac.[3], phos., plb.,

puls., ran-g.[12], rhus-t., sabad.[3], samb.[3], sars.[3], sec., sep., sil., sin-n.[2, 7, 12], sol-a.[12], stram., stront-c.[12], sulph.[3], tab.[2, 11, 12], thuj.[3], verat.[3, 6, 11, 12, 16], verat-v.[2, 6, 12], viol-o.[3], vip.[3, 6]

convulsions–apoplectic

paralysis-one-sided

weakness–apoplexy

threateninq[2]

aster., bell., COFF., fl-ac., glon.[2, 10], ign., kali-n.[10], laur.[2, 12], prim-v.[12], stront-c.[2, 8]

ARMS holding away from body am.[3]

psor., spig., sulph.

ARSENICAL poisoning

camph., carb-v.[2, 3, 8, 12], chin., chin-s.[2, 12], dig.[2], euph.[12], ferr., graph., HEP.[2, 3, 8, 12], iod., ip., lach.[2, 3, 12], merc., nux-m.[12], nux-v., ol-j.[3], phos.[2], plb.[2], samb., sulph.[12], tab.[2, 12], thuj.[7], verat.

paralysis-poisoning

ARTERIOSCLEROSIS[8]

adren., **am-i.**[6, 8], am-van., aml-ns.[6],
ant-ar., arg-n.[10], **arn.**[3, 6, 8, 10], ars.[6, 8],
ars-i.[6, 8], aster.[14], **aur.**[3, 6, 8, 10], aur-br.[6],
aur-i.[6, 8], aur-m-n.[6, 8], **bar-c.**[6, 8, 10],
bar-i.[6, 10], bar-m., bell-p.[10, 14], benz-ac.[6],
cact., cal-ren.[6], **calc.**[3, 6], calc-ar.[3],
calc-f.[6, 8, 14], card-m.[8], chin-s., chlol.[7],
con.[6, 8], crat.[6, 8], **cupr.**[6, 8], ergot.,
fl-ac.[3, 6], form.[3], form-ac.[6], fuc.[10],
glon.[6, 8], hed.[10, 14], hyper.[10],
iod.[3, 6, 10], **kali-i.**[6, 10], kali-sal.,
kres.[10, 14], lach.[8, 10], lith-c., mag-f.[10],
mand.[14], naja[10], **nat-i.**, nit-ac.[6,] phos.,
plb.[3, 6, 8, 10], **plb-i.**[6, 8, 10, 12], polyg-a.,
rad-br.[10], rauw.[10], **sec.**[3, 6, 8, 10], sil.[10],
solid.[6], **stront-c.**[3, 6, 8], **stront-i.**[6, 8],
stroph-h., sumb., **tab.**[3, 6], thlas.[6], thyr.,
vanad.[6-8], **visc.**[3, 6, 14], zinc-p.[6]

hypertension

ASCENDING agg.

acet-ac., acon., agar.[3, 6], aloe,
alum., alum-sil.[1'], **alumn.**[2], **am-c.**,
anac., **ang.**[2, 3], ant-c., **arg-m.**, arg-n.,
arn., **ARS.**, ars-s-f.[1'], asar., aur.,
aur-ar.[1'], aur-i.[1'], aur-s.[1'], **bar-c.**,
bar-m., **bar-s.**[1'], bell., **bor.**, **BRY.**,
but-ac.[8], **cact.**[2, 8], cadm-s., **CALC.**,
calc-ar.[1'], **calc-p.**, calc-sil.[1'], cann-i.,
cann-s., canth., **carb-v.**, **carbn-s.**,
caust., chin., **COCA**, coff., **con.**[2, 3],
conv., **cupr.**, dig., dios., dros.,
euph., **ferr.**[2, 3], gels., gins.[11], **glon.**,
graph., hell., hep., hyos., ign.,
iod.[3, 6, 11], kali-ar., kali-c., **kali-i.**,
kali-n.[1], kali-p., **kalm.**, kreos., lach.,
led., lyc., mag-c., mag-m., meny.,
merc., mosch., mur-ac., nat-ar.,
nat-c., **nat-m.**, nat-n.[3, 6], nat-p.,
nit-ac., nux-m., **nux-v.**, olnd.[3, 6],
ox-ac., par., petr., ph-ac., **phos.**,
plat., plb., prot.[14], **puls.**[3], ran-b.,
rhod.[2], rhus-t., **ruta**, sabad., **sabin.**[2],
seneg., sep., sil., **spig.**, **SPONG.**,

squil., **stann.**, staph., sul-ac., **sulph.**,
tab., **tarax.**, thuj., **valer.**[2], verb.,
vip-a.[14], **zinc.**, zinc-p.[1']

ailments from[12]

calc-p.

am[3]
allox.[14], am-m., arg-m., bar-c., bell.,
bry., canth., coff., **con.**, ferr., lyc.,
meny., nit-ac., plb., **rhod.**, rhus-t.,
ruta, sabin., stann., sulph., **valer.**,
verb.

high agg.

acon., agar.[3], bell.[3], bry., **CALC.**[1, 7],
carb-v.[3], **COCA**[1, 7], conv., merc.[3],
nat-m.[3], **olnd.**, onos.[3], rhus-t.[3], **spig.**,
sulph.

mountain
Höl

ATROPHY[3]

ars., bar-c., chin., cupr., hep., kali-c.,
nux-v., phos., plb., sec., stann.

paralysis–atrophy

glands, of

anan., ars., **aur.**, bar-c., carb-an.,
cham., chim.[2], chin., **CON.**, **IOD.**,
kali-ar., kali-c., **KALI-I.**, kali-p.,
kreos., lac-d., **nit-ac.**, nux-m.,
ph-ac., plb., sars., **sec.**, sil., **staph.**,
sul-i.[1'], verat.

myatrophy

autumn see seasons

AVIATOR'S DISEASE[7]

ars.[8], bell., bor., **coca**[7, 8], psor.

BALL, sensation of an internal

acon., **arg-n.**, arn.[3], asaf., atri[6], **bell.**,
brom., bry., calc., **cann-i.**, caust.,
cham.[3], chin.[3], cob.[3], coc-c., coloc.,
con., crot-t., cupr., gels.[3], graph.,
HEP.[7], **IGN.**, kali-ar.[3], kali-c., kali-m.[3],
lac-c.[3], **lach.**, **lil-t.**[3, 6], mag-m.,
merc-d.[3], merc-i-r.[3], mosch.[3], nat-m.,
nat-s.[3], nit-ac.[3], nux-m., par., phos.[3],
phyt., plan.[3], plat., **plb., puls.**[3], raph.,
rhus-t., ruta, **sabad.**[3], senec., **SEP.**,
sil., spig., staph., stram., sulph., tab.,
teucr.[3], ust.[3], valer.

knotted
plug
shot

hot[3]

carb-ac., phyt.

BASEDOW'S disease[8, 10]

adren.[7], aml-ns.[8], anh.[14], antip.[8],
aq-mar.[14], aran-ix.[14], ars., ars-i.,
atra-r.[14], aur., bad., bar-c.[8], **bell.**,
brom., **cact.**[8], **calc.**[8], calc-f.[10, 14],
cann-i.[8], chin.[10], chin-ar.[10], chr-s.[8],
cimic.[14], colch.[8], con., cupr.[10],
cupr-a.[10], cyt-l.[14], echi.[8], ephe.[8],
elaps[10], **ferr.**[8], ferr-i.[8], ferr-p.[8],
ferr-s[10], **fl-ac.**, flor-p.[10], fuc.[8], **glon.**[8],
hed[10, 14], **iod.**, jab[8], kali-c.[6], lach.[10],
lycps., mag-c.[10], mag-f.[10], nat-m.[6, 8, 10],
nux-v.[7], op.[10], phos.[10], **pilo.**[8], **rauw.**[14],
saroth.[8, 14], scut.[8], sec.[10], sel.[14], spong.,
stram.[8], thal.[14], thala.[14], **thyr.**[8, 14],
thyreotr.[14], tub.[10]

BATHING, washing **agg.**

aesc., aeth., **AM-C.**, am-m.,
ANT-C., ant-t., **apis**[6], **aran.**, ars.[2, 3],
ars-i., ars-s-f.[1'], **bar-c.**, bar-s.[1'], **bell.**,
bell-p.[8], bor., bov., bry., **CALC.**,
CALC-S., calc-sil.[1'], **canth.**, caps.[1'],
carb-v., carbn-s., caust., cham.,
CLEM., con., crot-c[8], **dulc.**, ferr.[8],
form.[3, 6, 8], **graph.**, hep.[2], **ign.**[2, 3],
kali-c., kali-m[1'], **kali-n.**, kali-s.,
kali-sil.[1'], kreos.[8], **lac-d.**, lach.[8], laur.,
lil-t.[8], **lyc.**, mag-c., **mag-p., mang.,**
merc., merc-c., **mez.**, mur-ac.,
nat-c., nat-m., **nat-s.**[8], **nit-ac.**,
nux-m., nux-v., op.[3, 6], **petr., phos.**,
phys.[3, 8, 12], puls., rat.[3], **RHUS-T.**,
rumx., sars., SEP., sil., **spig.**, stann.,
staph., **stront-c.**, sul-ac., **SULPH.**,
thuj.[3], urt-u.[8], zinc., zinc-p.[1']

ailments from[12]

nux-m., phys., rhus-t.

am.

acon., agar., **alum., alumn.**[2],
am-m., ant-t., **apis**, arg-n[3, 6], ars.,
ASAR., aur., **bor.**, bry., bufo[1'],
calc.[2], cann-i., **caust.**, cham.,
chel., euphr., fl-ac., form., hell.[2],
hyper.[3, 6], kali-chl., **lac-c.**, laur.,
LED., mag-c., mez., mur-ac.,
nat-m.[3, 6], nux-v., phos.[3], phyt.,
pic-ac., psor., PULS., rhod.,
sabad., sep., **spig.**, staph., thlas.[3],
thuj.[3], zinc.

affected part, of; and moistening[15]

alum., **am-m.**, ant-t., ars., **ASAR.**,
bor., bry., **caust.**, cham., **chel.**,
euphr., laur., mag-c., mez.,
mur-ac., nux-v., **PULS.**, rhod.,
sabad., sep., **spig.**, staph., zinc.

aversion to, dread of

AM-C., am-m., ANT-C., aq-mar.[14], bar-c., bar-m., **bell.**, bell-p.[7], **bor.**, bov., **bry.**, **calc.**, calc-sil.[1] , **canth.**, **carb-v.**, caust.[3], **cham.**, **CLEM.**, coloc.[3], **con.**, dulc., **hep.**[2], kali-c., kali-m.[1'], **kali-n.**, kali-sil.[1'], **laur.**, lyc., mag-c., mag-p.[3], mang.[3], merc., **mez.**, mur-ac., nat-c., nat-p., nit-ac., nux-m., nux-v., ol-an.[3], phos., **phys.**[2, 11], **PSOR.**, **puls.**, **RHUS-T.**, sars., **SEP.**, sil., **SPIG.**, stann., **staph.**, **stront-c.**, sul-ac., **SULPH.**, thuj.[3], **zinc.**

cold bathing agg.

acon.[1'], **AM-C**[2, 6], am-m.[2], **ANT-C.**, **ANT-T.**[1', 7], apoc.[7], ars.[3], ars-i.[6], **bar-c.**, **bell.**, bell-p.[7, 9], **bor.**[2], bov.[2], **bry.**[2], bufo[2], **CALC.**[2], calc-sil.[1], **canth.**[2], **caps.**, **carb-v.**[2], carbn-s., **caust.**, **cham.**[2], chim.[7], cimic.[7], **CLEM.**[2, 3], **colch.**, **con.**[2], **dulc.**[2, 3, 6], elaps, **form.**, glon[3], **IGN.**[2, 3], **kali-c.**[2], **kali-m.**[3], **kali-n.**[2, 6], **kreos.**, **lac-d.**, lach.[7], **laur.**[2], lyc.[2, 6], mag-c.[2], **MAG-P.**, **merc.**[2, 6], mez.[2, 3], mosch.[3], mur-ac., nat-c.[2], **nit-ac.**, **nux-m.**[2], nux-v.[2, 5-7], phos., psor.[1'], **puls.**[2], **RHUS-T.**, ruta[7], sars., **sep.**, sil.[3, 6], **spig.**[2], stann.[2], **staph.**[2], **stront-c.**[2], sul-ac.[2], **SULPH.**[2, 5, 7], thyr.[14], **TUB.**, **zinc.**[2]

ailments from[12]

mag-p., phys.

am.

agar[8], aloe[8], alum[6], ambr.[8], **apis**[3, 6, 8], **arg-n.**, **arn.**, asar., aster.[14], aur.[1', 3, 6], **aur-m.**, bell-p.[3], berb-a.[14], bism., **bry.**[3, 6, 8], bufo[8], calc-f.[14], **cals-s.**, camph[8], cann-i.[8], cann-s.[3], caust.[3], cupr.[8], fago.[8], **fl-ac.**, hed.[10, 14], hyper.[3, 6], ind.,

iod., **led.**[3, 6, 8], mag-s.[9, 14], meph., **nat-m.**, **phos.**[8], phyt.[3], pic-ac.[1', 6, 8], **psor.**[6], **puls.**[3, 8], sec.[3], sep.[5], spig.[6], sulph.[3], syph.[7]

desire for

aloe[6], **apis**[6], asar.[6], aster., caust.[6], chel.[6], fl-ac.[11], **hyper.**[6], iod.[6], **led.**[6], meph., nat-m., phyt., puls.[6], sep.[6]

desire for[11]

tarent.

face bathing agg.

fl-ac.[1'], plan.[3]

am.
  asar., **calc-s**, lac-d.[3], mez., nat-m[2], phos.[3], sabad.

hot bathing agg.[3]

APIS, arg-n., bell., bry., **carb-v.**, GELS., IOD., LACH., NAT-M., op., **puls.**, sec., **sulph.**

am.[3]
  anac., **ARS.**, hep., rhus-t., sil., thuj.

lukewarm bathing agg.[3]

acon, **ang.**[2, 3], phos.

sea agg., bathing in the

ars., lim.[8, 12], **mag-m.**, med.[7], nat-m.[3], **rhus-t.**, sep., **zinc.**[2, 3, 7]

ailments from[12]

    ars., mag-m., rhus-t.

am.[7]
med.

warm bathing agg.[1', 3, 6]

    acon.[5], ant-c.[1'], **apis**, ars-i.[6], bell.[5], caust.[1'], iod.[6], **lach., op.**[3, 6], phos.[3, 6], sulph.[3]

am.[8]
    ant-c., bufo, flav.[14], lat-m.[9, 14], mim-p[14], rad-br., sec.[6], **stront-c.**, thea

feet, of[14]

pneu.

bed see hard bed

BENDING, turning agg.[3]

    am-m., anac.[14], ang., ant-t., arn., **bell.**, bov., **bry.**, calc., camph., caps., carb-an., carb-v., cham., **chin., cic.,** cocc., coloc., **con.**[3, 8], cycl., dros., dulc., euph., guaj., **hep., ign.,** iod., ip., lach., laur., mag-c., merc. mez., mur-ac. **nat-m.**, nit-ac., nux-v.[3, 8], petr., ph-ac., plat., plb., puls.[3, 8], ran-b., rhod., **rhus-t.**, sabad., **sabin.**, samb., **sel.**, spig., **spong., stann.,** staph., thuj., verat., visc.[14], **zinc.**

affected part agg.[3]

    acon., am-c., **am-m.**, anac., ang., **ant-c.**, ant-t., arg-m., **arn.**, asaf., aur., bar-c., **bell.**, bor., bov., **bry., CALC.**, camph., caps., carb-an., carb-v., caust., cham., **chel., chin.,**

cic., cina., cocc., **coff.**, con., croc., cupr., cycl., dig., dros., dulc., graph., hep., hyos., **IGN.**, iod., ip., **kali-c.**, lach., laur., led., **lyc., mag-c.**, merc., mez., mur-ac., **nat-m.**, nit-ac., **nux-v.**, olnd., par., petr., ph-ac., plat., plb., **puls.**, ran-b., rhod., **rhus-t.**, ruta, sabad., sabin., samb., **sel., sep., spig., spong.**, stann., staph., sulph., tarax., teucr., thuj., valer.. verat., zinc.

drawing up

am.[3]
    acon., am-m., anac., arg-m., arg-n., **BELL.**, bov., calc., cann-s., caust., **cham., chin.**, colch., **coloc.**, guaj., hep., kali-c., lach., mag-c., mag-p., mang., meny., **merc., merc-c.**, mur-ac., nux-v., petr., **plb., puls.**, rheum, rhus-t., sabad., sabin., **squil.**, teucr., **thuj.,** verat.

backward agg.[3]

    am-c., **anac.**, ant-c., aran-ix.[14]. asaf., atra-r.[14], aur., **bar-c., calc.**, caps., carb-v., caust., chel., cina., coff., **con.**[3, 4], cupr., dig., dros.[3, 4], dulc.[3, 4], **ign., kali-c.**, kali-i.[4], kreos.[4], lac-c., lach.[4], lith-c.[3], mag-c.[4], mang.[4], nat-m., nat-s.[4], **nit-ac.**, nux-v., ph-ac.[4], **plat.**[3, 4, 6], plb., **puls.** [3, 4], rhod.[3, 4], rhus-t.[3, 4], ruta[4], samb.[4], **SEP.**[3, 4], stann., **sulph.**, teucr., thuj., tong.[4], valer.[3, 4], zinc.[4]

and forward agg.[3]

    asaf., **chel.**, coff., nux-v., thuj.

am.[3]
    acon., ant-c.[4], **bell.**[3, 6, 10],
    bism.[3, 6, 7, 10], bry.[4],
    calen.[4], cann-s., **cham.**, chin.,
    crimic.[3, 6], **DIOS.**[3, 6, 10],
    fl-ac.[3, 6], hep.[3], iod.[44], kali-c.,
    kreos.[3], lac-c., **lach.**, mag-m.[14],
    mand.[10, 14], med.[3], merc.[4], nux-v.,
    puls., rhus-t.[3], sabad.[3, 4], sabin.,
    sep.[4], spong.[4], squil.[4], **thuj.**,
    verat., zinc.[3], zinc-o.[4]

stretching am.

bed agg., turning in[2]

    acon., agar., am-m., anac., **ars.**,
    asar., **bor.**, **BRY.**, calc., **cann-s.**,
    caps., **carb-v.**, **caust.**, chin., cina,
    cocc., **con.**[2, 8], cupr., dros., **euph.**,
    ferr., graph., **hep.**, kali-c., lach.,
    led., **lyc.**, mag-c., merc., **nat-m.**,
    nit-ac., **nux-v.**[2, 8], petr., **phos.**, plat.,
    plb., **PULS.**[2, 8], ran-b., **rhod.**,
    rhus-t., ruta, **sabad.**, sabin., **samb.**,
    sais., **sil.**, **staph.**, **sulph.**, thuj.,
    valer.

double agg.[8]

    dios.

am.[6, 8]
    aloe[8], arg-n.[6, 7], bov.[6], caust.[6],
    chin., colch.[6], **coloc.**[6, 8, 10],
    mag-c.[6, 10], **mag-p.**, mand.[14],
    plb.[6]

bent holding

doubling up

forward agg.[3]

    aesc.[7], asaf., **bell.**[8], chel., **coff.**,
    kalm.[8], mag-m.[14], mang.[4],
    nux-v.[3, 8], thiop.[14], thuj.

am.
    apis[1'], **aur.**, coloc.[7], gels.[8],
    kali-c.[8, 14], **teucr.**

inward agg.[3]

    am-m., **ign.**, staph., verat.

am.[3]
    am-m., **bell.**

right agg., to[3]

    spig.

sideways agg.[3]

    bell., bor., **calc.**, canth., chel.,
    chin., cocc., **kali-c.**, lyc., **nat-m.**,
    plb., stann., staph.

am.[3]
    meny., **puls.**

BENT HOLDING the part **agg.**[3]

    hyos., lyc., **spong.**, teucr., valer.

am.[3]
    bov., bry., **coloc.**, nat-m., puls.,
    rhus-t., squil., sulph., verat.

bending-double

doubling up

BESNIER–BOEK–SCHAUMANN,
morbus[14]
aq-m., **aran-ix.**, asar., beryl.,
hip-ac., **hist.**, kres., mand.,
parathyr., thiop., v-a-b.

BINDING UP, bandaging am.[3, 6]

apis, arg-n.[3], bry., chin.[3], gels., mag-m.[3], mang.[3], mim-p.[14], puls., rhod., sil., tril.[3]

BLACKNESS of external parts

acon., agar., all-c.[12], alum., am-c., ang.[3], **ant-c.**, ant-t.[3, 4], **anthraci.**, apis, **arg-n.**, arn., **ARS.**, ars-i., asaf., asar., aur., bapt.[3], bar-c., bell., bism., both.[7, 11, 12], brass.[11, 12], brom.[3], bry., calc., **calc-ar.**[2], camph., canth., **caps.**[2, 4], carb-ac.[3, 12], **carb-an.**, **carb-v.**, carbn-o.[11], caust., cham., **chin.**, chin-ar., chr-ac.[2], chr-o.[12], cic., cina, cocc., com.[6], **con.**, **crot-h.**, **CUPR.**, cycl., **dig.**, dros., **echi.**, elaps[3], ergot.[12], euph., euph-c.[6], gels.[3], **ham.**, hell.[4], hep.[3], hyos., ign.[2, 3], iod., ip., **kali-p.**[1', 2, 12], kreos., kres.[13], **lach.**, lyc., mag-c., mag-m.[3], **MERC.**, **merc-c.**[3], **merc-cy.**[6], mur-ac.[4], nat-m., nit-ac., **nux-v.**, **OP.**, **ph-ac.**, **phos.**, phyt., plb., puls., ran-a.[12], ran-b.[3, 4], ran-s.[11], **rhus-t.**, ric.[12], ruta sabad., **sabin.**[4], **samb.**, sars., **SEC.**, sep., sil., solid.[3], spig., spong., squil., stann., staph.[3], stram., sul-ac.[3, 4, 12], sulph.[3, 4], **tarent.**[2, 3, 11], ter.[2], thuj., **VERAT.**, **vip.**[4, 6], **vip-r.**[4]

inflammation-internally-gangrenous

cold

ant-t., **ARS.**, asaf., bell., **canth.**, caps., **carb-v.**, chin.[2], con., crot-h., **euph.**, **lach.**, merc., **PLB.**, ran-b., **SEC.**, sil., squil., sul-ac., sulph., tarent-c., **ter.**[2]

diabetic[3]

ars.[6, 10], con., **kreos.**[6, 10], kres.[10, 14], lach., **sec.**[2, 6, 10], solid.

hot

acon., ars., bell., mur-ac., op.[3], **sabin.**, **sec.**

moist

brom.[3], **carb-v.**, **CHIN.**, **hell.**, lach.[6], ph-ac., phos.[3], tarent., **vip.**[3, 6]

senile

adren.[6], all-c.[2, 7, 8, 12], am-c.[2, 8], **ars.**[2, 6, 8, 12], **carb-v.**, chin.[2], con.[2], crot-h.[6], cupr.[7], echi.[6], ergot.[6], euph.[2], **kreos.**[6], **LACH.**[2, 6], ph-ac.[2], plb.[2, 6], **SEC.**, sul-ac.[8], vip.[6]

traumatic[2, 3, 8]

am-m.[2], **arn.**, calen.[2], **hyper.**[2], **LACH.**, **sul-ac.**[2, 8]

BLOOD too **quick**, sensation of circulation of[16]

ars.

thin, sensation as if[7, 11]

hell.

BREAKFAST agg., **before**

alumn.[2], croc.[8]

after b. agg.

agar., **am-m.**, ambr., anac., ars.,
bell., bor., **bry., calc.**, calc-sil.[1'],
carb-an., carb-v., carbn-s., **caust.,**
CHAM., chin., **con.**, cycl., **dig.,**
euph., form., **graph.**, grat.[3], **guaj.**[3],
hell., ign., iris.[3], **kali-c., kali-n.,**
laur., lyc., mag-c., mang., **nat-c.,**
nat-m., nat-s.[3], nit-ac., nux-m.,
NUX-V., par., petr., ph-ac., **PHOS.,**
plb., puls., rhod., rhus-t., sars.,
sep., sil., stront-c., **sulph.,**
thuj., valer., verat., **ZINC.**, zinc-p.[1']

after b. am.

acon.[3], alum.[3], am-c.[3], **am-m.**[2, 3],
ambr.[3], anac.[3], ars.[3], **bar-c.**[2, 3],
bov.[2, 3], bry.[3], **calc., cann-s.**[2, 3],
canth.[3], **carb-an.**[2, 3], carb-v.[3], caust.[3],
chel.[2, 3], chin.[3], cina[3], **croc.**, ferr.,
graph.[3], hell.[3], **hep.**[2, 3], **ign.**[2, 3],
iod., kali-c.[3], **lach.**[2, 3, 6], **laur.**[2, 3],
lyc.[2, 3], mag-c.[3], mag-m.[3], merc.[3],
mez.[2, 3], nat-c.[3], nat-m., nat-p.[1'],
nat-s.[1', 3, 8], nit-ac.[3], **nux-v.** [2, 3, 6],
petr.[2, 3], phos.[3], **plat.**[2, 3], **plb.**[2, 3],
puls.[3], **ran-b.**[2, 3], ran-s.[3], rhod.[3],
rhus-t.[2, 3], **sabad.**[2, 3], **sep.**[2, 3],
squil.[2, 3], **staph., stront-c.**[2, 3],
sulph.[2, 3], **tarax.**[2, 3], teucr.[3], valer.,
verat.[3], **verb.**[2, 3], zinc-p.[1']

BREATHING agg.[3]

acon., agar., alum., am-c., **am-m.,**
anac., ant-c., arg-m., arn., ars.,
asaf., asar., aur., **bell.**, bism., bor.,
bov., **BRY., calc., cann-s., caps.,**
cham., chin., **cina**, clem., cocc.,
COLCH., coloc., con., croc., cupr.,
dig., dros., dulc., euphr., graph.,
hep., hyos., **kali-c.**, kali-n., led.,
lyc., **mag-c.**, merc., mez., **mur-ac.,**
nat-c., **nat-m., nit-ac.**, nux-v.,

ph-ac., plat., **puls.**, ran-b., rhod.,
rhus-t., sabad., sars., **sel.**, seneg.,
SEP., sil., **SPIG.**, squil., stann.,
sul-ac., **sulph.**, thuj., verat.

Cheyne-Stokes' respiration

acon., **acon-f.**[7, 8, 12], am-c.[6],
ang.[6], antip.[7, 8, 12], atro[7, 8, 12], bell.,
camph[6], cann-i.[6], carb-v.[7, 8], chlol.[7],
coca [7], cocain.[7, 8], crot-h.[6], **cupr.**[6],
cupr-ar.[6], **dig.**[6], grin.[7, 8, 12],
hydr-ac.[6, 10], **ign.**, iod.[6], ip.[6],
kali-cy.[7, 8, 12], lach.[6], **laur**[6], led.[6,]
lob.[6], nux-v., olnd.[6], **op.**[1, 7],
morph.[7, 8], parth.[7, 8, 12], **saroth.**[7, 8],
spong., sul-ac.[3], sulph.[3], vanad.[7],
verat.[6]

deep b. agg.[3]

ACON., agn., am-m.[2, 3], arg-m.,
arn., asaf., **bell., bor.**, brom., **BRY.,**
calad., calc., **canth.**, caps., carb-an.,
caust., cina, dros., dulc., fl-ac.,
graph., hell., hep., hist.[14], hyos.,
ign., ip., **kali-c., kali-n.**, kreos.,
lach., **lyc.**, mag-m., mang., **merc.,**
merc-c., mosch., nat-c., nat-m.,
nux-m., nux-v., **olnd., phos.**, plb.,
puls., ran-b.[3], **ran-s.**, rheum,
RHUS-T., rumx.[3], **sabad., SABIN.,**
sang.[3], seneg., sep., **sil.**, spig.,
spong., **squil.**, stram., sulph.[3],
thuj., valer., verb.

am.
acon., agar.[3], asaf., bar-c., **cann-i.,**
chin., **colch., cupr.**, dig., dros.,
ign., iod., **lach.**, meny., mygal.[3],
nat-m.[3], olnd., osm., puls., **seneg.,**
sep., **spig., STANN.**, staph.,
sulph.[3], ter., verb.[3], viol-t.

desire to

acet-ac., achy.[14], acon., agar.[3], alum., alumn., am-br., ami-ns.[3, 6], ant-c.[6], apis[3], **aur.**, bapt., bor., brom., **BRY., CACT., CALC.,** calc-p.[6], camph.[6], cann-i.[6], **caps., carb-ac., carb-v., card-m., caust.,** cedr., **chin.,** cimx., coca, croc., **CROT-T.**[1, 7], **cupr.**[3, 6], **dig.,** euon., eup-per., **glon.,** hell.[3], hydr., **IGN., ind., ip.**[3, 6], kali-bi.[3], **kali-c., kali-n.**[3, 6], **kreos., LACH., lact.,** laur[3], lil-t., **lob.**[3, 6], **lyc.,** mag-p.[3], med.[2], **merc.,** mez., mosch., **NAT-S.,** nux-m., **op.**[3, 6], **par., phos., plat.**[3], podo., poth., prun., ran-b., rhus-t.[3], sabin.[3], samb., **sang., SEL., seneg.,** sep., sil.[3, 6], squil.[3], stann., stram., **SULPH.,** tab.[3], ther., tub[1], verb., xan.

exspiration agg.[3]

agn., ambr., anac., ang., ant-c., ant-t., **arg-m.**[2, 3], ars.[2, 3], asaf., aur., bry., cann-s., carb-v., caust., cham., chel., chin., **chlor.**[2], cic., cina, clem., coff., **COLCH., dig., dros.,** dulc., euphr., **fl-ac., ign., iod., ip.**[2], kreos., laur., led., mang., mur-ac., nat-c., nux-v., **olnd.,** ph-ac, **PULS.,** rhus-t., ruta, sabad., **sep., SPIG.,** spong., squil., stann., **staph.,** tarax., verat., **viol-o., viol-t.,** zinc.

am.[3]

ACON.[2, 3], agar., am-m., anac., ang., arg-m., arn.[2, 3], asaf., asar., bar-c., **bor., BRY.**[2, 3], calc., cann-s., canth., caps., carb-an., caust., cham., chel., chin., cina, clem., croc., cycl., euphr., guaj., hell., hep., ip., kali-c., kali-n., kreos., lyc., **meny.,** merc., mosch., nux-m., olnd., op., plat., plb., ran-b., ran-s., **RHUS-T.,** sabad., **SABIN.,** sars., sel., seneg., sep., spig., spong., **squil.,** stann., sul-ac., sulph., tarax. valer., verat.

inspiration agg.[3]

ACON.[2, 3, 8], **agar.,** agn., alum., am-c., am-m., **anac.,** ang., **ANT-C., arg-m.,** arg-n.[7], **arn.**[2, 3], ars., asaf., **asar.,** aur., bar-c., **bell., bor.,** bov., **BRY.**[3, 8], **calc.,** camph., cann-s., canth., **caps.,** carb-an., carb-v., caust., **cham., chel.,** chin., cic., cina, clem., coloc., con., croc., **crot-h.,** cupr., cycl., dulc., euphr., **guaj.,** hell., hist.[10], hyos., ign., iod., **ip., kali-c., kali-n., kreos.,** laur., led., lob., **lyc.,** mag-c., mag-m., **meny., merc.,** mez., mosch., mur-ac., nat-c., nat-m., nit-ac., nux-m., **nux-v.,** olnd., op., par., petr., ph-ac., phos.[3, 8], plat., plb., **puls., ran-b.**[3, 8], ran-s., rhod., **RHUS-T.,** ruta, **sabad., SABIN.,** sars., **sel., seneg., sep., sil., spig.**[3, 8], **spong., SQUIL.,** stann., **staph.,** stront., sul-ac., sulph., tarax., **teucr.,** thuj., **valer.,** verat., verb., viol-t., zinc.

am.[3]

ant-t., asaf., bar-c., bry., cann-s., caust., **chin.,** cina, **COLCH.**[3, 8], **cupr., dig.,** dros., dulc., **IGN.**[3, 8], iod., **lach.,** mang., meny., nux-v., **olnd.,** ph-ac., **puls.,** ruta, sabad., sep., **SPIG.**[3, 8], squil., **stann.,** staph., tarax., verat., verb., viol-o., viol-t.

hot air, ailments from i. of[12]

carb-v.

BRITTLE BONES

asaf.[3], bufo[3], **calc.,** calc-p.[3], cupr.[3], fl-ac.[3], lyc.[3], **merc.**[3], par.[3], ph-ac.[3], ruta[3], **SIL.**[3], **sulph.**[3], **symph.,** thuj.[3]

caries-bone

BROMIDES, abuse of[3, 6]

am-c.[2], camph.[2], cham., lach., mag-c.[2], op.[2], phos., zinc-p.

BUBBLING

Gefühl von
ambr., ant-c., asaf., bell., berb., caps.[3, 11], colch., coloc.[3], ip., junc-e.[7], laur.[3], lyc., mang.[16], nux-v., **puls.**, **rheum**, spig., squil., sulph.[3], tarax.

BURNS

acet-ac.[2, 7, 8, 12], **acon.**[2, 3, 4, 7, 8], agar., aloe[10], alum., alumn.[2], ant-c., arist-cl.[10, 14], arn.[2, 7, 8], **ARS., bar-c.**[4], **bell.**[4], **bry.**[4], calc., calc-p.[7], calc-s.[2, 8, 12], **calen.**[2, 7, 8, 12], camph.[7, 8], **CANTH.**, carb-ac., **carb-v., carbn-s.**[2, 12], **caust.**, chin.[4], cic.[2], crot-h.[2], cycl., des-ac.[14], echi.[6], euph., ferr.[4], gaul.[7, 8], grin.[7, 8, 10], **ham.**[2, 7, 8, 12], **hep.**[2, 7, 8, 12], hoit.[14], hyos[4, 10], **hyper**[2], **ign.**[4], jab.[7, 8, 12], **kali-bi.**[7, 8, 12], kali-c.[4], kali-m.[2, 12], **kreos.**, lach., mag-c., **mag-m.**[4], **merc.**[2, 4], **nat-c.**[4, 12], **nux-v.**[4], op.[4], par.[4], passi.[12], petr.[2, 7, 8, 12], phos.[4], pic-ac.[8, 12], **plan.**[2, 12], plat.[4], plb., **puls.**[2, 4], ran-b.[7], **rhus-t.**, ruta, sabad[4], **sec.**, sep.[4], **sil.**[12], spira.[12], **stram., sul-ac.**[4], **ter.**[2, 7, 8], thuj.[4], **urt-u.**[2-4, 6-8, 10, 12], verat.[4]

ailments from[12]

caust., kali-m., plan., rad-br., urt-u.

x-ray, from[3, 7]

calc-f.

CACHEXIA

acet-ac.[6], arg-m.[14], arg-n.[7, 11, 12], arn.[12], **ARS.**, ars-i.[6], bad.[2], bond.[11], calc.[12], caps.[2], carb-ac.[11], chim., chin.[1', 4, 11, 12], clem., **coc-c.**[2],cund.[2, 6], fl-ac.[6, 7], **form.**[2], hydr.[6], iod., **kali-bi.**, mang.[6], merc.[11, 12], merc-ns.[11], morph.[11], mur-ac.[11], nat-m., **NIT-AC.**, phos.[12], phyt.[6], pic-ac.[12], plb.[11], sec.[6, 12], seneg.[2], thal.[14], thuj.[1'], vip.[11], y-ray[14]

cancerous–cachexia

emaciation

CAGED in wires, twisted tighter and tighter

CACT.

CANCEROUS affections

acet-ac., alum., alumn., anan.[8, 12], anil.[12], **ant-m.**[8], **apis**, apoc.[7], **ambr.**, arg-m.[1'], arg-n.[10], **ARS.**, ars-br.[8], **ars-i., aster., aur.**, aur-ar.[1', 8, 12], aur-i.[1', 14], **aur-m.**, aur-m-n.[7, 8], aur-s.[1'], **bapt.**[7, 8, 12], bar-c.[1', 3], bar-i.[7, 12], bell.[2], bism., **BROM., bry.**[7, 12], **bufo, cadm-s., calc., calc-i.**[7, 8, 12], calc-ox.[8, 12], **calc-s., calen.**[2, 8], calth.[12], **carb-ac., CARB-AN., carb-v., carbn-s.,** carc.[8, 9], caust., chel.[12], cholin.[8], **cic.**[8, 12], cinnm.[8, 12], **cist., cit-ac.**[2], cit-l.[12], clem., **CON.,** cory.[7], crot-h.[12], **cund.**[2, 3, 7, 8, 12], cupr., cupr-a.[8], cur.[12], dulc., elaps[12], eos.[8], epiph.[12], eucal.[7], euph.[8, 12], euph-he.[12], ferr-i.[12],

ferr-p.[2], ferr-pic.[7], form.[8]. form-ac.[8],
fuli.[8], **gali.**[7, 8, 12], gent-l.[7], **graph.,**
gua.[7, 8], **ham.**[8, 12], hep., hippoz.[2, 12],
hydr., hydrin-m.[12], iod.[3, 7, 8, 12],
kali-ar., kali-bi., kali-chl.[3],
kali-cy.[2, 7, 8, 12], **kali-i.**[3, 8, 12], **kali-p.**[7],
kali-s., kreos., kres.[10], **lach., lap-a.,**
lob-e.[12], **LYC.,** maland.[8], matth.[12],
med.[7, 8], **merc., merc-i-f.,** methyl.[12],
mill.[2, 12], **morph.**[2], nat-m., nectrin.[12],
NIT-AC., ol-an.[12], **op.**[12], orni[12],
oxyg.[12], ph-ac., **PHOS., PHYT.**
pic-ac.[12], psor.[12], rad-br.[3, 8],
rumx-a.[8], **sang.**[7, 8, 12], sarcol-ac.[10],
scir.[8, 12], sed-r.[8], **semp.**[7, 8], sep.,
sieg.[10], sec.[3], **SIL.,** silphu.[12], squil.[4],
strych-g.[8], sul-ac., **sulph.,** symph.[3, 8],
tax.[8], tarax.[7, 14], **ter.**[2], **thuj.,**
trif-p.[7, 12], viol-o.[12], visc.[10, 14],
x-ray[9, 14], zinc.

Hodgkin's disease

leukaemia

sarcoma
tumors

bones, of[8, 12]

aur-i.[8], con.[2], hecla[12], **phos.,** symph.

cachexia, emaciation, with

acon.[7], **hydr.**[2], pic-ac.[12], thuj.[1']

cicatrices, in old[1', 7]

graph.

colloid cancer[2]

lach., phos.

contusions, after[2]

con.

encephaloma see tumors

epithelioma

abr.[8, 12], acet-ac., alum.[1', 6],
alumn.[1', 2, 8], arg-m., arg-n., **ars.,**
ARS-I., ars-s-f.[1'], aur., aur-ar.[1'],
bell., brom., calc., calc-p., calc-sil[1'],
carb-ac.[6], carb-an.[2], chr-ac.[8],
cic.[6, 8, 12], clem., **CON., cund.**[2, 6, 8, 12],
euph.[8], fuli.[8], **hydr., hydrc.**[6],
kali-ar.[6, 8, 12], kali-chl.[12], kali-m.[6],
kali-s., kreos., lap-a.[2, 3, 6, 8, 12],
lob-e.[8], **LYC.,** mag-m.[14], mag-s.[12],
merc., merc-c.[2], methyl.[12], nat-cac.[8],
nat-m.[2], nectrin.[12], nit-ac.[2], phos.,
phyt., puls.[2], rad-br.[8], raja-s.[14],
ran-b., scroph-n.[8], sep., **sil.,**
strych-g.[8], sulph., thuj., uran-n.[2]

fungus haematodes see tumors—
angioma

glands, of

aur-m., buni-o.[14], **CARB-AN., CON.,**
sieg.[10], strych-g.[8], sul-i.[1'], syph.[7]

lupus, carcinomatous

agar., alum., alumn., ant-c.,
arg-n., **ARS., ars-i.,** aur-m., **bar-c.,**
calc., **carb-ac., carb-v., carbn-s.,**
caust., **cist.,** graph., hep., **hydrc.,**
kali-ar., **kali-bi.,** kali-c., **kali-chl.,**
kali-s., **kreos.,** lach., **LYC.,**
nit-ac., phyt., psor., sep., **sil.,**
spong., staph., sulph., **THUJ.**

in rings
sep.

melanoma

arg-n., card-m., **lach.**, ph-ac.

pains see pain–cancerous affections

sarcoma

scirrhus

alumn., **anac.²**, arg-m., arn.², **ars.**,
ars-s-f.¹′, **aster.**, bell-p.³, **calc-s.**,
calen.², **CARB-AN., carb-v.,**
carbn-s., clem.¹′, **CON.**, cund.²,
graph., hydr., lap-a., nux-v.², petr.³,
phos., phyt., sep., **SIL.**, squil.¹⁶,
staph., **sulph.**

ulcers of glands

arn., **ARS.**, ars-i.¹, aur., **bell.,**
BUFO, calc., carb-an., carb-v.,
caust., clem., **CON.**, cupr., dulc.,
hep., kali-ar.¹′, kali-c., **kreos.**, lyc.,
merc., merc-i-f., nit-ac., ph-ac.,
phos., rhus-t., **sep., sil.**, squil.¹,
sul-ac., **SULPH.**, zinc.

of skin

ambr., ant-c., **anthraci.**, apis,
ARS., ars-i., ARS-S-F.¹′, aster.⁸,
aur., aur-ar.¹′, aur-i.¹′, **AUR-S.¹′,**
bell., **BUFO**, calc., **calc-s.,**
carb-ac., carb-an., carb-v.,
carbn-s., caust., chel., chim.⁸′ ¹²,
chin-s.²′ ⁴′ ¹¹, clem., **con., crot-c.,**
cund., dor.¹¹, dulc., **ferr.³**, fl-ac.⁶,
fuli.⁸, **gali.⁸**, graph., **HEP.,**
hippoz., hydr., kali-ar., kali-bi.¹′,
kali-c., **kali-i., kreos., lach., LYC.,**
lyss., mang., merc., **mill.²**,
mur-ac., **nit-ac.**, petr., **ph-ac.,**
phos., phyt., rhus-t., rumx., sars.,
sep., SIL., spong., squil., **staph.,**
sul-i.¹′, **SULPH.**, tarent-c.⁸, **thuj.**

CARIES of bone

ANG., anthraco.², arg-m.², **arn.²,**
ars., **ASAF., Aur.**, aur-ar.¹′, aur-i.¹′,
aur-m., aur-m-n., bell., both.¹¹, bry.,
calc., calc-f., calc-hp.⁸, **calc-p.,**
calc-s., caps., carb-ac., caust.²,
chin., cinnm.², **cist.**, clem., con.,
cupr., dulc., euph., ferr., **FL-AC.,**
graph., **guaj., guare.**, hecla⁶, **hep.,**
iod., kali-bi., **KALI-I.**, kreos., lach.,
LYC., mang.¹′ ⁸, **MERC., mez.,**
nat-m., **nit-ac.**, ol-j.², op., petr.,
ph-ac., phos., psor.², **puls.**, rhod.,
rhus-t., ruta, sabin., sal-ac.²′ ¹², sec.,
sep., SIL., spong., **staph.**, stront-c.¹⁰,
sulph., symph.⁸, syph.¹′ ⁷, tarent.²,
tell.³, ter.², **THER.**, thuj., tub-k.¹²

brittle bones

necrosis bone

softening bones

periosteum, of

ant-c., **ASAF.**, aur., bell., **chin.,**
cycl., hell., **merc.**, mez., **PH-AC.,**
puls., rhod., rhus-t., ruta, sabin.,
sil., staph.

CARRYING, ailments from⁷

carb-ac., caust., ruta¹²

am.³
ant-c., ant-t.⁸, ars., **cham.⁸**, coloc.,
ferr., ip., kali-c., nat-c., nat-m.,
ph-ac., sep.

back agg., on the

alum.

head agg., on the

    calc.

CARTILAGES, affection of[6] *

    ARG-M.[1', 2, 6, 7, 12], cimic., guaj.,
led., merc., nat-m.[2], olnd., plb., ruta,
sil.[1', 6]

enchondroma

inflammation–c.
swelling–c.

ulcers of

    merc-c.

CATALEPSY

    abies-c.[12], acon., aether[11, 12], **agar.,**
aran., **art-v.,** asaf.[6] bell.,
camph-br.[8], cann-i., canth.[11],
caust.[6], cham., chlol., **cic., cocc.,**
coff., con., crot-c.[8], crot-h.[6], **cupr.**[6],
cur., ferr., gels., GRAPH.,
hydr-ac.[2, 4, 6, 8], hyos., ign., indg.[12],
iod.[11], **ip.,** lach., laur.[4], **mag-m.**[6],
merc.[4, 8], **morph.**[8], **mosch.**[4, 6, 12],
nat-m., nux-m., ol-an.[6], **op., petr.,**
ph-ac., pip-m.[6, 12], **plat.,** plb.[11],
raph.[12], reser.[14], sabad.[8], spong.[12],
staph., stram., stry.[11], sulph., tab.[12],
tanac.[11] thuj., **valer.**[6], verat., **zinc.**[6]

Vol. I: *automatisms*

    gestures
    sits
    unconsciousness–conduct

afternoon[11]

    grat.

evening in bed

    cur.

anger, from[2]

    bry., **cham.**

fright, after

    acon., bell., **gels.,** ign., **OP.**

grief, after

    ign., **ph-ac.,** staph.

jealousy, from

    hyos., LACH.

joy, from

    COFF.

love, from unrequited

    hyos., **ign.,** lach., **ph-ac.**

menses, before[8]

    mosch.

during

    plat.

religious excitement, from

    stram., sulph., verat.

sexual excess, from[2]

chin., nux.

excitement, from

con., plat., stram.

worm affections, in[1']

sabad.

CATHETERISM, ailments from[6]

arn., mag-p.[6, 12], nux-v.

CAUTERY (with arg-n.), antidote to[12]

nat-m.

CHANGE of position agg.

acon., **bry., CAPS., carb-v.,**
caust., **chel.,** con., **EUPH., FERR.,**
lach., lyc., petr., ph-ac., **phos.,**
plat., plb., **PULS.,** ran-b., rhod.,
rhus-t., sabad., **samb.,** sil.,
SYPH.[3], thuj.

am.
agar., apis[8], arn.[3, 6], ars., buni-o.[14],
caust.[8, 15], cench.[1'], **cham., dulc.[3],**
IGN., meli., nat-s., ph-ac., plb.[3],
puls., **RHUS-T., sep.[3],** staph.[3],
syph.[3], tab.[3], teucr., valer., zinc.

desire for change of position[3, 6]

acon., alum.[3, 4, 6], **arn.[4, 6], ars.[2, 3, 6],**
bapt., bell.[3, 4, 6], **bry.[3, 4, 6],** caust.,
cham., **eup-per.,** ign., lyc.[3, 4, 6],
nat-s., **rhus-t.[3, 6],** sil.[3, 4, 6], tarax.[3, 4, 6],
zinc., **zinc-val.**

symptoms, constant ch. of[8]

apis, berb., carc.[10], cimic.[1', 7],
crot-t.[1'], **ign.[3, 8], kali-bi.[1', 7, 8],**
kali-c.[1'], **kali-s., lac-c.[7, 8],** lil-s.[1'],
lil-t., **mang.,** paraf., phyt., podo.[1'],
puls.[7, 8], sabin.[1'], sanic.[7, 8],
tub.[1', 7, 8], valer.[1']

alternating

contradictory

metastasis

rapid[3, 6]

ambr., ant-c.[1'], arn., benz-ac.,
berb., caul., caust., cimic., kalm.,
led., meph.[11], plat.[3], plb.[3], puls.,
sal-ac.[6], sul-ac.[6], tub., **valer.**

temperature agg., of

acon., act-sp.[2, 7], aesc.[1'], alum.,
alumn.[2], ant-c.[8], **ant-t.[2, 7], ARS.,**
bar-c.[3, 6], bufo[3], calc.[6], **calc-p.[3, 6],**
carb-v., caust., dulc.[3, 6],
FL-AC.[2, 7], graph., ip.[3, 7, 8],
kali-i.[3], **lach.[2, 3, 7, 8],** lyc., **mag-c.,**
meli.[3], merc-c.[3], nit-ac.[6],
nux-v.[1, 7], phos.[1, 7], phys.[11], **puls.,**
RAN-B., ran-s., rhod.[3, 6],
rhus-t.[1, 7], rumx.[3, 6], sabad.[3],
sabin., sang.[3, 6], sep.[3], sil.[1', 3, 6],
spong.[1, 7], sul-i.[3], sulph., verat.,
VERB.

ailments from[12]

nat-c., ran-b.

weather see weather–change

CHILDBED, ailments from (1897) ✶

cimic., sep., stram.

convulsions–puerperal

faintness–puerperal

CHILDREN, affections in
(Kent's Rep. 1897) ✶

abrot.[6], acet-ac.[12], **ACON.,** aeth.,
agar., **all-c.,** alum.[3, 6], **ambr.,**
ang.[2, 3], **ant-c., ANT-T.,** apis[6], arn.,
ars., asaf., **aur., bar-c., BELL., BOR.,**
bry., **CALC.,** calc-f.[14], **calc-p.,**
camph., canth., **CAPS.,** caust.[3],
CHAM., chel.[2], chin., chlol.[2],
chlorpr.[14], **cic.,** cic-m.[12], **cina,**
clem., coc-c.[6], **cocc., cocc-s.**[2], coff.,
con., **croc.,** cupr., dig., dros., euph.,
ferr., ferr-p.[3, 6, 7], **gels.,** graph., hell:,
hep.[3], **HYOS.,** ign., iod., **IP.,**
kali-br.[2, 12], kali-c., **kali-m.**[2],
kali-p.[2], **kreos., lach.,** laur., **lyc.,**
mag-c., mag-p.[2], meph.[14], **MERC.,**
mill.[2], **mosch.**[2], mur-ac., nat-c.,
nat-m.[2, 6], **nux-m., nux-v., OP.,**
ped.[12], phos.[6], phyt.[8], plb., **podo.,**
psor., PULS., rheum, rhod.[3], rhus-t.,
rib-ac.[14], ruta, sabad., **sabin.,**
samb.[3, 6], sec., seneg., senn.[4], sep.,
SIL., spig., **spong., squil.,** stann.,

staph., stram.[6, 12], sul-ac., **SULPH.,**
ter.[2], **teucr.,** thuj., thyr.[14], verat.,
viol-o., viol-t., zinc.

dentition
development, arrested

emaciation–children

growth

Vol. I: *feces-urinating*

biting nails[3, 7]

acon., am-br.[7], arn.[7], ars., **ARUM-T.,**
bar-c., calc.[3, 15], cina, hura[3],
hyos.[5, 7], **lyc.,** lyss.[3], med.[3],
nat-m.[7, 15], nit-ac.[3], phos.[3], plb.[3],
sanic.[7], senec., **sil.**[5, 7], stram.,
sulph.[5, 7]

delicate, puny, sickly[3, 6]

brom., calc-p., **caust.**[2], irid.[12],
lyc.[2, 3, 6, 12], mag-c.[12], phos., psor.[2, 12]

emaciation–pining boys

fingers in the mouth, put

calc, cham., IP., kali-p.[15], lyc.[5],
nat-m.[15], sil.[15], tarent.[7]

growing too fast[8, 12]

calc.[7, 8], **calc-p.**[8], ferr.[3], ferr-a.[6, 8],
iod.[3, 6], irid., kreos.,
PH-AC.[2, 3, 4, 6-8, 12], **phos.**[1'-3, 6-8, 12]

growth

CHILL, feels better before

psor.

CHINA (without quinine cachexia
[ ] /cinchonism)

ant-t.[6], aran.[2], arn.[2, 6], ars.[2, 4, 6],
bell.[2, 4], calc.[2, 4, 6], carb-v.[2, 4, 6], cham.[2]
coff.[2], eup-per.[2], ferr.[2, 6], hell.[2], HEP.[2],
iod.[2, 6], ip.[2, 4, 6], lach.[2, 4, 6], led.,
meny.[2, 4], merc.[2, 4, 6], nat-c.[2], nat-m.[2, 6],
nux-v.[2, 6], ph-ac.[6], puls.[2, 6], rhus-t.[2],
salv.[3], sel., sep.[2, 6], sulph.[2, 6], thea[3],
verat.[2, 4, 6]

CHLOROSIS

abrot.[2, 6], absin.[2, 12], acet-ac., alet.,
alum., alum-p.[1'], alumn., am-c.,
ambr.[2], ant-c., ant-t.[2], aq-mar.[6],
arg-m., arg-n., ARS., ars-i.,
ars-s-f.[1'], aur-ar.[12], bar-c., BELL.,
bry.[12], cadm-met.[14], CALC.,
calc-ar.[1'], CALC-P., carb-an.,
carb-v., CARBN-S., caust., cham.[12],
chin., chin-ar., chlor.[12], cina[2],
cob-n.[14], COCC., coch.[2], con., cupr.,
cycl., dig., FERR., FERR-AR., ferr-i.,
FERR-M., ferr-p., ferr-s.[2], franz.[12],
GRAPH., guar.[2], hell., helon., hep.,
ign., ip.[2], kali-ar., kali-bi.[6], kali-c.,
kali-fcy., kali-p., kali-perm.[6],
kali-s., lac-c.[6], lach.[12], LYC., lyss.,
MANG., med.[7], merc., mill.[2, 12],
nat-c., nat-hchls.[12], NAT-M., nat-p.,
NIT-AC., nux-v., olnd., petr.,
ph-ac., PHOS., phyt.[2], pic-ac.,

PLAT., plb., PULS., sabin.,
sacch.[11, 12], SENEC., SEP., sin-n.[2, 12]
spig., staph., sul-ac., SULPH., thuj.,
ust., valer., vanad.[7], xan.[2], zinc.

symptoms agg. alternate days

alum.

winter, in

ferr.

CHOREA

abrot.[2], absin.[8], acon., AGAR.,
agar-ph.[12], agarin.[8], agre.[14], ambr.[2],
aml-ns.[2, 12], ant-c.[12], ant-t., apis,
arg-n., arn.[12], ars., ars-i., ars-s-f.[1'],
ART-V., asaf., aster., atro.[2], aven.[8],
bell., bufo, cact., CALC., calc-i.[1'],
calc-p.[8, 12], cast.[2, 12], caul., CAUST.,
cedr., cham., chel., chin.[1], chlol.,
CIC., CIMIC., CINA, cocain.[8],
cocc., coch.[2], cod.[2, 12], coff., con.,
croc., crot-c., crot-h., CUPR.,
cupr-a.[8, 10, 12], cupr-ar., cypr., dios.,
dulc., eup-a.[8], ferr., ferr-ar.,
ferr-cit.[6], ferr-cy.[8], ferr-i., ferr-r.[8],
ferr-s.[2, 12], form., gels.[2], guar.[2],
hipp., hyos., IGN., iod., ip., kali-ar.,
kali-br., kali-c., kali-i., kali-p.,
kali-s.[2, 12], lach., lat-k.[8, 12], laur.,
levo.[14], lil-t., lyss.[10], mag-p.,
mand.[14], mang.[7], merc., mez., mill.[2],
morph.[2, 12], mur-ac.[12], MYGAL.,
nat-m., nit-ac., nux-m., nux-v.,
ol-an.[6], op., passi.[6], ph-ac., phos.,
phys.[2, 6, 8, 10, 12], phyt.[2], picro.[8], plat.,
plb., psor., puls., rhod., rhus-t.,
russ.[12], sabin., santin.[8], scut.[8, 12],
sec., sep., sil., sin-n.[2, 12], sol-n.[8, 12],
spig.[8], stann., stict.[2], STRAM.,

stry.[8], stry-p.[6, 8], sul-ter.[12], sulfon.[8], **sulph., sumb.,** tanac.[8, 12], **TARENT.,** tarent-c.[12], **ter.**[2, 13], thal.[11, 14], thiop.[14], thuj., **tub.**[7], valer.[6], verat-v., visc., **zinc.,** zinc-ar.[8], **zinc-br.**[8, 12], zinc-cy.[6, 8, 12], zinc-p.[1'], zinc-val.[6, 8], ziz.[2, 6, 8]

side, crosswise left arm and right leg[8]

    agar., cimic., **stram.**[2]

  right arm and left leg[8]

    tarent.

left

  cimic., cupr., rhod.

one sided

  calc., cocc., **cupr.,** nat-s., phys., tarent.[7]

right

  ars., caust., nat-s., phys., tarent., zinc.[15]

side lain on

  cimic.

daytime

  art-v., tarent.

morning

  arg-n.[15], mygal.

afternoon

  nat-s.

noon[15]
  arg-n.

evening agg.

  zinc.

night

  arg-n., CAUST.[1, 7], cupr.[1']

  am.[2]
  art-v., tarent.

anxiety, from[6]

  stram.

begins see face

children who have grown too fast

  phos.

  ch.-puberty

climacteric period, during[6]

  cimic.

coition (woman), after

  agar., cedr.

cold bath, after

  rhus-t.

dentition, in second

bell.⁸, **calc.²**

dinner, after

zinc., ziz.²

dry weather

caust.

eating, after

ign.

emotional

agar., arg-n.⁶, cimic.¹', **ign., laur.,**
nat-m.⁶, **op., phos., tarent.²**

exercise am.

zinc.

face, agg. in⁸

caust., cic., **cupr.².⁸,** hyos.,
mygal., nat-m., zinc.

begins in f. and spreads to body

sec.

falling, with²

calc.

fear, from⁷

calc.

fright, from

acon., agar., arg-n.⁶, **calc., CAUST.,**
cimic.⁸, cupr., **cupr-a.²,** cupr-ar.⁶,
**gels., ign., kali-br., laur., nat-m.,
op.,** phos., **stram.,** tarent.⁸, **zinc.**

grief, after

cimic.⁸, **cupr-a.²,** ign., tarent.⁸

hyperaesthesia, with excessive²

tarent.

imitation, from

caust., cupr., mygal., **tarent.**

light agg.

ign.⁸, ziz.²

loss of animal fluids, from

chin.

lying on back am.

cupr., cupr-a.², **ign.**

masturbation, from

agar.⁸, **calc.,** chin., cina²

menses, before⁶

caul.

during

caul.⁶, caust.¹'·⁷, **ZINC.**

after, am.[2]

sep.

moon, at full[15]

nat-m.

at new[6]

cupr.

motions agg.[2]

cupr-a., ziz.

backward, with[2]

bell.

gyratory, with[7]

stram.

rhythmical, with[8]

agar., caust., cham., cimic., lyc., **tarent.**

music am.[7, 8]

tarent.

noise agg.

ign.[8], ziz.[2]

numbness of affected **parts, with**[18]

nux-v.

nymphomania, with[2]

tarent.

periodic

cupr., cupr-a.[2], nat-s.

every seven days[2, 7]

croc.

pollutions, with[2]

dios.

pregnancy, during

bell.[8], **caust., chlol.**[2]**, cupr.**

puberty, in[6, 8]

agar.[6], asaf.[8], caul.[1', 2, 8], **cimic.,** ign.[8], puls.

punishment, from[2]

ign.

rest, during

zinc.

rheumatic

CAUST., cimic., kali-i., rhus-t., spig.[8], stict.

run or jump, cannot **walk must**

bufo, kali-br., nat-m., **stram.**[2]

sight of bright colors am.[8]

tarent.

sleep, during

cupr.[6], tarent.[8], **ziz.**[2, 6, 8, 12]

am.
AGAR., cupr.[8], hell., ziz.

spinal

asaf., cic., cocc., cupr., mygal., nux-v.

strabismus, with[2]

stram.

suppressed eruptions, from

caust., cupr.[6, 8], SULPH., zinc.

thinking of it, when

caust.

thunderstorm, before

agar., rhod., sep.

during

phos.

touch agg.[9]

ziz.

uterine[2]

caul., CIMIC., croc., ign., lil-t., nat-m., puls., sec., sep.

waking, on[2]

chlol.

wet, after getting

rhus-t.

wine agg.

zinc.

worms, from

asaf.[8], calc., cina, santin.[8], spig.[8]

clear weather see weather–clear

CHRONIC DISEASES,
to begin treatment[8]

calc., calc-p., **nux-v.,** puls., **sulph.**

CHRONICITY[3]

alum., arg-n., ars., calc., caust., con., kali-bi., kali-i., lyc., mang., phos., plb., psor., **sep., sulph.,** syph., tub.

CLOTHING, intolerance of

agar.[3], **am-c.**, aml-ns.[3], **apis,**
ARG-N., arn., asaf., asar., **bov.,**
bry., CALC., caps., carb-v.,
carbn-s., caust., cench.[1', 7], chel.[3],
chin., clem.[3], coc-c.[1', 3], coff., con.,
CROT-C., crot-h., dios.[6], euph.[11],
glon.[3], **graph., hep.**, ign., kali-bi.,
kali-c., kali-i.[3], kali-m.[2], kali-n.,
kreos., **lac-c.**[7], **LACH.**, lil-t.[3, 6],
LYC., merc.[3, 4, 6, 11], merc-c.[3],
nat-m.[3], nat-s., nit-ac.[3], nux-m.[3],
NUX-V., olnd., **ONOS.**, op., phos.[3],
polyg-h.[2, 7], psor.[3], **puls., ran-b.,**
sanic., sars., sec.[3], **sep., spig.,**
SPONG., stann., sulph., **tarent.,**
tub.[3], verat-v.[3], vip.[3]

covers–agg.

warm–desire

woolen

phos., psor., puls., **sulph.**

loosing, am.

am-c., arn., asar., ars.[2], **bry., CALC.,**
cann-i., caps., carb-v., caust., chel.,
chin., coff., **hep., LACH., LYC.,**
mag-m.[16], **NIT-AC., NUX-V.**, olnd.,
op., **puls.**, ran-b., **sanic., sars., sep.,**
spig., spong., stann., sulph.

pressure of, am.[3]

fl-ac., nat-m.

cloudy weather see weather–cloudy

COAL GAS, from

acet-ac.[7, 8], am-c.[8], arn., bell.[2, 8],
bor.[7, 8], bov., **carbn-s.**, carb-v., coff.[8],
ip.[2], lach.[7], **op.**[2, 7, 8, 12], phos.[12], sec.[3]

death–carbon

sewer–gas poisoning

COAT of skin drawn over inner parts,
sensation of

ant-t.[3], ars.[3], bar-c.[3], brom.[3], bry.[3],
calc.[3], caust., cina[3], cocc., dig.[3], dros.,
hep.[3], merc., nat-m.[3], nux-m., ph-ac.[3],
phos., pip-n.[3], **puls.**, sulph.[3]

COBWEB, sensation of a[2, 3]

alum.[3], alumn.[2], **bar-c., bor.**, brom.[3],
calc., chin.[3], **graph.**, mag-c., ph-ac.,
phos.[3], plb., **ran-s.**, sul-ac., sumb.[3, 11]

COITION, during*

alum.[3, 4], anac., asaf., bar-c.,
berb.[4], bor.[4], **bufo**[3], calad., calc.[4],
canth., carb-v.[4], caust.[4], clem.[4],
ferr., **graph., kali-c.**, kreos., lyc.,
nit-ac.[4], **nux-v.**[4], petr.[4], plat.,
plb.[4], **sel.**, sep., tax.[4], thuj.

after

AGAR., agn., alum.[4], am-c.,
ambr.[6], anac., anan., **apis**, arg-n.,
asaf., bar-c., berb.[4], bor., **bov.,**

bufo[3], **calad.**, **CALC.**, calc-i.[1]',
calc-s.[8], calc-sil.[1]', canth.,
carb-an.[4], carb-v.[3], **cedr.**, **chin.**,
con., daph.[4], dig.[4], eug.[4], **graph.**,
kali-bi.[3], **KALI-C.**, **KALI-P.**,
kreos.[3, 4], led.[4], lyc., mag-m.,
merc.[3, 4], mez.[4], mosch., **nat-c.**,
nat-m., **nat-p.**, nat-sil.,[1]', **nit-ac.**,
nux-v., **petr.**, **ph-ac.**, **phos.**, plb.,
puls.[3], rhod., **sel.**, **SEP.**, **SIL.**,
staph., sul-ac.[4], tab.[4], tarent.,
ther.

am.[3, 6]
    CON., merc.[3], **staph.**

interrputed agg.[3]

bell.

COLD in general **agg.**

abrot.[15], acet-ac.[1]', achy.[14], **acon.**,
act-sp.[3], adon.[6], aesc., **agar.**, **agn.**[7],
alum., alum-p.[1], **alum-sil.**[7], alumn.,
am-c., am-m.[1]', anac.[2, 3, 16], **ant-c.**,
ant-t.[3], **apoc.**, **aran.**, aran-ix.[10, 14],
arg-m., arg-n., arist-cl.[9, 10], arn.,
ARS., ars-i.[1', 3], asar., **aur.**, aur-ar.[15],
aur-s.[1]', **bad.**, **BAR-C.**, bar-m.[1, 7],
bar-s.[1]', **bell.**, bell-p.[9, 10, 14],
benz-ac.[15], **bor.**, **bov.**, brom.[3, 7, 11],
bry., cadm-s., **CALC.**, **CALC-AR.**,
CALC-F., **CALC-P.**, calc-s.,
CALC-SIL., **CAMPH.**[1'-4, 5, 8, 11],
canth.[1, 7], **CAPS.**, **carb-an.**, **carb-v.**,
carbn-s., card-m.[1]', **carl.**[11], cast.[3],
caul.[1', 7], **CAUST.**, **cham.**, chel.,
CHIN., **chin-ar.**, chin-s.[3], **cic.**,
cimic., cinnb., **cist.**, clem.,
coc-c.[1]', **cocc.**, coch.[12], **coff.**[1, 7],
colch., coll.[8], **coloc.**, **con.**, cop.[11],
crot-c.[8], **cycl.**, cyt-l.[9, 10, 14],
dig., **DULC.**, elaps, **eup-per.**[3, 7],
euphr.[7], **FERR.**[1, 7], **ferr-ar.**, ferr-p.[11],
flav.[14], **form.**[7, 8, 11], franz.[11], gins.[11],
GRAPH., **guaj.**, gymno., ham.[1]',
hed.[10], **hell.**, helon., **HEP.**, hydr.,

hyos., **HYPER.**, hypoth.[14], **ign.**,
iod.[11], **ip.**, **KALI-AR.**, **kali-bi.**,
KALI-C., kali-i.[6, 11], kali-m.[1]',
KALI-P., kali-sil.[7], **kalm.**, kreos.,
lac-ac.[11], **lac-d.**, lach., laur., **led.**,
lob.[8], **LYC.**, lycps., **MAG-C.**[1, 7],
mag-m.[1, 7], **MAG-P.**, mand.[14],
mang., med.[1]', meny., **merc.**, **mez.**,
mit.[11], moly-met.[14], **MOSCH.**,
mur-ac.[1], **NAT-AR.**, **nat-c.**[1, 7],
nat-m., **nat-p.**, nat-s.[1]', nat-sil.[1]',
NIT-AC., **nux-m.**, **NUX-V.**,
oci-s.[9, 14], onop.[14], **ox-ac.**, **petr.**,
ph-ac., **PHOS.**, phys.[11], **phyt.**,
pimp.[11], **plb.**[1, 7], podo.[7], polyg-h.[11],
polyg-pe.[12], psil.[14], **PSOR.**, ptel.[11],
puls., pyre-p.[11], **PYROG.**, raja-s.[14],
RAN-B., rheum, **rhod.**, **RHUS-T.**,
rib-ac.[14], **RUMX.**, ruta, **SABAD.**,
samb., saroth.[10], **sars.**[1, 7], sec.[11], sel.[8],
senec., seneg., **SEP.**, sieg.[10], **SIL.**,
sol-n.[11], sol-t-ae.[3], **SPIG.**, spong.,
squil., **stann.**, staph., stram.,
STRONT-C., stry.[11], **sul-ac.**, **sulph.**,
sumb., tab.[8], **tarent.**, teucr., thala.[11],
ther., **thuj.**, **tub.**, valer.[15], verat.[2, 3, 8],
verb., vichy[11], **viol-t.**[1, 7], x-ray[14],
xero.[8], **zinc.**

am.[2]
acon.[2, 3], aesc.[1', 6], all-c.[8], aloe[1', 3, 6],
alumn., am-m.[6], **ambr.**, anac., **ant-c.**,
ant-t.[2, 3], apis[1', 3, 6], **arg-n.**[3, 6], arn.,
asar., aur.[2], aur-i.[1]', bar-c., bell.,
bell-p.[8], beryl.[14], bor.[2, 8], **bry.**[1', 2, 3, 6, 8],
calad., calc., **cann-i.**, carb-v., caust.,
cham., chin., **cina**, coc-c.[1]', cocc.,
colch., coloc., **croc.**, cycl.[3], **dros.**,
dulc., **euph.**, fago.[8], ferr.,
FL-AC.[2, 3, 7], **glon.**[3], graph.,
guaj.[3, 7], hell., hep., hist.[9], **HYOS.**,
iber.[14], ign., **IOD.**[2, 3, 6-8], **ip.**[2], kali-c.,
kali-i.[3], kali-m.[3], **lac-c.**[1]', lach.,
laur., **led.**[2, 3, 6-8, 12], lil-t.[3, 6],
lyc.[2, 3, 6-8], mag-m.[6], mag-s.[9],
med.[3, 7], merc., mez., moly-met.[14],
mur-ac., nat-c., **nat-m.**[2, 3, 6], **nat-s.**[3],
nit-ac.[2, 4], nux-m., nux-v., onos.[8],
op.[2, 3, 8], ph-ac., **phos.**[2, 8], **plat.**,
PULS.[1'-3, 6, 7], rhus-t., sabad., **sabin.**,
sang.[3], sec.[1'-3, 8], **sel.**, seneg., sep.,
sil., spig., spong., staph., sulph.[2, 3, 6],
teucr.[2, 8], **thuj.**[2, 4], trios.[14], verat.

air agg.

abrot., acon., aesc., **AGAR.,
ALL-C.,** alum., alum-p.[1'],
alum-sil.[1'], **alumn.,** am-br.[2],
am-c., ammc., anac.[2, 3], ant-c.,
apis[3], apoc.[1'], **aran.,** arn., **ARS.,**
ars-s-f.[1'], asar., astac.[2], **AUR.,**
aur-ar.[1'], aur-s.[1'], bac.[8], **BAD.,**
bapt.[2], **BAR-C.,** bar-m., bar-s.[1'],
bell., bor., bov., brom.[11], **bry.,**
bufo[2, 3], cadm-s., **CALC.,
CALC-P.,** calc-sil.[1'], calen.[2],
CAMPH., canth., caps., **carb-ac.,
carb-an., carb-v.,** carbn-s., **carl.[11],
CAUST.,** cham., chin., chin-ar.,
cic., **CIMIC.,** cina, **CIST.,** clem.[6],
coc-c.[2], coca, cocc., coff., **colch.,
coloc., con.,** cupr.[7, 8], cur.[8],
cycl.[2, 3], dig., DULC., elaps,
euph.[8], **ferr.,** ferr-ar., ferr-p., fl-ac.,
graph., guaj.[8], ham.[1'], **HELL.,
HEP., hyos., HYPER., ign.,** ind.[2],
ip., KALI-AR., kali-bi., **KALI-C.,**
kali-m.[1'], kali-p., **kreos.,** lac-c.[11],
lac-d., lach., lappa[3], laur., **LYC.,**
lycps., lyss.[2], **mag-c.,** mag-m.,
MAG-P., mang., med.[2], meny.,
merc., merc-i-r.[2], mez., **MOSCH.,**
mur-ac., **nat-ar.,** nat-c., nat-m.,
nat-p., nat-s.[3, 7], nat-sil.[1'], nit-ac.,
nit-s-d.[2], **NUX-M., NUX-V.,
osm.,** ox-ac.[1'], par., **petr., ph-ac.,
phos.,** phys.[3], physal.[3], **plan.,**
plat.[3], plb.[3, 8], psil.[14], **PSOR.,**
ptel.[11], **puls., RAN-B., RHOD.,
RHUS-T., RUMX.,** ruta, **SABAD.,**
samb., sars., sel.[6, 8], senec.[11],
seneg., **SEP., SIL.,** sol-n., spig.,
spong., squil., staph., stram.,
**STRONT-C., sul-ac., sulph.,
sumb., tarent., thuj.,** tub.[8],
urt-u.[3, 8], **verat., verat-v.[2],** verb.,
viol-o.[3, 8], viol-t., visc.[8], **zinc.,**
zinc-p.[1'], **zing.[2]**

am.[8]

acon.[7, 8], aesc.[6, 8], aeth..
all-c.[1', 8], aloe[6, 8], **alum.[6, 8],**
am-m.[6, 8], ambr.[2, 6, 8], **aml-ns.,**
anac.[2], anan.[2], ang.[6], **ant-c.[2, 6, 8],**

ant-t.[2, 8], **apis[6, 8],** aran.[6],
aran-ix.[14], **arg-n.[6-8],** arist-cl.[14],
asaf.[6, 8], **asar.[2],** aur-i.[1'], bapt.[1', 3],
bar-c., bar-i.[1'], bell-p.[14],
beryl.[14], **bry.[1', 2, 6, 8], bufo[1', 8],**
cact., calad.[1', 2], calc.[2, 8],
calc-f.[14], cann-i.[2, 8], **carb-v.[2],**
cham.[2], **chin.,** cina[2], cit-v.[2],
clem., **coc-c.[2, 6],** coca,
colch.[2], com., conv., crat.,
croc.[2, 8], dig., dios., **dros.[2, 8],**
dulc.[8], euon-a., euph.[2],
euphr., foll.[14], gels., **glon.[1', 6, 8],**
graph., hed.[14], iber.[14], ign.[2],
IOD.[2, 6, 8], ip.[2], kali-bi.[6],
**kali-i.[1', 2, 6, 8], kali-s.[1', 6, 8],
lach.[2, 6, 8], led.[2, 3], lil-t.[6, 8],**
luf-op.[14], **LYC.[2, 6, 8], mag-c.,**
mag-m.[1', 6, 8], med.[1'], meph.[14],
merc.[2], merc-i-r., mez.,
mosch.[6, 8], naja, **nat-m.[2, 6, 8],**
nat-s., nep.[13, 14], **nit-ac.[2, 3],**
nux-v.[2], ol-an., **op.[2, 6],** phos.[2, 8],
pic-ac.[1', 8], pitu[14], plat.[2, 3, 8],
psil.[14], **PULS.[2, 6, 8],** rad-br.[3, 6],
rauw.[14], rhus-t.[2, 8], **sabad.,**
sabin.[2, 8], **sec.[1', 2, 6, 8], sel.[2],**
seneg.[2], **sep.[2, 6, 8],** stel.,
stront-c.[6], stry-p., **sulph.[2, 6, 8],**
syph.[1'], **tab.[6, 8], tarent.,**
tere-ch.[14], teucr.[2], thala.[14],
thuj.[2], tub.[7], tub-r.[14], vib.,
visc.[14]

windows open, must **have[1']**

aml-ns.[8], apis[6], **arg-n.[6-8],**
bapt.[6, 8], bry.[1'], calc.[8], camph.,
carb-v.[7], **carbn-s.,** glon., graph.,
iod.[6], **ip.[6], lach.[1', 8],** lyc.[6], med.[8],
puls.[1', 8], sabin., sec.,
sulph.[1', 6, 8], tub.

aversion to[6]

am-c., **aran., ars.,** bart.[11], bell.,
bry., **calc.,** caps.[6, 11], caust.,
cham., chin., graph., grat., **hep.,
kali-c.,** nat-c., nat-m., nux-m.,
nux-v., petr., sel., **sil.,** sulph.,
tub.

desire for

achy.[14], aloe, **apis**, arg-n.[1', 6],
asaf., asar., **aur.**, camph.[1'],
carb-v., cic.[11], **croc.**, gran.[11],
iod., kali-s.[1'], lil-t., **puls.**[1', 6], **sec.**,
sul-i.[1'], sulph.

open air see air–open–desire

inspiring of, agg.[3]

aesc., alum., **am-c.**, ant-c., **ars.**,
aur., **bell.**, **bry.**, **calc.**, camph.,
CAUST., cham., **cimic.**, cina, cist.,
dulc., **hep.**, hydr., **HYOS.**, **ign.**,
kali-bi., **kali-c.**, **MERC.**, mosch.,
nat-m., **nux-m.**, **NUX-V.**, par.,
petr., phos., psor., puls., **rhod.**,
rhus-t., **RUMX.**, **SABAD.**, sars.,
sel.[14], seneg., **sep.**, sil., spig.,
staph., **stront-c.**, sulph., syph.,
thuj., verat.

becoming cold

acon., aesc., **agar.**, **alumn.**, am-c.,
ant-c., arg.-n., **arn.**, **ARS.**, ars-i.,
asar., **AUR.**, aur-s.[1'], **bad.**,
BAR-C., bar-m., bar-s.[1'], bell.,
bor., bov., **bry.**, **calc.**, **calc-p.**,
calc-sil.[1'], **camph.**, canth., **caps.**,
carb-an., **carb-v.**, **carbn-s.**, **caust.**,
cham., chin., chin-ar., cic., **cimic.**,
clem., **cocc.**, **con.**, **dig.**, **dulc.**,
elaps, **ferr.**, ferr-ar., ferr-p.,
graph., hell., **HEP.**, **hyos.**, **hyper.**,
ign., ip.[3], **KALI-AR.**, **KALI-BI.**,
KALI-C., kali-p., kali-s., **kreos.**,
lach., **LYC.**, **mag-c.**, mag-m.,
mag-p., mang., **med.**, meny.,
merc., merc-i-r., mez., **MOSCH.**,
mur-ac., **nat-ar.**, nat-c., nat-m.,
nat-p., nicc., nit-ac., nux-m.,
NUX-V., petr., **PH-AC.**, **phos.**,
psor., puls.[3], **PYROG.**, **RAN-B.**,
rhod., **RHUS-T.**, **rumx.**, ruta,
SABAD., samb., sars., **SEP.**,
SIL., spig., spong., squil., staph.,

stram., **stront-c.**, **SUL-AC.**,
sulph., **sumb.**, **tarent.**, **thuj.**,
verat.[2, 3], verb., viol-t., **zinc.**

ailments from[12]

kalm., phyt.

when heated[12]

kali-s.

am.
acon., aesc.[3], agn., all-c.[3], aloe[3],
alum., alumn.[2], am-c.[3], am-m.[3],
ambr., anac.[2, 3], ang.[3], ant-c.,
ant-t., **apis**[3], **arg-n.**, arn., asaf.[3],
asar.[2, 3], aur., bapt.[3], bar-c., bell.,
bov., brom.[3], **bry.**, calad.,
calc.[2, 3], calc-i[1'], cann-i.[2], cann-s.,
carb-v., caust.[2, 3], **cham.**, chin.[2, 3],
cina[2, 3], clem., coc-c.[3], cocc.,
coff., colch., coloc., croc., **dros.**,
dulc., euph., **fl-ac.**[3], **glon.**,
graph.[2, 3], guaj.[3], hell., ign.[2, 3],
IOD., ip., kali-bi.[2], kali-c.[3], kali-i.[3],
kali-s.[3], kalm.[3], **lac-c.**, **lach.**,
led., lil-t.[3], **LYC.**, mang., **merc.**,
mez., mur-ac., nat-c., **nat-m.**,
nit-ac., **nux-m.**[2, 3], nux-v.[2, 3], olnd.,
op., **petr.**, ph-ac., phos., plat.,
PULS., rhus-t.[2, 3], sabad., **sabin.**,
sars., **sec.**, sel., seneg., sep.[2, 3],
sil.[2, 3], spig., spong., staph.,
sulph., teucr., thuj., verat.

after, agg.

acon., agar., **alum.**, alum-p.[1'],
alum-sil[1'], **alumn.**, am-c.,
anac.[2, 3], **ant-c.**[2, 3], ant-t., arg-n.,
arn., **ARS.**, ars-s-f.[1'], aur.
aur-s.[1'], **BAR-C.**, bar-s.[1', 3], **BELL.**,
bor., **BRY.**, **CALC.**, **CALC-P.**,
calc-s., calc-sil.[1'], camph.,
carb-v., **carbn-s.**, caust.[2, 3],
CHAM., **CHIN.**, cimic.[3], **coc-c.**[2],
cocc., **coff.**, colch.[1', 3], **coloc.**, **con.**,
croc., cupr., cupr-s.[2], **cycl.**, dig.,

dros., **DULC.**, ferr., ferr-ar[1]',
FL-AC.[3], **GRAPH.**, guaj.[3], **HEP.**,
hydr.[3], **HYOS.**, hyper., ign., **ip.**,
kali-ar.[1]', **kali-bi.**, **kali-c.**,
kali-m[1]', kali-p., **kali-sil.**[1]', kalm.,
led., **lyc.**, mag-c., **mang.**, **med.**,
MERC., nat-c., **nat-m.**, nat-p.,
nat-sil.[1]', **nit-ac.**, **nux-m.**,
NUX-V., op., **petr.**, **ph-ac.**,
PHOS., phyt.[1]', plat., polyg-h.[3],
psor., **PULS.**, **PYROG.**, **RAN-B.**,
RHUS-T., ruta, sabin., **samb.**,
sang.[1]', sars., sel., **SEP.**, **SIL.**,
SPIG., **stann.**, staph., stront-c.,
SUL-AC., sul-i.[1]', **sulph.**, **tarent.**,
thuj., tub.[1]', valer., **verat.**, **xan.**[2],
zinc-p.[1]'

uncovering

ə part of body agg.

agar.[3], am-c.[3], **bar-c.**, **bell.**,
calc.[3], cham., **hell.**, **HEP.**, ip.[2],
led.[1], **nux-v.**[3], ph-ac., **phos.**[3],
psor.[3], puls., **RHUS-T.**, **sep.**,
SIL., tarent.[3], thuj.[3], zinc.[3]

uncovering-single part

back[7]

pilo.

extremities

aur., **bry.**, con., **HEP.**, **nat-m.**,
RHUS-T., **SIL.**, squil., stront-c.,
THUJ.

feet

alum[3], am-c.[3], ars.[3], **bar-c.**,
bufo[3], cham., clem.[3], **con.**,
cupr.[1], kali-ar.[3], kali-c.[3],
lach.[3], lyc.[3], mag-p.[3], nit-ac.[3],

nux-m.[3], **NUX-V.**[3], phos.[3],
phys.[3], **puls.**[1], sep.[3], **SIL.**,
stann.[16], zinc.[3]

hand out of bed

acon.[3], **BAR-C.**, canth., **con.**,
HEP., merc.[3], phos., **RHUS-T.**,
sil.

head

am-c.[16], arg-n.[3], **BELL.**, **hep.**[3],
hyos.[3], led., nux-v.[3], puls.,
rhus-t.[3], **SEP.**, **SIL.**

heated, when[1]'

acon.[3], **bell-p.**[7], bry.[3], kali-ar.,
ran-b.

perspiration, during[3, 7]

ACON. ars-s-f.[1]', calc-sil.[1]',
dulc.[7], sul-i.[1]'

sitting on cold steps[3, 8]

chim., **nux-v.**, rhod.[3]

dry weather see weather—cold dry

feeling in blood vessels

abies-c.[3], **ACON.**, ant-c., ant-t.,
ARS., bell.[6], lyc., op.[3], plb.[3],
RHUS-T., sulph.[6], **verat.**

bones

aran., ars., berb.[1], calc., elaps,
eup-per.[3], kali-i.[3], lyc., merc.,
pyrog.[3], sep., sulph., **verat.**, zinc.

inner parts

anh.[10], ars., **calc., hura**[7]**, laur.,**
lyc., meny., nux-v., par., sep.,
sulph.

single parts[10]

agar., aran., aran-ix., buth-a.,
elaps, helo.

heat and cold

alum., alum-p.[1]', ang.[3], **ant-c.,**
ant-t.[7], arn.[7, 8], **ars-i.,** asar.[3],
aur-s.[1]', bar-s.[1]', calc.[3], calc-s.[1]',
caps.[3], **carbn-s., caust.,** cina[3],
cinnb., **cocc.,** cor-r.[3], ferr.[3, 6],
flav.[14], **FL-AC.,** glon.[3], **graph.,**
ip., kali-c., **lach.,** lyc., mag-c.[3],
mag-m., **merc.,** nat-c., **nat-m.,**
nux-v.[7, 16], **ph-ac.,** phys.[3], **psor.,**
puls., **ran-b.,** rob.[7], sanic.[3], **sep.,**
sil., sul-ac.[3], **sulph., syph.**[1'-3, 7],
tab.[3], thala.[14], **tub.**[7, 15]

hot days with cold nights[3]

acon., dulc., merc-c., rumx.

one part cold, with heat of another[3]

apis, bry., cham.

place agg., entering a

ARS., bell.[8], calc-p., **camph.**[2, 8],
carb-v., caust., con., **dulc., ferr.,**
ferr-ar., graph., hep., ip.[3],
KALI-AR., kali-c., kali-p.,
kali-sil.[1]', mosch., nux-m., **nux-v.,**
petr., phos., **psor., puls., RAN-B.,**
rhus-t., sabad., **SEP.,** sil., spong.,
stront-c., **tub., verb.**

take c., tendency to *****

ACON., aesc.[6], agar.[6], all-c.[6],
ALUM., alum-p.[1]', alum-sil.[1]',
alumn.[1]', am-c., am-m., anac.,
ant-c., ant-t., aral.[6], aran.[6], **arg-n.,**
arn., ars., ars-i., ars-s-f.[1]', **bac.**[7],
BAR-C., bar-i.[1]', bar-m.[6], bar-s.[1]',
bell., benz-ac.[3], bor., **BRY.,**
calad.[6], **calc.,** calc-i.[1]', **CALC-P.,**
calc-s., calc-sil.[1]', **calen.**[7], camph.,
caps.[10], carb-an.[6], **carb-v.,**
carbn-s., caust., **CHAM.,** chin.,
chin-ar., cimic.[1', 6], cinnb.[6], cist.[6],
clem.[6], coc-c., cocc., coff.,
colch.[1]', coloc., **con.,** croc.,
crot-h.[4], cupr., cycl.[6], dig., dros.,
DULC., elaps[6], eup-per.[1]',
euphr.[6], **ferr.,** ferr-ar., ferr-i.,
ferr-p., **form.,** gast.[11, 12], **gels.,**
goss., **graph.,** ham., hed.[10, 14],
HEP., hyos., hyper.[6], ign., iod.,
ip., kali-ar., **kali-bi., KALI-C.,**
KALI-I.[1], kali-p.[1], kali-s.,
kali-sil.[1]', **lac-d.,** lach.[4, 6], led.,
LYC., m-arct.[3], m-aust.[3], mag-c.[10],
mag-m., **MED.**[7]**, MERC.,** mez.,
naja[3]**, NAT-AR., nat-c., NAT-M.,**
nat-p., nat-sil.[1]', **NIT-AC.,**
nux-m., NUX-V., ol-j.[3, 6], op.,
osm.[12], **petr., ph-ac., phos.,** plat.,
PSOR., puls., rhod.[6, 12], **rhus-t.,**
RUMX., ruta, sabad., sabin.,
samb., sang., sars., sel.,
senec.[1', 6]**, SEP., SIL.,** solid.[3],
spig., stach.[11], stann., staph.,
sul-ac., sul-i.[1]', **sulph., thuj.**[2, 6],
TUB., valer., verat., verb.[6],
zinc.[6]

faintness–cold

paralysis–cold

ailments from[12]

coloc., kali-c., rhod.

spring, in[12]

all-c.

feet, from c.[7]

con., **sil.**

becoming cold—a part—feet

menses, during[3]

bar-c., graph., mag-c., senec.

wet weather see weather—cold wet

COLDNESS of affected parts[3]

alum-sil.[1'], **ang.,** ars., bry., calc., caust., cocc., colch., crot-h., dulc., graph., lach., **led.,** meny., merc., **mez.,** petr., plat., plb., rhod., **rhus-t., sec.,** sil., thuj.

lain side morning in bed, on[16]

arn.

one side of body in septic fever[16]

meny., **puls.,** rhus-t.

COLLAPSE

acet-ac., acetan.[8], acon.[3, 8, 10, 11], aconin.[11], adren.[7], aeth.[3], **AM-C.,**

ampe-qu.[11], amyg., **ant-t.**[3, 8], apis, aran-ix.[10], arn.[3, 8], **ARS., ars-h.,** bar-c., **CAMPH.,** cann-i., canth., **carb-ac.,** carb-an.[2, 10], **CARB-V., CARBN-S.,** cench.[11], **CHIN.**[2], cina, cit-l.[2, 11], colch.[3, 8], colchin.[11], con.[3], crat.[8], **crot-h.,** crot-t., **cupr.,** cupr-a.[8, 11], **cupr-ar.,** cupr-s., cyt-l.[2, 9-11], **dig.**[8], diph.[8], dor., euon., hell., home.[11, 12], **hydr-ac.**[3, 6-8], **hyos.**[2], iod., ip.[3], jab., kali-br.[6], kali-chl.[11], kali-chr.[11], kali-cy.[11], kali-n., **lach.**[6, 11], lat-m.[9], **laur.,** lob.[8], lob-p.[8], lol.[11], lyc.[6], **med.,** merc., merc-c., merc-cy.[3, 8], merc-ns.[11], merc-pr-a.[11], morph., **mosch.**[2], mur-ac.[8], naja, nicot.[8, 12], nit-s-d.[11], olnd., op., ox-ac., **phos.,** phys., pitu.[9], plb., sabad.[10], santin.[11], scam.[11], **sec., seneg.**[2], sep.[3], stram., sul-ac., **sulph.**[3], tab.[3], tarent.[10], tarent-c.[6], tax., **verat.,** verat-v.[3], vip., **zinc.**[6, 8]

faintess

weakness—sudden

diarrhoea, after

ant-c.[2], **ARS., CAMPH., CARB-V.,** ric.[11], **VERAT.**

fainting-diarrhoea

needle, prick of a[16]

calc.

paralysis, at beginning of general

con.

sudden

ARS., colch.[2], phos.

weakness-rapid, sudden

vomiting, during

ars., ric.[11], verat.[2]

after

ARS., lob., phys., ric.[11], **verat.**

COMPLEXION (color of eyes, face, hair), **dark,** · (Kent 1897)

acon.[1, 7], alum., anac., arn., ars., aur.[2, 6, 12], brom.[12], bry., calc., calc-i.[6], caps.[6], CAUST., cham.[12], **chin.**[2, 12], cina[3, 6, 7, 15], coff.[2, 12], con.[12], graph.[12], IGN., iod.[6, 12], KALI-C., kreos., lac-c.[2], lach.[3], lyc.[12], lycpr.[12], mag-p.[6], mur-ac.[12], nat-m., NIT-AC., nux-v., PHOS.[1, 7], pic-ac.[12], PLAT., PULS.[1, 7], RHUS-T.[7], sang.[12], sec.[6], sep., staph.[7], sulph., thuj.[12], viol-o.[12]

eyes[12]

aur., graph., iod., lach., lycpr., mur-ac., nit-ac.

rigid fibre, with[2]

acon., anac., arn., ars., bry., caust., kalm., nat-m., **nit-ac.,** NUX-V., **plat.,** puls., **sep.,** staph., sulph.

blue eyes and **dark** hair [15]

lyc., nat-m., sep.

fair, blonde, light (Kent 1897)

agar., **apis,** aur.[12], bell.[4, 6, 12], bor., **brom.,** bry., **CALC., caps.,** cham.[12], chel.[12], clem.[12], cocc.[6, 12], coloc.[12], con.[12], cupr.[12], cycl.[12], dig.[12], **graph., hep.,** hyos., ip.[4, 12], **kali-bi.,** kreos.[12], lob., lycps.[12], merc., mez.[12], nat-c.[6, 12], op.[12], PETR., PHOS., PULS., **rhus-t.,** sabad., sel.[12], sep.[4, 12], **sil.,** spig.[12], SPONG., stann-i.[3, 6, 12], sul-ac.[12], **sulph.,** thuj.[12], vario.[12], viol-o.[12]

eyes[12]

bell., brom., caps., lob., puls., spong.

lax fibre, with[2]

agar.[7], **bell., BROM., CALC., caps., cham.,** clem., cocc., con., dig., **GRAPH.,** hyos., **kali-bi.,** lach., **lyc., merc., rhus-t.,** sil., SULPH.

relaxation

red hair[2, 12]

calc-p.[15], lach., phos., sep., sulph.[7, 12]

CONGESTION of blood

ACON., act-sp.[2], AESC., agar.[3], agn.[3], **aloe, alum.,** alum-p.[1'], alum-sil.[1'], am-c., am-m., ambr., aml-ns.[3], ang.[3], anis.[2], ant-c., ant-t.[3], **anthraci.**[2], apis, aq-mar.[14], arist-cl.[9], **arn.,** ars.[1', 3], asaf., aster.[14], **aur.,**

aur-ar.[1'], aur-i.[1'], aur-s.[1'], bar-c.,
bar-i.[1'], **BELL.**, **bor.**, bov., brom.[3],
bry., **CACT.**, calad.[3], **calc.**,
calc-hp.[12], calc-sil.[1'], camph.,
cann-s., canth., carb-an., **carb-v.**.
carbn-s., caust., cham., chel.,
CHIN., chin-s.[4], cinnb.[7], clem.,
cocc., **coff.**, colch., coloc., con.,
conv., croc., cupr., cycl., dig., dulc.,
erig.[6], eucal.[6], euphr.[3], **FERR.**,
ferr-i., ferr-p., **ferr-s.**[2, 6], fl-ac.[3, 6],
gels.[1', 3], **GLON.**, **graph.**, guaj., **ham.**,
hell., hep., hir.[14], hydr.[6], hydr-ac.[11],
hyos., hypoth.[14], ign., iod., ip.[3],
jab.[12], kali-c., kali-i.[6], kali-n.,
kreos.[6], **lach.**, laur., led., **lyc.**,
mag-c., mag-m., mand.[10], mang.,
MELI., merc., merc-c.[3], mez., **mill.**[2-4],
mosch., nat-c., **nat-m.**, nat-s.[3],
nit-ac., nux-m., **NUX-V.**, op., petr.,
ph-ac., **PHOS.**, plat., plb., podo.[6],
psor., **PULS.**, raja-s.[14], **ran-b.**, rhod.,
rhus-t., sabin., samb., **sang.**[3, 6],
sars.[3], sec., sel.[3], **seneg.**, **sep.**, **sil.**,
spig., **spong.**, squil., staph.,
stram., **stront-c.**[6], **stront-i.**[6], sul-ac.,
SULPH., tarax., ter.[3], thuj., valer.,
verat., verat-v., **VIOL-O.**, zinc.[3]

heat, flushes of

orgasm of blood

plethora

coldness of legs, with[15]

bell., **nat-m.**, **stram.**

haemorrhage, after[1']

mill.

internally

aloe, **apis**, ars., aur-i.[1'], bar-i.[1'],
CACT., **camph.**, canth., **colch.**,
conv., cupr., **glon.**, **hell.**, **MELI.**,
phos., sars.[1'], sep., **verat.**, verat-v.

sudden[3]

acon., bell., glon., verat-v.

CONSTIPATION am.

calc., carb-v.[3], merc., **psor.**

CONSTRICTION, sensation of **external**

abrot., **acon.**, **aesc.**, aeth.,
aether[11], **agar.**, **all-c.**, all-s.[11],
alum., alum-sil.[1', 8], **alumn.**[2],
am-c., am-m., **ammc.**, **aml-ns.**,
anac., ang.[3], ant-c., **ant-t.**, **apis**,
aral., arg-m., arg-n., arn., **ars.**,
ars-i., **arum-t.**, asaf., **asar.**, atro.[11],
aur., **bar-c.**, bar-s.[1'], bell., berb.,
bism., bor., bov., brom.[3], **bry.**,
cact., cadm-s.[3], calc., **calc-p.**,
cann-i., cann-s., canth., **caps.**,
carb-ac., carb-an., carb-v.,
carbn-o [11], **carbn-s.**, caust., cham.,
chel., chin., **CIMIC.**, cina, coc-c.[3],
COCC., coff., colch., **coloc.**, con.,
croc.[2, 3], crot-h.[3], **cupr.**, dig.,
dios., **dros.**, dulc., euphr., **ferr.**,
gels., **glon.**, **GRAPH.**, guaj., **hell.**,
hep., hist.[9, 10], hydr-ac., **HYOS.**,
IGN.[2], **iod.**, **ip.**, kali-c., kali-n.,
kreos., **lach.**, laur., led., lil-t.,
lob., **lyc.**, mag-c., mag-m., **mag-p.**,
manc.[3], mang., meny., **MERC.**,
merc-c., **merc-i-r.**, **mez.**, mosch.,
mur-ac., naja, nat-c., nat-m.,
nat-n.[3], **NIT-AC.**, nitro-o.[11],
nux-m., **NUX-V.**, oena.[3], olnd.,
op., **ox-ac.**, **par.**, petr., **ph-ac.**[2],
phos., phys.[3], pic-ac.[1'], **plat.**,
PLB., puls., ran-b., ran-s., rheum,
rhod., **RHUS-T.**, ric.[11], russ.[11],
ruta, sabad., sabin., sars., sec.,
sel., **sep.**, sil., sin-n.[11], spig.,
spong., squil., **STANN.**, staph.,
STRAM., **stront-c.**, **sul-ac.**,
sulph., tab., thuj., **verat.**,
verat-v.[11], verb., viol-o.[3], viol-t.,
visc.[9], zinc.

as if caged with wires twisted
tighter and tighter

CACT.

small areas, of[9]

hist.

internal

acon., aesc., agar., agn., **alum.,**
am-c., ambr., aml-ns., anac., ang.[3],
ant-c., ant-t., arg-m., **arn.,** ars.,
ars-i., asaf., **asar.,** aur., **bapt.,** bar-c.,
BELL., benz-ac., bism., bor., bov.,
brom., bry., bufo[3], **CACT., calad.,**
calc., camph., cann-i., cann-s.,
canth., caps., carb-an., carb-v.,
carbn-s., caust., **cham., chel.,**
CHIN., chlol., cic., cina, **clem.,**
cocc., coff., colch., **COLOC., con.,**
croc., crot-h., crot-t., cub., **cupr.,**
dig., dios., **dros.,** dulc., euph., ferr.,
glon., graph., guaj., hell., hep.,
hyos., **IGN., iod., ip.,** kali-c., kali-n.,
kreos., **lach., laur., led.,** lyc.,
mag-c., mag-m., **MAG-P.,** mang.,
meny., merc., merc-c., mez., **mosch.,**
mur-ac., **naja,** nat-ar., nat-c.,
NAT-M., NIT-AC., nux-m.,
NUX-V., olnd., op., ox-ac., par.,
petr., **ph-ac., phos., PLAT., PLB.,**
PULS., ran-s., rheum, rhod., rhus-t.,
ruta, sabad., **sabin.,** samb., **sars.,**
sec., sel., seneg., **sep.,** sil., **spig.,**
spong., **squil.,** stann., staph., still.,
STRAM., stront-c., **sul-ac., SULPH.,**
sumb., tab.[3], tarax., teucr., **thuj.,**
valer., **verat., verat-v.,** verb.,
viol-t., zinc.

bones, of

am-m., anac., aur., chin., cocc.,
coloc., con., graph., kreos., lyc.,

merc., nat-m., **NIT-AC.,** nux-v.,
petr., phos., **PULS.,** rhod., **rhus-t.,**
ruta, sabad., sep., sil., stront-c.,
SULPH., zinc.

glands, in[3]

ign., iod.

joints, of[3]

acon., am-m., **ANAC.,** apis[6], **AUR.,**
calc., carb-an., chin., coloc., ferr.,
GRAPH., kreos., lyc., meny.,
NAT-M., NIT-AC., nux-m., nux-v.,
petr., ruta, sil., spig., squil., stann.,
stront-c., sulph., zinc.

orifices, of; sphincter spasm

acon., alum., alum-sil.[1'], ars., ars-i.,
bar-c., **BELL., brom., CACT.,** calc.,
calc-sil.[1'], carb-v., **chel.,** cic., cocc.,
colch., con., crot-h., dig., dulc., ferr.,
form., graph., hep., **hyos.,** ign., iod.,
ip., **LACH., lyc., MERC., merc-c.,**
mez., **nat-m., NIT-AC., nux-v.,** op.,
phos., plat., **plb.,** rat., rhod.,
RHUS-T., sabad., sars., sep., **SIL.,**
staph., STRAM., sulph., sumb.,
tarax., **thuj., verat., verat-v.**

band, sensation of a

acon., **alum.,** alum-p.[1'], alumn.,
am-br., **ambr., ANAC.,** ant-c., ant-t.,
arg-n., arn., ars., ars-i.[1'], ars-s-f.[1'],
asaf., **asar.,** aur., aur-ar.[1'], aur-i.[1'],
aur-s.[1'], **bell.,** benz-ac., brom., bry.,
CACT., calc., cann-i., **CARB-AC.,**
carb-v., **carbn-s.,** caust., **CHEL.,**
chin., coc-c., **cocc.,** colch., coloc.,
CON., croc., dig., dios.[3], gels.,
graph., hell., hyos., iod., kreos.,
lach.[3], laur., lyc., mag-m., **mag-p.,**
manc., mang.[16], **merc., merc-i-r.,**
mosch., **nat-m.,** nat-n.[3], **NIT-AC.,**

nux-m., nux-v., olnd., op., ox-ac.[3], petr., **phos.**, pic-ac.[1'], **PLAT., PULS.**, rhus-t.[3], sabad., sabin., sang., sars., **sec.**[3], sep.[3], **SIL., spig.**, stann., **stram.**[3], sul-ac., sul-i.[1'], **SULPH.**, tarent., til., zinc., zinc-p.[1']

belt, sensation of a[6]

cact., chin., phos., rhus-t., visc.[9]

CONTRACTIONS, strictures, stenoses, after inflammation

acon.[2, 3], **agar.**, alum., **alumn.**[2], ant-c., arg-m., **arn.**[2, 3], **ars.**[2, 3], asaf., **bell., bry.**, calc., **camph.**, canth., caust., chel., **chin., CIC., clem., cocc.**, con., dig., dros., dulc., euph., guaj.[3], hyos.[2, 3], **ign.**[2, 3], lach., led., meny.[3], **MERC., mez.**, nat-m., nit-ac., **NUX-V.**, op.[2, 3], petr., **phos.**, plb., **psor., puls.**, ran-b., **RHUS-T.**, ruta, sabad., sep., **spong.**, squil., staph., stram., sulph., teucr., thuj., **verat.**[2, 3], zinc.

CONTRADICTORY
and alternating states

abrot.[7], **aloe**[7], ambr.[3], **carc.**[7], cimic.[3, 7], croc., **IGN.**, kali-c.[1'], **nat-m., plat.**[1], plb.[3], **PULS.**, sanic.[7], **sep.**[7], **staph.**[7], **thuj.**[1], **TUB.**[7]

alternating states

change-symptoms

metastasis

CONVALESCENCE, ailments during[3, 6]

ail.[7], **alet.**[2, 7], am-c.[1'], apoc.[1'], aur.[7], **aven.**, bac.[7], cadm-met.[14], **CALC.**[2, 7], **calc-p.**, caps.[1'], **cast.**[3, 6, 7, 10], **CHIN.**[3, 6, 7, 10], **chin-ar.**[3, 6, 7], coca[6, 7], cocc.[7], cupr.[7, 11], **cur.**[7], cypr.[7], **ferr.**[3, 6, 10], ferr-a.[6], gels.[3], guar.[7], **kali-c.**, kali-m.[1'], kali-p.[3, 7], laur.[1'], lob.[7], mang.[1'], med.[7], meph., **nat-m.**, nat-p.[7], okou.[14], op., ph-ac., phos.[3], prot.[14], psor.[1', 3, 6, 7], **scut.**[7], **sel.**[1', 3, 6], **sil.**[2, 7], sul-ac., sul-i.[10], **sulph.**[1', 3, 6, 10], syph.[1'], **TUB.**[7], tub-a.[7], zinc.[3, 6, 7]

reaction, lack-convalescence

weakness–fever

fever, ailments from[12]

lyc.

infectious diseases, ailments from[6]

form-ac., gels.[3], psor., puls., sulph. thuj., tub., vario.

metapneumonic[7]

calc., carb-v., **kali-c.**, lyc., phos., sang., sil., sulph.

never well since pneumonia[7]

kali-c.

meningitis, after[7]

calc., sil.

parturition, after[2]

graph.

postdiphtheric[7]

alet., cocain., cocc., fl-ac., **helon.**[2], **lac-c.**[2]

postinfluenzal[7]

abrot., cadm-met.[14], okou.[14], scut.[7, 12], sulfonam.[14], tub.

rheumatism after tonsillitis[3]

echi., guaj., lach., phyt.

typhoid, ailments from[1']

carb-v., pyrog.[12], sulph.

CONVULSIONS

absin., acet-ac., **acon.,** aconin.[12], aesc., aesc-g.[11], aeth., aether[11, 12], agar., agar-pa.[11], agar-se.[11], agre.[14], alco.[11], **alet.**[2, 12], alum., alum-p.[1'], alum-sil.[8], am-c., am-caust.[11], am-m.[6], ambr., **aml-ns.**[2, 6], amyg.[11], ang.[3, 4, 6], anis.[8], **ant-c., ant-t., anthraci.**[2], antip.[8], **apis, aran.,** arg-m.[6], **arg-n.,** arist-cl.[9], **arn., ars.**[1], **ars-s-f.**[1', 2], **ART-V.,** arum-m.[2], **asaf.,** aster., **ATRO.,** aur., aur-ar.[1'], aur-fu.[4], bar-c., **bar-m.,** bar-s.[1'], bart.[11], **BELL.,** ben-n.[2, 11, 12], bism.[4], both.[11], bov.[3], brom.[6], bruc.[4], **bry., BUFO,** buth-a.[9], cact., **CALC.,**

calc-i.[1'], **camph.,** cann-i., cann-s., **canth., carb-ac.,** carb-an.[4], carbn.[12], carbn-h.[11], **carbn-s.,** cast.[3, 8, 12], caul.[3], **CAUST., CHAM.,** chen-a., chin., **chlf.**[2, 8, 12], chlor.[12], **CIC.,** cic-m.[8, 11], **cimic.**[6], **CINA,** cit-ac.[4], clem., coca, coc-c., **cocc.,** cod.[11, 12], coff., colch., colchin.[12], coloc., **con.,** convo-s.[9], cop., cortico.[9, 10], cortiso.[9, 10], croc., **crot-c., crot-h.,** cryp.[11], cub., **CUPR., cupr-a.**[8, 11], **cupr-ar.,** cupr-s.[11], cur., **cypr.**[6, 12], cyt-l.[8, 9, 11, 12], dat-m.[11, 12], dat-s.[11], **dig., dios.**[3, 6], dor.[2], dulc., euon.[8, 12], **eupi.,** fagu.[11], ferr., ferr-ar., ferr-m.[4, 11], ferr-s.[12], form., frag.[12], **gels., glon.,** gran.[11], **graph.,** grat.[1'], guare.[11], **hell., hydr-ac., HYOS.,** hyper.[8], **ign.,** indg.[6], iod., **ip.,** iris-fl.[8, 12], jasm.[11, 12], jatr.[4], juni.[11, 12], **kali-br., kali-c., kali-chl.,** kali-cy.[11], kali-i., kali-m.[1'], kali-ox.[11, 12], kali-p.[6], kalm., keroso.[11, 12], lach., lact.[4, 11], lat-m.[9], laur., linu-c.[11], linu-u.[12], **LOB.,** lol.[11], lon-x.[8, 11, 12], **lyc., lyss mag-c.,** mag-m., **mag-p.,** mag-s.[9], manc., mand.[9], med.[3, 12], meli., meph., **merc., merc-c.,** merc-d.[11], merc-ns.[11], merc-p-r.[11], methyl.[12], mez.[6], mill.[3], morph.[8, 11, 12], **mosch., mur-ac.,** nat-f.[9], **nat-m.,** nat-s., **nicot.**[8, 12], nit-ac., nitro-o.[11], **NUX-M., NUX-V.,** oena., ol-an.[3, 4, 6], ol-j.[6], olnd., **OP.,** ox-ac., passi.[8, 12], petr., **phos., phyt.,** pic-ac.[6], pitu.[9], plat., **PLB.,** plb-chr.[8, 12], **podo.**[3, 6], psor., **puls.,** pyre-p.[12], ran-b.[6], ran-s., **rat.**[6], rauw.[9], rhus-t., ric.[11], rob., rumx-a.[11, 12], russ.[11, 12], ruta, sabad., sal-ac.[6], samb., **santin.**[8, 11, 12], scol.[12], **sec.,** sep., **sil.,** sin-n., sium[12], **sol-c.**[8, 19], **sol-n.,** spig., spirae.[19], squil., stann., staph., **STRAM.,** stront-c., stroph-h.[3], **STRY., stry-s.**[6], sul-ac.[6], sul-h.[12], sul-i.[1'], **sulph.,** tab., tanac.[4, 11], tax., **ter.,** thal.[14], thea, thuj.[6], thymol.[9, 14], **tub.**[7], **upa.**[8, 12], upa-a.[8], valer., **vario.**[2], **verat.,** verat-v., verb.[6], verbe.[8], vesp.[1'], vib.[3], vip., zinc., zinc-cy.[12], zinc-m.[11, 12], zinc-o.[8], zinc-p.[1'], **zinc-s.**[8, 12], zinc-val.[3, 6], zing.[2], ziz.

Vol. I: *anger, anxiety, cheerful, clinging, cursing, delirium, impatience, insanity, irritability, lamenting, laughing, moaning, morose, prostration, rage, restlessness, shrieking, striking, stupefaction, stupor, unconsciousness, weeping, wildness.*

Vol. III: *Menses-copious, painful, scanty. Metrorrhagia. Pollutions. Sleep-comatose, convulsions, disturbed, sleepiness, sleeplessness, yawning.*

one-sided

apoc., **art-v.**, bell., brom.[6], **calc-p.**, caust., chin-s.[4], cina[8], dulc., elaps, gels., graph., hell., **ip., plb.**

left side of body

bell.[4], **calc-p.**, chin-s.[4], colch.[11], cupr., elaps, graph., **ip.**, nat-m., nit-ac.[4], plb., sabad.[4], stram.[4], **sulph.**

to right[2, 16]

sulph.

paralyzed side

phos., sec.

paralysis of the other

apis, **art-v.**, bell., hell.[1], lach.[6], phos.[6], **stram.**

right side of body

bell., caust., chen-a.[1], **LYC.**, **nux-v.**, sep.[4, 16], tarent.[6]

left paralyzed

art-v.

to left

visc.

daytime[2]

art-v., kali-br.

morning

    arg-n., art-v., **calc., caust.,** cocc.,
crot-h., kalm., **lyc., mag-p.,**
nux-v., plat., sec., sep., sulph.,
tab.

4–16 h
calc.

5 h[11]
plb.

9–10 h
nat-m.[2], plb.[11]

afternoon

    arg-m., stann.

evening

    alum., **alumn.**[2], **CALC., caust.,**
croc., gels. graph.[4], kali-c.[4], laur.,
merc-ns., nit-ac.[4], **op.,** plb-chr.[11],
stann., stram., sulph.

air, in open

    caust.

20 h
ars.

21 h
lyss.

night

    arg-n., ars., **art-v.,** aur., bufo,
calc., calc-ar., **caust., cic., cina,**
cupr., dig., **hyos.,** kali-c., kalm.,
lach.[4], lyc., **merc., nit-ac.,** nux-v.,
oena., **OP., plb.,** sec., **SIL., stram.,**
sulph., zinc.

midnight

    bufo, cina, **cocc.,** santin., zinc.

after
    nit-ac.

3 h[2]
stram.

absences see Vol. I unconsciousness–
frequent

Addison's disease, in

    calc., iod.[2]

alternating with excitement of mind

    STRAM.

rage

    STRAM.

relaxation of muscular system[11]

    acet-ac.

rigidity[11]

    stry.

unconsciousness

    agar., aur.

amenorrhoe, in[2]

    art-v.

anger, after

bufo, **CHAM.**, cina, **CUPR.**[2], **kali-br.**, lyss., **NUX-V.**, op., plat., sulph.

epilepsy from[2]

art-v., **CALC.**

vexation

anxiety, from[6]

stram.

apoplectic

bell., crot-h., cupr., lach., nux-v., stram., **verat-v.**[2]

begin in the abdomen

aran., **bufo**

arm

arum-t.[2], **bell.**

left[7]

sil.

back

ars.[4], sulph.

calf muscles[16]

lyc.

face

absin., **bufo,** cina, dulc., **hyos., ign., lach.,** santin., **sec.**

left side

lach.

fingers[2]

cupr-a.

and toes

cupr., cupr-a.[2]

head

cic.

legs[2]

cupr-a.

toes[2]

cupr-a., hydr-ac.

bending elbow am.

nux-v.

head backwards, from

NUX-V.

biting, with

croc.[4], **cupr.**[2], lyss., **tarent.**[2]

bone in the throat, from

cic.

bright light, from

bell., **canth.**[2], lyss., nux-v., op., **STRAM.**

light agg.

cerebral softening

bufo[2], **caust.**

changing in character

bell., ign., **puls., STRAM.**

children, in

absin.[8], acon., **aeth.,** agar., agre.[14], **ambr., aml-ns.**[2], ant-t.[2, 4], **apis,** arn.[1', 2], ars.[2], **ART-V.,** asaf.[4], **BELL.,** bry., bufo[8], **calc., calc-p.**[1', 3, 6], **camph., camph-br.**[6, 8], canth.[4], caust., **cham., chlol.**[2, 8], **cic.,** cimic.[2], **CINA,** cocc., **coff.,** colch.[2], **crot-c.,** cupr., **cupr-a.**[2], cypr.[3, 6, 8], dol., **gels.,** glon.[8], **guare.**[2], **HELL., hep., hydr-ac., hyos., ign., ip., kali-br.**[2, 7, 8], kali-c., kali-p.[3, 6], kreos.[2, 8], **lach.,** laur., **lyc., mag-p.,** meli.[2,8], merc.[1', 2], mosch.[8], nux-m.[4], **nux-v.,** oena.[3, 6, 8], **OP.,** passi.[12], ph-ac.[6], phos.[6], plat., **santin.**[8], scut.[8], sec., **sil., stann.**[2, 3, 4, 6, 8], **STRAM.,** sulph., ter.[2], **VERAT.,** verat-v.[2], **ZINC.,** zinc-cy.[6], zinc-s.[8], **zinc-val.**[3, 6]

infants, in[2]

art-v., bell., bufo, **cham., cupr., HELL.**[1', 2], **hydr-ac., mag-p.,** meli.

newborns, in[2]

art-v., bell.[2, 4], **cupr.,** nux-v.[4]

strangers, from approach of

lyss., op., tarent.[6]

chill, during

ars., **camph.**[2], **lach.,** merc., nux-v.

climacteric period, during

glon.[6], **lach.**[2, 7]

clonic

acon., **AGAR.,** alum-p.[1'], am-c., am-m., ambr., anac., ang.[3], ant-c., ant-t., **anthraci.**[2], **arg-m.,** arg-n.[3], arn., **ars., art-v.,** asar.[1] (non: asaf.), aster., aur., **bar-c.,** bar-m., bar-s.[1'], **BELL.,** bor., bov.[3], brom.[6], **bry., BUFO, calc.,** calc-i.[1'], **calc-p.,** camph., cann-s., canth., carb-v., carbn-o., **carbn-s.,** caul.[3], **caust., CHAM.,** chin., **chin-s.,** chlf.[2], **CIC.,** cimic., **cina,** clem., cocc., coff., coloc., **con.,** croc., **CUPR.,** dig., dulc., graph., guaj., hell., hep., **HYOS., ign.,** iod., **ip.,** kali-ar., kali-bi.[3], **kali-c.,** kali-m.[1'], **kalm.,** kreos., lach., lat-m.[9], laur., **lyc., LYSS.,** mag-c., mag-m., **mag-p.,** mang., med.[12], meny., **merc., mez.,** mosch., mur-ac., mygal., nat-c., nat-f.[9], **nat-m.,** nit-ac., **nux-m.,** nux-v., **oena.**[3], ol-an.[3], olnd.[1], **OP.,** petr., ph-ac., phos., phys., **plat., PLB.,** podo.[3], puls., ran-b., ran-s., rheum, rhod., rhus-t., russ.[11], ruta, sabad., samb., sars., **sec.,** sel., seneg., **SEP., sil.,** spig., spong., squil., **stann.,** staph., **STRAM., stront-c.,** stry.[3], **stry-s.**[6], sul-ac., **sulph.,** tab.[3], tarent., tarax., teucr., thuj., thymol.[9], valer.[3], verat., verat-v., visc., **zinc.,** zinc-p.[1'], zinc-val.[3, 6]

alternating with tonic

bell.[1', 3, 6], **cimic.**[2], con.[3, 6], **ign.**[3, 6], **mosch.**[3, 6], nux-v.[6], plat.[3, 6], sep.[3, 6], stram., **tab.**[2], verat-v.[3, 6]

closing a door, on

stry.

noise

coition, during

bufo

after

agar.

cold air, from

ars., bell., **cic., indg.**[2], merc., **nux-v.**

drinks, from

caust.[4], cupr., lyc.[4]

water am.

caust., lyc.[4]

cold, becoming

bell., **caust.,** cic., **mosch.**[1], nux-v.

coldness of the body

anan.[1], bell.[8], **camph.,** caust., cic., **hell.,** hydr-ac.[6, 8], hyos., mosch., nicot.[8], **OENA.,** op., stram., **verat.**

feet, of

bell.[8], **cupr.**[2]

hands, of[2]

cupr.

head hot, feet cold[8]

bell.

of one side of body

sil.

colic, during

CIC.[2], cupr.[2], plb., sec.[2]

commotion of the brain, from[2]

ARN., CIC., **hyper.,** nat-s.

compression on spinal column

tarent.

congenital[2]

hell., **kali-br.,** verat.

consciousness, with

ang.[3], ars., aur-ar.[1'], bar-m.[1'], bell., calc., camph., **canth.,** caust., CINA, grat., **hell.,** hyos., **ign.**[3], ip., kali-ar., **kali-c.,** lyc., **mag-c.,** merc., mur-ac., **nat-m.,** nit-ac., **nux-m., nux-v., phos., plat.,** plb., sec., **sep.,** sil., **STRAM.,** stry., sulph.

without

absin., acet-ac., acon., **aeth.,**
agar.[2], agre.[14], aml-ns.[2], ant-t.,
ARG-N., ars., aster., aur., **bell.,**
BUFO, CALC., calc-ar., calc-p.[2],
calc-s., camph., CANTH.,
carb-ac., **caust.,** cham., chin.,
CIC., cina, **cocc.,** crot-h., **cupr.,**
cupr-a.[8], cupr-ar.[8], cur.[2], dig.,
ferr., glon., hydr-ac., **HYOS.,**
ign.[1',2,4], **ip., kali-c.,** lach.,
laur., led., lyc., merc., **mosch.,**
nat-m., nit-ac., nux-v., **OENA.,**
op., phos., **plat., PLB.,** sec., **sep.,**
sil., stann.[2,4], staph., **stram.,**
sulph., tanac., **tarent.,** verat.,
vesp.[1'], **VISC.**

contradiction, from

aster.

cough, during[2]

bell., **calc.,** ign., meph., stram.[2,11],
sulph.

after
cupr., ip., verat.[2]

whooping cough, in[2]

brom., calc., cupr.[2,8], hydr-ac.,
ip.[1',2], KALI-BR.[2,8]

croup, in[2]

lach.

cyanosis, with[2]

cupr., cupr-a.[8], **hydr-ac.[2,6,8],** verat.

delirium tremens, in
hyos.

dentition, during

acon., **aeth.,** art-v., arum-t.[z], **bell.,**
CALC., calc-p.[2], caust.[2], CHAM.,
cic., cina, coff.[3,6], colch.[2], cupr.,
cupr-a.[2], cypr.[2,6], gels.[3,6], hyos.,
ign., ip.[2], KALI-BR.[2,3,6], kreos.,
lach.[2], **mag-p.[1'-3,6,7], meli.[2],** merc.,
mill.[2], nux-m.[3,6], passi.[6], **podo.,**
rheum[3,6], sin-n.[2], **stann., stram.,**
sulph.[4], thyr.[14], **verat-v.[2,3,6],**
zinc.[2,3,6]

diarrhoea am.

lob.

downwards, spread

cic., sec.

draft agg.

ars., cic.[1'], **lyss., NUX-V., STRY.**

drawing-up of legs, alternately[9]

cyt-l.

drinking, after

ars., art-v.[2], bell., **hyos., stram.[3]**

water[15]

calc., canth.

drugs, after[2]

acon., **ARN.**

drunkards, in

anthraci.², glon., **hyos.², nux-v., ran-b.**

eating, while

  plb.

  after

    aster.², **calc-p.²,** cina, grat., hyos., nux-v.⁶

emission of semen, during

    art-v., grat., **nat-p.**

    from²
    lach.

epileptic

    absin., acet-ac., acon.³, **aeth., agar.,** agre.¹⁴, alco.¹¹, all-c.¹¹, **alum.,** alum-p.¹ʹ, alum-sil.¹ʹ, alumn.², **am-br.², ⁸, ¹²,** am-c., **ambr.²,** ambro.¹², **aml-ns.², ⁶, ⁸, ¹²,** amyg.¹², **anac., anag.², ¹²,** ang.³, anil.¹¹, anis.⁸, ant-c.³, ant-t.³, antip.¹², apis³, aran-ix.¹⁰, **ARG-M., ARG-N.,** arn.³, **ars., art-v.,** asaf.³, **aster., atro.², ⁸, ¹²,** aur.³, aur-br.⁸, ¹², aven.⁸, **bar-c., BAR-M.,** bar-s.¹ʹ, **bell.,** ben-n.¹², bism.⁶, bor.⁸, bry.³, **BUFO,** caj.², ¹², **calc., CALC-AR., calc-p., calc-s.,** calc-sil.¹ʹ, camph., cann-i., **canth., carb-an.,** carb-v., carbn-s., **cast.², cast-eq.², ¹²,** caste.¹⁴, caul.⁶, **CAUST., cedr., cham.³, ⁴,** chen-a.¹², **chin., chin-ar.², ¹²,** chin-s., **chlol.²,** chlorpr.¹⁴, **cic.,** cic-m.⁸, ¹¹, ¹², **cimic.², ⁸, ¹²,** cina, cinnm.², **cocc.,** coloc.³, **con.,** convo-s.⁹, ¹⁴, cori-r.¹¹, **crot-c., crot-h., CUPR.,**

cupr-a.², ⁸, ¹¹, cupr-ar., cur., cypr.², ¹², dat-m.¹², des-ac.¹⁴, dig., dros.², ³, ⁴, ¹², dulc.³, fago.¹¹, fagu.¹², ferr.³, **ferr-cy.⁸,** ferr-p.⁸, **form., gels., glon.,** graph.¹ʹ, **hell.,** hell-v.¹², hep.⁸, hydr-ac., **HYOS., hyper.², ictod.², ign., indg.,** iod., **ip.³,** irid.⁸, kali-ar.¹ʹ, kali-bi.¹ʹ, ², ¹², **kali-br.,** kali-c., **kali-chl., kali-cy.⁸, ¹¹, ¹²,** kali-m.¹ʹ, ⁸, ¹², **kali-p.², ⁸,** kali-s., kres.¹⁰, ¹⁴, **lach., laur.,** led.³, levo.¹⁴, lith-br.¹², lol.⁶, **lyc., lyss., mag-c., mag-p.,** mand.¹⁴, **med.,** meli.⁸, ¹², merc., methyl.⁸, mill.¹², mosch., mur-ac.³, naja, **nat-m.,** nat-s., nicot.¹², nit-ac., nitro-o.¹², nux-m., **nux-v., OENA.,** oest.⁸, onis.¹², onon.¹², **op.,** paeon.¹⁰, passi.⁶, ⁸, ¹², perh.¹⁴, petr.², ³, **ph-ac., phos.,** phys.¹⁰, ¹², picro.⁸, **plat., PLB.,** polyg-pe.¹², **psor., puls.,** ran-b., ran-s.³, ⁴, rauw.¹⁴, rhus-t.³, rib-ac.¹⁴, ruta³, **salam.⁶, ⁸,** santin.⁸, ¹², **sec.,** sep., **SIL.,** sin-n.², **sol-c.⁸, ¹²,** sol-n.⁴, spirae.⁸, ¹², **stann.,** staph., **stram., stry.,** sulfon.¹², **SULPH.,** sumb.⁸, ¹⁰, ¹², **syph.,** tab., tanac.¹², tarax.³, **tarent., ter.², ¹²,** thea¹¹, thiop.¹⁴, thuj.³, ¹², tub.⁸, valer.³, ⁸, verat., verat-v.⁶, verb.⁷, ⁸, verbe-h.¹², vip., **VISC., zinc.³, ⁶, ¹⁰,** zinc-cy.⁸, ¹², zinc-o.¹⁰, zinc-p.⁶, **zinc-val.⁶, ⁸, ¹², ziz.², ⁸, ¹¹, ¹²**

Vol. I: *anxiety, delusions, dementia, fear, indifference, laughing-spasmodic, prostration, rage, unconsciousness.*

Vol. III: *Masturbation-m.*
Menses-pale, scanty. Sleep-
restless.

aura/Aura
Vol. I: *absent–minded, anger,*
anxiety, confusion, delusions--
small, dullness, eccentricity,
excitement, foolish, forgetful ,
imbecility, irritability, lascivious,
laughing–spasmodic, sadness,
sighing, speech–unintelligible

Vol. II: *shock electric-like,*
epilepsy

shuddering

abdomen to head

indg.

absent[3]

ars., art-v.[3, 6], atro., bell., camph.,
canth., cham., cic., cupr., cupr-ar.,
dios., hydr-ac.[3, 6], lach.[3, 6], nat-s.,
oena.[3, 6], plb., podo., tarent.,
valer., zinc.[3, 6], zinc-val.[6, 8]

arms, in

bell.[6], calc., **calc-ar.**[1], **lach.,**
sulph.

left arm, in

calc-ar.[2, 7], cupr.[2, 6], **sil.**[2, 6, 8],
sulph.[6, 7]

forearms, in[7]

bell., calc., sulph.

auditory disturbances[3, 6, 8]

bell., calc.[8], cic.[3, 6], hyos.[3, 6],
sulph.

back, in[4]

ars., sulph.

and left arm[7]

calc-ar., sulph.

creeping down spine[2]

lach.

blind

cupr.

cold air over spine and body

    agar.

cold feet, with

    cina[6], lach.[2]

coldness, with[3]

    cina, sil., sep.[16]

between scapulae[16]

    sep.

running down spine

    ars.

    on left side

    sil.

confusion[2, 3, 6]

    lach.

congestion of blood to head[6]

    calc-ar., op., sulph.

descending[8]

    calc.

drawing in limbs

    ars.

---

in left chest[16]

    nit-ac.

ear noises[7]

    hyos.

epigastrium to uterus, legs[2, 7]

    CALC.

eructations[2, 6]

    lach.

expansion of body, sensation of

    arg-n.

eyes, sparks before

    hyos.

turned upwards to left

    bufo

face, chewing motion

    calc.

formication in[6]

    nux-v.

twitching[3]

    laur.

fear[2]

aml-ns., arg-n., cupr., nat-m.

fingers and toes, in[2]

cupr.

formication[3]

bell., calc., nit-ac., **nux-v.**

general nervous feeling

arg-n.. **nat-m.**

hand, in right[2]

❧ cupr.

hands to head, from[2]

sulph.

head, from[3]

caust., lach., stram., sulph.

trembling sensation

caust.

headache[2]

bell., calc., **calc-ar.,** cann-i.,
caust.[2, 6], cina[2, 16], **lach.**[2, 6], staph.,
zinc.

heart, from

CALC-AR., lach., naja, nat-m.[3],
op.[3], sulph.[3]

heat, flushes of

calc-ar.[7], indg.[8]

heel to occiput, right

stram.[1]

jerk in nape

bry.[2], bufo

knees, in

cupr., cupr-a.[7]

ascending[6, 8]

cupr.

legs, in[6]

lyc., plb.

right leg to abdomen, from[6]

lyc.

limbs, in[3]

bell.[3, 7], calc.[3, 7], cina, cupr.,
lyc.[3, 8], plb., sil., sulph.

left[3]

cupr., sil., sulph.

morose[6]

zinc., zinc-val.

mouse, running like a

ars.[6], aur.[6], **BELL., CALC.,** ign.,
nit-ac., sep.[6], **sil.,** stram.[6], **sulph.**

mouth wide open

bufo

nausea[2]

cupr., **sulph.**

numbness of brain

bufo, indg.[8]

palpitation

absin.[3, 6], ars., **calc., calc-ar.,**
cupr., ferr.[3], **lach.,** nat-m.[6]

pupils dilated

ARG-N., bufo

ravenous appetite

calc., HYOS.

perspiration scalp

caust., hell-v.[12]

restlessness

arg-n.[1'], bufo[2], caust.[3, 6]

sadness

art-v.[2], zinc.[6], zinc-val.[3]

shocks

ars., **laur.**

shoulders, pain between[3, 6, 8]

indg.

shrieking

CIC.[2, 3, 6], **cupr.**[2, 3, 6, 8],
hydr-ac.[6, 8], stram.[3, 6]

solar plexus, from

art-v., bell., **bufo**[1, 7], **calc.**[1, 7],
caust., CIC., cupr., **indg.,**
NUX-V., sil., SULPH.

to head

calc.[7], **sil.**[2]

speech, unintelligible[6]

bufo

stomach, in

art-v., bell., bism.[3, 6], bufo,
calc., calc-ar.[3], **caust.**[7], **CIC.,**
cupr., **HYOS.,** indg., **NUX-V.,**
sil., SULPH.

to head

CALC.

teeth, grinding of[2]

sulph.

throat, narrow sensation[3, 6]

lach.

tongue swelling[3, 6]

plb.

trembling

absin.[3, 6-8], arg-n.[7], aster.[8]

urging stool[7]

calc-ar.

uterus, in

bufo

to stomach

bufo

to throat

lach.

vertigo

ars., **calc-ar., caust., HYOS.,** indg.[3, 6], **lach., plb.,** sil.[3, 6], **sulph., tarent.,** visc.[3, 6]

visual disturbance

bell.[3, 6, 8], calc.[8], hyos.[3, 6], lach.[3], sulph.[6, 8]

voice, loss of

calc-ar.

vomiting

cupr., op.

warm air streaming up spine

ars.

waving sensation in brain

cimic.

ailments during e. attack

Vol. I: *delirium laughing-spasmodic*

shrieking weeping-c.

biting tongue

art-v., bufo, camph., **caust.,** cocc., **cupr., oena., op.,** sec., stram.[1'], tarent., valer.

eyes turned upwards to right[2]

hydr-ac.

downwards[4]

aeth.

face, bluish

absin.², agar.², atro.², **bell.²**,
cic., cina², ⁴, **CUPR., hyos.**,
ign.⁴, **ip.**, nux-v.², **oena., OP.²**,
phys., plb.², stry., **verat.²**

pale²

am-c., ars.², ⁴, bell., calc.,
caust., chin., cic.², ⁴, cina, **cupr.**,
ip., lach.², ⁴, mosch.⁴, nat-m.,
plb., puls., sil., stann.², ⁴, sulph.,
verat.

red

aeth.², ⁴, ⁸, **bell.²**, ⁴, bufo,
camph.², ⁴, caust.², **CIC.²**, ⁴,
cina², cit-ac.⁴, cocc.⁴, **cupr.²**,
GLON., ign.², ⁴, ip.², ⁴, lyc.², ⁴,
nux-v.², **oena., OP.**, stram.², ⁴
•

yellow

cic.², ⁴, plb.²

froth, foam from mouth

aeth.⁴, ⁸, agar., ars., **art-v.**,
aster.², bell., **bufo**, camph.,
canth., **caust., cham.**, cic.², ⁶, **cina**,
cocc., colch., **cupr.**, gels., **glon.**,
hydr-ac.⁶, **hyos.**, ign.², **ind.²**,
lach.², laur.², ⁴, lyc.², lyss., med.²,
oena., op., plb.², **sil.²**, ⁴, staph.,
stry., sulph., tax., vip.⁶

involuntary discharges²
•

cocc.

urination²

art-v., **BUFO, caust.**, cocc.,
cupr., **HYOS.**, lach.², nat-m.²,
nux-v., **oena., plb.**, stry., **zinc.**

pupils contracted²

cic., **op.**, phyt.

dilated²

aeth.⁴, ⁸, **bell.**, carb-ac., cic.,
cina, cocc., oena., plb., verat-v.

shrieking²

bufo, cedr., **CIC.²**, ³, ⁶, ⁸, crot-h.,
cupr.², ³, ⁶, ⁸, hydr-ac.⁶, ⁸, **HYOS.**,
ign., **ip., kali-bi.**, lach., **lyc.**,
nit-ac., **nux-v., oena.**, op., **sil.**,
stann., stram.², ³, ⁶, sulph.,
verat-v.

teeth, grinding of

bufo, HYOS., sulph. tarent.

throwing (body) backwards²

camph.

forwards²

cupr.

winking of eyes

kali-bi.

ailments after e. attack

Vol. I: *delirium, laughing–spasmodic, memory–loss, mildness, rage, speech–incoherent, unconsciousness.*

weakness-c

blind

sec.

ear noises

caust.

headache

calc.[2]**, caust.,** cina, cupr., kali-br.[15]

hiccough[8]

cic.

prostration[8]

aeth., **chin-ar.**[2, 8]**, cic.,** hydr-ac., sec., sil., **stry.,** sulph.

ravenous appetite[16]

calc.

restlessness[8]

cupr.

urine, copious

caust.[4]**, cupr.,** lach.[4]

vomiting

acon., **ars.,** bell.[8]**, calc.**[2]**,** colch., **cupr.,** glon.

epileptiform

absin.[2, 3, 6]**,** acon., aeth., **AGAR.,** alum., alum-sil.[1']**,** am-c., aml-ns.[2, 3, 6]**, anac.,** ant-c., ant-t., arg-m.[1]**, ARG-N.,** arn., **ars.,** art-v.[6]**,** asaf., aur., aur-ar.[1']**, BELL.,** bism.[3, 6]**,** bry., **bufo, CALC.,** calc-i.[1']**,** calc-p.[3, 6]**,** calc-s., **camph.,** canth., carbn-s., caul.[3, 6]**, CAUST.,** cedr., **cham.,** chin., **chin-ar.**[2]**,** chlorpr.[14]**, CIC., CINA, cocc.,** coloc., con., **convo-s.**[9, 14]**,** cortico.[9]**, CUPR.,** cur., dig., dros., dulc., ferr., ferr-ar., gal-ac.[7]**, gels., GLON.,** graph.[1']**,** hell., **hydr-ac.**[6]**, HYOS., hyper.,** hypoth.[14]**,** ign., indg.[3]**,** iod., **ip.,** kali-br., **kali-c.,** kali-i.[2]**,** kali-m.[1', 3, 6]**,** kali-s., **lach.,** laur., led., lob.[3, 6]**,** lol.[6]**, lyc.,** mag-c., mag-p.[3]**, med.,** merc., mosch., mur-ac., **nat-m., nit-ac., nux-m., nux-v.,** oena., op., passi.[6]**,** petr., ph-ac., phos., **phys.**[2]**, plat., PLB.,** prot.[14]**, psor., puls., ran-b.,** ran-s., rauw.[14]**,** rhus-t., ruta, salam.[6]**, sec., sep., sil.,** stann., staph., **STRAM.,** stry., sul-i.[1']**, SULPH.,** tarax., **tarent.,** teucr., thuj., valer., verat., verat-v., verb.[3]**,** verbe-h.[6]**,** vip.[3, 6]**, VISC.,** zinc., zinc-cy.[12]**,** zinc-p.[1', 3, 6]**, zinc-val.**[3, 6]

errors in diet

cic.

eructations am.

kali-c.

eruptions fail to break out, when

ant-t., CUPR., ZINC.

exanthemata repelled or do not
appear, when

ant-t., apis[1, 8], ars.[8], bry., **camph.,
cupr., cupr-a.[2], gels., hep.[2], ip., op.[8],
stram., sulph., ZINC.,** zinc-s.[8]

excitement, from

acon., **agar.,** art-v.[6], **aster., bell.,**
cann-i.[11], **cham.,** cic., cimic., **coff.,
cupr., gels., HYOS., ign., kali-br.,
nux-v., OP.,** plat., **puls.,** sec.,
tarent., **zinc.[2]**

nervousness

religious[2]

verat.

exertion, after

alum., alumn.[2], **calc., glon.,** kalm.,
lach., lyss., nat-m., petr., sulph.

extension of body am., forcible

nux-v., stry.

extensor muscles

CINA

eyelids, while touching

coc-c.

falling, with

agar., alum., alum-p.[1'], am-c.,
ars., aster., BELL., bufo[1'], **calc.,**
calc-i.[1'], **calc-p.,** camph.[4], canth.,
caust., cedr., CHAM., chin-ar.[2],
cic., cina, cocc., **con., CUPR.,**
dig., dulc., **HYOS.,** ign., **iod.[1],** ip.,
lach.[4], laur., lyc., lyss.[2], merc.,
nit-ac., **OENA.,** op., petr., ph-ac.,
phos., plb., sec., sep., sil., **stann.,**
staph., **stram.,** sulph., verat., zinc.

backwards

ang.[2], **bell.,** camph.[2], canth., chin.,
cic., cic-m.[11], **ign., ip.,** kalm.[2],
nux-v., **oena., OP.,** rhus-t., spig.,
stram.

forward

arn., **aster.,** calc-p., canth., cic.,
cupr., ferr., rhus-t., sil., sulph.,
sumb.

left side

bell., caust., lach., sabad., sulph.[7]

right side

bell.

runs in a circle to

caust.

sideways[2]

bell., **calc.**, con., nux-v., sulph.

fear, from[6]

acon., arg-n.[7], **CALC.**[2, 7], **caust.**,
cupr.[6, 7], glon., kali-p., **op.**, sil.

fingers, spread[7]

sec.

fluids, from

bell., canth., hyos., **LYSS., STRAM.**

forcible aroused from a trance, when

nux-m.

fright, from

acon., agar., apis, **arg-n., art-v.,**
bell.[6, 7], **bufo, CALC., caust.,** cic.,
cina[6], **cupr., gels.**[2, 7], glon.[6],
HYOS., IGN., INDG., kali-br.,
kali-p.[2], laur.[7], lyss., nat-m.[7], **OP.,**
plat., sec., sil.[7], **stram.,** sulph.,
tarent., verat., **zinc.**

of the mother (infant)

bufo[2], **OP.**

grief, after

ars.[2, 7], art-v., **hyos.,** ign., indg.[7],
nat-m., nux-v.[5], **op.,**

haemorrhage, with

chin., hyos., ip.[15], **plat., sec.**

after[3]
ars., bell., calc., cina, con., ign.,
lyc., nux-v., puls., sulph., verat.

heat, during the

ars.[3], **bell.**[2, 3], camph.[3], carb-v.[3],
caust.[2], **cic., cina,** cur., **ferr-p.**[2],
hyos., ign.[2], **nat-m.**[2], **NUX-V.,** op.,
sep.[3], **STRAM.,** verat.[3]

hydrocephaly with[2]

arg-n., art-v., calc., kali-i., merc.,
nat-m., stram., sulph., zinc.

hydrophobia with[2]

bell., canth., cur., gels., stram.

hypochondriasis with[8]

mosch., stann.

hysterical

absin., acet-ac.[2], acon.[4, 11], **alum.,**
alum-p.[1'], ambr.[3, 6], **apis,** ars.,
ASAF., asar.[2, 3, 6, 8], **aur.,** aur-ar.[1'],
aur-s.[1'], **bell., bry., calc.,** calc-s.,
cann-i.[2], cann-s., cast.[8], caul.[2, 6, 8],
caust., cedr., cham., chlf.[2], **cic.,**
cimic., cocc., coff., coll., CON.,
croc., cupr.[1', 7, 8], dig.[3], **gels.,**
graph.[1'], hydr-ac.[2, 8], hyos., **IGN.,**
iod., ip., kali-ar.[1'], kali-p.[3, 6, 8],

lach., lact.[4], **lil-t.**[3, 6], lyc.,
mag-c.[3, 6], **mag-m.**, meph.[3, 6],
merc., **mill.**[2], **MOSCH.**, nat-m.,
nit-ac., **nux-m.**, nux-v., oena.[6, 8],
op., petr., phos., **plat.**, plb., puls.,
ruta[3], sec., **sep., sol-c.**[8],
stann.[3, 4, 8], staph., **stram.**, sul-i.[1'],
sulph., sumb., tarent., thyr.[12],
valer., **verat., verat-v.**, visc.[3],
zinc., zinc-p.[1'], **zinc-val.**[3, 6, 8, 12]

before menses[6]

hyos., ign., lach.

indigestion, from

IP.

indignation, from

staph.

injuries, from

ang.[2], arn., art-v., **cic.**, con.[8],
cupr.[8, 10], cupr-a.[10], **HYPER.,**
meli.[8], **nat-s., op.**, oena., puls.[2],
rhus-t., sil.[10], sulph., **valer.**

head, of the[2]

ARN., CIC., cupr., hyper., led.,
meli.[7], nat-s.

commotion

intermittent

absin.

internal

acon., agar., alum.[3], am-c., ambr.,
anac., ang.[3], ant-c.[3], ant-t.[3], arg-m.,

arn., ars., **asaf.**, asar.[3], bar-c.[3], **bell.,**
bism., bor.[3], bov., **bry.**, calad., **calc.,**
camph., canth., caps., carb-an.[3],
carb-v., CAUST., cham., cina,
COCC., coff., colch., coloc., con.,
cupr., dig., dulc.[3], euph.[3], **ferr.,**
graph., hep.[3], **HYOS., IGN.**, iod.,
ip., kali-c., kali-m.[1'], kali-n.[3], kreos.,
lach.,laur., led., **lyc.**, mag-c.,
mag-m., merc.[3], **mosch.**, mur-ac.,
nat-c., nat-m., nit-ac., nux-m.,
NUX-V., op., petr., ph-ac., **phos.,**
plat., plb., **PULS.**, rhod., rhus-t.[3],
sabad., sars.[3], **sec.**, seneg., **sep.**, sil.,
spong., **STANN., staph.**, stram.,
stront-c., sul-ac., sulph., teucr.,
thuj., valer., verat., **zinc.**, zinc-p.[1']

interrupted by painful shocks

stry.

isolated groups of muscles, of[8]

acon., **cic.**, cina, cupr., ign., nux-v.,
stram., stry.

jealousy, from[2, 8]

lach.

labor see parturition

laughing, from[2]

coff., cupr.

with
coff., graph.

leucorrhoea, with[2]

caust., lach.

light agg.

> bell., LYSS., op., nux-v., STRAM.
>
> *bright light*

love, from disappointed

> hyos., ign.[1']

lying on side, on

> puls.
>
> convulsively turned on the back

> cic.
>
> on abdomen with spasmodic jerking of pelvis upward[16]

> cupr.

masturbation, from

> bufo, calad., **calc.,** dig., elaps, kali-br., **lach.,** naja, nux-v., **PLAT.,** plb., sep., sil., stram., **sulph.**

meningitis, in cerebrospinal[2]

> ant-t., apis, arg-n., crot-h., glon., hell., tarent., verat.

menses, before

> bell.[2], brom.[2], **bufo,** carb-v., caul.[6], **caust.,** cimic.[2], **cupr.,** hyos., kali-br., mag-c.[6], mag-m.[6], oena., plat.[2], **puls.,** sulph.[2]

during

> apis, **arg-n., art-v.**[2], **bell.,** bufo[1', 7], **caul.,** caust., **cedr., cimic., cocc., coll., cupr.,** gels., glon.[3, 6], **hyos., ign., kali-br.,** kali-m.[6], **lach.**[1, 7], mosch.[6], **nat-m.,** nux-m., **nux-v., OENA.,** phys., **plat.,** plb., **puls., sec.,** stram., **sulph.,** tarent., **zinc.**

after

> kali-br.[7], syph.

instead of

> oena.

suppressed, from

> bufo, calc-p., cocc., cupr., **gels.,** mill.[2, 8, 15], **puls.**

mental exertion, after

> bell., cann-i.[11], **glon.**

mercurial vapors, from

> stram.

metastasis

> cupr.

mirror, from a[10]

> lyss.

miscarriage, after

> ruta

moon, at full[2, 6-8]

    CALC., caust.[6]**, nat-m.**[2]

   new m., at[2, 7, 8]

    bufo[2, 7]**, caust.**[2, 6, 8]**, cupr., kali-br., sil.**[2, 4, 6, 8, 11]

mortification, from

    calc., cham.[1']**, staph.**[2]

motion agg.

   ars., bell., **cocc.,** graph., **nux-v., stry.**

nervousness, from

   arg-n.

  excitement

newborns see children

noise, from

   ang.[4]**,** ant-c., arn., **cic.,** ign., **lyss., mag-p.**[2]**,** nux-v., stry.

   arrests the paroxysm

    hell.

odors, from strong

   bruc.[4]**, lyss.** (non[1]: sil., stram., sulph.)

old age, in[10]

   plb.

pain, during

   ars.[11]**, bell.,** coloc., ign., kali-c., lyc., nux-v., plb-chr.[11]

   renewed at every[2]

    bell.

palpitation, after

   glon.

paralysis, with

   arg-n., bell., **CAUST.,** cic., cocc., cupr., **hyos.,** lach., laur., **nux-m., nux-v., phos.,** plat., **plb., rhus-t.,** sec., **stann., tab.,** vib., zinc.

  followed by see paralysis–convulsions

paresis, followed by[8]

   acon., **elaps,** lon-x., plb.

parturition, during[8]

   acon.[4, 8]**,** aeth., aml-ns., arn., **bell.**[3, 4, 8]**, canth.,** cham.[3, 4, 8]**, chin.**[1'], chin-s.[3, 15]**,** chlf.[2]**, chlol., CIC.**[2, 3, 8], cimic.[3, 8, 15]**,** cinnm.[2]**,** cocc.[3]**,** coff.[2, 4, 8]**, cupr.**[2, 7, 8]**, cupr-ar.,** gels., glon., **hydr-ac.**[8, 12], **HYOS.**[2, 3, 7, 8, 15]**, IGN.**[3, 4, 8], ip.[3, 4, 8]**, KALI-BR.**[2, 8]**,** merc., merc-d., mosch.[3]**, oena.,** op., pilo., **plat.**[2, 3, 4, 8]**, sec.**[1', 6]**,** sol-n., spirae., stram.[3, 8]**, VERAT-V.**[3, 8], **zinc.,** ziz.[2, 8]

after[2]

cupr.[7], **mill., plat.**

periodic

agar., ars., bar-m., calc., **cedr.,**
chin.[2], chin-s., cupr., ign., indg.,
lach.[2], lyc., nat-m., nux-v.[2], plb.[2],
sec., stram., vip[3]

every 5 or 6 days[2]

lyc.

7 days
agar., chin-s., **indg., kali-br.[2],**
nat-m.

10 days[2]
kali-br.

14 days
cupr., **kali-br.[2],** oena.

15 or 20 days[2]
tarent.

21 days[2]
camph.[1'], **cupr.[2], ferr.,** stram.,
cupr., op.

perspiration during

ars., **bell., BUFO,** camph.,
nux-v., op., sep.

cold

camph.[1'], **cupr.[2], ferr.,** stram.,
verat.[2]

after
acon., ars., **pry.[2],** cedr., cupr.,
sec., stry.

pregnancy, during

acon.[8,] aeth.[8], aml-ns.[8], arn.[8],
bell.[2, 3, 4, 8], canth.[3, 8], cast.[12], **cedr.,**
cham., chlol.[3, 8], cic., cimic.[3, 8],
cina[4, 11], coff.[8], croc.[3], **cupr.,**
cupr-ar.[3, 8], gels.[2, 3, 8], glon[6, 8],
hell.[3], **hydr-ac.[8], hyos.,** ign.[3, 8],
ip.[1', 2, 8], kali-br.[8], lyc., lyss.[8, 12],
mag-c.[6], mag-m.[6], merc-c.[8], merc-d.[8],
mill., mosch.[4], nux-m.[4], **oena.[2, 3, 8],**
op.[3, 8], pilo.[8], pitu.[9], plat.[3, 4, 8],
rhus-t.[2], sec.[3], sol-n.[8], spirae.[8],
stram.[3 4, 8], stry.[3], **verat-v.[2, 3, 8],**
zinc.[3, 8]

pressure on a part, from

cic.

on spine

tarent.

on stomach

canth., cupr., cupr-a.[11], nux-v.

puberty, at

caul.[2, 6], caust., cupr.[1', 6], hypoth.[14],
lach.[3], puls.[3, 6], zinc.[6], zinc-val.[3, 6]

puerperal

acon.[2], ambr., **ant-c.[2],** ant-t.[2, 15],
apis, **arg-n.,** arn.[2], ars., art-v.,
atro.[2], BELL., benz-ac.[2], **CALC.[3],**
canth., carb-v., caul.[8], caust.,
cham., chin.[3], chin-s.[2, 12], chlf.[2, 12],
chlol.[2, 12], **CIC.,** cimic., cinnm.[2],
cocc., coff., crot-c., **crot-h.[2], cupr.,**
gels., glon., hell., helon.[2],
hydr-ac., **HYOS., ign., ip., jab.[2],**
KALI-BR.[2], KALI-C.[2, 3], kali-p.[2],
lach., laur., lyc., lyss., mag-p.,

merc.[2], merc-c., mill.[2, 12], mosch.,
nat-m.[2], nux-m., nux-v., oena.,
op., ph-ac.[2, 3, 12], phos.[1], pilo.[12],
plat., puls., sec., sol-n.[12],
STRAM., sulph.[3], ter., thyr.[12],
verat., verat-v., zinc.

blindness, with

aur-m., cocc., cupr.

haemorrhage, with

chin., hyos., plat., sec.,

perspiration and fear, with[7]

stram.

shrieking, with

hyos., iod., lach.[2]

punishment, after

agar.[1', 7], cham., cina, cupr.[7], IGN.

reproaches, from

agar.[1' 6], ign.[6]

riding in a carriage am.

nit-ac.

rubbing am.

phos., sec., stry.[7]

running, after

sulph.

sexual excesses, from[2]

bufo[2], kali-br., phos.

excitement

art-v.[8], bar-c.[3], bufo, calc.[3, 8],
KALI-BR.[2], lach., plat., stann.[8],
sulph.[8], visc.[3]

shining objects, from

bell., LYSS., STRAM.

bright light

shock, after

aesc.[1'], op.

shrieking, with[2]

acon.[4], aml-ns., ant-t.[4], apis, art-v.,
bell.[4], calc.[4, 6], camph., canth.[4],·
caust.[2, 4], cedr., cic.[2, 4, 6], cina[2, 4],
crot-h.[2, 4], cupr., HYOS.[1', 2, 4], ign.,
ip.[2, 4], lach.[2, 4], lyc.[4], merc.[2, 4],
nux-v.[2, 4], nit-ac., oena.[6], OP.[2, 4, 6, 11],
stann., stram., sulph.[2, 4], verat-v.,
vip.[4], zinc.

sleep, during

arg-n.[6], bell.[2, 6], bufo, calc.[4],
caust., cham.[6], cic., cina[4], cocc.[6],
cupr., cupr-ar.[6], gels.[2], hyos.,
ign., kali-c., lach., mag-c.[4, 6],
merc.[4], oena., op., puls.[4, 6],
rheum[2], rhus-t.[4, 6], sec., sil.,
stram., tarent.[3, 6]

loss of, after

COCC.[1]

on going to[6]

arg-m., sulph.

sleeplessness, with or after[3]

alum., art-v.[2], bell., bry., calc.,
carb.-an., carb-v., **cic.**[2], cupr.,
cypr.[2], hep., hyos.[3, 4], ign., ip.,
KALI-BR.[2], kali-c., merc., mosch.,
nux-v., passi.[6], ph-ac., phos., puls.,
rheum, rhus-t., sel., sep., sil.,
stront-c., thuj., verbe-h.[6], zinc.[6],
zinc-val.[6]

small pox fails to break out, when

ANT-T.

speak, on attempting to

lyss.

strange person, sight of

lyss., op., tarent.[6]

stretching out parts am.

sec.

of limbs before c.

calc.

during c.[16]

bell.

sudden

ars.[6], **bell.**[2, 8], hydr-ac.[6], mez.[6],
oena.[6], stry., **verat-v.**[2]

suppressed discharges, from

asaf., cupr., stram.

eruption

agar., ant-c.[2], bry., calc., camph.[2],
caust., cupr., cupr-a.[2], hyos.[2],
ip.[2], kali-m.[2], psor.[8], **stram.**,
sulph., urt-u.[2], zinc.

footsweat, after

SIL.

mother milk

agar.

perspiration[6]

sil.

secretions and excretions

stram.

suppuration, during

ars., **bufo,** canth., lach., **tarent.**

swallow, during attempt to

LYSS., mur-ac., nux-m., nux-v.[11],
stram.

swing, letting legs, exites c.

calc.

syphilitic

aur.², iod.², **kali-br.²·⁸, KALI-I.²,**
merc-c², mez.², **nit-ac.**

tetanic rigidity

abel.¹⁴, absin., acet-ac.¹¹, **acon.,**
aconin.¹², aesc., agar-ph.¹¹, agre.¹⁴,
alum., **am-c.,** am-m.³, **aml-ns.²,**
amyg.²·¹¹·¹², **anac.,** ang.²·³·⁴·⁶·¹²,
ant-t.², aran-ix.¹⁴, **arn., ars.,** asaf.,
atro.²·¹², bell., ben-n.¹¹·¹², both.¹¹,
bruc.⁴, bry.³·⁴, **calc.**³·⁶·⁷·¹⁰,
calc-f.¹⁴, calc-p.³·⁶, **calen.⁶·¹²,**
camph., cann-i., cann-s., **canth.,**
carbn.¹², carbn-h.¹², carbn-o.,
carbn-s.¹², **cast.²·¹²,** caust., **cham.,**
chin-s., chlf.¹², **chlol., CIC.,**
cic-m.¹², cimic.³, cina³, **cocc.,**
con., cori-m.¹¹, cortico.⁹,
crot-h.²·¹², **cupr.,** cupr-a.¹⁰
cupr-ar., **cur.,** dig.³·⁶, dros.,
dulc.¹¹, **gels.,** grat.⁴·¹², **hell.,**
hep., **hydr-ac., hyos., HYPER.,**
ign., ip., jasm.¹¹·¹², juni.¹²,
kali-bi.¹¹, **kali-br.²·¹²,** kali-c.³,
kali-cy.¹¹, kali-n.¹¹, kreos.,
kres.¹⁰, **lach., laur.,** led., linu-c.¹¹,
lob., lyc., lyss., mag-c.³·¹⁰,
mag-m.¹⁴, **mag-p.,** meph.¹⁴,
merc., methys.¹⁴, **mill.²·¹²,**
morph.¹¹·¹², **mosch.,** mur-ac.,
nat-f.¹⁴, nicot.¹², nux-m.³,
NUX-V., oena., ol-an.³, **OP.,**
ox-ac.¹², passi.⁸·¹², **PETR.,** phos.,
phys., phyt., PLAT., plb., puls.,
pyre-p.⁷, rhod., **rhus-t¹,** santin¹²,
scor.¹¹·¹², **sec.,** seneg., **SEP.,**
sium¹², sol-c.¹², **sol-n.,** solin¹²,
stann.³·⁶, **stram., stry.,** stry-p.⁶,
sul-ac.¹¹, sul-h.¹², sulph., tab.¹²,
tanac.¹¹, **ter.²·¹²,** teucr., **ther.,**
thyr.¹², upa.⁷·⁸·¹², valer.³, verat.,
verat-v., verin.¹², vib-p.¹², zinc.

dashing cold water on face am.

ben-n.

injured parts become cold as ice
and spasms begin in the wound

LED.

traumatic²

acon., **arn.²·⁷, chlol.,** cic., cur.,
hell., hydr-ac., **HYPER.,** nux-v.,
stram.⁷, tetox.⁷, teucr.¹²

trismus, with²

ant-t., bell., cupr-a., oena., stram.,
verat-v.

wiping perspiration from face agg.

nux-v.

wounds in the soles, finger or
palm

bell., HYPER., led.

thunderstorm

agar., **gels.**

tight grasp am.

nux-v.

tightly binding the body am.

mez.

tonic

acon., agar., alum., alum-p.[1'],
alum-sil.[1'], am-c., am-m., ambr.[3, 6],
anac., **ANG.**[3, 6], ant-t., apis, arg-m.,
arn., ars.[3], asaf., asar., **BELL.**, bor.,
bry., **BUFO, calc.**, camph., cann-s.,
canth., caps., carbn-o., **caust.**,
cham., chin., chlf.[2], **CIC.**, cina, clem.,
cocc., coloc., con., cupr., **cur.**[3, 6],
cycl., dig., **dros.**[3], dulc., euph., **ferr.**,
ferr-ar., graph., guaj., hell.[3],
hep., hydr-ac.[2], hyos., **hyper.**[3, 6],
ign., ip., kali-c., lath.[6], laur., led.,
lyc., mag-p., mang., med.[2], meny.,
merc., mez., **mosch.**, nat-c., nat-m.,
nit-ac., nux-v., olnd., op., **PETR.**,
ph-ac., **phos., phys.**[3, 6], phyt.[3, 6],
PLAT., plb., puls., rhod., rhus-t.,
sabad., sars., **sec.**, seneg., **SEP.**, sil.,
spig., spong., stann., **stram.**, stry.[3],
stry-s.[6], sumb., **sulph.**, tab.[3, 6], thuj.,
verat., verat-v.[6], visc.[9], zinc.,
zinc-p.[1']

tooth extraction, after[7]

bufo

touched, when

acon., **bell., carbn-o., CIC.**, cocc.,
lyss., mag-p.[2], nux-v., stram., stry.

turning the head

cic.

in bed[11]

chen-a.

unjustly accused, after being

staph.[1, 7]

mortification

uraemic

apis[3], apoc., ars.[3], **carb-ac.**[8], chlf.[15],
cic.[8], crot-h., **cupr.**, cupr-ar., **dig.**,
glon.[8], hell.[8], hydr-ac., **KALI-BR.**[2, 8],
kali-s., merc-c., **mosch.**, oena.[8],
op.[8], pilo.[8, 12], **plb.**, stram.[7], **ter.**,
urt-u.[8, 12], **verat-v.**[3]

vaccination, after

SIL., thuj.[8]

vexation, after

agar.[6], ars., bell., calc., camph.,
cham.[6], **CUPR., ign., ip.**, nux-v.,
staph.[1, 7], sulph., verat.[6], zinc.[6]

anger

vomiting, during

aeth.[6, 8], **ant-c.**[2], **CUPR.**[2], guar.,
ip.[2], oena.[2], op., upa.[8]

am.
agar.

waking, on

bell., lyss.[2], **ign.**[2]

warm bath agg.

    apis, glon., nat-m., op.

warm room, in[1']

    op.

water, at sight of

    bell., **LYSS., STRAM.**

waving of arms[9]

    cyt-l.

weakness, during

    hura[11], kali-c.[6]

    weakness-c

    nervous

        sep.

wet, from becoming

    calc., **cupr.,** rhus-t.

worms, from

    art-v.[2], asaf.[4], bar-m.[2], **bell.**[2], **cham.**[2], **cic.**[2, 8], **CINA,** cupr.[6], cupr-o.[6], **hyos., ign.,** indg.[2, 6, 8], kali-br.[6, 8], sabad., **santin.**[8], sil., spig.[8], **stann.,** stram.[2], sulph.[8], tanac.[8], **ter.,** teucr.[8]

yawning

    graph.

CONVULSIVE movements

    acon., **agar., alum.,** alum-p.[1'], ang.[3], ant-t., apis, **arg-n.,** arn., ars., ars-i., **asaf.,** bar-c., bar-i.[1'], **BELL.,** brom.[3], bry., **bufo,** cact., **calc.,** calc-i.[1'], **camph.,** cann-s., **canth., caust., CHAM.,** chin-s., **CIC.,** cina, **COCC.,** coff., **con.,** croc., **CUPR.,** cupr-ar., dig., dulc., **hell., HYOS., IGN., iod., IP.,** kali-ar., lach., laur., lyc., m-arct.[3], **mag-p.,** meny., merc., mosch., **mygal.,** nat-c., nux-m., **nux-v.,** olnd., **OP.,** phyt.[3], **plb.,** petr., ph-ac., phos., plat., ran-b.[3], ran-s., **rheum,** rhus-t., **ruta,** sabad., samb., **SEC.,** spig., spong., **squil., stann.,** staph., **STRAM.,** sulph., tab.[3], **tarent., verat., zinc.**

beginning in extremities[3]

    verat.

    face[3]

    dulc.

COPPER fumes agg.

    camph., **ip.,** lyc., **merc.,** nux-v. op. **puls.**

vessels of, agg.[7]

    hep.

CORYZA am. general symptoms[3, 7]

    thuj.

suppressed c. agg.[3]

acon.[2], am-c., **am-m.**, ambr., ars., **BRY.**, calad., **CALC.**, carb-v., caust., cham., **chin.**[3, 12], cina, con., **dulc.**[3, 6], **fl-ac.**, graph., hep., ip., **kali-bi.**[3, 6], kali-c., kreos., **LACH.**[2, 3, 6], laur., lyc., mag-c., mag-m., mang., merc., mill.[6], nat-c., nat-m., **nit-ac.**, nux-m., **NUX-V.**, par., petr., phos., **puls.**, rhod., sabad., samb., sars., **sep.**, **sil.**, spig., spong., stann., stram., sul-ac., sulph.[3, 6], teucr., thuj., verat., zinc.

COVERS agg., intolerance of [3, 6]

acon., aloe, **apis**, asar., **camph.**, **cham.**, ferr., ign.[3], **iod.**, kali-i., led., med.[7], merc.[16], mur-ac., op., phos., **puls.**, rhus-t., **sec.**, **sulph.**, tab.[3], verat.

clothing-intolerance

warm-wraps

am. and desire for[3, 6]

ars., aur., bell.[6], clem., colch., **hep.**, **nux-v.**, **puls.**, rhus-t., **samb.**, sil., **squil.**, **stront-c.**, tub.[3]

aversion to[3]

calc-s., camph., led., sec.

kicks off[6]

BRY.[7], camph., **cham.**, iod.

in coldest weather[7]

hep., sanic., sulph.

CRAMPS of muscles (1897)

acon., agar., alum., am-c., am-m., **ambr.**, **ANAC.**, **ANG.**[3], arg-m., **arn.**, ars., asaf., asar., aur., bar-c., **BELL.**, bism., bor., bov.[3], bry., bufo[3], **CALC.**, camph., **cann-s.**, caps., carb-an., carb-v., carbn-s.[11], **cast.**[2], **caust.**, cham., chin., cic., cimic.[3, 6], **CINA**, clem., **cocc.**, colch., **coloc.**, **con.**, croc., cupr., dig., dios., dros., **dulc.**, euph., **euphr.**, ferr., gels., **glon.**, **graph.**, hell., hep., hyos., **ign.**, iod., ip., **iris**[2], jab., **kali-br.**[2], **kali-c.**, kali-n., kreos., lach., **LYC.**, mag-c., mag-m., **mag-p.**[3, 6], mang., meny., **MERC.**, mez., mosch., **mur-ac.**, nat-c., nat-m., **nit-ac.**, nux-m., nux-v., olnd., **op.**[2, 3, 6], par., petr., ph-ac., phos., **phyt.**[3, 6], **plat., plb.**, puls.[3, 6], ran-b., rheum[3], rhod., **rhus-t.**, ruta, sabad., samb., sang.[3], **sec.**, **SEP.**, **SIL.**, spig., **spong.**, squil., **stann.**, staph., stram., stront-c., sul-ac., **SULPH.**, tab.[2, 3, 6], **thuj.**, **valer.**, verat., **verb.**, vib., viol-o., viol-t., zinc.

night on waking[16]

sulph.

CROSSING of limbs agg.[3]

agar., alum., ang., arn., **asaf.**, aur., bell., bry., **dig.**, kali-n., laur., lyc., mur-ac., nux-v., phos., plat., rad., rheum, rhod., **rhus-t.**, squil., valer., verb.

am.[3]
abrot., ant-t., rhod., **SEP.**

CYANOSIS

absin.[11], acetan.[12], acon., agar.,
alum., **am-c.**, amyg.[11], ang.[3], anil.[11],
ant-ar.[6], ant-c., **ant-t.**, **arg-n.**, arn.,
ars., asaf., asar., aur., bar-c., **bell.**,
ben-n.[11, 12], bism., both.[11], bry.,
calc., calc-p.[3], **CAMPH.**, canth.[3],
carb-an., **CARB-V.**, carbn-o.[11,]
caust., cedr., cham., chel., chin.,
chin-ar., cic., cina, cocc., cod.[11],
con., crot-h[6], **CUPR.**, cupr-ar.[6],
DIG., dros., ferr., glon.[3, 11], hep.,
hydr.-ac.[6, 11], hyos., ign., iod.[3], **ip.**,
kali-c.[3], **kali-chl.**, kali-n.[11], **LACH.**,
LAUR., led., lyc., mang., merc.,
merc-c.[3], meth-ae-ae.[11], mez.[3],
mosch., mur-ac., **naja**, nat-m.,
nat-ns.[12], nit-ac., nux-m., nux-v.,
OP., ox-ac.[3, 6], petr.[11], ph-ac.,
phenac.[12], phos., phyt.[3], plb., puls.,
ran-b., **rhust-t.**, ruta, sabad., **samb.**,
santin.[11], sars., **sec.**, seneg., sil.,
spong., staph., stram., stry.[11],
sul-ac., sulfon.[12], sulph., thuj.,
VERAT., **VERAT-V.**[3, 6], vip[11], xan.,
zinc.[3]

fever, during[11]

arund., crot-h.

infants, in

arn., ars., **bor.**, **cact.**, **camph.**,
carb-v., chin., **DIG.**, **LACH.**, **LAUR.**,
naja, op., **phos.**, psor., rhus-t., sec.,
sulph.

DARKNESS agg.[3]

acon., **am-m.**, anac., ang., **arg-n.**[3],
ars.[3, 8], bar-c., **CALC.**[3, 8], camph.,
cann-s., **carb-an.**[3, 8], **carb-v.**[3],
caust.[3], con., **gels.**[3], **lyc.**[3], nat-m.,
phos.[8], **plat.**, **PLB.**, puls.[3], **rhus-t.**,
staph., **STRAM.**[3, 6, 8], **stront-c.**,
sul-ac., valer.[3], zinc.[6]

am[2, 3]

acon.[2, 3, 6], agar., agn.[3], am-c.,
am-m., **anac.**, anh.[9, 14], **ant-c.**,
arn., **ars.**, **asar.**, **bar-c.**, **bell.**[2, 3, 6, 7],
bor., bry., **CALC.**[2, 3, 6], camph.,
carb-an., **caust.**, **cham.**, **chin.**[2, 3, 6],
cic., **cina**, **clem.**, coc-c.[2], coca[8],
cocc.[3], **coff.**, colch., **CON.**[2, 3, 8],
croc., **dig.**, dros., **EUPHR.**[2, 3, 6, 8],
GRAPH.[2, 3, 6, 8], hell., hep.,
hyos.[2, 3, 6], **ign.**, kali-c., kali-n.,
lach., **laur.**, **lyc.**, mag-c., **mag-m.**,
mang., merc., mez., mur-ac., **nat-c.**,
nat-m., **nit-ac.**, nux-m., **nux-v.**,
petr., **ph-ac.**, **PHOS.**[2, 3, 8], **puls.**,
rhod., rhus-t., ruta, sang.[8], **sars.**,
sel., **seneg.**, **sep.**[2, 3], **sil.**[2, 3], **spig.**,
staph., **stram.**, **sulph.**, tarax.[3],
tarent.[2], thuj., valer., verat., zinc.

DEATH, apparent; asphyxia (1897)

acet-ac., acon.[3], **ant-t.**, arn., bell.,
camph., carb-v., **carbn-s.** chin.,
chlor., **cochl.**, **coff.**, coloc, crot-h.[4],
hydr-ac.[4], laur., merc., nit-ac., **op.**,
ph-ac., phos., rhus-t., **sin-n.**, stram.,
sul-h.[12], tab.

carbon monoxide poisoning, from[4]

acon., bell., op.

coal gas

drowned persons, of[4]

lach.

frozened persons, of[4]

acon., ars., bry., carb-v.

haemorrhages, after[4]

chin.

hanged, strangled persons, of[4]

op.

injuries, after

arn.

lightning-stroke, after

lach.[4], nux-v.

neonatorum, in asphyxia of

acon, am-c.[3, 6, 8], **ANT-T., arn.,
bell., CAMPH.,** chin., crot-h.[3, 6],
hydr-ac.[3, 6, 8], hyos.[3, 6], **laur.,
op.,** sul-h.[8], upa.[8], vip.[3, 6]

DEBAUCH, agg. **during**[3]

acon., bell., **op.**

after a, agg.[3]

acon., agar., **am-m.,** ang., **ant-c.**[3, 6],
arg-m., ars.[6], bell., **bry.**[3, 6], calc.,
CARB-V.[3, 6], chin., **cocc., coff.**[3, 6],
dulc., **ip.**[3, 6], kali-c., kali-n., kreos.,
lach.[3], **laur.,** nat-c.[3, 6], nat-m.,
nit-ac., nux-m., **NUX-V.**[1', 3, 6, 7],
OP., ph-ac., phos., **puls.**[3, 6], rheum,
rhus-t., samb., sars.[1'], **spong.,** squil.,
staph.[6], **stram.,** sul-ac.[3], sulph.[3, 6],
teucr., valer.

ailments from[12]

arg-n., carb-v., dig., nux-v., sel.

eating–overeating

feeling as after[11]

caj., conin., kreos., lyc., op., ox-ac.

DENTITION, difficult*

ACON.[2, 3, 8, 12], **aeth.**[2, 8, 12], am-c.[3],
ant-c.[2], **ant-t.**[2], apis[2], arn[2],
ARS[2, 3], arund.[12], **bell.**[2, 3, 8], **bism.**[2],
BOR.[2, 3, 8, 12], bry.[2, 3, 12], **CALC.,**
calc-f.[10], **CALC-P., canth.**[2],
caust.[2, 8, 12], **CHAM.,** cheir.[8], **chlol.**[2],
chlor.[12,] cic., cimic[12], **cina**[2, 3, 12],
coff.[2, 3, 7, 8, 12], **colch.**[2, 3], **coloc.**[2],
cupr., **dol.**[2, 12], dulc.[2], ferr.[2, 3],
ferr-p.[2, 6], **gels.**[2, 6, 8, 12], **graph**[2],
hecla[8, 12], **hell.**[2], hep., hyos., **ign.,**
ip[2, 3], kali-br.[8], kreos., lyc.[2],
mag-c.[2, 3], **MAG-M.**[2, 3, 12],
mag-p.[2, 8, 10, 12], **meli.**[2], **merc.**[2, 3, 8, 12],
merc-c.[3], mill.[12], nat-m.[12], nit-ac.[3],
nux-m.[2, 3], **NUX-V.**[2, 3, 8], op.[3],
passi.[8, 12], **phys.**[2, 12], **phyt.,** plat.[12],
plect.[12], **podo., psor**[2], puls.[3, 8],
rheum, rhus-t.[2, 3], scut.[12], sec., sep.,
SIL., sol-n.[8], stann., **STAPH.**[2, 8, 12],
stram.[2, 3], sul-ac.[2], **SULPH.**[2, 3, 8],
syph.[12], **ter.**[8, 12], til.[12], tub.[3], tub-k.[12],
verat.[2], **zinc.**[2, 3, 8, 12], zinc-br.[8, 12]

convulsions–d

weakness – d.

Vol. III: *sleeplessness–d.*

ailments from[12]

cham., mag-c., mag-p., rheum,
stann., staph.

wisdom teeth

calc., cheir., ferr-pic.[7], **fl-ac.,
mag-c., SIL.**[1, 7]

diarrhoea, with

acet-ac.[8], **acon., aeth., apis,** apoc.[6, 7], **arg-n., ars.,** arund.[8], **bell.,** benz-ac., bor., **CALC.,** calc-a.[8], **calc-p.,** canth., carb-v., **CHAM.,** chin., **cina, coff.,** colch., **coloc.,** corn., cupr., **DULC., FERR.,** ferr.-ar., **gels.,** graph., hell., **hep.,** ign., **ip.,** jal.[8], **kreos., mag-c., mag-p.**[2], **merc.,** nux-m., olnd.[8], ph-ac., **phyt.**[2, 8], **podo., psor., RHEUM,** sep., **SIL.,** sul-ac., **sulph.,** zinc.

slow

aster.[14], **CALC.,** calc-f.[6], **CALC-P., fl-ac.,** mag-c., mag-m., merc.[6], nep.[14], phos.[6], **SIL.,** sulfa.[14], **sulph.**[6], thuj.[6], **tub.**[7]

DESCENDING agg.

acon., alum., am-m., **arg-m.,** bar-c., bell., berg[3], **BOR.,** bry., canth., carb-v.[3], coff., **con., ferr., GELS.**[3, 8], **lyc.,** meny., nit-ac., phys.[3], plb., **rhod.,** rhus-t., **ruta,** sabin., sanic.[3, 8], sep.[3], **stann.**[1, 7], stram.[3], sulph., **verat.,** verb.

am.[2]

acon., alumn., am-c., anac., **ang.,** ant-c., arg-m., arn., **ARS.,** asar., **aur., bar-c.,** bell., **bor., BRY.,** calc., **cann-s.,** canth., carb-v., caust., chin., coff., **cupr.,** dig., dros., **euph., graph., hell.;** hep., **hyos., ign.,** kali-c., **kali-n., lach.,** led., **lyc.,** mag-c., mag-m., **meny., merc.,** mosch., mur-ac., **nat-c.,** nat-m., **nit-ac.,** nux-m., **nux-v., par., petr.,** ph-ac., phos., plat., plb., ran-b., **rhus-t.,** ruta, sabad., **seneg., sep.,** sil., **spig., SPONG.**[2, 8], **squil., stann., staph.,** sul-ac., **sulph., tarax., thuj.,** verb., **zinc.**

DEVELOPMENT, arrested[3]

agar., bac.[8], **bar-c.**[1', 3, 8], bor.[1'], **calc.**[8] **CALC-P.**[3, 8], caust.[8], chin., cupr.[11], des-ac.[14], kali-c., kreos.[8], lac-d.[8], med.[8], nat-m.[1', 3, 8], nep.[14], ph-ac.[3, 8], **phos.,** pin-s.[8], **sil.**[3, 8], sulfa.[14], sulph., thyr., vip.[11]

DIARRHOEA am.

abrot.[1'], bry.[7], nat-s.[1'], ph-ac.[1', 7], **zinc.**

yellow am.[9]

saroth.

DISCHARGES am.[3]

Ausscheidungen am. ars., **bry.**[3, 6], calc., camph., cimic.[3, 6], cupr.[6], dulc.[6], graph.[6], ip., **LACH.**[3, 6, 8], lyc., mosch.[6, 8], nux-v.[3, 6], ph-ac., **PULS.**[3, 6], rhus-t., sep.[3, 6], sil., stann.[8], **SULPH.**[3, 6], thuj.[6], verat., zinc.[3, 6, 8]

DISTENTION blood vessels

acon., aesc.[3], agar., alum., alum-p.[1'], alum-sil.[1'], **am-c.,** ambr.[3], ant-t.[3], apoc.[1'], **arn.,** ars., aur.[3], **aur-m.**[7], aur-s.[1'], **bar-c., bar-m.,** bar-s.[1'], **BELL.,** bov.[3], bry., calc., calc-f., calc-sil.[1'], **camph., carb-v., carbn-s.,** caust.[3], celt.[11], **chel., CHIN.,** chin-ar., **chin-s.,** cic., clem.[3], cocc.[3], coloc., con., **croc.,** cycl., dig., **FERR.,** ferr-ar., ferr-i.[1'], ferr-p., fl-ac.[3], **graph., ham.,** hep.[3], **HYOS.,** kreos.[3], **lac-d.**[7], lach., laur.[3], **led., lil-t.**[3], lyc., mag-c.[3], meny., merl., mosch., nat-c.[3], nat-m., nit-ac.[1'],

nux-v., olnd., op., ph-ac., **phos.,**
pilo.[11], **plb., podo., PULS.,** rheum[3],
rhod., rhus-t., ruta[3], sars., sec., sel.[3],
sep., sil., spig., **spong.,** staph.,
stront-c., sul-ac.[3], **sulph., THUJ.,**
vip., zinc.

evening

PULS.

fever, during

agar., bell., camph., **CHIN.,** chin-s.,
HYOS., LED., PULS.

motion, on[16]

spong.

DOUBLING UP of the body[3, 6]

acon.[3], aloe[3], ant-t., **ars.,** calc.[3],
caps.[3], caust., cham.[3], chin., cimic.,
cocc., coloc., dros.[3], graph.[3],
kali-c.[3], li-t.[11], lyc.[3], mag-c.[3], mag-p.,
merc-c.[3], pareir.[3], plb.[3], puls.[3],
rheum[3], rhus-t., sabin., sec., **sep.**[3],
sin-n.[11], sulph., thuj.[3]

bending-double

bent holding

DRAWING UP the limb, flexing **agg.**[3]

agar., alum., am-m., anac., **ant-t.,**
asar., bell., bor., carb-an., carb-v.,
cham., chel., chin., coff., dig., dros.,
dulc., ferr., guaj., hep., ign.,
kali-c., mag-c., merc., mur-ac.,
nat-m., nux-m., nux-v., olnd., par.,
petr., plat., puls., rheum, rhod.,

RHUS-T., sabad., sabin., **SEC.,**
stann., staph., thuj., verb., zinc.

am.

alum., am-c., am-m., anac., ang.,
ant-c., arg-m., arn., aur., bar-c.,
bell., bov., **bry., CALC.,** cann-s.,
caps., carb-v., caust., cham., **chin.,**
cina, clem., **coloc.**[6], con., croc.,
crot-h.[3, 6], dig., dros., dulc., ferr.,
graph., guaj., **hep.**[3, 6], ign., kali-c.,
lach.[3, 6], laur., lyc., **mang., meny.,**
merc., mur-ac., nat-m., nux-v.,
petr., phos., plat., plb., puls., rheum,
rhus-t., **ruta,** sabin., sel., **SEP.**[3, 6, 8],
sil.[3, 6], spig., spong., stann., staph.,
SULPH.[3, 8], **THUJ.**[3, 8], valer., verat.

DRINKING agg.[3]

acon.[-2], **aeth.**[3, 6], anac., **arg-n., ars.,**
aur.[2], **bell.**[3, 7, 8], bry., **CALC.,**
CANTH., caps., cham., **chin., cina**[3, 6],
cocc.[2-4], colch., coloc., con., **crott.**[3, 6],
cupr., dig.[2], **eup-per.**[6], ferr.[3, 6],
gink-b.[14], grat.[6], hell.[4], **hyos.**[3, 4, 6],
ign., **IOD.,** kali-c., **LACH.,** laur.,
med.[2], **merc.**[2, 3], **merc-c.,** nat-ar.[2],
nat-m., **nux-v.**[3, 6], **phos., phyt.,**
podo., puls[2], rhus-r., rhus-t., sabad.,
sabin., **sel.**[2], sep., **sil.,** squil., **stann.,**
stram.[3, 6], sul-ac., **verat.**

after d. **agg.**[3]

acon., ambr., anac., ang., ant-t.,
arn., **ARS.,** asaf., asar., aur., **bell.,**
bry., cann-s., **canth.,** caps.,
CARB-V., caust., cham., **chin.,**
cic., cina, **cocc.,** colch., coloc.,
con., **croc.,** cupr., dros., **ferr.,**
graph., hell., **hep.,** hyos., ign., ip.,
kali-c., lach., laur., lyc., **MERC.,**
mez., mosch., mur-ac., **NAT-C.,**
nat-m., nit-ac., **NUX-V.,** op., petr.,
ph-ac., phos., plb., **PULS.,** rhod.,
rhus-t., ruta, sabad., sabin., sec.,
sel., sep., **SIL.,** spig., squil.,

staph., stram., **SUL-AC.**[3, 6],
SULPH., tarax., teucr., thuj.,
verat.

am.[3, 6]
acon., alum.[3], bapt.[3], bar-c.[3],
bism.[3], brom.[3], **bry.**[3], carb-an.[3],
CAUST., cist., coc-c.[3], crot-h.[3],
cupr.[3], ferr.[3], graph.[3], ip.[3],
lac-c.[3], lob., lyc.[3], mosch.[3],
nat-m.[3], nit-ac.[3], nux-v.[3], olnd.[3],
phos., psil.[14], psor., rhus-t.[3], sep.[3],
sil., spig.[3], **spong.**[3], sulph.[3],
tarax.[3]

aversion to drink in spite of thirst[6]

cann-i., canth., stram.

rapid, hasty, agg.[3, 6]

ars., **hell.**[6], hep.[6], ip., nat-m.,
NIT-AC., nux-v., SIL., sulph.,
verat.[6]

DROPSY from **abuse of quinine**[8]

apoc.

albuminuria, with[2]

AUR-M.[1, 2], **chin., eup-pur., helon.,**
hep.

alcoholism, from[8]

ars., fl-ac.[1', 8], sulph.

eruption, from suppressed[2]

APIS, apoc., **ars.,** asc-c., dig., dulc.[8],
hell., sulph.

exanthema, from suppressed[3]

apis[5], ars., hell.[3, 8], rhus-t., sulph.,
zinc.[8]

external

abel.[14], acet-ac., acetan.[8],
acon.[3, 8], adon.[3, 6], adren.[6], aeth.[2],
aether[8], agar., alco.[11], all-c.[2],
am-be.[6], am-c.[3], ambr.[3, 6],
ammc.[2], anac-oc.[2], anag.[2],
ANT-C., ant-t., anthraci.[2], **APIS,**
apoc., arn.[8], **arg-n.**[1', 2], **ARS.,**
ars-i., **ARS-S-F.**[2], asaf.[2], **asc-c.,**
asc-t.[2], aspar.[2], aur., aur-ar.[1'],
aur-i[1'], **aur-m., aur-m-n.**[2], aur-s.[1'],
bar-m.[2], bell., bism., bor-ac.[12],
bov.[3, 6], **brom.**[2], bry., cact.,
cain.[7,8], **caj.**[2], calad., **calc., calc-ar.,**
calc-p.[3], **calc-s.**[2], calc-sil.[1'],
camph., cann-s.[3], **canth.,**
carb-v.[2], **carbn-s., card-m.,** casc.[2],
cedr., cham.[2, 11], chel., **chen-a.**[2],
chim.[2], **CHIN.,** chin-ar., **CHLOL.**[2],
cinnb., cinnm.[2], coca, **coch.**[2],
coff.[3, 6], **COLCH., coll.,** coloc.,
con., conv., convo-a.[4], cop.,
cortiso.[14], **crat.**[3, 6, 8], **crot-h., DIG.,**
dulc., elat.[2, 8], erig.[2], eup-pur.,
euph., **ferr.,** ferr-ar., **ferr-i.,** ferr-p.,
ferr-s.[2], **fl-ac.**[1', 2], **form.**[2], frag.[12],
gamb.[2], **GRAPH.,** grat.[2], guaj.,
ham.[2], **HELL., helon.**[2], **hep.**[2, 4],
hippoz.[2, 12], hom.[12], **hydr.**[2], hyos.,
iber.[2], **ictod.**[2], **IOD.,** iris[2], jat-m.[12],
just.[3], kali-ar., **kali-c.,** kali-chl.[12],
kali-i., kali-m.[2], kali-n., kali-p.,
kali-s., **kalm.**[2, 3], kreos.[4], **lac-d.,**
lact.[2], **lach.,** lat-k.[12], **laur.**[2, 3], **led.,**
lept.[2], **liat.**[3, 7, 8], lith-c.[3, 6], lob.[3],
lyc., lycps.[3, 6], mag-m.[3, 6], **MED.,**
MERC.[1, 7], **merc-c.**[2, 8], mez.,
mur-ac., **naja**[2], nat-ar., nat-c.,
nat-m.[1'-3, 12], nat-s.[1', 2], nat-sal.[12],
nit-ac., nux-m., OLND., OP.,
oxyd.[8], ped.[12], phos., pic-ac., plat.,
plb., prun.[2, 3, 6-8], psor.[2], **puls.,**
pyrog.[3,6], ran-b.[2], rauw.[14], reser.[14],
rhod., rhus-t., **ruta,** sabad.[2],

sabin., **sal-ac.**[2, 6], **samb.**, sars.,
sec., senec.[1'], **seneg., sep.**, sil.,
solid.[3, 6], **SQUIL.**, staph.[3], stram.,
stront-c.[3, 4], stroph-h.[6], **sulph.**,
TER., **teucr.**, **thyr.**[7, 12], til.[3], toxi[12],
uran-n.[2, 8], urea[11], **urt-u.**[2, 3],
verat., verat-v.[2], **verb.**, vesp.[12],
vip.[3, 4, 6], zinc., **zing.**[2]

morning

chin., **nat-c.**

forenoon[3]

apoc., aur., just., kali-chl., phos.,
sep., sil.

old people, in[7]

KALI-C.

serum oozing, with[8]

ars., lyc., rhus-t.[3, 8]

haemorrhage, after[3]

apoc., chin.

heart disease, from[2]

adon.[8], aml-ns., **apis**[2, 8], **apoc.**[2, 8],
arn.[8], **ARS.**[2, 8], **ars-i.**[8], asc-c.[8],
AUR-M.[1', 2, 8], bry., cact.[2, 8], **calc-p.**,
chin-ar., **chlol.**, coffin.[8], **colch.**[2, 6],
COLL.[2, 7, 8, 12], conv.[8], cop., **crat.**[8],
crot-h., **dig.**[2, 8], digin.[8], **fl-ac.**, **hell.**,
iod.[8], kali-c.[1'], **kali-m.**, kalm.[8],
LAC-D.[1', 2], **LACH.**, liat.[8], **LYC.**[1', 2],
lycps.[6], merc-d.[8], merc-sul., **nat-m.**,
ph-ac., phos., **prun.**, rauw.[14], **sep.**,
squil., stroph-h.[8, 12], ter.

internal

acet-ac.[6, 8, 12], acetan.[8], **acon.**[3, 4, 8, 12],
adon.[6, 8, 12], agn., alco.[11], am-be.[8, 12],
am-c., ambr., ampe-qu.[8, 12], anag.[12],
ant-ar.[6], ant-c., **ant-t.**, anthraco.[4],
APIS, apisin.[6], **apoc.**, apoc-a.[12],
arg-m., arg-n.[11], arg-p.[8], arn., **ARS.**,
ars-i., asc-c.[8, 12], aspar.[12], aur.,
aur-ar.[1'], aur-i.[1'], **aur-m.**, bar-m.[4],
BELL., benz-ac.[8], **blatta**[6],
blatta-a.[8, 12], brass.[8, 12], **bry.**, bufo[12],
cact.[8, 12], **cain.**[8, 12], caj.[12], **calc.**,
calc-ar.[6, 8, 12], calc-s.[12], camph.,
cann-s., canth., caps., carb-v.,
CARD-M., casc.[12], chel.[4], chen-a.[12],
chim.[12], **CHIN.**, **chin-ar.**, chin-s.[12],
chlol.[12], cina, cit-l.[12], coca[11], coch.[8],
coffin.[8], **COLCH.**, coloc., **con.**,
conv.[6, 8], cop.[8], **crat.**[6, 8], crot-h.[4],
DIG., **dulc.**, elat.[8, 12], equis.[12],
ery-a.[12], euonin.[12], eup-pur.[6, 8, 12],
euph., **ferr.**, ferr-ar., ferr-i.[1'],
ferr-p., **fl-ac.**[6, 8, 12], form.[12], gali.[8],
graph.[6, 12], grat.[12], guaj., **HELL.**,
hep., hyos., iber.[12], ictod.[12],
ign.[3], iod., **ip.**, iris[8], iris-g.[8, 12],
jatr.[8], junc-e.[12], **juni-c.**[6, 8, 12],
kali-a.[6, 8, 11, 12], **kali-ar.**, kali-bi.[6],
kali-bit.[6], **kali-c., kali-i.**[6, 8, 12],
kali-m.[12], **kali-n.**[4, 6, 8], kali-p.,
kali-s., **kalm.**[6, 12], lac-d.[8, 12], lach.,
lact., laur., **led., liat.**[8, 12], lith-c.[6],
lyc., lycps.[6], med.[1'], **merc.**,
merc-c.[6], merc-d.[6, 8], merc-sul.[6, 12],
mez., mur-ac., nat-a.[6], nat-m.[1', 12],
nast.[8], nit-ac., **nit-s-d.**[6, 8],
nux-m.[11], nux-v.[3], olnd.[4], onis.[8],
op.[3, 4, 11], **oxyd.**[8, 12], ph-ac.,
phase.[6, 8, 12], phos., **pilo.**[8], **plb.**[4, 12],
prim-v.[12], prun.[6, 8, 12], psor.[8], puls.,
querc.[8], ran-b.[12], **rhod.**[4], **rhus-t.**,
ruta[4], sabad., **sabin.**[4], sacch.[11, 12],
samb., **samb-c.**[8], sanic.[12], sars.,
sec.[4], senec.[12], **seneg., sep.**, sil.,
sol-n.[8], **solid.**[6, 8], spig., spong.,
squil., stann., stigm.[12], stram.,
stroph-h.[6, 8, 12], stry-ar.[8], sul-i.[1'],
SULPH., tarent.[11], **ter.**[1], teucr.,
teucr.-s.[8], thlas.[8, 12], thyr.[12], toxi.[8],
ur-ac.[8], urea[12], urea-n.[6], urt-u.[6],

verat., vesi.[12], vince., viol-t., zinc.[3], zing.[12], ziz.[12]

joints, of[6]

apis, arn., **bry.**, canth., cedr., chin., chin-s, iod., kali-m., **ran-b.**, samb.

kidney disease, from[8]

ampe-qu., ant-t., **apis.**[2, 6, 8], apoc.[1', 6, 8], **arg-n.**[6], ars.[6], **asc-c.**[2, 8], aspar., aur.[6], **calc-p.**[2], **chim.**[2, 8], **COLCH.**[2, 6], coloc.[2], crot-h.[2], **dig.**, digin., eup-pur.[2, 6, 8], **hell.**[6], helon., lac-d., liat.[8, 12], **merc.**[6], **merc-c.**, merc-d., nit-ac.[6], phos.[6], plb., rauw.[14], **sal-ac.**[2], senec.[1'], **solid.**[6], ter.[6, 8], ur-ac.

liver disease, from[2]

apoc.[8], ars.[8], ars-s-f.[1'], asc-c.[8], aur.[8], **AUR-M.**[1', 2], **CALC.**, card-m.[1', 2, 8], cean.[8], chel.[8], **chim.**[2, 8], **chin.**, cop., cupr., **ferr.**, **fl-ac.**[1', 2], iris, kali-ar.[1'], **kali-m.**, lac-d.[1', 8], **LACH.**, lept., liat.[8], **LYC.**[1', 2, 8], merc., merc-sul., mur-ac.[8], **nat-m.**, **nux-v.**, polym.[8], tarax.[9]

motion am.[16]

nat-c.

newborn, in[8]

apis, carb-v., coffin., dig., lach.

overexertion agg.[3]

apis

painful[16]

dulc.

pregnancy, in[2]

apis, apoc., ars., aur-m., colch., dig., dulc., hell., helon., **jab.**, lyc., merc.[11], merc-c., sanic.[12], uran-n.

scarlatina, after[2]

acet-a.[8], acon.[8], **ambr.**, APIS[2, 8], apoc.[8], **ARS.**[2, 8], asc-c.[2, 8], **AUR-M.**[1', 2], bar-c., **bar-m.**[1', 2], **calc.**, **colch.**[1', 2, 8], coloc., cop., **crot-h.**, dig.[8], **dulc.**[2, 8], **HELL.**[2, 8], **hep.**[2, 8], juni-c.[8], **LACH.**[2, 8], merc.[2], **nat-m.**, nat-s., **phos.**[1', 2], pilo.[8], squil.[8], **stram.**[2, 12], **TER.**[2, 8], verat-v., zinc.

spleen disease, from[8]

cean., **LACH.**[2], liat., querc.[8, 12], squil.[8, 12]

thirst, with[8]

acet-ac., acon., **apoc.**[1', 8], ars.

without[8]
apis, hell.

urine, with supressed[1]

aral-h., **hell.**[2, 8]

weakness-dropsy

DRY sensation **in internal parts**[3]

acon., **ALUM.**[3, 6], am-m., arg-m., arn., ars.[3, 6], **asaf.**[3, 6], **asar.**, bar-c.[3, 6], **bell.**[3, 6], **bry.**, calad., camph.[3, 16], cann-i.[6], cann-s., canth., caps., carb-v., caust., chin., cic., cina,

cinnb.[3, 6], cocc., coff., con.[3, 6], croc.,
dros., euph., ferr., ign., kali-c.,
m-arct., m-aust., meny., merc.,
mez., mosch., **nat-m.**[3, 6], **NUX-M.**[3, 6],
nux-v., olnd., par., petr., phos.[3, 6],
plb., **puls.**[3, 6], rheum, **RHUS-T.**[3, 6],
ruta, sabad., sec.[3, 6], seneg., sil.[3, 6],
spig., squil., stann., staph., **stram.**[3,6],
sul-ac., sulph.[3, 6], tarax., teucr.,
thuj.[3, 6], valer., **verat.**, viol-o.,
viol-o., viol-t., **zinc.**[3, 6]

joints, in[3, 6]

canth., croc., **lyc.,** m-arct.[3],
NUX-V., ph-ac., **PULS.**

dry weather see weather–dry

DRYNESS of usually moist internal
parts[3]

acon.[3, 6], agar., agn., alum., am-c.,
am-m., ambr., anac., ang., ant-c.,
ant-t., apis[3, 6], arg-n.[3, 6], arn., **ars.**[3, 6],
asaf., asar., atro.[6], aur., **bar-c.**[3, 6],
BELL.[3, 6], bor., bov., bry., **CALAD.**[3, 6],
CALC.[3, 6], **camph.**[3, 6], **cann-i.**[6],
CANN-S., canth.[3, 6], caps., carb-ac.,
carbn-o., caust.[3, 6], **cham.,** chel., chin.,
cic., cina, clem., cocc.[3, 6], coff., colch.,
con.[3, 6], cor-r.[6], croc.[3, 6], cupr., cycl.,
dig., dros., dulc., euph., euphr., ferr.,
gels.[3, 6], **graph.**[3, 6], guaj., hell., hep.,
hist.[9], **hyos.,** ign., iod., ip., **kali-bi.**[3, 6],
kali-i.[3, 6], kali-n., kreos., lach., laur.,
led., **lyc.,** mag-m., **mang.,** meny.,
merc., mez., mosch., mur-ac., nat-c.,
NAT-M.[3, 6], **nit-ac.**[3, 6], **NUX-M.**[3, 6],
nux-v.[3, 6], olnd., op., **par., petr.,** ph-ac.,
PHOS.[3, 6], plat., plb., **puls.**[3, 6], ran-b.,
ran-s., rheum, **rhod., rhus-t.**[3, 6], ruta,
sabad., sabin., samb. sang.[3, 6], sars.,
sec., sel., **SENEG.**[3, 6], **SEP.**[3, 6], **sil.,**
spig., spong., squil., stann., staph.,
stram.[3, 6], **stront-c.,** sul-ac., **sul-i.**[3, 6],

SULPH.[3, 6], tarax., **thuj., verat.**[3, 6],
verat-v.[3, 6], **zinc.**

DUST in internal parts, **feeling** of[3]

am-c., ars., **bell., CALC.,** chel.,
cina, cocc., crot-c., dros., hep.,
ign., ip., op., **ph-ac.,** plat., rheum,
sulph., teucr., zinc.

DWARFISHNESS

ambr.[3], aster.[14], bac.[12], **BAR-C.,**
bar-m., bor.[7], **calc., CALC-P., carbn-s.,**
carc.[9], **con.**[3], iod., lyc., mag-m.[3, 6],
med., merc., merc-pr-a.[12], nat-m.[7],
nep.[14], **ol-j.,** op.[3], ph-ac.[7], sec., **sil.,**
sulfa.[14], **SULPH., SYPH.**[1', 2, 3, 7],
thyr.[12], **tub.**[2, 7], zinc.

EATING, before

acon., alum., am-c., am-m., **ambr.,**
anac., ang.[3], arn., ars., **ars-i.,**
ars-s-f.[1'], bar-c., bar-i.[1'], bell., bov.,
bry., **calc.,** calc-i.[1'], **cann-s.,**
carb-an., carb-v., carbn-s., caust.,
cham., **chel., chin.,** colch., **croc.,**
dulc., euphr., **ferr., FL-AC.**[3], **graph.,**
hell, hep., **ign., IOD.,** kali-c., **lach.,**
LAUR., mag-c., mang., meny.,
merc., mez., mosch., **NAT-C.,**
nat-p., nit-ac., nux-v., olnd., petr.,
PHOS., plb., puls., ran-b., **rhus-t.,**
sabad., sabin., sars., seneg., sep.,
sil., spig., squil., stann., staph.,
stront-c., sulph., tarax., valer.,
verat., verb.

while

aloe, alum., **AM-C.,** am-m.,
ambr., anac.[3], ang.[3], ant-c., ant-t.,

arg-m., arn., ars., aur., aur-ar.¹′,
aur-s¹′, **bar-c.**, bar-s.¹′, bell.,
bism., **bor.**, bov., **bry.**, **calc.**,
calc-f.⁷, calc-sil.¹′, cann-s.,
canth., **carb-ac.**, **CARB-AN.**,
CARB-V., **carbn-s.**¹, **caust.**,
cham., chin., **cic.**, clem., **cocc.**,
coff., colch., **CON.**, cycl., dig.,
dros., dulc., euph., ferr., **graph.**,
hell., **hep.**, ign., iod., kali-bi.³,
KALI-C., kali-n., kali-p., lach.,
laur., led., **lyc.**, mag-c., **mag-m.**,
mang., merc., mur-ac.³, **nat-c.**,
nat-m., **NIT-AC.**, nux-m., nux-v.,
olnd., petr.¹, ph-ac., **phos.**, plat.³,
plb., **puls.**, ran-b., ran-s., rauw.¹⁴,
rhod., rhus-t., **rumx.**, ruta,
sabin., samb., sars., sec., **sep.**,
sil., spig., spong., squil., staph.,
stram., sul-ac., **SULPH.**, tarax.,
teucr., thuj., valer., verat.,
verb.³, zinc.

am.
aloe, **alum.**, alumn.², am-m.,
ambr., **ANAC.**, aq-mar.¹⁴, arn.,
aur., **auran.**², bar-c.⁴, bell.,
buth-a.¹⁴, cadm-met.¹⁴, cadm-s.,
calc-p., cann-i., **caps.**, carb-an.,
carb-v., cham., **chel.**, chin.,
cimic.¹⁴, cocc., **croc.**, cur.²,
cyn-d.¹⁴, dig., dros., ferr., fl-ac.⁷,
graph., **IGN.**, iod., **LACH.**, laur.,
led., lyc., mag-c., mang., merc.,
methys.¹⁴, **mez.**, nat-c., nit-ac.,
nux-v., onop.¹⁴, par., perh.¹⁴,
ph-ac., phos., phyt.³, plat.²′³,
prot.¹⁴, puls., rheum, rhod.,
rhus-t., sabad., sabin., **sep.**, sil.,
spig., spong., squil., stann.,
staph., sul-ac., sulph., tarax.,
thymol.¹⁴, v-a-b.¹⁴, **ZINC.**

after

abies-n., acon., aesc.⁸,
AETH.³′⁸, **agar.**, agn., all-c.,
ALOE, alum., alum-p¹′,
alum-sil.¹′, am-c., **am-m.**, ambr.,
ANAC., ang.³, ant-c., ant-t.,
apis, apoc., arg-m.³, **arg-n.**, arn.,

ARS., **ARS-S-F.**¹′, arum-t.²,
asaf., asar., aur., aur-ar.¹′,
aur-s.¹′, **bar-c.**, bar-i.¹′, bar-s.¹′,
bell., **bism.**, bor., bov., **BRY.**,
bufo, cain., calad., **CALC.**,
calc-i.¹′, **CALC-P.**, **calc-sil.**¹′,
camph., cann-s., canth., caps.,
carb-an., **carb-v.**, **carbn-s.**,
CAUST., cham., **chel.**, **chin.**,
chin-s.², chion.⁸, chloram.¹⁴,
cic., cina, cinnb.¹′, clem.,
coc-c., **cocc.**, **coff.**, colch.,
COLOC., **CON.**, croc., **crot-t.**,
cycl., dig., dros., dulc.,
eup-per., euph., euphr., **ferr.**,
ferr-ar., **ferr-i.**, ferr-p., **gran.**,
graph., grat., guat.⁹′¹⁴, hell., hep.,
hyos., ign., **indg.**, iod., ip., **jug-r.**,
kali-ar., **KALI-BI.**, **KALI-C.**,
kali-m.¹′, kali-n., kali-p., kali-s.,
kali-sil.¹′, kreos., **LACH.**, laur.,
led., **LYC.**, mag-c., mag-m.,
manc.², mang., meny.³, meph.³,
merc., **mez.**, mosch., mur-ac.,
nat-ar., **nat-c.**, **NAT-M.**, nat-s.,
nat-sil.¹′, **nit-ac.**, nuph.², nux-m.,
NUX-V., ol-an.⁸, olnd., op.,
ox-ac., par., **petr.**, **ph-ac.**, **PHOS.**,
phyt., plat., plb., **podo.**, **psor.**,
ptel., **PULS.**, **ran-b.**, ran-s.,
raph.², rauw.¹⁴, **rheum**, rhod.,
rhus-t., **RUMX.**, ruta, sabad.,
sabin., samb., sang., sars., sec.,
sel., seneg., **SEP.**, **SIL.**, spig.,
spong., squil., stann., staph.,
stront-c., stry.⁸, sul-ac., sul-i.¹′,
SULPH., **tarax.**, teucr., thea⁸,
thuj., tril., trom.¹, valer., verat.,
verb., viol-t., **ZINC.**, zinc-p.¹′

agg. long after e.³

grat., kali-i., kreos., murx., **phos.**,
PULS.

am.
acet-ac.⁸, acon., agar.²,
aloe, alum., alumn., am-c.,
am-m., ambr., amor-r.¹⁴, **anac.**,
ang.²′³, arn., ars., ars-i., **aster.**²,
bar-c., bar-i.¹′, bell-p.¹⁴, **bov.**,

brom., **bry.**, buth-a.[9, 10],
cadm-met.[9, 10], cadm-s.[8], calc.,
calc-f.[10, 14], calc-i.[1'], **calc-s.**,
cann-i.[2], **cann-s.**, caps.[8], carb-an.,
carbn-s., **caust.**, cham., **chel.**.
chin., cimic.[8], cist.[6, 8], con.[3, 8],
cupr.[3, 8], dicha.[10, 14], dios., euphr.,
ferr., ferr-a.[8], fl-ac., gamb., goss.[7],
graph., guat.[9], hed.[9, 10], hell.,
hep., hom.[8], **ign., IOD.**, kali-bi.,
kali-br., kali-c., **kali-p.**[8], **kali-s.**,
kalm.[6], kreos.[2], lac-ac.[2, 6], lach..
laur., lith-c., lyss.[2], mag-c.[3],
mag-m., mand.[10], mang., med.[7],
meny., merc., mez., mosch.,
NAT-C., nat-m.[3, 8, 16], **nat-p.**,
nicc., nux-v., **onos.**, ox-ac.[3],
paeon., petr., **PHOS.**, pip-n.[8],
plan., plat.[2], plb.[3], psor.[8], **puls.**,
ran-b., rhod., rhus-t., **sabad.**,
sars., **SEP.**, sil., spig., **SPONG.**,
squil., stann., **stront-c.**, sul-i.[1'],
sulph.[1'], verat., zinc.[3, 6, 8],
zinc-p.[1']

fast

ars., **ip.**, led., **nux-v.**, sulph.

overeating agg.[3, 6]

acon.[3], aeth.[3], alum.[3],
ANT-C.[3, 6, 8], **ant-t.**, arg-n.[7],
arn.[3], ars.[3], asaf.[3], bry.[3], calc.[3],
carb-v., caust., chin.[3], **coff.**[3, 6, 7],
hep.[3], ign.[3], **IP.**, lyc.[3], mag-c.[3],
nat-c., nat-p.[3], nux-m.[3],
nux-v.[3, 6, 8], **PULS.**[3, 6, 8], staph.,
sulph.[3], tub.[1']

ailments from[12]

all-s., ant-c., bry., dios., nux-m.

children, in[3, 6]

aeth., nat-p.

satiety, to

bar-c., bar-s.[1'], **calc.**, carb-v.,
chin.[3], **LYC.**, nat-c., nat-m.,
nux-v., phos.[16], **PULS.**, sep., sil.,
sulph., zinc.[16]

am.
ars., **iod.**, phos.

small quantity agg., a[3]

alet., am-c., arg-n., bar-c., bell.,
BRY., canth., carb-an., **carb-v.**,
chin., con., crot-t., cycl., ferr.,
hep., **ign.**, kali-bi., **kali-c.**, kali-s.,
led., lil-t., **LYC.**, merc., nat-m.,
nat-p., **NUX-V.**, petr.[3], **PHOS.**,
puls., rhod., rhus-t., sars., **sep.**,
sulph., thuj., verat., zinc.

am.[9, 14]
guat.

EFFICIENCY increased[6]

agar., ars., coca, coff., kola, lach.,
nat-p., op., pic-ac., pip-m., stram.

vigor—increased

ELECTRIC STATES, ailments from[12]

nat-c.

ELECTROSHOCK, ailments from[12]

morph.

ELEPHANTIASIS[8]

anac.[8, 12], **ars.**, calo., card-m., **elae.**,
graph., ham., hell.[2], hippoz.[12],
hydr., iod., lyc., **myris.**, sil.[8, 12],
still.[2, 12]

arabum[12]

ars., elae., **hydrc.**[2, 12], myris., **sil.**[2]

EMACIATION

ABROT., **acet-ac.**, adren.[7], **agar.**,
alco.[11], **alet.**[2, 12], **alum.**, alum-p.[1'],
alum-sil.[1'], alumn., am-c.,
am-caust.[11], am-m., **ambr.**, ambro.[12],
anac., ant-c., ant-i.[8], ant-t., **apis**,
apoc.[1', 11], aq-mar.[14], **arg-m.**, **arg.-n.**,
arn., **ARS.**, **ARS-I.**, ars-met.[2, 11],
ars-s-f.[1'], arum-i.[11], asc-t., astra-e.[14],
aur.[2], aur-ar.[1'], aur-m., bar-a.[11],
BAR-C., bar-i.[1'], **bar-m.**, bar-s.[1'],
bell.[2], ben-n.[11], benz-ac.[2, 11],
beryl.[14], bism.[3], bor., both.[11],
brach.[2, 11], **brom.**[1', 2], **bry.**, **bufo**,
buni-o.[14], **cact.**, **CALC.**, calc-ar.[6],
calc-f.[10, 14], calc-hp.[6], **CALC-I.**,
calc-m.[11], **calc-p.**, **calc-sil.**[1', 8],
camph., cann-s.[11], **canth.**, **caps.**[2],
carb-an.[2, 3, 6, 8], **carb-v.**, carbn-o.[11],
carbn-s., carl.[11], **caust.**[2, 3, 6, 8, 12].
cench.[1'], cere-b.[11, 12], **cetr.**[2, 8],
cham., **chel.**, **CHIN.**, chin-ar.,
chin-s.[2, 4, 11], chlol.[11], **chlor.**, **chion.**,
cic.[14], cimic.[10], cina, **cist.**[2, 6], **clem.**,
cob-n.[14], coca[2, 11], **cocc.**, **colch.**,
coloc., con., cor-r., **crot-c.**, crot-t.,
cub.[2, 11], cund.[2, 6], **cupr.**, dig.,
digin.[11], dros., dulc., echi.[11],
euphr.[2], **FERR.**, **ferr-ar.**, **ferr-i.**,
ferr-m., ferr-p.[8], **fl-ac.**, fuc.[11],
gamb.[2], gels.[11], glyc.[8], gran.[4, 11],
GRAPH., **guaj.**, hed.[10], **HELL.**,
helon., **hep.**, **hippoz.**, hura[11], **hydr.**,
ign., **IOD.**, **ip.**, jug-c.[11], kali-ar.,
kali-bi., **kali-br.**[2, 6, 11], **kali-c.**,
kali-i., **kali-p.**, kali-s., kali-sil.[1'],

kali-t.[11], **kreos.**, kres.[10, 13, 14],
lac-ac.[2], lac-c.[2], **lac-d.**[2], **lach.**,
lat-k.[11], **laur.**[2], led.[3, 8], lil-t.[11], **lith-c.**[2],
luf-op.[10, 14], **LYC.**, **lycps.**[2], lyss.[2],
mag-c., mag-m., mag-p.[12],
mang.[3, 6, 8], med.[1', 7], **merc.**,
merc-c.[8, 11], mez., moly-met.[14],
morph.[11], **mur-ac.**[2, 3, 6, 11, 16],
myos-a.[6], **myos-s.**[2], naja[11], **nat-ar.**,
nat-c., **NAT-H.**, **NAT-M.**, nat-n.[6],
nat-p., **nat-s.**, nat-sil.[1'], **nicc.**[2],
NIT-AC., nit-s-d.[6], nuph.[11], nux-m.,
NUX-V., **ol-j.**, **op.**, ox-ac.[11],
parathyr.[14], pers.[14], **petr.**, **ph-ac.**,
phel.[2], **PHOS.**, **phyt.**[6, 8], pic-ac.[2],
pin-s.[6], pip-m.[11], **plan.**[2], **PLB.**,
plb-a.[8], plb-i.[8], **podo.**[2], **psor.**, **puls.**,
pyrog.[3, 6], raph.[4, 11, 12], **rheum**[2],
rhus-g.[11], **rhus-t.**[3, 8], rhus-v.[4, 11],
ric.[8], **rumx.**[2], ruta, sacch.[11], samb.,
sanic.[3, 8, 12], saroth.[14], **sars.**, **sec.**,
SEL., **senec.**[2], sep., **SIL.**, spig.,
spong., **STANN.**, **stann-i.**[6], staph.,
still.[11], **stram.**, **stront-c.**,
sul-ac.[1', 2, 6, 11], sul-h.[11], sul-i.[1'],
sulfa.[14], **SULPH.**, sumb.,
syph.[1'-3, 7, 8], tab.[3, 4, 11], **tarent.**, **ter.**,
teucr.[2], thal.[10, 11, 14], **ther.**[2, 7],
thuj.[2, 3, 6, 8, 11], thuj-l.[14], thyr.[3, 14],
TUB., tub-r.[14], uran., uran-n.[6],
vanad.[7, 8], **verat.**, **verat-v.**[2], vesp.[11],
vip.[4, 6], voes.[11], x-ray[14],
zinc.[1'-3, 6, 8, 12], zinc-m.[11, 12],
zinc-val.[12]

cachexia

affected parts, of

ars., bry., calc.[3], **carb-v.**, **caust.**[8],
cupr.[16], dulc., **GRAPH.**, **LED.**, lyc.,
mez., nat-m., **nit-ac.**, nux-v., ph-ac.,
phos., plb., **PULS.**, **SEC.**, sel., sep.,
sil.

appetite with e., ravenous

abrot., acet-ac.[8], ars.[3], ars-i.[8],
bar-c.[6, 8], bar-i.[1'], **CALC.**, calc-f.[14],
chin.[6], cina[3], con.[8], **IOD.**, luf-op.[14],

lyc.[3, 6], NAT-M., PETR., phos., psor., sanic.[6-8], sil.[6], **sulph.**, thyr.[8], **tub.**, uran.[7], uran-n.[6]

children, in

abrot., ars-i., **bar-c., bar-i.**[1, 7], **CALC.**, calc-p., caust., **chin.**, **CINA, IOD.**, lyc., **mag-c.**, **NAT-M.**, nux-v., petr., **sil.**, sul-i.[1'], **sulph.**

cancerous see cancerous–cachexia

children, in; marasmus

abrot., ACET-AC.[2, 7], aeth.[2], alum., ant-c., **apis**[2], **arg-n.**, arn.[4], **ARS.**, **ARS-I.**, ars-s.[8], ars-s-f.[12], **ARUM-T.**[2], aur.[3], bac.[8], bar-c., bell.[4], **CALC.**, **CALC-P.**, calc-sil.[1', 7, 8], **carb-v.**, caust., cham.[4], chin., cina, coca[12], con.[7], **ferr.**[1', 2, 4], hecla[7], hep.[4], **hydr.**, **IOD.**, kali-c., kali-i.[12], **kreos., lyc.**, **mag-c.**, med.[1'], **NAT-M., nux-m.**, **nux-v.**, ol-j., op., petr., **phos., plb.**, **podo.**[2, 8], **psor., puls., sanic.**[7, 8], sars., sep., **SIL.**, staph.[2], sul-i.[1'], **sulph.**, ther.[2], thyr.[8], **tub.**[7, 8]

downwards, spreads

calc.[1', 7], cench.[1'], lyc., nat-m., psor.[1'], sanic.[3, 6], sars.

grief, after

petr., ph-ac.

insanity with

arn., ars., calc., chin., graph., lach., lyc., nat-m., nit-ac., nux-v., phos., puls., sil., sulph., verat.

loss of animal fluids, from

CHIN., LYC., SEL.

old people

ambr., anac.[3, 6], **BAR-C.**, carb-v.[3, 6], chin.[3], chin-s.[4], **fl-ac.**[3, 6], **IOD., LYC.**, nit-ac.[3, 6], op.[3], rhus-t.[3, 6], **sec., sel.**, **sil.**[7]

pining boys

AUR., LYC., nat-m., ph-ac.[2], **TUB.**

children–delicate

single parts, of

bar-c.[3], bry., calc., caps., carb-v., **caust.**[3], con., dulc., graph., **iod.**, led., **mez.**, nat-m., nit-ac., ph-ac., **plb.**[3], **puls.**[3], sec.[3], **sel.**, sil., **sulph.**[3]

upwards

abrot., arg-n.

EMISSIONS agg., SEMINAL*

abrot.[6], agar., **alum.**, ars., aven.[6], **bar-c.**, bor., bov., bufo[6], **calc.**, cann-i.[6], cann-s., carb-ac.[6], carb-an., carb-v., **caust.**[1, 5], **chin.**, cob., con.[5, 6], dig., ferr-br.[6], **iod.**, **KALI-C.**, led., **lyc.**, merc., mez., nat-c., **NAT-P., NUX-V.**, petr., **ph-ac., phos., pic-ac.**, plat.[6], plb., **psor.**, puls., ran-b., rhod., sabad., **SEL., SEP., sil.**, stann.[6], **staph.**, stram.[6], **sulph.**, thuj.

ailments from[12]

staph.

am.[2]
agn., **calc-p.**, **lach.**, **zinc.**[2, 7]

EMPTINESS, sensation of (Kent 1897)

alum.[3], am-c.[3], am-m[3], ant-c.[3],
ant-t.[3], arg-m[3], arn.[3], astra-m.[12],
aur.[1', 3, 6], bar-c.[3], bry.[3], calad., calc.[3],
caps.[3], carb-an.[3], carb-v.[3], caust.[3],
cham.[3], **chin.**[3], cina[3], **COCC.**, coff.[3],
coloc.[3], croc.[3], cupr.[3], dig.[3, 6], dulc.[3],
euph.[3], glon.[3, 6], graph.[3], hep.[3],
hydr.[3, 6], **IGN.**, iod.[3], ip.[3], **KALI-C.**,
kali-n.[3], lach.[3], laur.[3], **LYC.**,
mag-c.[3], mang.[3], med.[3], meny.[3],
merc.[3], mez.[3], **mur-ac.**, nat-c.[3],
nat-m.[3], nux-v.[3], olnd., op.[3], par.[3],
petr.[3, 6], **PHOS.**[3, 6], plat.[3], plb.[3],
podo.[3, 6], **PULS.**, rhus-t.[3], ruta[3],
sabad.[3], **SARS.**, seneg.[3], **SEP.**, spig.[3],
squil.[3, 6], **STANN.**, staph.[3], stram.[3],
sul-ac.[3], **sulph.**, tab.[3, 6], tell.[3],
teucr.[3], verat.[3], verb.[3], vib.[6], vinc.[12],
zinc.[3, 6], **zing.**

fainting, with sensation of
(Kent 1897)

SEP.

general[11]

ail., apoc., aur.[3, 11], cob-n.[9],
hydr-ac., kali-c.[3, 11], merc., **SEP.**,
zing.

EXERTION agg., physical

acon., **agar.**, agn.[1', 7], allox.[14],
ALUM., **alum-p.**[1'], alum-sil.[1'],

alumn., am-c., am-m., **ambr.**,
ammc.[4], **anac.**, ant-c., **ant-t.**,
apis, apoc., **arg-m.**, **arg-n.**,
arist-cl.[9], **ARN.**, **ARS.**, **ARS-I.**,
ars-s-f.[1'], asaf., asar., aur., aur-ar.[1'],
aur-i.[1'], aur-m[1'], aur-s.[1'], **bar-c.**,
bar-i.[1'], **bar-s.**[1'], bell-p.[10], **benz-ac.**,
berb.[3], beryl.[14], **bol-la.**, bor.,
bov., brom.[3], **BRY.**, buni-o.[14],
buth-a.[9, 10, 14], **cact.**, **CALC.**,
calc-ar.[1'], calc-c-f.[9, 10, 14], **calc-p.**,
CALC-S., calc-sil.[1'], **cann-s.**,
carb-an.[3], **carb-v.**, **caust.**, **chel.**,
chin., chin-ar., chin-s.[4], cic., cina,
coca[6, 12], **COCC.**, coff., **colch.**,
CON., croc., **crot-h.**, cur.[6], cycl.,
DIG., dulc.[1'], erig.[10], euphr., **ferr.**,
ferr-ar., **FERR-I.**, ferr-p., fl-ac.[3],
flor-p[14], **GELS.**, graph., **guaj.**, **ham.**,
hell., **helon.**, **hep.**, ign., **IOD.**, ip.,
kali-ar., **kali-bi.**, **kali-c.**, kali-m.[1'],
kali-n., **kali-p.**, kali-s., kali-sil[1'],
kalm., kreos., **lac-d.**[7], **lach.**, lact.[4],
LAUR., led., lil-t., **lob.**, **lyc.**,
lycps., m-arct.[4], mag-p.[1'], meny.,
merc., **merc-c.**, **mur-ac.**, murx., naja,
NAT-AR., **NAT-C.**, **NAT-M.**, **nat-p.**,
nat-sil.[1'], nit-ac., nux-m., **nux-v.**,
olnd., **ox-ac.**, paro-i.[14], petr.[4], **ph-ac.**,
phos., **PIC-AC.**, plat., **plb.**, **podo.**,
prot.[14], **psor.**, **puls.**, **rheum**, rhod.,
RHUS-T., **ruta**, sabad., **sabin.**,
sacch-l.[12], **sang.**, sarcol.-ac.[9], sars.,
sec., **SEL.**, **SEP.**, sil., sol-n., **SPIG.**,
SPONG., squil., **STANN.**, **STAPH.**,
stront-c.[3], stroph-h.[3], stroph-s.[14],
sul-ac., sul-i.[1'], **SULPH.**, tab.[3],
tarent., tax.[14], tell.[14], thuj., **tub.**,
v-a-b.[14], **valer.**, verat., **zinc.**,
zinc-p.[1']

ailments from[12]

agar., alum., ars., calc., carb-an.,
carb-v., cimic., cocc., con., epiph.,
kali-c., mill., nat-c., ovi-p., rhus-t.,
ruta, sanic., scut., sel., sil., sulph.,
ter.

am.
agar.[3], alumn.[8], brom.[8], canth.,
cycl.[3, 6], fl-ac.[3, 7], helon.[6], **hep.**[3], **ign.**,
kali-br.[3], kali-c.[14], **LIL-T.**[3, 6], nat-m.,
phys.[3], plb., rauw.[9, 14], **RHUS-T.,**
SEP., sil., stann., thlas.[3], tril.

in open air[9]

rauw.

impossible
calc-i.[1']

EXOSTOSES

am-c.[4], **arg-m., AUR., AUR-M.**, calc.,
CALC-F., calc-p.[2], crot-c., daph.[12],
dulc., ferr-i.[2], **fl-ac.**, graph.[2], hecla,
kali-bi.[7, 8, 12], **kali-i.**, lap-a.[7, 8],
maland.[7, 8], **MERC.**[2, 3, 7, 8, 11], **merc-c.,**
merc-p.[8], **mez., nit-ac.**, ph-ac.[3, 4],
PHOS., plb.[4, 12], **puls.**, rhus-t., **ruta,**
sars.[2], **SIL.**, staph.[1'], still.[7, 8], sul-i.[3],
sulph., syph.[1', 3, 7], **zinc.**[4, 7, 8], zinc-m.[7]

FAINTNESS, fainting

abies-c., acet-ac., acetan.[8, 12],
ACON., aesc., aeth.[6], aether[11],
agar., agar-em.[11], alco.[11], alet.[8],
all-c., aloe[6], **alum.**, alum-p.[1'],
alum-sil.[1'], alumn., am-br.[11], am-c.,
am-m., ambr., **aml-ns.**[2, 8],
amyg.[2, 11, 12], anac., ant-c., ant-m.[2],
ant-t., apis, **apoc.**[6], apom.[7, 11],
arg-n., arn., ARS., ars-h., **ars-i.,**
ars-s-f.[1', 11], ars-s-r.[2, 11], asaf., asar.[2],
atro., bapt., bar-c., bar-i.[1'], **bar-m.,**
bar-s.[1'], bell., ben-n.[11], benz-ac.,
berb., beryl.[9], bism.[6], bol-la.[11],
bol-s.[11], bor., **both.**[11], bov., brom.[1'],
BRY., bufo, cact., **CADM-S.**[3], calad.,
calc., calc-ar.[1'], calc-i.[1'], calc-m.[11],
calc-p., calc-sil.[1'] calo.[11], **camph.,**
cann-i., **cann-s., canth.**, carb-ac.,
carb-v., **carbn-o., carbn.s.**, carl.[11],

cass.[11], cast.[2], cast-eq., **CAUST.,**
cedr., cench., cere-s.[11], **CHAM.,**
chel., chim., **CHIN., chin-ar.**, chin-s.,
chlol., chlor.[1], cic., **cimic.**, cina,
cinnm.[2], cinch.[11], cit-v.[12], **COCC.**[1, 7],
coch.[2], coff.[6], colch., **coll., coloc.,**
con., conin.[11], conv.[6], convo-d.[11],
cot.[11], croc., **crot-c., CROT-H.,**
crot-t., culx.[1'], cupr., cupr-a.,
cupr-ar.[2, 11], cupr-s., cur., cycl.,
cyt-l.[9, 11], **DIG.**, digin.[11], digox.[11],
dios., dros., dubo-h.[11], dubo-m.[11]
dulc., elaps, ery-a.[11], eucal.[2, 11],
eup-pur., **euph.**[2, 11], euph-c.[11], **ferr.,**
ferr-ar., ferr-i., ferr-p., **form.,**
gamb., gels., gent-c.[11], **GLON.,**
gran.[11], **graph.**, grind., hedeo.[11],
hell., hell-f.[11], **HEP.**[1, 7], hippoz.,
hura, **hydr.**[1', 12], hydr-ac., **hyos.,**
IGN., IOD., iodof.[2], **IP.**[1, 7], iris,
jab., jal., jasm.[11], jug-c., kali-ar.,
kali-bi., kali-br., kali-c., kali-cy.,
kali-m.[1'], kali-n., kali-ox.[11], kali-p.,
kali-sil.[1'], kalm., **kreos.**, lac-ac.,
lac-d.[2], **LACH.**, lat-k.[11, 12], **laur.,**
led., lept., **lil-t., lina.**[8, 12], lob.[12],
luf-act.[11], lup.[11], **lyc.**, lycps.[2], lyss.,
mag-c., **mag-m.**, magn-gl.[12],
magn-gr.[12], manc., mang., merc.,
merc-c., merc-cy., merc-d.,
merc-i-f.[3], merc-ns.[11], merc-pr-r.[11],
mez., mom-b.[11], **MOSCH.**, mur-ac.,
naja, narc-po.[11], narc-ps.[11],
nat-hchls., nat-m., nat-ns.[12],
nat-p.[11], nit-ac., nitro-o.[11], **NUX-M.,**
NUX-V., oena., ol-an., olnd., **op.,**
ox-ac., paeon.[2], pana.[11], parth.[12],
petr., ph-ac., phase.[8], **phos.**, phys.,
phyt.[2, 3, 11], picro.[11], pip-m.[11], plan.,
plat.[6], **PLB., PODO., psor.**, ptel.,
PULS., puls-n.[11], ran-a.[11], ran-b.,
ran-s., raph.[11], rhodi.[11], rhus-t.,
rob., ruta, sabad., sacch.[11],
sal-ac.[2], **sang.**, sapin.[11], **sars.**, sec.,
senec.[12], **seneg., SEP.**, sieg.[10], **sil.,**
sin-n., sol-t.[11], sol-t-ae., **spig.,**
spong.[8, 12], stann.[2, 6], staph.,
STRAM., stroph-h.[3], stry., sul-ac.,
sul-i.[1', 11], **SULPH., SUMB., tab.,**
tanac.[11], tarent., tax., **ter.**[2, 11], thea[11],
ther., thuj., thyr.[8, 12], til., **tril.**[6, 8],
tub.[1'], uran-n.[2], ust., valer., **VERAT.,**

verat-v., verin.[11], vesp., **vib.**, viol-o., vip., wies.[11], zinc., zinc-m., zinc-p.[1'], zing.

Vol. I: *unconsciousness*

convulsions-consciousness

collapse

morning

alumn., **ARS.**, bor.[4, 16], **carb-v.**, **cocc.**, **con.**, culx.[1'], dios., kali-c.[4], kali-n.[4], **kreos.**, lach.[4], med., nat-m., nit-ac.[4], **NUX-V.**, petr.[4], plb., puls., **sang.**, sep.[4], staph.[4], stram., stry., **SULPH.**

7 h
dios.

8 h[11]
dios., ped.

8–9 h
phos.

air, in open

mosch, nux-v.

bed, in[2]

carb-v.[16], **con.**

eating, before

calc.

during

lach.

am.
nux-v.

house, on entering

petr.

rising, on

BRY., calc.[16], **CARB-V.**, **COCC.**[1, 7], **iod.**, **kreos.**[1], **lac-d.**[7], **lach.**, nat-m.[16], petr.[4], sep.

quickly from stooping or turning head

sang.

stool, during

phys

waking, on[11]

graph.

forenoon

kali-n.[4], phos., sep., staph., stram.

9 h[11]
ped.

10 h[14]
ven-m.

in phthisis[2, 7]

kali-c.

11 h
  ind., **lach.**, **SULPH.**

11–12 h[6]: zinc.

standing erect, on

  dios.

walking in open air, on

  lycps.

noon[16]

  bov., cic.

afternoon

  anac., **asar.**, bor., dios., phys.[11], seneg.[4], sulph.

13 h
  lycps.

14 h after chill

  gels.

16 h after mental exertion[11]

  rhodi.

17.30 h
  nux-m.

evening

  aesc-g.[7], alet., am-c., asaf., **calc.**[1, 7], coff.[4], glon., **hep.**, kali-n.[4, 16], **lac-d.**[2, 7], lach.[4], lyc., lycps., mosch., **nat-m.**[1, 7], nux-v., phos., rhus-t.[4], **sep.**

18 h
  glon.

19 h
  lycps., seneg.

20–21 h
  nux-v.

21 h
  mag-m., meli., rhus-t.

cardiac depression, from

  lycps.

exertion, on

  nat-m.

stiffness of fingers and arms, with[16]

  petr.

stool, during[11]

  sars.

undressing, on

  chel.

night

  am-c., ars.[4], bar-c., calc.[4], carb-v.[4], dios.[11], graph.[4], **mosch.**[1, 7], nit-ac., nux-m., **nux-v.**[2, 4, 7], sep.[4], **sil.**, ther., vip.[4]

midnight

  sep.

3 h
  dios.

abortion, after[11]

rosm.

Addison's disease, in[2]

calc.

after-pain, after every

hep., **nux-v.**

agg. after f.[3]

acon., ars., chin., **mosch.,** nux-v., **op.,** sep., stram.

air, in open

mosch.[2, 4], nit-ac.[16], **nux-v.**[2]

am.[11]
bor.[4], crot-c., dios., trif-p.

amenorrhoea, in[2]

glon.

anaemia, in[2]

acet.-ac.[1'], ferr-i.[1'], **mosch., spig.**

anger, after

cham.[7], **gels.,** nux-v.[2, 5], phos.[5], staph.[2, 5], vesp.[1']

angina pectoris, in[2, 7]

arn.[2], hep., **spong.**

cardiopathy

heart
pain—heart

praecordial, anguish with[2, 7]

aml-ns., merc-i-f.[7], plb.[11], tab.

anguish, after[2]

nux-v., verat.

ascending hill, on

agar.

mountains, on[7]

coca

stairs

aether[7, 11], **anac.,** iod., lycps., plb.

asthma, from[7]

ars., atro.[2], berb., kreos., lach., morph.

bed, in

caust., dios.

bending head backwards am.[15]

ol-an.

blood, at sight of

ALUM.[7], nux-m., **verat.**[7]

Vol. I: *blood–wounds*

unconsciousness–blood

f.–wounds

blowing an instrument, when[16]

kali-n.

breakfast, before[2]

calc.

after
bufo, naja

breath am., deep

asaf.

cardiopathy, in[2, 7]

arn.[7], ars., cact., chel., dig., kali-p., lycps., **spig.**

angina pectoris

palpitation

weakness of heart, from[15]

ars., dig., hydr-ac., lach., laur., verat.

chill, before[2, 7]

ars.

during
acon.·, ars., asar., calc.[2, 7], calen.[4], coloc.[7], kali-c.[4], morph.[7], sapin.[7, 11], **SEP.,** stram.[2, 7], valer.[2, 7]

chilliness with[2]

zing.

church, in[2, 7, 11]

ign.[1', 7], merc-i-f.

crowded room

kneeling

climacteric period, during[2, 7]

ACON., chin.[6], cimic.[6, 8], cocc., coff., crot-h.[8], ferr.[8], glon.[6, 8], hydr-cy., kali-c., LACH.[2, 6-8], mosch., nit-ac., nux-m.[6, 8], nux-v.[6], phys.[2], sep.[6, 8], sulph.[2, 6-8], tab.[6], tril.[8], valer., **verat.,** viol-t.

close room, in

acon.[1, 7], asaf., ip., **lach., PULS.,** tab., vesp.[1']

coition, during[8]

murx., orig., **plat.**[6, 8]

after
AGAR., ASAF.[1, 7], dig., nat-p., sep.

clothes, from tight[16]

kali-n.

cold, from taking

petr., **sil.**

water am.

    glon., vip.[4]

weather, from

    sep.

coldness of skin, with[2]

    camph., carb-v., **chin., laur.,** mosch., **tab., verat.**

colic, during intestinal[2]

    asaf., **cast., coll.**[7]**, coloc.,** hydr.[7]**, manc., nux-m.,** stram.

constriction of chest, with

    acon., ars.[16]

convulsions, after[2]

    ars-s-f., **verat.**

cough, during

    ars., cadm-s., cina, coff., **cupr.,** ip.[15]**, phos.**[2, 7, 15]

between spells[2, 7]

    ant-t.

crowded room, in

    am-c., ambr., **ars.,** bar-c., con., **ign.**[1, 7]**, lyc.,** nat-c., **nat-m., nux-m.**[1, 7]**, nux-v.**[1, 7]**, phos., plb., PULS.,** sulph.

    church

street

    asaf.

dark places, in

    stram.

diarrhoea, before

    ars., sulph., sumb.

during[7]
    ars., crot-t.[2]**, cupr-a.**[2]**, nux-m.**[2]**,** paeon., podo., **puls.**[2]**,** verat.

after
    aloe[6], ars., colch.[6]**, NUX-V.**[2, 7]

    collapse-diarrhoea

dinner, during

    asaf., lyc., **mag-m., nux-v.**

after, when taking exercise in open air

    am-m., **kali-c.**[2, 7]**, nux-v.**[2, 7]

diphtheria, in[2, 7]

    brom., canth., kali-m.[7]**, lach.**[7]**, sulph.**

discouraged, when

    ars.

drowsy, with

    ars.

drug, on thinking of

    asaf.

eating, before

    asaf., bufo., ind., phos., ran-b.[1], sulph.

    hunger

after

    bar-c., bufo, **caust.**[1, 7], dios.[2, 7], **kali-bi.**[2, 7], kali-c.[2, 7], **mag-m.,** nux-v., ph-ac., plan., sang., sil.[3], sul-ac.[3]

egg, on smelling freshly beaten

    colch.

emission, after seminal

    ASAF., ph-ac.

epistaxis, from [2, 7]

    acon., cann-s., croc.[7], crot-h., **ip., lach.**

    before[2, 7]
    carb-v.

    with[7, 15]
    calc.[3], cann-s.[3], carb-v.[15], croc., lach.

eructation, from

    arg-n., CARB-V.[2, 7], nux-v.[2, 7]

after
    arg-n.[2, 7], **nux-v.**
    am.
    mag-m.

excitement, on

    acon.[1, 7], am-c., **asaf.,** aster.[7], camph., **caust., cham.,** cocc.[3], **COFF., IGN.,** kali-c.[3], **LACH.,** mosch.[6], **nat-c., nux-m., OP., ph-ac., SUMB., verat.**[1, 7], vesp.[1']

exertion, on

    arn.[7], ars., calc., **calc-ar.**[2], **carb-v., caust., cocc.,** ferr.[1'], hyper., **iod.**[2], **lach.**[2], **lob.**[2, 7], mosch.[6], nat-m., nux-v., plan., plb., **rhus-t.**[7], senec., **SEP.,** sulph., **ther.,** verat.

eyes closing agg.[3]

    ant-t.

face, with blue[7]

    morph.

    pale[2]

    acon.[7], berb.[7], **cimic., ip., LACH.**[2, 7], **lob.,** nat-m.[7], nux-v.[7], puls.[7], **stram., tab.**

    red

    acon.[7], **ptel.**[2]

falling, with[2, 7]

    ars., camph., stram.

backward[2, 7]

lac-d.

to left side[2, 7]

mez.

fasting am.[1']

alum-sil.

fever, before[4]

ars.

during
acon., arn., ars.[4], bell.,
eup-per.[2], ign.[2, 7], nat-m.,
nux-v., op., phos., puls.[2], SEP.

intermittent[2, 7]

phos.

puerperal[2, 7]

cimic., **coloc.**

after[2, 7]
sal-ac.

frequent

ARS., bapt.[2, 7], camph.[2, 7],
carbn-s.[2, 7], hyos.[2, 7], merc.[2],
merc-cy.[2, 7], murx.[2, 7], op.[2, 7], phos.,
SULPH.

fright, after

ACON., gels., ign., lach., nux-v.[5],
OP., phos.[5], staph.[5], verat.[1, 7]

fruit am., acid

naja

gastric affections. in[2]

alumn., ARG-N.[2, 7], bufo, dios.,
dor.[2, 7], elaps, kali-bi.[2, 7], mag-m.,
mez., nat-s.[2, 7], sang., SULPH.

pain-stomach

grief, from[7]

ign., staph.

haematemesis, from[7]

ARS.

haemoptysis, after[16]

sil.

haemorrhages, nose bleeding, from[2]

acon., cann-s., crot-h., ip., lach.

post partum[2, 7]
cann-s., croc., IP.[7], TRIL.[7]

rectum[2, 7]

ign., nux-v.

uterine[2, 7]

apis, CHIN., coc-c.[7], kreos.,
merc., phys., tril.[12]

headache, during

ars.[11], calc.[2, 7], carb-v.[2, 7], cast.[2],

gels.[2, 7], glon., graph.[7], hippoz.[2], lyc.[7, 16], mez.[16], mosch.[3, 7], nat-m.[7], sil.[2, 7], stram., **sulph.**[2, 7], **ter.**[2], verat., zing.

heart, with pressure about

cimic., **manc.**[2], petr., plb.

angina pectoris

cardiopathy

pain–heart

heat, with flushes of[2]

crot-t., sep.[15], **SULPH.**

heat then coldness, with

SEP.

from[7]
ant-c.[2], berb., nux-v., petr.

heated, when[3, 4]

tab.

hunger, from

cocc.[2, 7], crot-c.[7, 11], culx.[1'], **phos., sulph.**

hysterical

acon.[8], am-c.[1', 7], arn.[2, 7], ars., asaf.[8], cench.[1'], **cham.,** cimic., **COCC.,** cupr.[8], **dig.**[2, 7], **IGN.,** kali-ar.[1'], lac-d., lach.[8], **mosch., nat-m., nux-m., nux-v.,** puls., **sep.**[2], stict.[2], sumb., ter.

injury, from shock in[2]

arn.[4], atro., **camph., cham.,** dig., **hyper.**

wounds

concussion of brain, from[2, 7]

hyos.

kneeling in church, while

SEP.

church

labor, during

cimic., cinnm.[2, 7], **coff., NUX-V., PULS., SEC., verat.**

after[7]
cann-s., croc.

leucorrhoea, with[2]

bar-c., cycl., **lach., nux-m.,** sulph.

lights, from being in a room with many

nux-v.

listening to reading, from[11]

agar-em.

looking steadily at any object
directly before eye

sumb.

upward[3]

tab.

loss of fluids, from

ars.[7], bar-c.[4], **carb-v.[2, 7], CHIN.,**
IP.[7], kreos.[7], merc.[7], nux-m.[7],
nux.v.[7], **PH-AC.[1, 7], TRIL.[1, 7],**
verat.[2, 7]

blood

chin.[6], ferr.[1'], **ip.[6],** op.[1', 6], tril.[6]

lying, while

berb.[2, 7], calad., **CARB-V.[2, 7],**
caust.[4], iod., lyc., sulph.
am.
alumn,, dios., hedeo[7]., **merc-i-f.,**
nux-v.
after

calad., mag-c.

on the side, while

lyc., sil.

meditating, mental exertion, from

calad., **calc.[2],** coff.[2, 7], **nux-v.[2, 7],**
par.[2]

meningitis, in[2]

ant-t., dig., glon.

menses, before

am-c.[6], cimic.[2], cocc., lach., **lyc.,**
murx., nat-m.[2, 6, 7, 16], **nux-m.,**
nux-v., **sep., thuj.**

during

acon.[2], apis, berb., **calc.[1, 7],**
cham., chin.[4, 6], cimic., **cocc.,**
glon.[2, 6, 7], **ign., LACH.,**
lyc.[3, 4, 6], mag-m., **mosch.,**
murx.[7], nat-m., nux-m.,
NUX-V., plb., **puls.,** raph.,
sars., **SEP.,** sulph., uran-n.[2, 7],
verat., **vib.[2],** wies.[7, 11]

from pain

cocc.[2, 7], kali-s., **lap-a.,**
nux-v.[2, 7], sars.[2, 7], sep.[2, 7]

after

chin.[1, 7], lach., lyc.[1, 7]

suppressed, from[8]

cocc.[4], kali-c., **nux-m.,** op.

metrorrhagia with[8]

apis, **chin.[4, 8],** ferr-m., **tril.**

moving, on

ARS., BRY.[2], COCC.[1, 7], croc.[7],
cupr., cupr.a.[11], **hyos.[2, 7],** kali-c.,
lob.[7], nat-hchls.[11], **nit-ac.,**

nux-v.[4], phys., spig.[7], **SPONG., verat.**

am.
  jug-c.

quickly

samb., sumb.[11]

music, on hearing

cann-i., sumb.

mydriasis, with[7]

morph.

nausea, before[11]

dig., glon., **verat.**[2]

during
ail.[11], alum., alumn.[2], ang.[2, 7],
arg.n., ars.[11], calad.[2, 7], calc.,
carb-an.[7], carbn-s., caust.[7],
cham., chel., **COCC.,** coff-t.[11],
fago., **glon.,** graph., **IP.**[2, 7],
kali-c.[2, 7], **LACH.,** lob.[2, 7], nat-m.,
NUX-V., op., petr.[7], picro.[7, 11],
plan.[2, 7], sep.[11], sul-ac., sulph.,
tab.[2, 7], valer.[2, 7], verat.,
vesp.[2, 7, 11]

after
kali-bi.

nervous[1']

cench.

noise, from

ant-c.[1'], asaf., bor.[1'], lyc.[1'], merc.,
nat-m.[1']

numbness, tingling, with[7]

ACON.[2], bor., nat-m., nux-v.

odors, from

ign., **NUX-V., PHOS.**[1, 7], sang.[11]

Vol. I: *sensitive-odors*

cooking food, of

COLCH., ip.

eau de Cologne am.[7, 11]
sang.

eggs, of[2]

colch.

fish, of

colch.

flowers, of

PHOS.[1, 7], sang.

perfume or vinegar, of[2, 7]

agar.

operations, on talking of[7]

alum.

pain, from

acon.[2, 3, 7], apis, ars.[3, 5], asaf.,
bism.[7], bol-la.[7, 11], **cham., cocc.,**
coff.[3], coloc., **gels.**[2, 7], **HEP.**[1, 7],

iod.[3], **nux-m., nux-v.**, phos.[7], phyt., ran-s.[3], sil.[3], stroph-h.[3], **valer., verat.**[1, 7], vib.[3], vip.[3]

Vol. I: *sensitive-pain*

abdomen, in

cocc., coll.[7], plb., **stram.**[7]

anus, in[16]

sulph.

ear, in

cur., hep., merc.

head, in[16]

mez.

heart, in

arn.[1] (non: aur.), **cact.**[2, 7], **LACH., manc.**[2]

angina pectoris.

heart

prick of a needle, from[16]

calc.

sacrum, in[11]

dios., hura

spermatic cords, in[2, 7]

calc-ar.

stomach, in

ars.[2, 7], **BISM., coll.**, cupr-s.[2], **dios.**[2], **nux-v.**, puls., ran-s., sin-n.[2], **sulph.**[2]

gastric

stool, during[2, 7]

cocc.

teeth, in

chin., **puls.**, verat.

testicles, in[2, 7]

laur.

palpitations, during

ACON.[2, 7], **am-c.**[2, 7], arg-n.[15], beryl.[9], cact., cimic., **cocc., hydr.**[2], iod., kalm.[2], **LACH., manc.**[2], **NUX-M.**, petr., sul-i.[1'], **verat.**

after[15]
am-c.

periodical

cact., **coll.**[2], fl-ac., lyc., nit-ac.[4], staph.[4]

every day[2, 7]

hydr.

perspiration, during

agar., ant-t.[2], apis, **ars., calc.**[2], carb-v., **hyos., ign., lob.**[2], morph.[7], **sep.**[2]

cold, with[2]

> bry., camph., caps., carb-v., chin., **DIG.**, hydr., lach.[7], **tab.**, ther., **verat.**[2, 7]

am.[2, 7]
> **olnd.**

after
apis[2, 7], arn.[3, 11], chin.[7], sal-ac.[2]

suppressed foot sweat, from[2, 7]

> **sil.**

pregnancy, during

> bell., kali-c.[7], nux-m., nux-v., puls., sec., sep., verat.[2]

slightest motion of child, from[2, 7]

> **lach.**

pressure in waist, by

> lac-c.[2, 7], merc.[7]

prolonged

> hydr-ac., laur.

puerperal

> coloc.[2, 7], cimic.[7]

pulse, with imperceptible[2, 7]

> chin., crot-h., morph.[7]

irregular[2, 7]

> **DIG.,** morph.[7]

slow[2, 7]

> **DIG.**

raising arms above head

> lac-d., lach., spong.

the head

> apoc., bry., ip.

read, when attempting to, while standing

> glon.

reading, after

> asaf., cycl., tarax.

restlessness, after

> calc.

riding, while

> berb., cocc.[7], grat., sep., sil.

after[11]

> berb., sep.

rising, on

> acon.[7], ambr., bry., calad., calc.[2, 7], cere-b.[11], chel., crot-h., cupr., ind.,

iod.[2], lach.[2, 7], merc-i-f.[3], phyt.[3], plb., ran-a.[11], vac.[2, 7], vario.[2, 7], **verat-v.**[2, 3, 7], vib.[3]

sitting up

from bed, on

acon., apoc.[1'], berb.[4], **BRY.,** calad., **calc.**[2], **carb-v., cina,** colch.[15], **iod.**[1, 7], nat-m.[16], op., **PHYT.,** rhus-t., rob., sep., trom.[11]

from a seat, on

carb-v.[16], staph., sumb., trom.

after[2]

CARB-V., iod.

running up stairs

sumb.

scolding, from[7]

mosch.

sexual excesses, after

dig.[2], ol-an.[6]

shock, from[2]

atro.

sitting, while

iod., kali-n., nat-s., nux-v.[4]

down, on[4]

bov., kali-n.

up, from

ACON., arn., **BRY.,** carb-v., chin.[6], **dig.**[6], dios., **ip., nux-v., PHYT.**[1, 7], **ran-b.**[2, 7], **sep.**[2, 7], sulph., verat-v., **vib.,** vip.[6]

rising

suddenly

ery-a., **verat-v.**

upright, while[7]

acon., calad.

sleep, after[2, 7]

CARB-V.

followed by, f.[2, 7]

nux-m.

loss of, by[2, 7]

syph.

sleeping on left side

asaf.

smoking, on

ign.[2, 7], ip.[2, 7], sil.

after

caust.[2, 7]**. lob.**[2]

snoring, with[7]

stram.

speaking, from

ars.

standing, while

ALUM., ALUMN.[2], apis, berb.[4],
bry., cur.[7], **dig.,** dios.[11], glon.[11],
kali-n.[4], lil-t., lyc.[4], **nux-m.,**
nux-v., phyt., rhus-r., sil., **sulph.,**
zinc.

in church during menses

lyc., nux-m., puls.

prolapse of uterus, from[7]

lil-t.

urinating, while[2, 7]

acon.

starting at something falling to the
floor, from[11]

merc.

stomach, sensation of something
rising from

am-br., **CALC.**[2, 7]

stool, before

ars., dig., glon., puls., sars.,
sulph.[2], sumb.

during
aloe, bor.[2, 7], colch.[2, 7], coll.,
crot-t.[7], **dulc.,** dios., **nux-m.,**
ox-ac., petr.[2, 7], plan.[2, 7], **puls.**[1, 7],
sars.[1, 7], spig.[4, 7], stann.[6], **sulph.,**
verat.[2, 7], verat-v.[6]

after
aloe[2, 7], apis[2, 7], **ars., ars-s-f.**[1'],
bol-la.[2, 7], **calc.**[1, 7], **cocc.,** colch.,
CON., crot-t.[2], cur., dig.[2, 7], dios.,
hydr.[2, 7], kiss.[11], **lyc.,** morph.,
nat-s., **nux-m., phos.**[1], phyt.,
plan., **PODO.,** sarr.[2, 7], sulph.,
ter., verat.

am. by[11]
rhodi.

odor of, from

dios.

urging, from

cocc.

stooping, on

elaps, sumb.

storm, before a[11]

petr.

sudden

ant-c.[1'], camph.[7], cham.[12],
hydr-ac.[6], kali-cy.[7], **phos.**, podo.[6],
ran-b.[1', 6, 7], rhus-t., **sep.**, valer.[6]

summer heat, from

ant-c., ip.

tendency to[2, 11]

aether, carbn-o., carbn-s., colch.,
cupr-s., dig., elpas, euph., iod.[4],
kali-ox., **magn-gl.**, nux-m.[4], ol-an.,
sol-t-ae., sulph., **sumb.**[7], tab., thea,
verat.[4]

temples with both hands, on rubbing

merc.

tetanic spasm, before[11]

sul-h.

after[11]
nux-v.

thunderstorm, before

petr., sil.

transient[2, 7]

mur-ac., nux-m.

trembling, with[7]

asaf.[11], caust.[6], **lach.**[2], nux-v., petr.

trifles, from

sep., sumb.[7]

turning the head, on

ery-a.[11], ptel.

urinating, during[6]

stann.

after
ACON., all-c., med.

uterine affection in[2]

cimic.[2, 7], cocc., murx.

vomiting, before[2]

ARS., crot-h., IP.

with[2, 7]
agar.[2], apom.[7], crot-t.[11], IP..
kali-c., nit-ac.[16], phyt., TAB.,
VERAT.

after
ARS., bism.[6], cocc.[2], dig., elaps,
gamb., kali-c.[16], NUX-V.[2], stict.[2],
verat.[2]

waking, on

CARB-V., dios., graph., lach., ptel.,
ther.[4]

walking, while

aether[7, 11], arn., **ars.**, berb.[4], bov.,
con.[2], cur., dor., ferr., get.[11],
merc.[5], nat-s., **verat-v.**

after

berb., **con.**[2, 7], **nux-v.**[4, 7], paeon.

continuing am.

anac.

downstairs, from going

ery-a.[11], stann.[2, 7]

in open air

berb.[4], bor.[4], caust.[16], lycps.,
mosch.[4], seneg., sep.

am.[4]
am-c.

rapidly am.

petr.

after

nux-v.

upstairs, from going[2, 7]

anac.

warm bath from

lach.

warm room, in

acon., ant.-c.[2, 7], calc-i.[1'], **ip.**,
kreos., **lach., LIL.-T.**[1], lyc., **nat-m.**,
nux-v., **PULS., SEP.**, spig., tab.,
trif-p.[7, 11], vesp.[1']

water on, am. by dashing cold[11]

glon.

weakness, from[2, 7]

ant-t.[4], **ars.**[2], carb-v.[3, 4], caust.[4],
chin.[3], **coca, ferr., hydr.**[2], **lach.**[2],
nux-m.[3], nux-v.[3], ran-b.[2], **sang.,**
verat.[2, 3]**, zing.**

loss of fluids

wet, after getting

sep.

wine agg.[11]

sumb.

wounds, from slight

verat.[1, 7]

writing, after

calad., **calc.**[2], mosch., op.

FANNED, desire to be[3]

apis, ars., bapt., **CARB-V.**[1', 3, 6, 7],
caust., chin.[3, 6], chlol.[7], chlor., glon.[1'],
kali-n., lach., lyc., med.[1', 3], nux-m.,
puls., **sec.**[3, 6], sulph.[2], tab., zinc.

being, am.[3, 8]

ant-t.[3], apis[3], **arg-n.**, bapt.[3],
CARB-V., chin., crot-h.[3], ferr.[3],
hist.[14], kali-n.[3], lach., med., sec.[3].
xan.[3]

sensation see air–draft–sensation

FASTING, while

acon.[3], aloe, alum., am-c., **am-m.**[1], **ambr.,** anac.[1], ars., **bar-c.,** bar-i.[1]', bov.[3], **bry.**[3], cact.[3], **CALC.,** calc-i.[1]', cann-i.[3], canth.[3], **carb-ac., carb-an.,** carb-v., caust.,**chel.,** chin., cina, **coc-c., CROC.,** ferr., ferr-p., **graph.,** hell., **hep.,** ign., **IOD., kali-c.**[1], **kreos., LACH.,** laur., lyc., mag-c., mag-m., merc., **mez.,** nat-c., nat-p.[1]', nit-ac., **nux-v.,** petr., **phos., PLAT., PLB.,** puls., **RAN-B.,** rhus-t.[3], **rumx., sabad., SEP., spig., STAPH., sulph., TAB., tarax.,** teucr., **valer.,** verat., **verb.**

agg. (1897)
acon., aloe, alum., am-c., am-m., ambr., anac., ars., bar-c., bov., bry., cact.[3], **CALC.,** cann-s., canth., carb-ac., carb-an., carb-v., cast.[3], caust., **chel.,** chin., cina, coc-c., **CROC.,** ferr., ferr-p., gran., graph., hell., hep., **ign., IOD., kali-c.,** kreos.[3], **lach.,** laur., lyc., mag-c., mag-m., merc., mez., **nat-c.,** nit-ac., nux-v., petr., phos., **plat.,** plb., **psor.,** puls., **ran-b.,** ran-s., rhod., rhus-t., **rumx., sabad., sep., spig., STAPH.,** stront-c., sulph., **tab., tarax.,** teucr., valer., verat., **verb.**

ailments from[12]

dios.

am. (1897)
agar., alum., alum-sil.[1]', am-m., ambr., anac., ant-c., arn., ars., asaf., bar-c., bell., bor., **bry.,** calc., calc-sil.[1]', caps., carb-an., carb-v., **caust., CHAM., chin.,** cocc., **CON.,** cycl., **dig.,** euph., ferr., graph., hell., hep., hyos., ign., iod., **kali-c.,**

kali-n., kali-p.[1]', kali-s.[1]', lach., laur., lyc., mag-c., mang., nat-c., **NAT-M.,** nit-ac., **nux-m.,** nux-v., par., petr., **ph-ac.,** phos., plb., puls., rhod., rhus-t., sabin., sars., sep., **sil.,** stann., stront-c., sul-ac., sulph., thuj., valer., verat.[3], **zinc.**

fat people see obesity

FATTY DEGENERATION of organs[8]

ars., **AUR.**[2, 8], **calc-ar.**[2], **cupr.,** kali-c., **lac-d.**[2], **PHOS.**[2, 8], vanad.

FEATHER-BED agg.

asaf., cocc., **coloc.,** led., lyc., **MANG., merc., psor., sulph.**

FEEL every muscle and fibre of her right side, as if she could

sep.

FEMALES' disease[3]

acon.[3, 4], agar., am-m., ambr., ang., ant-t., apis[3], arn., ars.[4], asaf., **BELL.**[3, 4], bor., **bry., CALC.**[3, 4], camph., canth., **CAPS., caust., CHAM.**[3, 4], **chin.**[3, 4], cic., cimic.[3], clem., **COCC.**[3, 4], con.[3, 4], **CROC.,** cupr., dig., euph., ferr., fl-ac., graph., hell., **hyos., ign.**[3, 4], iod., ip.[3, 4], kali-c., lach.[3, 4], laur., led., mag-c.[3, 4], mag-m.[4], mang., merc., merc-c., **mosch.**[3, 4], mur-ac., nat-c., **nat-m.,** nux-m.[3, 4], nux-v., op.,

perh.[14], **PLAT.**[3, 4], plb., **PULS.**[3, 4],
rheum, **rhus-t.,** sabad., **SABIN.**[3, 4],
sec., sel., seneg., **SEP.**[3, 4], sil., spig.,
spong., stram., sul-ac., sulph., thuj.,
valer., verat., viol-o., vip.[3]

FEVER agg., **before**[3]

acon., ant-c., ant-t., **arn., ARS.,**
bar-c., bell., bry., **calc.,** caps.,
carb-v., caust., **CHIN., cina,** cocc.,
ferr., graph., hep., hyos., ign., **ip.,**
kali-c., kali-n., lach., lyc., mag-c.,
merc., nat-c., nat-m., nit-ac., nux-v.,
ph-ac., phos., **PULS.,** rhod., **rhus-t.,**
ruta, sabad., sabin., samb., sep., sil.,
spig., **sulph., verat.**

during, agg.[3]

acon., agar., alum., am-c., am-m.,
ambr., anac., ang., **ant-c.,** ant-t.,
arn., **ARS.,** aur., bar-c., bell., bor.,
bov., **bry.,** calad., **calc.,** canth.,
caps., carb-v., caust., **cham., CHIN.,**
cina, cocc., coff., con., croc., dig.,
dros., dulc., euph., **ferr.,** graph.,
hell., hep., hyos., ign., iod., **ip.,**
kali-c., kali-n., kreos., lach., laur.,
led., **lyc.**[3, 12], mang., merc., mez.,
mosch., mur-ac., nat-c., **nat-m.,**
nit-ac., nux-m., **NUX-V., op.,** petr.,
ph-ac., **phos.,** plat., **puls.,** ran-b.,
rheum, rhod., **rhus-t.,** ruta, sabad.,
samb., sars., sec., **SEP.,** sil., spig.,
staph., stram., stront-c., sul-ac.,
sulph., tarax., teucr., thuj., valer.,
verat., zinc.

after, agg.[3]

ant-c., ant-t., arn., **ARS., bell.,** bry.,
carb-v., **CHIN.,** cina, dig., **hep.,**
kali-c., nat-m., **nux-v.,** phos., puls.,
sep., sil., verat.

convalescence

FISTULAE[12]

alum., aur-m., bac., bar-m.,
berb.[3, 12], bry.[6], bufo[2], cact.,
CALC.[3, 6, 12], **calc-f.**[3, 6], calc-hp.[6],
calc-p.[3, 6, 12], calc-s.[6, 12], **calen.,**
carb-v.[6], **caust.**[3, 12], con.[6], cop.,
cund., eucal., **fl-ac.**[3, 6-8, 12], **hep.**[2, 6],
hydr., iris, kreos.[6], lach.[6], **lyc.**[3],
maland., mez.[1'], **nat-s.**[2],
nit-ac.[3, 6, 8, 12], ol-j., petr.[3, 6, 12],
phos.[1', 2, 3, 6, 12], puls.[3, 6], pyrog.,
querc., **SIL.**[1', 2, 3, 6, 8, 12], stront-c.[6],
sulph.[1', 3, 6], syph.[1'], thuj.[6], **tub.**[6],
tub-k.[12]

abscesses

bones, of[6, 10]

ang., **asaf.,** aur.[6], bufo[2],
calc-f.[3, 6, 7, 10], calc-hp.[3, 6], calc-p.[10],
calc-sil.[10], fl-ac.[10], **hep.**[2, 3, 6], lyc.[6],
merc.[6], **nat-s.**[2, 12], **ol-j.**[2], phos.[3, 6, 10],
SIL.[3, 6, 10]

glands, of

cist.[6], lyc.[6], merc.[6], nit-ac.[6], **phos.,**
phyt.[6], **sil., sulph.**

joints, of

calc., hep., ol-j., **PHOS., SIL., sulph.**

operation of, after[1']

berb., calc., calc-p.[1', 12], caust.,
graph., sil., sulph., thuj.

ulcers of skin with

agar., ant-c., ars., **asaf.,** aur., bar-c.,
bell., berb.[3], **BRY., CALC., calc-f.**[3],
calc-m.[6], **calc-p.,** calc-s., carb-ac.,
carb-v., carbn-s., **CAUST.,** chel.,

cinnb., clem., **con., fl-ac., hep.,**
hippoz., kreos., **lach.**[4], led., **LYC.,**
merc., mill.[2], nat-c., **nat-m.,** nat-p.,
nit-ac., petr., ph-ac.[3, 4], **PHOS.,**
PULS., rhus-t., ruta, sabin., sel.,
sep., **SIL.,** stann.[4], **staph.,** stram.,
sulph., ter.[3], **thuj.**

FLABBY feeling

acon., agar., am-m., ambr., ant-t.,
arg-m., arn., **ARS.,** asar., **bar-c.,**
bell., bov., bry., **CALC., calc-p.,**
calc-s., calc-sil.[1'], canth., **CAPS.,**
carb-an., carb-v., **CAUST., cham.,**
chel., chin., chin-ar.[1'], cic., cina,
clem., coff., **CROC., cycl., dig.,**
euph., euphr., **ferr., fl-ac.,** graph.,
hep., **IGN.,** iod., **ip., kali-ar., kali-c.,**
kali-n., kali-p., kali-s., laur., **LYC.,**
mag-c., mag-m., meny., merc.,
mosch., mur-ac., **NAT-C.,** nit-ac.,
nux-m., **nux-v.,** olnd., par., petr.,
PHOS., plat., psor., puls., rhod.,
rhus-t., **sabad.,** sabin., seneg., **sep.,**
sil., spong., **staph.,** stront-c.,
SULPH., tarax., teucr., tril.[12], thuj.,
VERAT., zinc.

relaxation–physical

hard parts, in

bar-s.[1'], caust., **merc.,** mez., **nit-ac.,**
nux-m.

internally

calc., kreos., **SEP.**

foggy weather see weather–foggy

FOOD and DRINKS

alcohol agg.*

acon., **agar.,** agav-t.[14], aloe[6],
alum., alumn., **am-c.**[3], am-m.,
anac., ang.[3], **ant-c.,** apom.[8],
aran-ix.[10, 14], **arg-n.,** arn., **ARS.,**
ASAR., aur.[8, 12], **BAR-C., bell.**,
berb.[2], bor., bov., cadm-s.,
calc., calc-ar., calc-f.[10],
calc-sil.[1'], **cann-i.**[8], **carb-ac.**[13],
carb-an., **carb-v., carbn-s.,**
card-m.[8], caust., **chel., chin.,**
chlol., cimic.[3, 8], **coca**[2, 8], cocc.,
coff., colch.[8], **con.,** cortiso.[9],
crot-h., dig., eup-per.[8], **ferr.**[2],
ferr-i.[12], fl-ac.[1', 3, 7], gels., **glon.**[2, 6],
gran.[12], grat.[1'], guar.[12], hed.[9],
hell.[3], hep., hydr.[8], hyos., **ign.,** ip.[8],
kali-bi., **kali-br.**[2], **LACH.,** laur.,
led., lob.[8], lyc., mand.[9, 10, 14],
merc.[2, 3, 4], naja, **nat-c., nat-m.,**
nux-m., **NUX-V., OP.,** petr.,
phos.[3], phyt.[7], **puls.,** querc.[8],
RAN-B., rhod., rhus-t., ruta,
sabad., **sang., SEL.,** sep., **sil.,**
spig., stram., stront-c., stroph-h.,
stry.[8], **SUL-AC., SULPH.,**
syph.[2, 7], tab., thuj., verat., zinc.

easily intoxicated

CON.[2, 7, 11, 12], naja[11], **zinc.**[2]

beer

ailments from[12]

agar., ars., aur., bry., cadm-s.,
calc., carb-v., chin., crot-h., dig.,
gels., lach., led., lob., nux-m.,
nux-v., op., querc., ran-b., sel.,
sep., stroph-h., sulph., ter., verat.

am.
dicha.[10], gels.[7]

aversion
> ail.[2], alco.[11], ang.[3], ant-t., ars.,
> ars-met.[2, 11], bell., bry.[6], calc.[13],
> calc-ar.[13], carb-v.[13], cham.[6], chin.[6],
> cocc.[6], **hyos.**, ign., lec.[13], manc.,
> mand.[10, 14], merc., nux-v., ph-ac.,
> phos.[13], phyt.[7], psor.[13], **rhus-t.**,
> sil.[8], spig.[6], spong.[6], stram.,
> **sul-ac.**[13], sulph.[6, 13], zinc.[6]

desire
> acon., agav-t.[14], ail.[6], alco.[11],
> aloe, am-c., ant-t., arg-m.[3], arn.,
> **ARS., ars-i., ASAR.,** aster.,
> **aur.,** aur-ar.[1'], aur-i.[1'], bov.,
> bry., bufo, calc., **calc-ar.,**
> calc-s., **CAPS., carb-ac.**[3, 8],
> carb-an., **carb-v.**[3, 6, 8], chin.,
> cic., **coca**[2, 6, 8, 13], cocc.[8],
> **CROT-H.,** cub., cupr.,
> ferr-p.[8, 13], fl-ac., gins., hell.,
> **hep.,** iber.[2], ign.[3], **iod.,**
> **kali-bi.**[8, 13], **kreos.,** lac-c.,
> **LACH.,** lec.[8], **led., lyc., med.,**
> merc., mosch.[2, 3, 8, 13], **mur-ac.,**
> naja, nat-m.[3], nat-p., nux-m.[3],
> **NUX-V.,** olnd.[6], **op., phos.,**
> plb., **psor., puls.,** rhus-t.[3], **sel.,**
> **sep.,** sil.[3], **sol-t-ae., spig.,**
> **staph.,** stront-c.[8, 13], stry-n.[7],
> **sul-ac., SULPH.,** sumb., **syph.,**
> tab., ter., ther., **tub.,** ziz.[2]

disgust for, but[14]

> thiop.

menses, before

> **SEL.**

ale agg.[2]

> **gamb., spong., sulph.**

> beer

> aversion.
> > ferr., **NUX-V.**

desire
> ferr-p., **med., sulph.**

almonds, desire for

> cub.

anchovies, desire for[3]

> verat.

> herring
> sardines

apples agg.[3]

> alum., ant-t.[3, 7], arg-n., ars.[5],
> ars-i.[3], bor.[16], chin.[5], con., mang.[16],
> merc-c., nat-s., ox-ac.[1'], phos.,
> puls., rumx., sep., sulph.[5], thuj.

> am.[11]
> ust.

> aversion.
> > ant-t.[13], guaj.[13], lyss.

> desire.
> > aloe, ant-t., fel[11], **guaj.,** menth.[6],
> > sulph., tell.

aromatic drinks agg., smell of[3]

> agn., puls.

> desire.
> anan.

ashes, desire for

> tarent.

> indigestible things

bacon am.

    ran-b., ran-s.

aversion[12]
    rad-br.

desire
    ars.[6, 7, 13], calc.[3], **calc-p.**, cench.,
    mez., rad-br.[3], **sanic.**, tell.[14], **tub.**

    fat ham.

bananas, aversion to

    bar-c.[2], elaps

desire
    ther.

beans and **peas** agg.

    ars., **BRY.**, **calc.**, carb-v., chin.,
    cupr., erig.[10], hell., kali-c., **LYC.**,
    nat-m., **petr.**, phos.[3], puls., sep., sil.,
    sulph.[5], verat.

beef, aversion to

    crot-c., merc.[7], ptel.[7]

smell[11]
    ptel.

beer agg.

        •

    act-sp.[2, 7], acon., **aloe**, alum.[3],
    ars., asaf., bapt.[2, 3, 7], bell., **bry.**,
    cadm-s., calc-caust.[6], carbn-s.,
    chel., chin., chlol., chlor.[13],
    coc-c., cocc.[3], coloc., crot-t.,
    euph., **ferr.**, fl-ac.[3], ign.,
    kali-bi., kali-m.[2], **led.**, **lyc.**[1, 7],
    merc-c.[3], mez., mur-ac.,
    nux-m.[8], **NUX-V.**[1, 7], **puls.**[1, 7],
    rhus-t., sec.[3], sep., **sil.**[1, 7],

    stann., staph., stram., **sulph.**[1, 7]
    teucr., **thuj.**[2, 3, 7], **verat.**[1, 7]

ale

easily intoxicated[2, 7]

    chim., coloc., ign.[6], kali-m.

new[7]

    chin., lyc., puls.

smell[3, 4]
    cham.

ailments from[12]

    kali-bi., rhus-t., thuj.

bad[12]
    nux-m.

am.
    aloe[3, 6], mur-ac.[2, 7], **verat.**[3]

aversion
    alum., alum-p.[1'], asaf., atro.,
    bell., bry., calc., carbn-s.[11],
    cham., CHIN., clem., cocc.,
    crot-t., **cycl.**, ferr., kali-bi.[13],
    merc.[1'], nat-m., **nat-s., NUX-V.**
    pall., ph-ac., **phos.**, puls.[3, 8, 13],
    rhus-t., sang.[3], sep., spig.,
    spong., **stann., sulph.**

morning
    nux-v.

evening
    bry., nat-m., sulph.

smell[11]
    cham.

desire
ACON., agar., aloe, am-c.,
ant-c., ant-t.[11], arn., ars., asar.,
bell., bry., calad., calc., camph.,
carbn-s., **caust.**, chel., chin.,
cic.[14], coc-c., **cocc.**, cod.[11],
coloc., cupr., dig., digin.[11],
graph., kali-bi., kali-i.[13], **lach.**,
mang., med.[7], **merc.**, mosch.,
nat-ar., **nat-c., nat-m.**, nat-p.,
nat-s., NUX-V., op., petr.,
ph-ac., **phel.**, phos., psor., **puls.**,
rhus-t., sabad., sep., **spig.**,
spong., staph., stram., **stront-c.**,
stroph-h.[3], **SULPH.**, tell.,
zinc.[1, 7]

morning[11]
nux-v., phel., **puls.**[2, 7]

forenoon[11]
agar., phos.

afternoon[11]

psor., sulph.

evening
coc-c.[11], **kali-bi.**[11], mang.[11],
med.[7], nux-v.[11], sulph.[11],
zinc.[1, 7]

bitter[8]
aloe, cocc., **kali-bi.**, nat-m.,
nux-v., puls.

chill, during[2, 11]

ant-c., **nux-v.**

colic, after[11]

ph-ac.

fever, during[11]

acon.[2, 11], nux-v., puls.

after[11]
puls.

thirst, without[2, 7]

calad.

biscuit, desire for

plb.

bitter drinks, desire for

acon., aloe[13], cod.[7, 11], dig., **nat-m.**,
ter., ther.[13]

bitter food, ailments from[12]

nat-p.

desire
cod.[2], dig., graph.[3, 6], **nat-m.**,
nux-v.[1', 7], sep.[1']

brandy, whisky agg.

agar., **ars.**, ars-met.[2], bell.,
calc., carb-ac.[13], chel.[3, 6, 13],
chin., cocc., fl-ac.[3], hep., hyos.,
ign., lach., laur., **led.**, med.[7],
NUX-V., OP., puls., **ran-b.**,
rhod., **rhus-t.**, ruta, spig.,
stram., sul-ac., **SULPH.**, verat.,
zinc.

and wine am.[2]

sul-ac.

ailments from bad[12]

carb-v.

am.
prot.[14], sel.[3, 6]

aversion
    ant-t.[2], **carb-ac.**[2, 11], ign., lob.[13],
    lob-e.[8], **merc.,** ph-ac.[3, 6],
    rhus-t., stram.[13], zinc.

brandy drinkers, in

arn.

desire (+ Kent 1897)

    acon., **agar.,** ail., alum., am-m.,
    anac., **ant-c.,** arg-n., **arn., ars.,**
    ars-met., asar.[6], aster., **bell.,** bor.,
    bov., bry., bufo, cadm-s., **calc.,**
    carb-ac., **carb-an.,** carb-v.,
    carbn-s., caust., **chel., chin.,** cic.
    coc-c.[13], coca, **cocc., coff.,** con.,
    crot-h., cub., ferr-p., fl-ac., gels.,
    hep., hyos., **ign., LAC-C., LACH.,**
    laur., **led., LYC., med.**[7], merc.,
    mosch., mur-ac., **nat-c., nat-m.,**
    nux-m., NUX-V., olnd., **OP.,**
    petr., phos., puls., RAN-B., rhod.,
    rhus-t., ruta, sabad., **sel., sep.,**
    sil., spig., staph., stram., stront-c.,
    sul-ac., SULPH., ther., **verat.,**
    zinc.

bread agg.

    ant-c., bar-c., **BRY.,** carb-an.,
    caust., chin., cina[2, 3], clem., coff.,
    crot-h., crot-t., cupr.[13], **hydr.**[2, 6, 8],
    kali-c., lith-c.[13], **lyc.**[2, 8], merc.,
    nat-m., nit-ac., nux-v., olnd.,
    ph-ac., phos., **PULS.,** ran-s.,
    rhus-t., ruta, **sars.,** sec., **sep.,**
    staph., sul-ac., **sulph.,** teucr.,
    verat.[2, 3], **zinc.,** zinc-p.[1'], zing.

black, agg.

    bry., ign., **kali-c., lyc.,** nat-m.,
    nit-ac., nux-v., **ph-ac.,** phos.,
    puls., sep.[3], sulph.

butter agg., and

    acet-ac.[2], carb-an., caust., **chin.,**
    crot-t., cycl., meny., nat-m.,
    nat-s.[3], **nit-ac.,** nux-v., phos.,
    PULS., sep., sulph.

ailments from[12]

    nat-m., zing.

am.[2, 3]
    caust., lact.[13], laur., **nat-c.**[2, 3, 13],
    phos.

aversion
    agar., aphis[8, 13], **CHIN., con.,**
    corn.[11], cur., **cycl.,** elaps,
    ferr-ar.[13], hydr.[13], ign., **kali-c.,**
    kali-p., kali-s., **lach.**[1, 7], lact.,
    lil-t., **lyc., mag-c.**[1, 7], manc.,
    meny., **NAT-M.,** nat-p., nat-s.,
    nit-ac., nux-m.[11], nux-v., ol-an.,
    ph-ac., phos., puls., rhus-t.[1, 7],
    sep., sulph.[1, 7], tarent.

black
    kali-c., lyc., merc.[6],
    nat-m.[3, 6, 11, 16], **nux-v.**[1, 7],
    ph-ac.[3, 6, 16], puls., sulph.

butter, and

    cycl.[1, 7], **mag-c.**[1, 7], meny.,
    nat-p., sang.[3]

pregnancy, during[2, 7]

    ant-t.[16], laur.[16], **sep.**

rye bread[7]

    lyc., nux-v.

desire
    abrot., aloe, am-c., **ars., aur.,**
    aur-ar.[1'], **bell.**[1, 7], bov.,

cann-i.[11], con., **cina, coloc.,**
cub., **ferr.,** ferr-ar., ferr-m.[13],
grat., hell., hydr., ign., lyc.[13],
mag-c., merc., nat-ar., **nat-c.**[1'],
nat-m., ol-an.[11], op., **plb.,**
puls.[1, 7], sec., sil., staph.,
stront-c., sumb.

evening
cast.[11], tell.[14]

boiled in milk

abrot.

butter, and

agar., **bar-m.**[13], bell., **ferr.,**
grat., hell., hydr., ign., **mag-c.,**
MERC., merc-sul.[2], puls.,
stront-c.[3]

dry
aur.[3], **bar-m.**

only
bov., grat.

rye bread

ars., carl., **ign.**[1, 7], plb.

white
aur.[3], bar-m.[3']

broth agg.

mag-c.

sensitive to the smell of

COLCH.

aversion[2, 3, 1]
arn.[1'-3 11]**, ars.**[2, 3]**,** bell.[2, 3],
cham., graph.[2, 3, 11, 16], kali-i.[11],
rhust-t., sil.[7, 16]

desire[1]
mag-c.

buckwheat agg.

ip., **phos.**[2, 3]**, PULS., sep.**[2, 3]**,** verat.

butter agg.

acon., ant-c., ant-t., **ars.,** asaf.,
bell., carb-an., **CARB-V.,** caust.,
chin., colch., **cycl.,** dros., euph.,
ferr., ferr-ar., hell., hep., ip.,
mag-m., meny., merc-c.[3], nat-ar.,
nat-c., nat-m., nat-p., nit-ac.,
nux-v., **phos., ptel., PULS., sep.,**
spong., sulph., **tarax., tarent.**[13]**,**
thuj.

bread–butter

ailments from[12]

carb-v.

aversion,
ars., carb-an.[13], carb-v., **CHIN.,**
cycl., hep.[8], mag-c., meny., **merc.,**
nat-m.[13], petr., **phos.,** prot.[14],
ptel.[1], **PULS.,** sang.

desire,
all-s., ferr.[3, 8], ign.[3], mag-c.[3],
mand.[9], merc., nit-ac.[6], prot.[14],
puls.[3]

buttermilk agg.[3, 16]

puls.

aversion[13]
cina

desire[3]
ant-t., chin-s., chion., elaps[3, 8, 13],
sabal., thlas.

cabbage agg.

ars., **BRY.**, calc., carb-v., **chin.**,
cupr., erig.[10], hell., kali-c., **LYC.**
mag-c., nat-m., **nat-s.**, **PETR.**,
phos.[3], podo.[1'], **puls.**, sep., sil.,
sulph.[5], verat.

ailments from[12]

petr.

aversion[13]
bry., carb-v., cocc., kali-c., lyc.,
petr.

desire[3]
acon.[11], **acon-l.**[7], alum.[13], **CIC.**,
con.

carrots agg.

calc., **lyc.**

cereals, aversion to

ars., phos.

charcoal, desire for

alum., **calc.**[2, 8, 13], **cic.**, con.,
ign.[8, 13], nit-ac., nux-v., **psor.**[8, 13]

indigestible

chlorosis, in[7]

alum.

cheese agg.[2, 3, 6]

arg-n.[5], ars.[3, 6], coloc.[2, 3, 6, 8],
nux-v., phos.[3], ptel., sanic.[3],
sep.[3], staph.[5]

old ch. agg.

ars., bry., coloc., hep.[3], nux-v.[3],
ph-ac., **ptel.**, **rhus-t.**, sanic.[3],
sep.[3]

spoiled ch. agg.[6]

ars., bry.[3, 6], ph-ac., rhus-t.

ailments from[12]

nit-s-d.

aversion
arg-n.[5, 7], **chel.**, chin.[3], **nit-ac.**[5, 7],
olnd.[1, 7], **staph.**[5, 7]

Gruyère[5,]
merc., sulph.

Roquefort[5, 7]
hep.

strong[t, 7]

hep., nit-ac.

desire
arg-n., aster., calc-p.[10], **cist.**,
coll.[13], ign., mand.[9, 10, 14],
mosch., puls., sep.[3, 6]

strong

arg-n., aster., ign.[6]

cherries, desire for

chin.

chicken agg.[1']

bac.[7], bry.

aversion[7]
bac.

chocolate agg.[2, 3, 5, 7]

    bor.[2, 7], bry.[2, 3, 7], calad.[2, 7], caust.[2, 3, 7], coca[3], kali-bi.[3], lil-t.[3], **lith-c.**[2, 7], **LYC.**, ox-ac.[3], prot.[14], **puls.**

    aversion
    osm., prot.[14], tarent.

    desire
    arg-n.[7], calc.[7], **carc.**[7], lepi., lyss., **sep.**[7]

cider agg.

    aster.[14], phos.[3]

    am.[3]
    bell.

    desire
    ben., benz-ac.[13], puls.[3], sulph.

cloves, desire for

    arum., chlor.

coal, desire for

    alum., calc., cic.[1, 7], ign.[13], psor.[13]

    indigestible

cocoa, aversion to

    osm.[2, 11], tarent.[2]

coffee agg.

    aeth., agar.[3], alet.[6], all-c., anac.[14], ars., arum-t., aster.,

aur-m.[1', 2], bell., bov., bry., **cact.**, calc., **calc-p.**, cann-i.[8, 13], **CANTH., caps.**, carb-v., caul.[2], **CAUST., CHAM.**, chin.[2, 3], cist., clem.[7], **cocc.**, coff.[13], colch., coloc.[2, 3, 13], cycl., fl-ac., form., glon., grat., guar.[8, 12], **hep., IGN., ip.**, kali-bi., kali-c.[8, 13], kali-n., **lyc.**, mag-c., mand.[9, 10, 14], mang., **merc.**, nat-m., **nat-s.**, nit-ac., **NUX-V.**, ox-ac., **ph-ac.**, plat., psor.[8, 13], **puls.**, rhust-t., sep., stann.[14], stram., sul-ac., sulph., **thuj.**, vinc.

    hot[13]
    caps.

    smell of c. agg.

        fl-ac.[3], lach.[3], **nat-m.**[3], osm.[3], sul-ac., tub.[3]

    sensitive to the

        arg-n., lach., sul-ac.

    climacteric period, during

        LACH.[7], **sul-ac.**[2]

ailments from[12]

    grat., nux-v., ox-ac., thuj.

am.
    acon., agar., aran-ix.[10], arg-m., **ars.**, brom.[3, 6], cann-i., canth., **CHAM.**, chel.[2, 3, 6], **coloc.**, dicha.[10], eucal., **euph.**[13], euph., fl-ac.[8, 13], glon.[3], hyos., **ign.**[3], lach., levo.[14], mag-c.[16], mosch.[3], nux-v.[3], op., phos.,

aversion
    acon.[13], alum-sil.[1'], **bell., bry.**, **CALC.**, calc-s., carb-v.,

caust.[13], **cham.**, chel., **chin.**,
cinnb.[3], coc-c., **coff.**, con.[13],
dulc., fl-ac., kali-bi.[2], kali-br.,
kali-i.[13], kali-n., lec.[13], lil-t.,
lol.[3, 6], **lyc.**, mag-p., mand.[9],
merc., nat-c., **nat-m.**, **NUX-V.**,
osm., ox-ac., ph-ac., **phos.**,
phys., puls.[7, 16], rheum, rhus-t.,
sabad., **spig.**, **sul-ac.**, **sulph.**[13]

morning[11]
lyc.

noon[11]
ox-ac.

smell[16]

sul-ac

sweetened[2]
aur-m.

unsweetened[3, 11]
rheum
desire
alum., alum-p.[1'], **ANG.**, arg-m.,
arg-n., **ars.**, ars-s-f.[1'], aster.,
aur., aur-ar.[1'], aur-s.[1'], bell.[3],
bry., calc.[5], calc-p., **caps.**,
carb-v., cham., chel., **chin.**,
chin-s.[5], colch., **con.**, **fl-ac.**[3, 6],
gran., grat.[12], kali-i.[13], lach.,
lec., lepi.[11], lob., **mez.**, mosch.,
nat-m., **nux-m.**, nux-v., pauli.[11],
ph-ac., puls.[5], sabin., **sel.**,
sol-t-ae., stroph-h.[3], sulph.,
xan.[3]

beans of[6]

chin.[2, 6, 7], nux-v., sabin.

black[2, 7, 11]
mosch.

burnt
alum., chin.

dysmenorrhoea, in[2, 7]

lach.

ground of[6, 7]
alum.

strong
bry.[2, 7], mosch.[7]

which nauseates

caps.[1, 7]

cold drink, cold water agg.

agar., **all-s.**[2], allox.[9], **alum.**,
alum-p.[1'], alum-sil.[1'], **alumn.**[2],
anac., **ant-c.**, apis, **apoc.**, arg-n.,
ars., ars-s-f.[1'], aur-ar.[1'], **bell.**,
bell-p.[7], bor., bry.[1'], cadm-s.[1'],
calad.[8], calc., calc-p.,
calc-sil.[1'], camph.[3], **CANTH.**,
caps.[1'-3], carb-an., **carb-v.**,
cham.[2, 3], **chel.**, chin.[2, 3], clem.,
cocc., coloc., **con.**[2, 6], **croc.**,
crot-t.[8, 13], cycl.[8, 13], **dig.**, dros.[8],
dulc., elaps[8], **FERR.**, ferr-ar.,
ferr-m.[13], ferr-p.[1'], **graph.**,
grat., hep.[3], hyos., **ign.**, kali-ar.,
kali-c., kali-i., kali-m.[1'], kali-p.,
kali-sil.[1'], **kreos.**[2-6], lach.[6],
lept.[3], lob.[3, 8], **lyc.**, **mag-p.**,
mang., merc., mur-ac., nat-ar.,
nat-c., nat-p., nat-sil.[1'], nit-ac.[6],
nux-m., **nux-v.**, oci-s.[9], op.[3],
ph-ac., puls., rauw.[9], **rhod.**,
RHUS-T., sabad.[8, 13], sars.,
SEP.[3, 6], **sil.**, **spig.**, spong.[3, 8, 13],
squil.[3, 6], staph.[3], stram.,
sul-ac., **sulph.**, tarent., **teucr.**,
thuj., verat.

heated, when

bell-p.[7, 9, 12], **bry.**[1', 7], **kali-ar.**,
kali-c., **nat-c.**, **rhus-t.**[1', 7], samb.

hot weather, in

bry., kali-c., nat-c.

am.
acon.[3, 6], acon-f., all-c., aloe,
ambr., anac., **ant-t.,** apis, arg-n.[3],
ars., **asar.,** aster.[14], **BISM.,** bor.,
brom.[3, 6], **BRY.,** calc., cann-s.[3],
carb-ac.[2], CAUST., cham., **clem.,**
coc-c., coff., **cupr., fl-ac.[3], jatr.[8],**
kali-c., laur., meph.[14],
moly-met.[14], **onos.,** op.[3], **PHOS.,**
phyt.[3, 6], pic-ac.[8], **puls.,** sel.[14],
SEP., stann.[14], sumb., tab.[3], thuj.,
trios.[14], verat., zinc., zinc-p.[1']

aversion to cold drinks

acon.[3], alum-p.[1'], ant-t.[13],
arn.[13], **ars.[13],** bram.[6], calad.,
calc-ar.[13], carb-an.[11], **chel.[3, 6],**
dig.[13], elaps[13], kali-i.[13], mag-c.[7],
nat-m.[13], nat-s.[13], nux-v.[13],
onos.[13], phel.[13], phos.[13], phys.,
stram.[13], verat.[13]

cold water, to

bell., brom., bry., **calad.,**
canth., caust., chel., chin.,
chin-ar., lyss.[1], nat-m., nux-v.,
phel., phos[13], phys., puls.[13],
rhus-t.[13], **SABAD.[13], stram.,**
sulph.[13], tab.

desire
abel.[14], achy.[14], **ACON.,** agar.,
agar-em.[8], ail., allox.[9], **alum.[13],**
alumn., am-c., am-m.[3], **ang.,**
ant-t., apis[3], apoc.[1', 8], **arg-n.,**
arn., **ARS.,** arum-t.[9], asim.,
asaf., aster., aur., aur-ar.[1'],
aur-s[1'], **bell.,** bism., bor.[13],
bov., BRY., cadm-s.[1', 7], **calc.,**
calc-ar., calc-s., camph.[2],
cann-i., cann-s.[3], **caps.,**
carbn-s., **caust.,** cedr., **cench.,**
CHAM., chel., **CHIN., chin-ar.,**

cimic., **CINA,** cinnb., clem.,
coc-c., **cocc.,** colch., corn.[2],
croc., cub., **cupr., cupr-a.[2],**
dig., **dulc., echi., EUP-PER.,**
euph., fl-ac., **glon., graph.,**
hell., ign.[3], kali-bi., kali-m.[3],
kali-n., **kali-p., kali-s.,** lap-a.,
led., lyc., lycps., mag-c.,
mag-p.[3], manc., **MERC.,**
MERC-C., mez., nat-ar.,
nat-c., nat-m., **nat-p.,**
NAT-S., nux-v., oci-s.[9], oena.,
olnd., onos., op.[8, 13], paro-i.[14],
ph-ac., PHOS., pic-ac., plat.,
plb., podo., polyg-h.[3], psor.,
puls., rauw.[9], **rhus-t.,** ruta,
sabad., sabin.[3], sacch-l.[3], sars.,
sec., sel.[3], **sep.,** spig., spong.,
squil., stann.[14], sulph., **tarent.,**
tell.[14], **thuj.,** ven-m.[14], **VERAT.,**
vip., vip-a.[14], zinc.

afternoon[11]

croc.

15 h[11]
caust.

evening[11]
oena.

night[11]
eup-per.

chill, during[1']

bry., carb-v., tub.

fever, during[1']

tub.

cold food agg.

acet-ac., acon.[3], agar., alum.,
alum-p.[1'], alum-sil.[1'], **alumn.[2],**
ant-c., arg-n., ARS., ars-s-f.[1'],
bar-c., **bell.[3],** bell-p.[9], **bov.,** brom.

bry., calad., calc., calc-f., **calc-p.,**
calc-sil.[1'], canth., **carb-v.,**
carbn-s., caust., cham., chel.,
cocc., coloc., **con.,** crot-t.[3], cupr.[3],
dig., **DULC.,** elaps[2], ferr.[3], fl-ac.[3],
graph., hell., **hep., hyos.**[3], ign.,
ip.[3], kali-ar., **kali-bi.**[3], **kali-c.,**
kali-i., kali-m.[1'], **kali-n.,**
kali-sil.[1'], **kreos., LACH.,** lept.[3],
LYC., mag-c., mag-m., mag-p.[3],
mang., merc., mez.[3], mur-ac.,
nat-ar., nat-c., nat-m., nat-p.,
nat-s., nat-sil.[1'], **nit-ac., nux-m.,**
NUX-V., par., **ph-ac.,** plb., **puls.,**
rhod., RHUS-T., rumx., sabad.,
sep., SIL., spig., squil.[3],
staph.[3, 13], stram.[3], sul-ac.[2, 3],
sulph., syph.[7], thuj., **verat.**

frozen

am.[2, 3]
acon., adlu.[14], agn.[3], alum.[3],
alumn.[2], am-c., **ambr.**[2, 3, 8, 13],
anac., ang., ant-t., apis[3], arg-n.[3],
ars., **asar., bar-c., bell.,** bism.[3],
bor., brom.[3], **BRY.**[2, 3, 8, 13],
calc., cann-s.[3], canth.,
carb-v., caust., cham., clem.,
coc-c.[3], **cupr.,** dros., **euph., ferr.,**
graph.[3], hell., **kali-c., lach.**[1'-3],
laur., lyc.[8, 13], mag-c., mag-m.,
merc., mez., nat-m., nux-m.,
nux-v., op.[3], par., **ph-ac.,**
PHOS.[2, 3, 8, 13], phyt.[3], **PULS.,**
pyrog.[3], rhod., rhus-t., sars.,
sep., sil.[2, 3, 8, 13], spig., squil.,
stann.[3], **sul-ac.,** sulph., tab.[3],
thuj.[3], verat., **zinc.**

aversion
acet-ac., alum-p.[1'], chel., cycl.,
kali-i.[13], phos.[13]

desire
abel.[14], am-c., ang.[3], **ant-t.,**
arg-n.[1'], **ars.**[3], asaf.[2], bell.[3],
bism.[3], **bry.**[3, 8, 13], caust.[3],
cham.[3], chin.[2], cina[3], cocc.[3],
croc.[3], cupr., cupr-ar., euph.[3],
ferr-p.[3], fl-ac.[7], **ign.**[1', 3], kali-p.[3],
kali-s., lach.[1'], lept.[3], **lyc.,**

merc.[3, 11], merc-c., nat-m.,
nux-v.[2], olnd.[3], **PHOS.,**
pic-ac.[13], pip-n.[3], plb.[3],
PULS., rhus-t[3], ruta[3],
sabad.[3], sars.[1']
sec.[3], **sil., thuj.,** ven-m.[14],
verat., zinc.

afternoon[11]

nat-m.

menses, during

am-c.

pregnancy, in[2]

verat.

cooked food agg.

ars.[14], podo.[1']

warm f.

sensitive to the smell of

ars.[1'], chin., **COLCH., dig.,**
eup-per., sep., stann.

aversion
am-c.[16], asar.[14], bell., bov., calc.,
chel., cupr., **graph.,** guare, ign.,
kreos.[2], lach., **lyc.,** mag-c.,
merc., petr., phos., psor., **sil.,**
verat., zinc., zinc-p.[1']

corn agg.[5]

chin., kali-c., puls., sulph.

meal
    calc-ar.

cucumbers agg.[6]

all-c., ars., puls.[6], sul-ac.[6, 16],
verat.

aversion[14]
    prot.

desire
    abies-n., **ant-c.,** verat.

delicacies, aversion to[13]

caust.[1'], petr., sang.

desire
    acon-l.[11], aeth.[3], **aur.,** bufo, calc.,
    CHIN., cub., cupr., cupr-ar[13], **IP.,**
    kali-c., mag-c., mag-m.[3], nat-c.,
    paull.[11], petr., psor., rauw.[9],
    rhus-t., sabad., sang., **spong.,**
    TUB.

drinks, aversion to

agar., agn., aloe, ang., **apis,**
arn., **bell.,** berb., bor.[3], bov.[3],
bry.[3], bufo, calad.[3], calc.[7, 13],
camph.[3], **canth.,** carb-an.,
caust.[3], cham.[3], chin., chin-s.[3],
chlor.[11], coc-c., cocc., coff.,
colch.[3], coloc.[13], corn., cupr.,
dros.[13], **FERR.,** graph.[1', 13],
hell.[3], **HYOS.,** ign., kali-bi.[8, 13],
lac-c., lach., lyc.[3, 13], **lyss.,**
merc., nat-m.[3, 13], **nit-ac.,**
NUX-V., phys., plb., plb-chr.[11],
puls., rat., sabin.[3], samb., sec.,
staph.[13], **stram.,** verat.[3]

children, in[3]

bor., bry.

headache, during

FERR.

heat, during

con.

desire
    cob-n.[9], lyc.[13]

capricious, but refuses when
offered[16]

bell.

without thirst[11]

bell., camph., coloc., wies.

dry food agg.

agar., bov.[3], **CALC.,** calad.[3], chin.,
ferr.[3], ign.[3], ip., kali-i.[3], **lyc.,**
nat-c., nit-ac., nux-v., ox-ac.[3],
petr., ph-ac., **puls.,** raph.[3], sars.,
sil., sulph.

aversion[3]
    merc.

desire
    alum.

eel, desire for[13]

med.

eggs agg.

anthraci.[7], **calc.**[3, 5, 7], calc-f.[6],
chin-ar., colch., **ferr.**, ferr-m.,
lyc.[3], merc-c.[3], **PULS.**[2, 3, 5, 6],
sulph.[3, 6]

smell of

anthraci.[7], **colch.**

ailments, from bad[12]

carb-v.

aversion
bell.[3], calc-f.[9, 10, 14], carc.[7, 10],
colch.[5, 7, 13], **ferr.**, kali-s.,
nit-ac., prot.[14], puls.[5, 7],
saroth.[10, 14], sulph.

hard boiled
bry.[3, 6, 16], prot.[14]

smell of

colch.

desire
calc., calc-p.[3, 6], **carc.**[7, 10],
hydr., nat-p., ol-an., olnd.[13],
prot.[14]

fried

nat-p.

hard boiled
CALC.

soft boiled

calc., nat-p.[13], ol-an., olnd.[13]

farinaceous food agg.

alum.[3, 6], **bry.**[3], carb-v.[3, 13], **caust.,**
chin.[2], coloc.[3], iris[3], kali-bi.[2, 3, 6],
kali-c.[3], lyc., mag-c.[3, 6], **nat-c.,**
NAT-M., NAT-S., nux-v.,
psor.[3, 13], **PULS.**[3], sulph., verat.[3]

starchy food

aversion
ars., nat-m.[3, 6], ph-ac.[13], phos.,
plan.[13], ptel.[3, 6]

flour

desire
calc-p.[8], lach., **nat-m.,** sabad.,
sumb.

fat agg.

acon., agn.[3], alet.[6], ant-c.,
ant-t., aran-ix.[10, 14], arg-n.[3],
ars., ars-s-f.[1'], **asaf.,** bell., bry.,
buni-o.[14], but-ac.[9], calc.[3, 8],
calc-f.[10], carb-an., **CARB-V.,**
carbn-s., **caust.,** chin., **colch.,**
convo-s.[9, 14], cupr.[13], **CYCL.,**
dros., erig.[10], euph., **FERR.,**
ferr-ar., ferr-m., GRAPH.[3],
ham.[3], **hell.,** hep., hir.[14], **ip.,**
jug-r.[7], kali-ar., kali-c.,
kali-chl., kali-m.[1', 3, 8, 12],
kali-n., kali-sil.[1'], **lyc.**[3, 8],
mag-c., **mag-m.,** mag-s.[10],
mand.[9, 10, 14], meny., merc.,
merc-c., merc-cy.[13], **nat-ar.,**
nat-c., nat-m., **nat-p.,** nat-sil.[1'],
nit-ac., nux-v., phos., podo.[1'],
psor.[3], **ptel., PULS.,** rob., ruta,
sep., sil., **spong.,** staph., **sulph.,**
TARAX., TARENT.[13], **thuj.,**
verat.

heavy food

oil
pork
rich

infants, in[9]

but-ac.

rancid
ars.[12], carb-v.[7, 12]

ailments from[12]

ars., carb-v.

aversion to fats and rich food

acon-l.[7, 11], ang., **ars.**, ars-s-f.[1'],
bell., **bry.**, calc., **calc-f.**[10],
carb-an., **carb-v.**, carbn-s.,
carc.[7, 10], **CHIN.**, chin-ar., **colch.**,
convo-s.[9], croc., **cycl.**, dros.,
erig.[10], ferr.[3], grat., guare., hell.,
hep., ip.[5, 7, 16], lyc.[13], lyss.,
mag-s.[9, 10], mand.[10, 14], meny.,
merc., nat-ar., nat-c., **nat-m.**,
nit-ac.[13], nux-v.[13], **PETR.**, phos.,
PTEL., PULS., rheum, rhus-t.,
rib-ac.[14], sang., sec., **sep., sulph.**,
tarent.[3], thyr.[14]

fat meat

desire.
ars., calc.[7], **calc-p.**[3, 6], **carc.**[7, 10],
hep., **mez.**[2-3, 6, 8], nat-c.[3], nat-m.[3],
NIT-AC., nux-v., prot.[14],
rad-br.[3], sanic.[3], **sulph., tub.**[3, 7]

bacon
fat ham

lard
fried

fat ham, desire for

calc-p., **carc.**[7], **mez., sanic., tub.**

ham

fat meat, aversion to

carb-v., hell., phos.

fish agg.

ars.[3], calad., carb-an.,
carb-v.[3-6, 8, 13], carb-ns.[1'],
chin.[3, 6], chin-ar., fl-ac.[3], kali-c.,
kali-s.[3, 6], lach.[6], lyc.[6], mag-m.[13],
medus.[3, 6], nat-s.[8, 13],
phenob.[13, 14], **plb., puls.**[3],
sep.[3, 6], thuj.[3], urt-u.[3, 6, 8, 13]

pickled[2, 3]
calad.

sensitive to smell of

colch.

shell-fish see shell-fish

spoiled.
all-c.[2, 7, 12], ars., bell.[3], **BERB.**[3],
carb-an.[2, 12], carb-v., chin.,
COP.[3], euph.[3], kali-c.[2], **lach.**[3, 6],
lyc.[3], **plb.**[2], puls., **pyrog.**[3, 6],
rhus-t.[2, 3], ter.[6]

aversion.
carb-v.[13], **colch., GRAPH.,**
grat.[7], guare., kali-i.[13], nat-m.,
phos., sulph., **zinc.**

salt
phos.

desire
calc-p.[10], mand.[9], **nat-m.**, nat-p.,
phos., sul-ac.[8]

flatulent food agg.

ars., **bry.**, calc., carb-v., **chin.,**
cupr., hell., kali-c., **LYC.**, nat-m.,
nat-p.[13], **PETR.**, puls., sep., sil.,
verat.

beans and peas

cabbage
sauerkraut

flour, aversion to

ars., ph-ac., **phos.**

farinaceous

desire.
  calc., lach., sabad.

food after eating a little, **aversion to**

bar-c., bry.[3], caust.[3], cham.[3],
cina[3], **cycl.,** ign.[3], lyc.[3], **nux-v.,**
prun.[3], **rheum,** rhus-t.[3], **ruta**[1, 7, 16],
sil., **sulph.**

hunger, with

act-sp., **agar.,** all-s.[2], **alum., ars.,**
bar-c., bry., carb-v., **carbn-s.,**
chin., chin-ar.[13], **chin-s., COCC.,**
dulc., grat.[2], hell., hydr., kali-n.,
lach., **NAT-M.,** nicc., **NUX-V.,**
olnd., op., **phos.,** psor., **rnus-t.,**
ruta[13], sabad., **sil.,** stann.[2],
sul-ac., sulph., tax., **tub.,** verb.

loathing of f. on attempting to eat

ant-t.[1'], petros.[7], **sil.**

pregnancy, in [2, 7]

ant-t., **laur., nat-m.**[2], **sep.**[16]

sudden, while eating

bar-c., ruta

tastes it, until he, then he is
ravenous

LYC.

thinking of eating, when

arg-m.[16], **ars.**[2], **CHIN.**[2], colch.[7],
mag-s., mosch.[2], sars.[2],
sep.[2, 7, 16], **zinc.**[2]

pregnancy, in[7]

sep.

fried food, aversion to

adel.[1'], mag-s.[9]

desire
  plb.

fried potatoes[9, 14]

cob-n.

frozen, agg.

arg-n., **ars.,** bry., **calc-p., carb-v.,**
coloc.[3], dulc., **ip.**[1, 7], psor.[3],
PULS., rumx.

am.[6]
  phos.

desire[6]
  arg-m., eup-per., nat-s., phos.

fruit agg.

acon., **aloe, ant-c.**, ant-t., **ARS.**,
ars-s-f.[1'], aster.[14], **bor., BRY.**,
calc., **calc-p., carb-v., caust.**[8],
CHIN., chin-ar., cist., colch.[3],
COLOC., crot-t., cub., elaps[2],
ferr., ign., iod.[3], **ip., iris,**
kali-bi.[8], kreos., lach., lith-c.,
lyc., mag-c., mag-m., merc.[2, 3],
merc-c.[3], **mur-ac., nat-ar.,
nat-c.**, nat-p., **NAT-S., olnd.,**
ox-ac.[3], **ph-ac.**, phos., **podo.,
psor., PULS.**, rheum, **rhod.,
rumx.**[8], ruta, samb.[2, 8, 13], **sel.,
sep.**, sul-ac., sulph.[3], tarax.,
tarent.[13], trom., **VERAT.**

sour
ant-c., ant-t.[1'], **cist.**[6], ferr.[1', 2, 6],
ip., mag-c.[6], ox-ac.[1', 6], **ph-ac.**,
podo.[6], **psor., sul-ac.**[2], ther.[2]

spoiled[1]
act-sp.

ailments from[12]

ars., rhod.

unripe[3, 12]
rheum

am.
lach.

sour[6]
lach.

aversion
aloe[13], **ant-t.**[13], **ars.**[5, 7, 13], bar-c.,
carb-v.[13], **carc.**[7, 10], **caust.**[13],
CHIN.[5, 7]. ferr-m.[13], ign.,
kali bi[13], kali br.[13], mag-c.[7],
phos.[13], **PULS.**[5, 7], **rumx.**[13],
sul-ac.[13]

green[7, 16]
mag-c.

desire
acon-l.[7, 11], aloe, **alum.**,
alum-p.[1'], alumn., **ant-t.**, ars.,
ars-s-f.[1'], asar.[14], calc-s.,
carb-v.[3, 6], **carc.**[7, 10], chin.,
cist., cub., gran., guaj.[3, 6], hep.,
ign., lach., lepi.[11], **mag-c.**,
mag-s.[9, 10, 14], med.[8], nat-m.,
paull.[11], **PH-AC.**, phos.[8], puls.,
staph.[3], **sul-ac., VERAT.**

green
calc.[11], calc-s., lepi.[11], **med.**

sour
adel.[11], ant-t.[1'], **ars.**, calc.,
calc-s., chin., **cist.**, cub., ign.,
lach.[6], **mag-c.**[6], thuj., **VERAT.**

garlic, agg. from the smell of[2, 3]

sabad.

aversion
prot.[14], **sabad.**

desire[3]
nat-m.

grapes agg.[5]

chin., verat.

gruel, agg.[5]

chin., puls., sulph.

aversion
ars., **calc.**

desire[3]
bell.

ham, aversion to[7]

puls.

desire
calc-p.[3, 7, 8], mez.[6], **uran-n.**[2, 7]

fat ham

hearty food, desire for[11]

rhus-t., ust.

heavy food agg.

bry., calc., **caust.**, cupr., **IOD.**, lyc., mag-c.[16], nat-c., **puls.**, sulph.

fat
rich

herring agg.[3, 7]

fl-ac., lyc., nat-m.[3]

sardines

aversion
phos.

desire
cist., **NIT-AC.**, puls., **verat.**

anchovies
sardines

highly seasoned food see spices

honey agg.

nat-c., **nat-m.**[2, 13], phos.[3]

aversion[7]
nat-c.

desire
sabad., verat.[3, 6]

hot drinks agg.[2]

am-c., ambr., anac., ant-t., apis[6], asar., **bar-c., bell., BRY.,**[2, 6, 8,]

calc., **carbv-v.**, caust., **cham.**, chion.[8, 13], cupr., euph., ferr., graph.[6, 8], hell., ign.[6,] kali-c., **lach.**[2, 6, 8], laur., **merc-i-f.**, **mez.**[2, 6], oena.[11], **ph-ac.**, **PHOS.**[2, 6, 8], **phyt.**[6], **PULS.**[2, 8], pyrog.[6, 8], sep., sil.[1'], stann.[6, 8, 13], sul-ac.

am.[3]: ars., chel.[6], lyc.[7], nux-v., sul-ac.

aversion
caust.[1', 13], cham.[6], chin.[1'], ferr., graph.[13], **kali-s., lyc.**[13], mang.[16], oena.[11], ptel.[3], **puls.**[6, 13]

desire[2]
ang., bell., **BRY.**, calad., casc., **cast-v.**[2, 13], cedr., chel., cupr., eup-pur., hyper., kali-i.[6], kreos., **LAC-C., lyc.**, med.[8, 13], **puls.**, spig.[8, 13]

hot food agg.

acon.[2], alum-sil.[1'], alumn.[2], **am-c.**[2], **ambr.**[2], **anac.**[2], ang.[2], **ant-t.**[2], apis[2], ars.[2], arum-t., **asar.**[2], **bar-c.**[2], **bell.**[2], bor.[2], bry., **calc.**[2], canth.[2], caps., carb-v., **caust.**[2], **cham.**[2], chin.[13], clem.[2], coff., **cupr.**[2], **euph.**[2], ferr., graph., **hell.**[2], kali-c.[2], **lach.**[2], **laur.**[2], mag-c.[2], mag-m.[2], **merc.**[2], **mez.**[2], nat-m.[2], **nat-s.**, nux-m.[2], nux-v.[2], par.[2], **ph-ac.**[2], **PHOS.**[2], phyt., **puls.**, rhod.[2], rhus-t.[2], sars.[2], **sep.**, sil.[2], squil.[2], **sul-ac.**[2], sulph.[2], thuj.[2], tub.[3], verat.[2], zinc.[2]

am.[2]
agar., alumn., ant-c., **ARS.**, bar-c., bell.[3], bov., bry., calc., canth., carb-v., caust., cham., chel.[3], **con., graph.**, hell., **ign.**, kali-c., **kali-n., kreos., LYC.**, mag-c., mag-m., **mang., mez.**, **mur-ac., nat-m.**, nit-ac., **nux-m.**, **NUX-V.**, par., ph-ac., **plb.**, puls.,

RHUS-T., sep., **sil., spig.,** sul-ac.,
sulph., thuj., **verat.**

aversion,
calc.[7], **CHIN.,** ferr., kali-s.,
merc-c., petr., pyrog.[13], sil.[1', 13],
verat.[13]

desire[2]
ang., ars., chel., cupr.[2, 13], cycl.,
ferr., LYC., ph-ac., **sabad.**[2, 13]

ice agg.[3]

arg-n.[7], **ARS.**[3], bell., bell-p.[3],
bry., calc-p., **CARB-V.**[3], hep.,
ip., kali-bi[3], kali-c., **nux-v.,**
puls.[3, 7], rhus-t.

ailments from ices[12]

arg-n., ars., bell-p., carb-v.,
puls.

ice-water[12]

carb-v., rhus-t.

desire
arg-m.[3], arg-n.[1'], **ars.**[3], **calc.**[7],
elaps, eup-per.[3], lept.[3], **med.,**
merc-c., merc-i-f.[13], nat-s.,
paro-i.[14], phos.[13], sil.[1'], **VERAT.**

ice-cream agg.[7]

arg-n., ars., kali-ar.[1'], puls.[1']

ailments from[12]

puls.

aversion[12]
rad-br.

desire
arg-n.[1'], **calc., eup-per., med.**[7],
PHOS., puls.[1'], rad-br.[12], **sil.**[1', 7],
tub., verat.

indigestible things agg.[3]

bry., calc., **caust.,** cupr., **IOD.,**
lyc., nat-c., **puls.,** sulph.

ailments from[12]

ip.

desire
abies-c.[3, 6], **alum.,** alumn., aur.[7],
bell, bry., **calc., calc-p.,** cic.[3, 6, 7],
con.[7], cycl., ferr.[6, 7], ign.[8], **LACH.**[7],
nat-m.[7], **NIT-AC.**[3, 5-7], **nux-v.**[3, 6, 7],
psor.[3], **SIL.**[3], **tarent.**[3]

ashes, charcoal, coal, lime,
paper, rags, sand, strange,
tea grounds

indistinct desire, knows not what

arn.[3], **BRY.,** cham.[3], chin., cina[3],
hep.[3], **IGN.,** ip., kreos.[3], **lach.,**
mag-m., PULS., sang., sil.,
sulph.[3], **ther.**

capricious appetite (hunger, but
knows not for what, or refuses
things when offered)

ail., ang.[2], ars., aster., bell.,
BRY., bufo, carbn-s., **cham.**[3],
CHIN., CINA, coca, fago., ferr.[3],
hep., ign., ip., kali-bi., kreos.,
mag-c., **mag-m.,** merc.[3], merc-i-f.,
petr., **phos.,** phys.[3], **puls.,** rheum[3],
sang., staph.[3], sumb., symph.[7],
tep., **ther., tub.,** zinc.

juicy things, aversion to[13]

aloe

desire
aloe., **ant-t.**[8], chin.[8], gran.,
graph.[3, 6], mag-c.[8], med.[8, 13],
nat-ar., nux-v.[1', 7], **PH-AC.,**
phos.[3, 8], puls., sabad.[3,] **sabin.,**
sars., staph.[3, 6], verat.

refreshing

lard, desire for

ars.

lemonade agg.

calc.[7], phyt., **sel.**

ailments from[12]

sel.

am.
bell.[2, 3], cycl.[3, 8, 13], phyt.[3]

desire
am-m.[3, 6, 8, 13], **BELL.,** calc.,
cycl., eup-per.[6], eup-pur.,
fl-ac.[3, 6], jatr., lach.[3, 6], **nit-ac.,**
puls., **sabin.,** sec., **sul-i.,** xàn.[3]

hot[2]
puls.

lemons, desire for

ars., **BELL.**[1', 2, 6, 7], ben-ac.[1], nabal.[1],
puls.[7], verat.

lime, slate pencils, earth, chalk, clay,
desire for

alum., alumn.[13], **calc.,** calc-p.[6],
chel.[3], cic., con.[3], ferr., hep.[3],
hyos.[3], ign.[3, 13], nat-m., **NIT-AC.,**
nux-v., oci.[3], psor.[13], sil.[3], sulph.[3],
tarent.[3, 7]

indigestible

liqueur agg.[1, 3]

ant-c., ars., bell., bov., **cann-i.,**
carb-v., cimic., led., **ran-b.,**
rhod., rhus-t., sel., sulph., verat.

desire[7]
med.

liquid food, desire for

ang., bell., bry., **calc-ar.,** caps.,
ferr., merc., ph-ac., **staph., sulph.,**
verat.

many things, desire for

CINA, kreos., phos.

indistinct desire

marinade, desire for[7]

ars., aster., **cist., fl-ac., hep., lac-c.,**
nat-p., ph-ac., **sang.**

meat agg.

all-s.[8], arg-n.[3], **ars.**[3, 8], bor.[8],
bry.[8], **calc.**[3], carb-an.,
carb-v.[3, 8], caust., **chin.**[3, 8],
colch., cupr., **ferr.**,
ferr-ar.[13], ferr-i.[13], ferr-p.[13],
graph.[3, 6], **kali-bi., kali-c.**[2],
kreos.[3, 6], lyc.[5], lyss.[1], mag-c.,
mag-m., med.[7], merc., nat-m.[8],
nux-v.[1', 7], **ptel., puls.**, ruta,
sel.[8], sep.[3], sil., staph., sulph.,
ter., ther.[13], verat.[8]

bad, agg
absin.[8], acet-ac.[8], all-c.[8], **ARS.,**
bell.[6], bry.[6], camph.[8], carb-an.[8],
carb-v., chin., **crot-h.,**
cupr.-ar.[8], gunp.[8], kreos.[8],
lach., ph-ac.[6], **puls., pyrog.,**
rhus-t.[6], urt-u.[8], **verat.**[8], vip.[6]

sausages

fresh, agg.
ars.[3, 13], **caust., chin.**[3], kali-c.[3]

smell of cooking, agg.

ars., colch.

pickled, agg.[3, 7]

carb-v.

am.
lat.[13], **verat.**[2, 3, 6, 13]

aversion
abies-c., adel.[11], agar., all-s.[13],
aloe[2, 3, 8, 11], **alum.**, alum-p.[1'],
alum-sil.[1'], alumn., am-c.,
am-m.[13], **ang.**, aphis, **arn., ars.,**
ars-s-f.[1'], asar.[14], aster., atro.[11],
aur., aur-ar.[1', 12], aur-s.[1'], bell.,
bor.[13], **bry.**, cact., **CALC.,**
calc-f.[10], **CALC-S.,** calc-sil.[1'],
cann-s., carb-v., CARBN-S.,
card-m.[8, 13], cary.[11], caust.,

cham., chel., chen-a.[2], **CHIN.,**
chin-ar., chin-b.[2], **coc-c.,**
colch.[8, 13], convo-s.[9], crot-c.,
crot-h.[8, 13], **cycl.**, der.[11], **elaps,**
ferr., ferr-ar., ferr-i., **ferr-m.,**
ferr-p., **GRAPH.**, hell., hydr.,
ign., kali-ar., kali-bi., kali-c.,
kali-m.[1'], kali-p., kali-s.,
kali-sil.[1'], kreos., lachn., lact.,
lap-a., lepi., **lyc.**, mag-c.,
mag-m.[13], mag-s., manc.,
meny.[13], **merc., mez.,**
morph.[7, 8], **MUR-AC.**, nat-ar.,
nat-c., **nat-m.**, nat-p., nat-s.,
nat-sil.[1'], nicc., **nit-ac.,**
NUX-V., ol-an., olnd.[13], op.,
PETR., phos., plan., **plat., ptel.,**
PULS., rad-br.[12], **rhus-t.**, ruta,
sabad., saroth.[10, 14], sec., sel.[13],
SEP., SIL., stront-c., **SULPH.,**
sumb., **syph., tarent.**, tep., ter.,
ther.[13], thuj., til., tril.[11], **tub.,**
upa., uran.[6], verat.[3], x-ray[9],
zinc., zinc-p.[1']

noon
ol-an., olnd.[13], sulph.

evening
sulph.

boiled
ars., calc.[6], chel., nit-ac.

dinner, during

nat-c.

fresh
thuj.[1, 7]

men, in[9]

x-ray

menses, during

plat.

pickled[6]
carb-v.

roast[3]
ptel.

smell of[11]
ars.

soup[3]
arn., cham., rhus-t.

spicy[7]
mag-c.

thinking of it, while
.

GRAPH.

desire
abies-c., aloe, anth.[11], aur.,
bell-p.[9], **calc.[7]**, **calc-p.**[3, 8, 10, 13],
canth., caust.[3], coca[3, 11], cocc.[3],
cycl., erig.[10], ferr., **ferr-m.**,
graph., hell., hydr.[13],
iod., **kreos., lil-t., mag-c.,**
mand.[9, 10, 14], med.[7], **meny.,**
merc., morph.[11], nat-m.,
nit-ac.[6], **nux-v.[7]**, sabad., sanic.,
staph.[7],sulph.[1, 7], thiop.[14], tub.,
viol-o.[3]

boiled[3]
caust.

children, in[7]

mag-c.

lean[3]
hell.

must have[7]

calc., nux-v., staph., sulph.

pickled[3, 6]
abies-c., ant-c., cori-r.[11],
hyper., **mag-c.[7]**

smoked,
calc-p., CAUST., kreos., **TUB.**

supper, at[11]

graph.

melons agg.

ars.[6, 7], fl-ac.[3], puls.[6], zing.[3, 6-8]

ailments from[12]

zing.

aversion [5, 7]
ars., chin., verat., zing.[13]

desire[6]
puls.

milk agg.

AETH., alum., alum-p.[1'],
alum-sil.[1'], alumn.[2], **ambr.,**
ang.[2, 3, 13], **ant-c.,** ant-t.,
arg-m., ars., ars-s-f.[1'],
brom., **bry., CALC.,**
CALC-S., carb-an., **carb-v.,**
carbn-s., **cham., chel., CHIN.,**
cic., **CON.,** crot-t., **cupr.,** ferr.[2],
hell., hom.[1] (non: ham.), ign.,
iris, kali-ar., kali-bi.[3], **kali-c.,**
kali-i., kali-n.[3], kali-p.,
kali-sil.[1'], lac-c.[10], **LAC-D.,**
lach., lac-v.[12], lact.[8], levo.[14],
lyc., mag-f.[10], **MAG-M.,**
merc.[1'], **nat-ar., nat-c., nat-m.,**
nat-p., **nat-s.,** nat-sil.[1'], **nicc.**[2, 8],
NIT-AC., nux-m., **nux-v.,**
ol-j., past.[12], **phos.,** podo.[8],
psor., puls., rheum[8], rhus-t.,
sabin., samb., **SEP.,** sil., spong.,
STAPH.[5, 7], stram., sul-ac.,
SULPH., valer., **zinc.,** zinc-p.[1']

cold[1']

hot[13]
  bry.

mother's[1', 3]

  cina[3], nat-c., SIL.

warm
  ambr.

ailments from[12]

  hom., mag-c., nat-c., nat-p.,
  nux-m.

boiled[12]
  sep.
cold
  calc-sil.[1'], kali-i.[12]

am.
  acon.[3], apis, ant-c.[3], aran.[14],
  arist-cl.[9], ars., chel.[2, 3, 6, 13],
  cina[3], crot-t.[3], ferr.[3], graph.[3],
  iod., lact.[13], merc.[3], mez.,
  ph-ac.[3], rhus-t.[3], ruta, squil.[3],
  staph.[3], verat.

hot[2]
  crot-t.

warm
  chel., graph.[1']

aversion.
  acon.l.[11], aeth., alum-p.[1'],
  am-c., ammc.[11], ant-t., arn.,
  ars.[3], bell., bov.[3], bry., cact.[13],
  calad., calc., calc-s., calc-sil.[1'],
  carb-v., carbn-s., carc.[7, 10],
  chin.[3], cina, con.[7], convo-s.[9],
  elaps[13], esp-g.[13], ferr.[1'], ferr-p.,
  guaj., guare., ign., iod.[3, 6],
  kali-i.[13], LAC-D., lach.[3], lec.,
  mag-c., mag-m.[13], merc.[3, 7],
  NAT-C., nat-m.[3], nat-p., nat-s.,
  nicot.[13], nit-ac.[3, 6, 13], nux-m.[3],
  nux-v., ol-j.[11, 13], past.[8, 13],.
  pers.[14], phos., podo.[13], puls.,
  rheum, rhus-t.[3, 13], sep., sil.,
  stann., STAPH.[5, 7], sul-ac.[3],
  sulph.

morning
  puls.

boiled
  phos.

cold[3]
  ph-ac., tub.

mother's
  ant-c., ant-t.[13], cina, lach.,
  merc., nat-c.[13], rheum[3], SIL.,
  stann., stram.

child refuses

  bor., calc., CALC-P., cina,
  lach., mag-c.[7], merc., sil.,
  stann.[7]

smell of
  bell.

desire
  anac., apis, aran.[14], ars., aur.,
  aur-ar.[1'], aur-s.[1'], bapt., bor.,
  bov., bry., calc., calc-sil.[1'],
  carc.[7, 10], chel., elaps, kali-i.,
  lac-c., lach.[3], lact.[13], lycps.[13],
  mag-c., mang., merc., nat-m.,
  nux-v., ph-ac., phel., RHUS-T.,
  sabad., sabal[3, 8], sabin.,
  sanic.[3], sil., staph., stront-c.,
  sulph., tub.[7], verat.[13], vip.[3, 6]

boiled
  abrot., nat-s.

cold
  adlu.[14], apis[3, 6], ph-ac., phel.,
  phos., rhus-t., sabad., staph.,
  tub.

hot
  calc., chel., graph., hyper.

sour
  ant-t.[3, 1i], mand.[9], mang.

warm
  bry.

mustard, desire for

ars., cic.[14], **cocc.,** colch., hep.,
lac-c.[2], mez., mill., nicc.

mutton agg.

bor.[16], lyss.[3], ov.

aversion
calc.[3], ov.

nuts, desire for

cub.

oil agg.

bry.[2, 3, 6, 13], **canth.[2, 3, 6],**
PULS.[1'-3, 6, 13]

onions agg.

acon-l.[12], alum.[3, 6], brom.[8],
kali-p.[3], **LYC.,** murx.[3, 6], nux-v.,
puls., sep.[3, 13], **thuj.[1, 7]**

ailments from[12]

thuj.

aversion
brom.[13], lyc.[13], nit-ac.[5], **phos.[13],**
prot.[14], **sabad.,** sep.[13],
thuj.[5, 7, 13, 16]

desire for raw

all-c., all-s.[13], bell-p.[9, 10], cop.[3],
cub., med.[7], staph.[5], **thuj.[3, 5, 7]**

oranges, aversion to[13]

elaps

desire
cub., elaps, med., sol-t-ae., ther.

oysters agg.

aloe, brom., bry., calc.[7],
carb-v.[3, 6, 8, 13], **coloc.[3], LYC.[1, 7],**
podo., puls.[3], sul-ac.

shell-fish

am.[3]
lach.

aversion
calc.[7], lyc.[13], **phos.**

desire
apis, brom., **bry., calc., LACH.,**
lyc., **LYCPS.[13],** nat-m., rhus-t.

pancakes agg.

ant-c.[3], **bry.,** ip., **kali-c., PULS.,**
verat.

paper, desire for[3]

lac-f.

indigestible

pastry agg.

ANT-C.[1, 7], arg-n., ars., **bry.[2, 3],**
carb-v., cycl.[3], ip., **kali-c.[2, 3, 13],**
kali-chl., kali-m.[3, 6, 8, 13], lyc.,
nat-s.[3, 6], **phos.,** ptel.[6], **PULS.,**
sulph.[3, 7], sumb.[11], **verat.[2, 3]**

sweets

ailments from[12]

puls.

aversion[2]
  ars., lyc.[13], **phos., ptel., puls.**[6, 13],
  sumb.[11]

desire
  bufo, **calc.**, chin., mag-m.[14],
  merc-i-f.[7], plb., puls.[1'], sabad.[3],
  sulph.[7]

peaches, after

    all-c.[8], **fl-ac.**[3, 6], glon.[3, 7, 8],
    psor., verat.[5]

  sensitive to the smell of

    all-c.

pears agg.

  bor., bry., merc-c.[3], nat-c.[3], puls-n.[7],
  verat.

pepper agg.

  alum.[1'], ars., **chin.**[2, 3], **cina,** nat-c.,
  nux-v.[2, 3, 7], sep., sil.

  desire for black

    lac-c., nux-v.[12]

  cayenne (red)

    merc-c.

pickles agg.[3]

  apis, ars., nat-m.[13], sul-ac., verat.

aversion
  abies-c., arund.[13]

desire
  abies-c., alum.[13], am-m.[13], **ant-c.,**
  arn.[13], ars.[13], carb-an.[13], chel.[13],
  cod.[13], ham., hep., hyper., ign.[13],
  kali-bi.[13], **lach.,** lact.[13], mag-c.[13],
  myric.[13], nat-ar., rib-ac.[14], sec.[13],
  sep.[13], **sul-i., sulph.,** verat.

plums agg.[3]

  mag-c.[3, 16], **merc.,** puls.[5], rheum[3, 11]

  ailments from[12]

    rheum

  aversion
    bar-c., elaps[2], sul-ac.[13]

  desire
    sul-ac.

  sauce
    arg-n.

pork agg.

  acon., acon-l.[12], **ant-c.,** ant-t.,
  ars., asaf., bell., **CARB-V.,**
  caust., clem.[3], **colch., CYCL.,**
  dros.[2, 3], **GRAPH.**[3], ham., **ip.,**
  nat-ar., nat-c., nat-m., PULS.,
  SEP., tarax., tarent.[13], thuj.

  smell of p. agg.[2, 3]

    colch.

  ailments from[12]

    puls. sep.

  am.[3, 6]
    mag-c.[2, 3, 6], nat-m., ran-b., ran-s.

aversion[7]
  ang., **colch.**, cycl., **dros.**, prot.[14],
  psor., puls., sep.[3]

desire
  calc-p.[3], **crot-h.**, **mez.**[3], nit-ac.[3, 6],
  nux-v.[3, 6], rad.[7], rad-b.[3], **tub.**

potatoes agg.

  alum., alum-p.[1'], **alumn.**[2], am-c.[3],
  am-m., **bry.**[2], calc., **coloc.**, gran.[3],
  mag-c.[7], mag-s., merc.[13], merc-c.,
  merc-cy.[13], **nat-s., puls.**[3], **sep.**,
  sil.[5], **sulph.**[3, 5], **verat.**

aversion
  alum., alum-p.[1'], camph., sep.[13],
  thuj.

desire
  calc-p.[3, 6], hep.[13], med.[7], nat-c.,
  ol-an., olnd.[3, 6, 13]

  fried
  raw

poultry, ailments from[12]

carb-v.

puddings agg.[2, 3, 6]

  ptel.

sweets

aversion
  ars., **phos., ptel.**

desire
  sabad.

pungent things, aversion to[13]

  fl-ac., sang.

---

spices

desire
  acon.[1'], ars., aster., caps.[3],
  caust.[1'], chin.[3], **cist., fl-ac., hep.,**
  lac-c., nat-p., nit-ac.[1'], nux-v.[1'],
  ph-ac., puls.[1'], **sang.,** sep.[1'],
  stry-p.[6], sulph.[1']

spices

rags, desire for clean

  alum., alumn.[13]

raw food, agg.

  ars., bry., chin., lyc., **puls.,**
  RUTA, Verat.

am.[3]
  ign.

desire
  abies-c.[3, 8], ail., all-c.[3], alum.[3],
  ant-c.[3], calc.[3], cub.[3], ign.[3],
  lycps.[13], sil., **SULPH.,** tarent.

  onions

ham
  uran-n.

potatoes,

  calc., cic.[1']

tomateos
  ferr.

refreshing things, aversion to[13]

  fl-ac., phos., rheum, sang.

desire
 allox.[14], aloe, ant-t.[3], **ars., calc.,**
 calc-f.[10], **calc-p.**[13], calc-s.,
 carb-an., **caust., chin., cist.,**
 cocc., fl-ac., hep.[3], iod.[3], mag-s.[14],
 nat-ar., **PH-AC., phos., puls.,**
 rheum, **sabin.,** sang., sars., sel.[3],
 thuj., til., **tub.,** valer., **VERAT.**

rice agg.[5]

 bry., puls., sulph., tell.[12]

desire for dry

 alum., mand.[9], ter., ther.[13]

rich, agg.

 ant-c., arg-n., ars.[3], **bry.,**
 buni-o.[14], calc.[7, 13], carb-an.,
 CARB-V., caust.[13], cupr.[13], cycl.,
 dros., ferr., iod.[13], **ip.,** kali-chl.,
 kali-m.[13], nat-c.[13], nat-m., **nat-s.,**
 nit-ac., phos., **PULS.,** sep., staph.,
 sulph.[13], tarax., thuj.

 fat
 heavy

 ailments from[12]

 kali-m.

rolls, desire for **stale**[16]

 aur.

salad agg.

 all-c.[3], ars., bry., **calc.,** caps.[3],
 carb-v., ip.[3', 6], lach., lyc., nux-v.[5],
 puls.[3, 5, 6], sulph.[5]

aversion
 mag-c.[7], prot.[14]

desire
 elaps, lepi.[11], lycps.[13],
 mag-s.[9, 10, 14]

salt agg.

 alum., ars., bell.[3], calc., **carb-v.,**
 coca[2], **dros.,** lyc., mag-m.,
 NAT-M.[3, 8], **nit-s-d.**[2, 8], nux-v.,
 PHOS., puls.[3], **sel.,** sil.[3]

ailments from[12]

 carb-v., nat-m., nit-s-d., sel.

am.
 halo.[14], mag-c.[2, 3, 6, 13], nat-m.[3, 6]

aversion
 acet-ac., allox.[9, 14], bufo[3], **carb-v.,**
 carc.[7, 10], card-m., chin.[3, 6], **con.**[13]
 COR-R., cortico.[9], **GRAPH.,**
 lyc.[7, 16], lyss.[7], **nat-m.,** nit-ac.[13],
 phos.[13], puls.[3, 6], **sel., sep.,** sil.

desire
 acet-ac.[13], **aloe,** aq-mar.[6],
 ARG-N., atro., **calc.,**
 calc-f.[9, 10, 14], **calc-p.,** calc-s.,
 CARB-V., carc.[7, 10], caste.[14],
 caust., cocc., **con., cor-r.,**
 galin.[14], halo.[14], **LAC-C.,**
 lycps.[13], **lyss., manc., med.,**
 meph., merc.[13], merc-i-f.,
 merc-i-r., **NAT-M., NIT-AC.**[1, 7],
 pers.[14], **PHOS., plb.,** prot.[14],
 sanic., sel., sulph., **tarent.,**
 tell.[14], teucr., **thuj.**[1, 7], **tub.**[1, 7],
 VERAT.

and dainties[7]

 ARG-N., calc., carb-v., caste.[14],
 med., plb.

pregnancy, during[2]

 nat-m., verat.

sand, desire for

sil.[3], **TARENT.**

indigestible

sardines agg.[7]

fl-ac., **lyc.**

herring

desire
cycl., **verat.**

anchovies
herring

sauces with f., desire for

arg-n.[13], nux-v.[11]

sauerkraut agg.

arist-cl.[9], ars., **BRY., calc.,**
carb-v., **chin.,** cupr., hell., **lyc.,**
nat-m., **PETR., phos., puls.,** sep.,
verat.

aversion
hell., sulph.[6]

desire
carb-an., cham., **lycps.**[13]

sausages agg.[8]

acet-ac., **ars.**[3, 8], bell.[7, 12], bry.[3],
puls.

spoiled
acet-ac.[12], **ARS., BELL.,** bry.,
ph-ac., rhus-t., verat.[3]

ailments from[12]

bell.

aversion
ars.[13], puls.[7]

desire[13]
acet-ac., calc-p.[6]

shell-fish agg.

bell.[3, 4], carb-v., **coloc.**[3], cop.[4],
euph.[3], levo.[14], **lyc.,** phenob.[14],
rhus-t.[3], ter.[3, 6], **urt-u.**

sight of food agg.

ant-t., **COLCH., kali-bi.,** kali-c.,
lyc., merc-i-f., mosch., ph-ac.,
sabad., **sil.**[3, 13], spig., squil.[3].
SULPH., xan.

aversion
ail.[2], **arr.**[2], **ARS.,** caust.[1'], chin.[1'],
colch.[13], dig.[8, 13], lyc.[13], **merc-i-f.**[2],
mang.[16], **mosch.**[2], nux-v.[13], ptel.[3],
sep.[3], **sil.,** squil., stann.[13]

smell of food agg.

ars., bell.[3], **cocc., COLCH.,**
dig., dros.[3], eup-per., **ip.,**
lach.[3], merc-i-f.[3, 6], nat-m.[3],
nux-m.[6], nux-v.[3], osm.[3], ph-ac.[3],
phos.[3], podo.[3, 6], ptel.[3], sang.[3],
sep., sil.[13], stann., sul-ac.[3],
sulph.[3], **thuj.,** xan.[3]

sensitive to the

arg-n., **ARS., cocc., COLCH.,**
eup-per., **ip.,** lach., **SEP.,**
stann.

aversion
ars., bell.[13], caust.[1]', **COCC.,
COLCH.**, dig.[8, 13], **IP.**, lyc.[13],
nux-v.[13], **podo., sep.**, stann.[8]

smoked food agg.

calc., sil.

desire
calc-p., **CAUST., kreos.**, puls.[3, 6]

snow, desire for

crot-c.

soft food, desire for[11]

alumn., pyrus, sulph.

solid f., aversion to

aether[11], ang., bell.[3], bry.[3], **ferr.**,
lyc., merc., **staph.**, sulph.[3, 16]

soup agg.[8, 13]

alum., alumn.[2], chin.[5], kali-c.,
staph.[5]

aversion
arn., ars., bell., carb-v.[5], cham.,
chin.[5], **graph.**, kali-c.[13],
kali-chl.[13], kali-i., merc-cy.[3],
nat-m.[5], ol-an.[11], puls.[5], **rhus-t.,**
staph.[5]

desire
calc-ar., kali-chl.[13], ol-an.[11],
staph.[2]

*liquid
warm food*

sour, acids agg.

ACON.[3], aloe[2], **ANT-C.**, ant-t.,
apis[2], **arg-n., ars.**, ars-s-f.[1]',
aster.[14], **bell.**, bor., brom.,
calad., calc.[3], **CARB-V.**[3, 8, 13],
caust., chin., cimic.[3], cub.,
dros., **ferr.**, ferr-ar., ferr-m.[13],
ferr-p., fl-ac.[7], **HEP.**[3], ip.[13],
kali-bi.[2], kreos., lach., mand.[10],
merc-c., merc-cy.[13], merc-d.[3, 13],
nat-c., nat-m., **nat-p.**, nux-v.,
ph-ac., phos., **psor.**[13], **puls.**[3],
ran-b., **rhus-t.**[3], sel., **sep.**,
staph.[1], sul-ac.[3], **sulph.**,
thuj.[1]'

sensitive to smell of

dros.

ailments from[12]

nat-m.

am.[3, 6]
arg-m., arg-n., lach.[3], ptel.[8, 13],
sang.[8]

aversion
abies-c., arund.[13], **bell.**, chin.[13],
clem.[3], **cocc., con.**[13], dros.[8, 13],
elaps[13], **ferr.**, ferr-m., **fl-ac.**[13],
ign., kali-bi.[3], lyc.[13], mand.[10],
nat-m.[13], nat-p.[3], nux-v., ph-ac.,
sabad., sulph.

desire
abies-c.[8], **ACON.**[3], alum.,
alum-p,[1]', alumn., am-c.,
am-m., **ant-c., ant-t., apis,**
arg-n., **arn., ars.**, ars-s-f.[1]',
arund., bell., bism.[3], bol-la.,
bor., brom., bry., calc., calc-s.
calc-sil.[1]', carb-an., **carb-v.**,
carbn.[11], carbn-s., **cham.**, chel.
chin., chin-ar., **cist.**, cod.[8, 13],
con., conv., **COR-R.**, corn.,

cub., cupr., cupr-a.[11], der.[11],
dig., dor.[2, 11], elaps, erig.[10,]
eup-per.[2], **ferr.**, ferr-ar.,
ferr-m., ferr-p., **fl-ac.**, gran.,
HEP., hipp., **ign.**, joan.[8],
kali-ar., kali-bi., **kali-c.**,
kali-p., kali-s., kreos., **lach.**,
lact.[8, 13], lyc.[13], **mag-c.**, mang.,
med., merc-i-f., **myric.**[6, 8, 11, 13],
nabal.[11], **nat-m.**, **ph-ac.**[8], phel.,
phos., plb., **podo.**, psor., ptel.,
puls., rauw.[9], rhus-t., **sabad.**,
sabin., sec., sep., spirae.[11],
squil., staph.[2], **stram.**, stry-p.[6],
sul-i., **sulph.**, thea, ther., thuj.,
ust., **VERAT.**, ziz.

and salt[7]

arg-n., **calc.**, calc-s., **CARB-V.**,
con., **COR-R.**, med., merc-i-f.,
NAT-M., **PHOS.**, plb., sulph.,
thuj., **VERAT.**

and sweets[7]

bry., calc., carb-v., **kali-c.**,
med., sabad., sec., sep.,
SULPH.

pregnancy, during[2]

verat.

spices, condiments, highly seasoned food agg.

bism.[3], ign.[3], kali-m.[3], naja[3],
NUX-V.[2, 3, 7, 8, 13], phos., sel.[3],
sep.[13], zin.c.[3]

am.[3, 6]
hep., nux-m.

aversion[13]
mag-s.[12], phos., puls.[3, 6], **sang.**,
tarent.

pungent

desire
abies-c.[3], alum.[6, 8], ant-c.[3, 6],
arg-n.[3], **ars.**[3], aster.[2, 11], calc-f.[9],
calc-p.[3, 6, 10], caps.[3], **carc.**[7],
chel.[3, 6], **CHIN.**, cic.[14], **fl-ac.**[1, 7],
hep., hyper.[3, 6], **lac-c.**,
mand.[9, 10, 14], mag-s.[9], meph.[2],
nat-m.[3, 6], nux-m.[8], **nux-v.**,
PHOS., puls., **sang.**, sep.,
staph.[3, 8, 13], stry-p.[6], **SULPH.**,
tarent., **zing.**[7]

pungent

starchy food agg.[8]

alum.[1, 7], bry.[7], **carb-v.**, chin.,
coloc.[1], lyc., **nat-c.**, nat-s.,
ox-ac.[1], sulph.

farinaceous food

aversion[13]
chin., lyc., **nat-c.**, nat-s., **sulph.**

desire
alum., atri.[7], calc., cic., **nat-m.**[13],
nit-ac., nux-v.

stimulants agg.[8]

agar.[1], ant-c.[1, 8], cadm-s., chion.,
fl-ac., **glon.**, ign., lach., led., naja,
nat-sil.[1], **nux-v.**[7, 8], op., thuj.[1],
zinc.

tonics

am.[8]
gels., glon.

desire[11]
alco., aloe[6, 11], ant-t., ars-s-f.[1],
aster., aur., aur-s.[1], calc-i.[1],·
caps.[7], caust.[3], chin.[6], crot-h.[3],
fl-ac.[6], gins., hep.[3], iber., iod.,

kali-i., naja, nat-p., nux-v.[7], **puls.**,
sol-t-ae., staph.[3, 6], sul-i.[1'],
sulph.[1', 6], sumb., tab., ziz.

strange things, desire for

bry., **calc., calc-p., chel., cycl.,**
hep., lyss.[13]**, manc., ter.**[2]

indigestible

pregnancy, during

chel., LYSS., mag-c.

strawberries agg.

ant-c., ox-ac., sep., thlas.[3]

aversion[5, 7]
chin.[5, 7, 16], ox-ac.[13], **sulph.**

sugar agg.[6]

arg-n.[1', 6, 7, 12], bell., **calc.**[2, 5, 7],
merc.[6, 8], nat-p.[8, 12], ox-ac.[1', 2, 6],
sang., **sel.**[1', 2, 6, 12]**, SULPH.**[2, 5],
thuj. zinc.

aversion[6]
ars., caust., chloram.[14], graph.,
merc., phos., rauw.[9], sin-n.,
zinc.

desire
am-c., am-m.[13]**, ARG-N., calc.,**
kali-c., lyc.[2, 6], op.[11], prot.[14],
sec., sulph.[6]

evening
arg-n.

sugared water

bufo[2, 7, 11], sulph.[11]

sweets agg.

acon., am-c., **ant-c., ARG-N.,**
ars.[3, 5], aster.[14], bad.[3], bell.[3],
calc., calc-f.[9, 10, 14]**, cham.,**
cina[3], cycl.[6], ferr.[3], fl-ac.,
graph., hep.[5]**, IGN., ip.**[2, 6, 8],
lach.[3]**, lyc.**[6, 8, 13]**, mand.**[9, 10, 14],
med.[7, 8, 13]**, merc.,** nat-c.,
nat-p.[3], nux-v.[5], ox-ac., phos.,
puls.[5, 6], sang.[3, 8, 13], sel., spig.,
spong.[12]**, sulph.,** thuj., zinc.,
zinc-p.[1']

delicacies

pastry
puddings

sensitive to the smell of[3]

aur., nit-ac., sil.

ailments from[12]

thuj.

am.
am-c.[14], bell.[3]

aversion
arg-n.[13]**, ars.,** bar-c., beryl.[9, 14],
caust., chloram.[14], erig.[14],
GRAPH., hipp., hippoz.[3'],
kali-c.[13], lac-c., lol.[8]**, lyc.**[13],
med.[7, 15]**, merc.,** nit-ac.,
nux-v.[5, 7, 16], petr.[13]**, phos.,**
puls.[5, 7], rad.[13], rad-br.[3, 7, 8],
rauw.[9], rheum[13], senec.[3]**, sin-n.,**
sul-ac.[13]**, sulph., zinc.,** zinc-p.[1']

desire
alf.[8, 13]**, am-c.,** aran-ix.[10, 14],
arg-m., **ARG-N., ARS.,**
ars-s-f.[1'], bar-c., bar-s.[1']**, bry.,**
bufo, cael.[14]**, calc., calc-f.**[9, 10, 14],
calc-s., carb-v., caste.[14],
cere-b[11]**, CHIN.,** chin-ar., **cina**[8, 13],

coca[8, 13], **cocain.**[8, 13], crot-h.[8, 13],
elaps, ferr.[3], **ip.,** joan.[8], kali-ar.,
kali-c., kali-p., **kali-s.,** lil-t.[3],
LYC., mag-m., mand.[9, 10, 14],
med., meph.[14], **merc.**[1, 7],
merc-d.[3'], nat-ar., **nat-c.,**
nat-m., nux-v., onop.[14], op.,
petr., **plb.,** rad-br.[12], **rheum,**
rhus-t., rib-ac.[14], **sabad., sec.,**
sep., sil.[2], **SULPH., tub.,**
x-ray[9, 14]

dainties[7]
  acon-l., arg-n., calc.

and salt[7]

  ARG-N., calc., carb-v.,
  caste.[14], **med., plb.**

and sour[7]

  bry., **calc., carb-v., kali-c.,**
  med., sabad., sec., sep.,
  SULPH.

tea agg.

abies-c.[13], **abies-n.**[3, 8, 12], **aesc.,**
agar.[3], ars.[3], aur-m.[1', 2], cham.[3, 6],
chin., cocc.[3, 6], coff., dios., **ferr.,**
fl-ac.[1'], hep.[3], kali-bi.[3], kali-hp.[8],
lach., lob.[8, 12, 13], **nux-v.**[1', 7, 8, 12, 13],
ph-ac.[3], puls.[3, 8, 13], **rhus-t.**[2, 12],
rumx., **SEL., SEP.**[2, 3], spig.[3],
thuj., verat.

ailments from[12]

abies-n., **chin.,** cocc., dios., lob.,
nux-v., sel., stroph-h., thuj.

am.
  carb-ac., dig., ferr., kali-bi.[3, 6],
  pyrus[13]

aversion
  carb-ac., carb-an.[13], chin.[13],
  dios.[13], ferr-m[13], kali-hp.[13], **phos**
  sel.[13], thea, thuj.[13]

desire
  alum.[8], aster., calc-s., **chin.**[5, 7],
  hep., hydr., lepi.[11], nux-v.[5, 7],
  puls.[7], pyrus, sel.[3 6], thuj.[7]

grounds
  alum.

  indigestible

thought of food agg.[3]

arg-n., bor., cann-s., carb-v., dros.,
graph., lach., lil-t., nat-m., **puls.,**
sars., **sep.,** thuj.

tomatoes agg.[3]

  lith-c., ox-ac.[1'], phos.

desire[7, 13]
  ferr.

tonics agg.[13]

  carb-ac.

  stimulants

aversion[13]
  sul-ac.

desire
  aloe, carb-ac., carb-an., caust.,
  cocc., nux-v., **rhus-t., ph-ac.,**
  puls, rheum, sul-ac., **valer.**

turnips agg.

  bry., calc-ar., **lyc., puls.,** sulph.[5]

aversion
  bry.[7, 16], puls.[13], sulph.[5, 7, 16]

veal agg.

ars., **calc.**, **caust.**, chin., **IP.,**
KALI-N., nux-v., **sep.**, sulph.,
verat., **zinc.**

ailments from[12]

kali-n.

aversion
merc.[3], phel., **zinc.**

vegetables agg.

alum., ars., **bry.**, calc.[7], cupr.,
hell., hydr.[2, 6, 8], **kali-c.**[2], lyc.,
mag-c.[2], **nat-c.**, **NAT-S.**,
petr.[3], verat.

decayed
carb-an.[2, 12], **CARB-V.**

aversion
bell., **hell.**, hydr., lyss.[13], **mag-c.**,
mag-m.[2], ruta

desire
abies-c.[8], adel.[11], all-c.[3], **alum.**,
alumn., ars., asar.[14], calc-s.,
carb-an., cham., **lycps.**[13],
m∍g-c.[1], **mag-m.**, onos.[13]

vinegar agg.

acon.[3, 6], aloe, alum.[1'],
ANT-C., ars., **bell.**, bor.,
calad., **carb-v.**[3, 8], caust., dros.,
ferr., ferr-ar., **graph.**[3], hep.[3],
kreos., lach., merc-c.[3], nat-ar.,
nat-c., nat-m., **nat-p.**, nux-v.,
ph ac., phos., **puls.**[3], ran-b.,
sep., staph., sul-ac.[3], **sulph.**

sensitive to the smell of

agar.

am.
asar., bry., ign., meny., op., **puls.**,
sang.[13], stram., tab.[6]

desire
apis, arn., ars., asar.[14], bell-p.[9, 10],
chel., **HEP.**, kali-p., lepi., puls.[7],
rib-ac.[14], **sep.**, sulph.

warm drinks agg.[13]

ambr.[2, 7, 8, 13], apis[1', 6], bry.[6, 8],
CARBN-S., chel., fl-ac.[1'],
graph.[6, 13], ign.[6], **lach.**[6, 8],
phos.[6, 8, 13], **puls.**[8, 13], pyrog.[6],
RHUS-T., sars.[1'], sep.[8], sil.[1'],
stann.[8, 13, 14], **sulph.**, verat.,
zinc-p.[1']

am.
alum., apoc.[1'], arg-n., **ARS.**,
bry., calc-f.[7], **carbn-s.**, **cedr.**,
chel., cupr.[6], **graph.**, guare.,
lyc., mang., nux-m., **NUX-V.**,
pyrus, **RHUS-T.**, sabad.[6, 8, 13],
spong., **sulph.**, verat.

aversion
bry.[13], caust.[13], **cham.**, **cupr.**[13],
graph.[13], kali-s.[8], **PHOS.**, **PULS.**,
pyrog.[13], rib-ac.[14], zinc-p.[1']

desire
ang., **ARS.**, ars-s-f.[1'], bell.,
BRY., **calad.**, carb-v., casc.,
cast.[11], cast-v., cedr., chel..
chin-ar.[1'], cocc.[3], cupr.,
eup-per., eup-pur., ferr.[3],
ferr-p.[7, 8], graph., hep.[1'],
hyper., kali-ar., kali-c.[14],
kali-i.[3, 6], kreos., **LAC-C.**, **lyc.**,
med.[7, 8], merc-c., pyrus, **sabad.**,
spig.[3, 8], **sulph.**, tub.[7]

angina pectoris, in[1]

spig.

chill, during

ARS., cedr., eup-per.

fever, during

casc., cedr., eup-per., lyc.

warm food agg.

acon., agn., all-c., alum.,
alum-p.[1'], alum-sil.[1'], am-c.,
ambr., anac., ang.[3], ant-t.,
ars.[3], asar., **bar-c., bell.,**
bism., bor., **BRY.,** calc.,
canth., **carb-v.,** carbn-s., caust.,
cham., clem., **coc-c., cupr.,** dros.,
euph., ferr., gran., guat.[14], hell.,
kali-c., LACH., laur., **mag-c.,**
mag-m., merc., **mez.,** nat-m.,
nit-ac., nux-m., nux-v., par.,
ph-ac., PHOS., PULS., rhod.,
rhus-t., sars., sep., sil., spig.,
squil., stann., sul-ac., sul-i.[1'],
sulph., thiop.[14], thuj., verat.,
zinc.

am.[13]
asar., kreos.[8, 13], **laur.,** lyc.[3, 7, 8, 13],
sabad.[1']

aversion
alum-p.[1'], **bell., calc., chin.,** cupr.,
GRAPH., guare., **ign., lach., lyc.,**
mag-c., mag-s., merc., **merc-c.,**
merc-cy[13], **nux-v.**[3], petr., **PHOS.,**
psor., **PULS., sil., verat.,** zinc.

desire
ang., **ARS.,** ars-s-f.[1'], **bry.**[3], cast.[3],
cedr.[3], **chel.,** china-ar.[1'], **cocc.,**
cupr., cycl., **ferr.,** kali-i.[3], **lyc.,**
med.[7], **ph-ac., sabad.,** sil.

soups
bry., **calc-ar.,** ferr., nat-m.,
phel.

soup

water agg.[13]

arg-n.[6, 13], ars., bry., calc.,
canth.[6, 13], chin-ar.[6], **cocc.,**
crot-t.,, dros., ferr-m., lach.,
lob., lyc., nux-m,., puls.,
sabad., sep., spong., stann.,
sulph.

seeing or hearing of[13]

lyss.

am.[13]
ars., **BRY.**

aversion.
apis, ars.[1', 13], **bell.,** berb.[1'], **brom.,**
bry., **calad.,** cann-i., **canth.,** carl.,
caust., cedr., chel.[13], **chin.**[1, 7],
chin-ar.[13], coc-c., coloc., elaps,
ham., hell., **HYOS.,** kali-bi.[1],
lach.[5, '], lyc., **lyss.,** manc.,
merc [13], merc-c., merc-cy.[13],
nat-m., NUX-V., onos., ox-ac.,
phel., **phys., puls., STAPH.**[5, 7],
STRAM., sul-ac.[5, 7], **tab.**[6], thea,
zinc., zing.[13]

cold drinks-cold water

wine agg.*

acon., acon-l.[12], agar., alum.,
am-m., **ant-c., arn., ARS.,** aur.,
aur-m., bell., benz-ac.[3, 6, 8, 13],
bor., bov., bry., cact., **calc.,**
calc-sil.[1'], carb-an., carb-v.,
carbn-s., **CHIN.**[1], chlol.,
chlor.[13], cob-n.[10], coc-c.,
COFF., coloc., **con.,** cor-r.,
des-ac.[14], eup-per.[1'], **fl-ac.,**
flav.[14], **gels., glon.,** hyos.[4],
ign., kali-chl., **lach., led.,**
LYC., mag-m.[14], **merc.**[2, 4], **naja,**
nat-ar., **nat-c., nat-m.,** nat-sil.[1'],

nux-m., NUX-V., OP., ox-ac.,
petr., phos.[16], prot.[14], puls.,
RAN-B., rhod., rhus-t., ruta,
sabad., sars.[1'], sel., SIL..
—staph.[3, 6], stront-c.,
sulph.[2, 3, 4, 5], thuj., verat.,
ZINC., zinc-p.[1']

champagne[7]

calc.

red[3, 6, 7]

fl-ac.

sensitive to the smell of

tab.

sour
ANT-C., ant-t., ars., ferr., sep.,
sulph.

sulphureted[2, 3, 7]

ars., chin., merc., PULS., sep.

ailments from[12]

coff., lyc., nat-m.

bad[12]

carb-v.

am.
acon., agar., ars., bell., brom.,
bry., canth., carb-ac., chel.,
chen-v.[2], coca[8, 13], cocc., con.,
gels., glon., graph., lach., mez.,
nat-m.[3], nux-v., onos.[3, 6], op.,
osm., phos., ran-b.[13], sel.,
sul-ac., sulph., thea

sour[2, 7]
ferr.

aversion
ACON.[13], agar., alum.[13], ars-m.,
carb-v.[13], carbn-s.[13], coff.[13], fl-ac.,
glon.[13], hyper.[13], ign., jatr.,
jug-r., lach., lact.[13], manc.,
mand.[9], merc., nat-m., nux-v.[13],
ph-ac., puls.[13], rhus-t.. SABAD.,
sil.[13], sulph., tub.[7], zinc., zinc-p.[1']

desire.
acon., aeth., arg-m., arg-mur.[11],
ars., asaf., bov., bry., calc.,
calc-ar., calc-s., CANTH.[13],
chel., chin., chin-ar., chlor.[3],
cic., colch., cub., eup-per.[1'],
fl-ac., hep., hyper., iod.[3, 6],
kali-bi., kali-br., kali-i., lach.,
lec., LYCPS.[13], merc., mez.,
nat-m., nux-v.[5, 12], op.[5, 13],
PHOS., puls., sec., sel., sep.,
spig., staph., sul-i.[3, 6], SULPH.,
sumb., ther., thiop.[14], vichy[11]

claret
calc-s., staph., sulph., ther.

FORCED through a narrow opening,
as if[3]

BAR-C., bell., bufo, carb-an., card-m.,
coc-c., cocc., dig., glon., lach., op.,
plb., puls., sulph., tab., thuj., tub.,
valer.

FOREIGN BODIES or grains of sand
were under the skin, sensation as if
small

COCAIN.

FORMICATION, externally

abrot.³, **ACON.**, acon-c.¹¹, acon-f.¹¹,
aconin.¹¹, aesc., aether¹¹, agar.,
agn.¹ʼ³, alco.¹¹, all-s., aloe³ʼ¹¹,
alum., alum-p.¹ʼ, alum-sil.¹ʼ,
alumn.², am-c., am-m., ambr., anac.,
ang.³, ant-c., ant-t., apis³, **aran.**²ʼ⁶,
arg-m. **ARG-N.**³ʼ⁶, **ARN.**, ars.,
ars-i., ars-s-f.¹ʼ, arum-t.⁷, arund.,
asaf., asar., aur., aur-ar.¹ʼ, aur-s.¹ʼ,
bar-c., bar-i.¹ʼ, bar-m., bar-s.¹ʼ, bell.,
bor., bov., bry., bruc.¹¹, bufo³,
cadm-s.¹ʼ, calad., calc., calc-p.,
camph., cann-i., cann-s., canth.²ʼ⁴,
caps., carb-an., carb-v., carbn-s.¹ʼ,
card-b.¹¹, **carl.**¹¹, **cast.**³ʼ⁶, **caust.**,
cedr.²ʼ³ʼ¹¹, cham., **chel.**, chin., cic.,
cina, cist., **clem.**, **cocc.**, **COLCH.**,
coloc., con., conin.¹¹, **croc.**,
cupr-s.², cur.⁷, dros., dulc., euon.⁴ʼ¹¹,
euphr., fago.¹¹, ferr., ferr-ma.⁴,
fl-ac.³, **gran.**, graph., guaj., guare.¹¹,
halo.¹⁴, ham.¹¹, hep., hist.¹⁰,
hydr-ac.², hyos., **hyper.**³ʼ⁶, ign.,
iod., ip., kali-ar., **kali-br.**³ʼ⁶, **kali-c.**,
kali-m.¹ʼ, kali-n., **kalm.**³ʼ⁶, kreos.,
kres.¹³, lach., lath.⁶, laur., led., **lyc.**,
m-arct.⁴, m-aust.³ʼ⁴, mag-c., **mag-m.**,
mang., **med.**¹ʼ, **merc.**, merc-c.,
merc-i-r.¹¹, **mez.**, morph.¹¹, mosch.,
mur-ac., nat-ar., **nat-c.**, **nat-m.**,
nat-p., nat-sil.¹ʼ, nit-ac., nit-s-d.¹¹,
nux-m., **NUX-V.**, ol-an.³, ol-j.¹¹,
olnd., onos., op., pall., par., petr.³ʼ⁶,
ph-ac., **phos.**, phys.⁶, **pic-ac.**, **PLAT.**,
plb., **puls.**, **ran-b.**, ran-s., rheum,
rhod., RHUS-T., rumx.³ʼ¹¹, **sabad.**,
sabin., samb., sars., **SEC.**, sel.,
seneg., **SEP.**, sil., **SPIG.**, spong.,
squil.⁴, stann., staph., stram.,
stront-c., sul-ac., sul-i.¹ʼ, **sulph.**,
tab.³ʼ⁶ʼ¹¹, tarax., **tarent.**, teucr.,
thuj., tub.¹ʼ, urt-u., valer., verat.,
verb., viol-t., **visc.**³ʼ⁶, **zinc.**, zinc-p.¹ʼ

internally

acon., acon-f., agar., agn., aloe³,
alum., alum-sil.¹ʼ, am-c., am-m.,
ambr., ant-t., apis³, arg-m., **arn.**,
ars., asaf., bar-c., bell., bor.³, bov.³,
brom.³, **bry.**, cadm-s.¹ʼ, calc., **canth.**,
caps.³, carb-an.³, carb-v., caust.,
cham.³, chel., **chin.**, cic., cina³, cocc.,
COLCH., coloc., con.³, cupr., dig.³,
dros., dulc., euphr., ferr.³, graph.,
guaj., hep., hyos., ign., iod., **ip.**³,
kali-ar.¹ʼ, kali-c.³, kali-n.³, kres.¹³,
lach.³, laur., led., mag-c.³, mag-m.³,
meny., merc., mez., mur-ac.³,
nat-ar., nat-c., **nat-m.**³, nat-p.,
nat-sil.¹ʼ, nux-m., nux-v.,
olnd.³, ph-ac., phos., **PLAT.**, plb.,
prun.³, **puls.**, rheum, rhod.,
RHUS-T., **sabad.**, sabin., **SANG.**,
sec., sel., seneg., sep., sil., spig.,
spong., stann., staph., sul-i.¹ʼ,
SULPH., tarax., teucr.³, thuj.,
verat.³, viol-o., **zinc.**, zinc-p.¹ʼ

bones

acon., arn., cham., colch., ign.²ʼ¹¹,
kali-bi.³, merc., mez.³, nat-c., nat-m.,
nux-v., ph-ac., plat., **plb.**, puls.,
rhod., **rhus-t.**, sabad., sec., **sep.**,
spig., sulph., zinc.

emissions, after seminal¹⁶

mez.

glands

acon., **arn.**, bell., calc., cann-s.,
canth., **CON.**, ign., m-aust.⁴, laur.,
merc., nat-c., ph-ac., **plat.**, puls.,
rhod., **rhus-t.**, sabin., **sep.**, **spong.**,
sulph., zinc.

painful sensation of crawling through whole body if he knocks against any part

spig.

suffering parts, of[16]

con.

FROSTBITE, ailments from[12]

zinc.

FULL feeling **externally**

aesc., aloe[1'], ars., aur., aur-m., caust., kali-n., laur., nux-m., par., phos., sul-i.[1'], verat.

blood-vessels, of[3]

ham., sang.

internally

ACON., AESC., agar., aloe[3], alum., alum-sil.[1'], am-c., am-m., aml-ns., anac., ant-c., **ant-t., apis,** arg-n.[3], **arn.,** ars., **asaf., asar.,** aur., aur-m.[1'], aur-s.[1'], **bar-c.,** bar-i.[1'], bar-m., bar-s.[1'], **bell.,** bor., bov., **bry.,** cact., calc., calc-i., calc-s.[1'], calc-sil.[1'], camph., cann-i., cann-s., **canth., caps., carb-an., carb-v., carbn-s.,** caust., cench.[1'], **cham.,** chel., **CHIN.,** cic., **CIMIC.,** coc-c.[11], cocc., coff.,

colch., coloc., com., **con.,** conv.[3], croc., **crot-t., cycl., dig.,** dirc.[11], **ferr.,** ferr-ar.[1'], gels.[3], **GLON., graph.,** guaj., halo.[14], **ham., hell.,** hyos., ign., iod., **iris, kali-c.,** kali-m.[1'], **kali-n.,** kreos., lach., laur., led., **lil-t.[3],** lob.[3], **lyc.,** mag-c., mag-m., mang., **MELI.,** meny., merc., mez., **MOSCH.,** mur-ac., **nat-ar.,** nat-c., nat-m., nat-s.[1', 3], **nit-ac., nux-m., nux-v.,** olnd., op., par., petr., ph-ac., **PHOS.,** phys.[11], **phyt.,** plat., plb., **psor., puls., ran-s.,** rheum, rhod., **RHUS-T.,** ruta, sabad., **sabin.,** sars., **sep.,** sil., spig., spong., stann., staph., stict., stront-c., sul-ac., sul-i.[1'], **SULPH.,** thuj., **valer.,** verat., verat-v., verb., vip.[6], zinc.

playing piano, after[1]

anac.

GAIT REELING, staggering, tottering and wavering[3]

acet-ac.[11], acon.[3, 6, 8], **AGAR.[3, 4, 6, 8, 11],** agro.[8], ail., **alum.[3, 6],** am-c.[4], anan.[2], ang.[8], ant-c., **arg-m.[3, 8],** arn., ars.[3, 11], ars-s-f.[2], **asar.[3, 8, 11],** aster.[8], astra-m.[8], aur., aur-s.[2], **BELL.[3, 4, 6, 8, 11],** bov., **BRY.[2, 3, 11],** calc., calc-p.[8, 11], **camph.,** cann-s.[3, 4], canth., **caps.,** carb-an., carb-v.[3, 11], **carbn-s.[8], CAUST.[3, 4, 6, 8,]** cham., chel., chin.[2, 3], cic.[3, 11], **COCC.[3, 4, 6, 8], coff.,** colch.[3, 8], **con.[3, 6, 8, 11],** croc., crot-h.[2], cupr.[3, 4], cupr-ar.[6], cycl., dig.[6], dros.[3, 11], dub-m.[8], dulc., euph., ferr., **gels.[3, 8], glon.[2, 3],** graph., hell.[3, 4], helo.[8], hydr-ac.[2, 4], hydrc.[6], **hyos.[3, 6], ign.[3, 4, 6, 8],** ip., kali-br.[3, 6], kali-c., kali-n., lac-ac.[8], lach.[4], lact.[11], **lath.[8], laur.,** led., lil-t.[8, 11], lol.[3, 6, 8], lyc.[11], mag-c., **mag-m.[3, 4],** mag-s.[6], mang.[3, 8],

merc.[3, 8, 11], **mez.**, morph.[11], mosch.,
mur-ac.[3, 8], **mygal.**[8], naja[11],
nat-c.[3, 6, 8, 11], nat-m.[3, 4, 6], nit-ac.,
nux-m.[3, 8], **NUX-V.**[3, 8], **olnd.**, onos.[3, 8],
OP.[3, 4, 6], **oxyt.**[8], paeon.[8], par.,
petr.[3, 4, 6], **ph-ac.**[3, 4, 6, 11], **phos.**[3, 11],
phys.[11], phyt.[2], pic-ac., plat.[4], plb.,
prun.[4, 6], puls., rheum, **rhod.**[3, 4, 6],
RHUS-T.[3, 4, 6, 11], ruta[3, 4, 6], sabad.[3, 4, 6],
samb., sars., **sec.**[3, 4], seneg., sep., **sil.**,
spig., spong., **STRAM.**[2-4, 6, 11],
stront-c., sulph.[3, 11], tab., tanac.[11],
tarax.[3, 11], teucr.[3, 4, 6], **thuj.**[3, 4, 11],
valer., **VERAT.**[3, 4], **verat-v.**, verb.[3, 4],
viol-o., viol-t.[3, 11], vip.[3, 4], visc., zinc.

gangrene see blackness

GLANDERS

acon.[8], **ars.**, calc., chin-s.[8], **crot-h.**[8],
hep.[8], hippoz.[8, 12], **kali-bi.**[8, 12], lach.[8, 12],
merc.[8], ph-ac., phos.[8], sep.[8], sil.[8],
sulph., thuj.[8]

GONORRHOEA, suppressed

acon.[3], agn., ant-t.[8], aur., benz-ac.,
brom., **calc.**, **CANTH.**[2], **chel.**[2], **clem.**,
coca[2], crot-h., daph., graph.[8], kali-i.[8],
kalm., **MED.**, merc., mez.,
NAT-S.[1', 2, 7, 8, 12], **nit-ac.**, phyt.[3],
psor.[8], **puls.**, sars., sel.[3], sep.[1'], sil.[1'],
staph., **SULPH.**[2, 3, 7], **THUJ.**, verat.,
viol-t.[2, 12], x-ray[8], zinc.

sycosis

GOOD HEALTH before paroxysms[7]

bry., carc., helon., nat-m.[3], phos.[3],
psor., sep.[3]

GROWTH in length too fast[8]*

calc.[7, 8], **calc-p.**, ferr.[3], ferr-a., iod.[3],
irid., kreos., **ph-ac.**[3, 8], **phos.**[3, 8]

children-growing

pains-growing

weakness-growing

young people, in[2]

hippoz., kreos.[12], **ph-ac.**[2, 12], **PHOS.**

HAEMORRHAGE

abies-n.[12], acal.[8], acet-ac., acon.,
adren.[6, 8], agar.[3, 4, 6], alet.[1'], aln.[12],
aloe, **alum.**, alumn.[8, 12], am-c.,
am-caust.[10], am-m.[4], ambr., **ammc.**[2],
anac.[3, 4], **ant-c.**, ant-t.[3, 4], anthraci.[8],
apis, apoc.[1', 6], **aran.**, arg-m.[4],
arg-n., **ARN.**, **ars.**, ars-h.[8], ars-i.,
arum-t.[6], asaf.[1', 4, 11], asar.[3, 4], aur.[12],
aur-m.[12], bapt.[6], **bar-c.**, bar-i.[1'],
bar-m., **BELL.**, bell-p.[6, 10], bism.[3, 4],
bor.[3, 4], **BOTH.**, **bov.**, brom.[6], **bry.**,
bufo[2], **cact.**, **CALC.**, calc-f.[6],
CALC-S., calc-sil.[1'], cann-s.[3, 4],
CANTH., **caps.**, carb-an., **CARB-V.**,
carbn-s., card-m.[1', 12], casc.[2, 12],
caust.[3], **cham.**, **CHIN.**, chin-ar.,
chin-s.[4, 8, 12], cina[3, 4], cinnb., **cinnm.**,
cit-l.[12], clem.[3, 4], cob.[12], coc-c.[6, 12],
cocc.[3, 4, 11], **coff.**, coff-t.[7], colch.[3, 4],
coll.[12], **coloc.**, con.[3, 4], **croc.**, crot-c.[7],
CROT-H., cupr., des-ac.[14], dig.,
dor.[6, 7], **dros.**, dulc., **elaps**, equis.[10],
erech.[7, 8, 12], ergot.[8, 12], **ERIG.**,
erod.[12], euphr.[3, 4], eupi.[12], **FERR.**,
ferr-ar., **ferr-i.**, **ferr-m.**[2, 12], **ferr-p.**,
ferr-s.[12], fic.[8, 10, 12], gal-ac.[8, 12],
ger.[8, 10, 12], glon.[10], **graph.**, **HAM.**,
HELL.[2], hep.[3, 4], hir.[7, 8, 10, 12, 14], hydr.[6],
hydrin-s.[8], **hyos.**, ign.[3, 4], **iod.**, **IP.**,

jug-c.[6], juni-c.[12], kali-c., kali-chl.,
kali-i., kali-m.[1'], kali-n., kali-p.,
kreos.[1], LACH., lachn.[2], l d., leon.[12],
lyc., lycps.[3, 6], m-arct.[4], m aust.[4],
mag-c.[3, 4], mag-m.[3, 4], ME .I.,
MERC., MERC-C., merc-c r.[8, 12],
mez., MILL., mosch., mur- .c.,
MURX.[2], nat-c., NAT-M., 1at-n.[6, 10],
nat-s.[6, 10], nat-sil.[8], NIT-A(.,
nux-m., NUX-V., op.[4, 8], p(r.[3, 4],
petr.[4], ph-ac., PHOS., plat plb.[3, 4],
psor., PULS., pyrog.[6], rat.[', 6, 12],
rhod., rhus-a.[12], rhus-g.[12], rhus-t.,
ruta[3, 4, 12], sabad.[3, 4], SABIN.,
sal-ac.[6], sang., sanguiso.[6], ars.,
scir.[12], SEC., sel.[3, 4], senec., SEP.,
sil., squil., stann., staph.[3, 4], stram.,
SUL-AC., sulfa.[14], SULPH., syph.[7],
tarax.[3, 4], ter., thlas.[6, 8, 12], thuj.,
til.[8], tril., urt-u.[12], ust.[6, 8], valer.[3, 4],
verat.[3, 4, 8], vib.[3], vinc.[4, 6], vip.[4, 6, 12],
vip-a.[14], wies.[12], x-ray[9, 14], xan.[8],
zinc.[3, 4, 6]

agg., slight h.[3]

bufo, **carb-an., chin.**, ham.,
HYDR., sec.

after h.[3]
CHIN., ferr., nat-m., ph-ac., sep.[1'],
sul-ac.[3]

ailments from[12]

senec., squil., stict., stront-c.

am.
ars.[3], bov., brom.[3], bufo[3], calad.[3],
card-m.[3], coloc.[3], ferr.[3], ferr-p.[3],
ham.[3], kali-n.[3], **lach.**[3], mag-c.[3],
meli.[3], sars., sel., tarent.[3], thiop.[14]

blood, acrid[4]

am-c., ars., bar-c., bov., canth.,
carb-v., graph., hep., **kali-c.**[3, 4, 6],
kali-n.[3, 4, 6], rhus-t., sars., **sil.**[3, 4, 6],
sul-ac.[3, 4, 6], **sulph.**[3, 4, 6], zinc

black[4]
am-c.[1', 4], arn., ars.[1'], asar.,
bapt.[1'], ben-n.[11], both.[7, 11], canth.,
carb-v.[1', 4], **chin., croc.,**
crot-h.[1', 3], elaps[1', 3], **ferr.**[4, 11]
fl-ac.[3], ham.[1'], kali-n., kreos.,
lach.[1'], led.[1'], **mag-c.**, mag-m.,
mag-s., nat-c., **nat-m.**[4, 11], nat-s.,
nit-ac., ol-an., op.[11], **puls.,**
sec.[1', 4, 12], stram., sulph.

bright red[4]
abrot.[3, 6], **ACON.**[2, 3, 6, 8], am-c.,
ant-t.[2, 4], **arn.**[3, 4], **ars.**[1', 2, 4], bar-c.,
bell.[3, 4, 6, 8], bor., bov., bry., calc.[4, 7],
canth., carb-an., carb-v.[3, 4],
chin., cinnm.[6], **crot-h.**[6], dig.,
dros.[2, 4], **dulc.**[2-4], erech.[7, 8],
erig.[3, 6-8, 10], **ferr.**[3, 4, 8], **ferr-p.**[2, 8],
graph.[2, 4], **ham.**[2], hyos.[2, 3, 4, 6],
IP.[2, 3, 4, 6, 8], kali-n.[3, 4, 6], **kali-p.**[2],
kreos., laur., led.[3, 4, 8], **m-aust.**,
mag-m., meli.[3, 6], **MILL.**[1'-3, 6-8, 10],
nat-c., **nat-m.**[2], nit-ac.[3, 4, 6, 8],
nux-m., **phos.**[1'-4, 6, 8, 10], plb.[3],
puls., rhus-t., sabad.,
sabin.[1', 3, 4, 6, 8, 10], sec., sep.,
sil., stram., stront-c., **sulph.**[3, 4],
tril.[2, 3, 6, 8], ust.[8], zinc.

with dark clots[3]

ferr., sabin., sang.

brownish[3, 4, 6]
ben-n.[11], bry., calc.[4], **carb-v.,**
con., ferr.[1'], puls.[4], rhus-t.[4],
sul-h.[11]

clots[4]
am-m., arn.[3, 4], ars.[1'], **bell.**[3, 4, 6],
bry., calc.[3], canth.[3, 4], carb-an.,
caust., **CHAM**[3, 4, 6], **chin.**[3, 4, 6],
con., croc.[3, 4, 6], erig.[8],
ferr.[1'-4, 8], ferr-p.[2], **hyos.**[3, 4],
ign.[3, 4], **ip.**[3, 4], **kali-m.**[1'-3, 6],
kali-n., **kali-p.**[2], lach.[1', 3],
mag-m., **merc.**[2, 3, 4, 6], **nat-m.**[2, 11],
nat-s., nit-ac.[3, 4, 6], nux-v.[3, 4],
ph-ac., phos.[1'], **PLAT.**[2, 3, 4, 8],
puls.[3, 4, 8], rat.[8], **RHUS-T.**[3, 4, 6],

rhus-v., **sabin.**[1', 3, 4, 8], sec.,
sep., **stram.**[3, 4], stront-c.,
sul-ac.[3, 6], sulph.[3, 11], **thlas.**[2],
ust.[3, 8], zinc.

dark[8]
    alum., anthraci., chin.,
    CROC.[2, 8], crot-h., **elaps,** ham.,
    kali-m.[1'], lach., mangi., merc.,
    merc-cy., mur-ac., plat., **puls.**[2],
    sec.[2], **sul-ac.,** ter., **thlas.,** tril.

dark[4]
    acon.[3, 4], agar.[3, 6], **am-c.**[1'-3, 4, 6],
    ant-c., anthraci.[7], arn., **asar.**[3, 4],
    bell.[4, 12], **bism.,** bov.[3, 6], bry.,
    canth.[3, 4], **carb-v.**[3, 4, 6], carbn-h.[11]
    carbn-o.[11], card-m.[3, 6], caust.[3],
    cham.[3, 4], **chin.**[3, 4], cocc., con.,
    croc.[3, 4], **crot-h.**[3, 6], cupr., cycl.[3],
    dig., dros., **ferr.**[1', 2, 4, 11], graph.,
    ham.[1', 3, 6], kali-m.[1'], kali-n.,
    kreos.[3, 4], **lach.**[3, 4, 6], led., lyc.,
    mag-c., merc.[3, 6], nit-ac.[1', 3, 4, 6],
    nux-m.[3, 4, 6], **NUX-V.**[2-4],
    ph-ac.[3, 4], phos., plat., **puls.**[3, 4],
    sec.[3, 4, 6, 12], sel., **sep.**[3, 4], **stram.**[3, 4],
    sul-ac.[1', 3, 6], sulph.[4, 11], **thlas.**[2],
    ust.[3, 6] verat.[3]

decomposed[3, 4]

    cic., **crot-h., lach., vip.**[4]

hot[3, 6]
    acon., anac.[11], **bell.,** dulc.[3], sabin.

non-coagulable, hemophilia

    adren.[6, 8], ail.[8], am-c., anthraci.,
    apis, aran.[2], **arn.**[3, 6], ars.,
    BOTH.[1, 7], bov.[6, 8], calc.[3, 6],
    calc-lac.[6], calc-p.[6], carb-an.[3, 6],
    carb-v., chin., chlol., chloram.[14],
    cortico.[9], croc.[6], **CROT-C., crot-h.,**
    dig., dor., **elaps, erig.**[1],
    FERR.[2, 6, 8], ferr-m.[6], **ham.**[2, 3, 6, 8],
    HIR.[7], ip.[6], **kali-p.,** kreos.[3, 6-8],
    LACH., LAT-M.[1, 7], led.[6],
    merc.[6, 8], mill.[6, 8], nat-m., nat-n.[6],
    nat-s.[3, 6, 10], **nat-sil.**[6, 8], **NIT-AC.,**

op.[11], ph-ac.[6, 10], **PHOS.,** puls.[6],
rad-br.[7], **sec.,** sil.[3, 6], **sul-ac.,**
sulph.[6, 11], ter.[2, 6; 8], vip.[3, 11], x-ray[7]

offensive[4]
    ars.[1', 4], bapt.[1'], **bell., bry.,**
    carb-an., carb-v., caust., **cham.,**
    chin., **croc.,** ign., kali-c., **kali-p.**[1'],
    merc., mur-ac.[3], phos., plat.,
    rheum, sabin.. sec.[1', 3, 4], sil.,
    sulph.

pale[3]
    apis[11], carb-ac., carb-an., carb-v.,
    ferr., graph.[1', 3], kreos., **phos.**[3, 11],
    sabad., sulph., tarent.[11]

ropy, tenacious[3, 4, 6]

    anthraci.[2], apis[2], **CROC.**[2-4, 6],
    cupr., kali-chl.[4], **kali-m.**[2], kreos.[3],
    lach.[3], mag-c., **merc.**[3, 6], naja[3],
    sec., ust.[3], verat.[3]

thick[4]
    agar.[3], bov.[3], carb-v., cham.[3],
    chin.[3], **croc.**[3], cupr.[3], **ferr-m.**[11],
    kali-n., kreos., lach., laur.,
    mag-c., mag-s., **nux-m.**[3, 4],
    plat.[3, 4], **puls.,** rhus-t.[3], sep.[3],
    sulph.

thin[3]
    ant-t.[11], ben-n.[11], both.[11], carb-v.,
    crot-h., ferr.[1'], ham., lach., laur.[3],
    nit-ac., phos.[3, 11], **sec.**[3, 12], sul-ac.,
    tab.[11], ust.

watery[4]
    alum., am-c., ant-t., **berb.,** bor.,
    bov., carb-v.[3, 4], crot-h., dulc.,
    ferr.[1', 4], **graph.,** hir.[12], kali-c.,
    kreos., lat-m.[12], laur., mang.[1'],
    nat-m.[1'], nat-s., nit-ac.[3, 4], phos.,
    prun., **puls.,** rhus-t., sabin.[3, 4],
    sec.[4, 12], stram., sulph.

mixed with clots[3]

    arn., bell., caust., puls., sabin.

climacteric period, in[7]

phos.

exertion, after

bell-p.[10], **mill.**, **NIT-AC.**[2]

exudates, hemorrhagic[2]

anthraci.

internally[3]

acon.[15], alumn.[2], **bell.**[3, 15], bry.,
cham., **chin.**[3, 15], cic., con., dulc.,
euph., ferr., ferr-p.[15], hep., hyper.,
iod., lach., laur., mill.[15], nux-v.,
par., petr., phos., plb., puls., rhus-t.,
ruta, sabin.[15], sec., sul-i.[1'], sulph.,
thlas.

mucous membranes, from[1']

calc-sil.

orifices of the body, from

anthraci.[7], aran., **BOTH.**, **chin.**,
CROT-H., elaps, **ip.**[1, 7], **lach.**,
PHOS., **sul-ac.**

passive, oozing[3]

ars-h.[11], bov., bufo, carb-v., **chin.**,
crot-h., ferr-p., ham., ph-ac., sec.,
tarent.[11], ter., ust.

vicarious[1']

abrot.[6], bry., ham., ip.[6], kali-c.[6],
phos., **sec.**

HAIR brushing back agg.[3]

carbn-s.[2, 3], puls., rhus-t.

combing agg.[3]

asar.[2], **bell.**[1'], **bry.**, chin., ign.,
kreos., nat-s., **sel.**

cutting agg.[3]

acon.[8], **BELL.**[2, 3, 6, 8], **glon.**[2, 3, 6, 8],
kali-i.[3, 6], lappa, led.[3], **phos.**[2, 3, 6],
puls., **sep.**

ailments from[12]

bell., glon.[6], kali-i.[6], led., phos.

distribution masculine in women[9]

cortico.

sensation of a

all-c.[3], **arg-n.**, **ars.**, bell.[3], caps.[3],
carbn-s., caust.[3], coc-c., croc.[3],
kali-bi., lac-c.[5], laur.[3], lyc., mosch.[3],
nat-m., nat-p., nux-v.[3], ptel.[3], **puls.**,
ran-b., rhus-t.[3], **sabad.**[3], **SIL.**, sulph.,
ther.[3], thuj.

touching agg.[3]

ambr., **APIS**[2, 3, 6], **ARS.**[2, 3], **bell.**[3, 6],
carb-v.[2, 3], chin.[3, 6], ferr.[3, 8], ferr-p.[7],
hep., ign.[3, 6], mez., nit-ac.[6],
nux-v.[3, 6], ph-ac., phos., **puls.**[3, 6],
rhus-t., **SEL.**[3, 6], sep.[3], stann.,
verat.[3], **zinc.**[2, 3, 6]

HAND on part **am.**, laying

bell., calc., canth., carb-an.[3], **croc.**, dros., **mang.**[1, 16], meny., mur-ac., nat-c., olnd., par., **phos.**, rhus-t., sabad., sep., sil.[16], spig., sulph., thuj.

magnetism

hand near part am.[16]

sul-ac.

agg.[16]
kali-n.

HANG DOWN, letting limbs, agg.

alum., am-c., ang.[3], bar-c.[3], **BELL.**[3], berb., **CALC.**, **carb-v.**, **caust.**, cina, con.[3], dig., hep., ign., lyc., m-aust.[3], nat-m., nux-v., ox-ac., par., ph-ac., phos., phyt., plat., plb., **puls.**, ran-s., ruta, **sabin.**, sil.[3], stann., stront-c.[3, 6], sul-ac., sulph., thuj., valer., **vip.**, vip-a.[14]

am.
acon., am-m., anac., ant-c., arg-m., arg-n., **arn.**, asar., **bar-c., bell.**, berb.[3], bor., **bry.**, calc.[3], camph., caps., caust., chin., cic., cina, **cocc.**, coff., colch., coloc., **CON.**, cupr., dros., euph., ferr., graph., hep., ign., **iris, kali-c.**, kreos., **lach., led.**, lyc., **mag-c., mag-m.**, mang.[3], merc., **mez.**, nat-c., nat-m., nit-ac., nux-v., olnd., **petr.**, phos., plb., puls., ran-b., rat.[3], **rhus-t.**, ruta, **sil.**, stann., sul-ac., sulph., teucr., thuj., verat., verb.

HARD bed, sensation of

acon., agar., alum.[3], **ARN., ars., BAPT.**[1, 7], bar-c., bry., caust., cham.[6], con., dros., eup-per.[6], euphr.[3, 11], fago.[11], **ferr., ferr-p.**, graph., hep.[4], ip., kali-c., lach.[3], lyc., mag-c., mag-m., manc., merc., **nat-s.**[3, 6], nux-m., nux-v., **op.**[1, 7], petr.[3, 7, 11], phos., plat., podo.[3], **psor.**[3, 6], puls., **PYROG.**[1, 7], **rhus-t., RUTA**[1, 7], sabad., **SIL.**, spong., stann., sulph., tarax., thuj., til.[3], verat.

HEAT, flushes of

acet-ac., **acon.**[1, 7], aesc., agar.[6, 11], agn., ail., **all-c.**[11], **aloe**[6], alum., alum-sil.[1'], **alumn.**, am-c., am-m., ambr., **AML-NS.**[1, 7], ang., ant-t., apis, apoc.[11], aran-ix.[10, 14], **arg-n.**[6, 7], arist-cl.[10], **arn.**, ars., **ars-i.**, arum-t., asar., aur., bapt., bar-a.[11], bar-c., **bell.**[1, 7], berb., bism., bol-la.[11], bor., bor-ac.[8, 12], bov., brom., bruc.[4], bry., bufo, buth-a.[9], **cact., CALC., calc-s.**, calc-sil.[1'], camph.[1'], cann-s.[4, 11], carb-an., **carb-v., carbn-s.**, carl.[11], **CAUST.**, cedr.[11], cench.[1'], **cham.**[1, 7], chel., chim.[11], **chin.**, chin-s., cic.[6], **cimic.**[6, 8, 10], cimx., **cina**[2, 7], clem.[11], **COCC.**, coff., **colch.**, coll.[3], coloc., corn., croc., **crot-h.**[1, 7], **crot-t.**[1, 7], cupr., cupr-am-s.[11], cyt-l.[10], dig., dros.[11, 16], dulc.[4], **elaps**, ery-a.[2, 7, 11], eucal.[7], eup-per., euphr.[11], fago.[11], **ferr.**, ferr-ar., ferr-i., ferr-p., fl-ac.[3, 6, 7], flav.[14], flor-p.[10, 14], frax.[7, 11], galin.[14], **gamb.**[1, 7], **GELS.**[3], **GLON., graph.**, guaj.[6], hep., helon., hura, hydr-ac.[7], hyos., **IGN.**[1, 7], **iod.**, ip.[1], **jab.**[6-8, 12], jug-r.[11], kali-ar.[1], **kali-bi.**[1], kali-br.[3, 6, 8], **KALI-C.**[1], **kali-i.**[1], kali-n.[4, 11], **kali-p.**[1], **kali-s.**, kiss.[11], **kreos.**, kres.[13], lac-ac., **LACH.**, lachn.[11], lat-m.[14], laur.[11], lil-s.[11], lipp.[11], lob., **LYC.**, lyss., m-aust.[4], mag-c.[4], mag-m., **MANG.**, med.[ε, 7],

MELI.[3], meny., meph.[6], **merc.,**
merc-i-r.[11], methys.[14], mit.[11],
morph.[11], mosch.[11], nat-ar., nat-c.,
nat-m., nat-p., **NAT-S.,** nep.[13, 14],
nicc-s.[8], nid.[14], **NIT-AC.,** nit-s-d.[2, 7, 11],
nux-v., ol-an.[6, 11], ol-j.[11], olnd., op.,
ov.[6, 8], **ox-ac., petr., ph-ac., PHOS.,**
pilo.[8], pip-m.[11], **PLAT.**[1, 7], plb.[11],
podo., **PSOR.,** ptel.[2, 7], **PULS.**[1, 7],
raph., rauw.[14], rumx., **rhus-t.,** ruta,
sabad., sabin., sal-ac.[6], samb.[4],
sang., saroth.[14], sec.[6], sed-ac.[8],
sel.[6, 14], seneg, **SEP., sil.,** sol-a.[1],
spig., **spong.,** squil.[6], stann.,
stront-c.[3, 6, 8], **SUL-AC., SUL-I.**[1'],
SULPH., SUMB., tab.[6, 11], tanac.[11],
ter.[7], teuer., thala.[14], **THUJ.,**
thyr.[3, 14], til.[11], trom.[2, 7], **TUB.,**
uran-n.[6], **ust.**[6-8], valer., verat-v.[8],
vesp.[8], vinc.[6, 8], vip.[11], visc.[14],
voes.[11], **xan.,** zinc., zinc-val.[6, 8]

weakness–heat

Vol. I: *anxiety–flushes*

daytime[11]

bar-c.[2], bism., bor., bry., **lach.**[2],
nit-ac., **petr.**[2, 12], **senec.**[2]

morning
bism., bor., ox-ac.[2]

eating, after

thuj.

forenoon agg.[11]

sabad.

11 h with hunger[2]

SULPH.

afternoon
ambr., bell., bor.[2], colch., con.,
fago.[11], laur., meny., **nat-p.**[1], plb.,
samb., **SEP.**

14 h[11]
ptel.

16–21 h[2, 7, 11]
arum-t.

evening
acon., all-c., arum-t., bor.,
carb-an., carb-v., **elaps**[1, 7], **lyc.,**
merc-c., nat-p., **nat-s.,** nit-ac.,
phos., **psor., SEP., stann.**[2, 7],
sulph.

19 h[11]
gins.

20 h with nausea

ferr.

20.30 h
arum-t., cimic.[11], cina, sep.

eating, after

carb-v , upa.[11]

falling asleep, before

carb-v.

night
arum-t.[2], bar-c., flav.[14], **kali-i.**[2, 7],
rhod.[2], **sep.**[2], spig., **sulph.**[2]

orgasme of blood–night

Vol. III: *sleeplessness–*
climacteric period

3 h[11]
fago.

feeling as if sweat would break out ·

bapt.

air, am. in open[11]

mosch.

alternating with anxiety[2, 7]

calc., dros., plat.

chills
acon., ang.[11], ars., asar., **calc.**[1, 7], **chin-s.**[1, 7], corn., iod., jug-c.[11], **kali-bi.**, kalm.[11], med., morph.[11], pin-s.[11], **sep.**, spig.

headache[2, 7]

lyss.

anger, after

petr.[2], phos.

back or stomach, from[1']

phos.

bed, in[11]

eupi.

chill, before

CAUST., sang.

after[2]
ail., cimx.,

chilliness, with

agar., am-br.[11], apis, **ars., carb-v., colch.,** corn., eup-per., kali-bi., lach., lob., **merc., petr.**[2, 7], plat., puls., sang.[2], sep., sulph., ter., thuj.

after[11]
corn., gast., gels., nat-p.[2, 11], nit-ac., **puls.**[2], rhus-t., sang.

climacteric[2, 6]

acon.[6, 8], **aml-ns.**[2, 6, 8, 12], **arg-n.**[2], aur.[6], **bell.**, bor-ac.[12], calc.[6, 8], con.[2], croc.[6], crot-h.[2], **dig.**, eucal.[2], ferr.[6], **glon.**[2, 6, 8], hydr-ac.[2], jab.[2, 6, 12], **kali-bi.**[2, 6, 12], **kali-br.**, kali-c.[6], **LACH.**[2, 6, 8], lyc.[2], **MANG.**[2, 12], nux-v.[6], ol-an.[6], ov.[6], ph-ac.[6], **plat.**[2], **sang.**[2, 6, 8, 12], **sep.**[2, 6, 8], **stront-c.**[6], **SUL-AC., SULPH.**[2, 6, 8], sumb., **ter.**[2], **ust.**[2, 6, 8], valer., vinc.[6], xan.[2], zinc-val.[6]

coitus, after[2, 7]

dig.

dinner, during

calc-s., nux-v.

after[11]
par., sumb.

downward

aesc.[2, 7], glon., sang., xan.[2]

down back[2, 7]

nat-c., sumb.

head to stomach

sang.

eating, while

bov.[2], calc-s., nux-v., psor.

after

alum., arg-n., carb-v., card-b[11], cinnb.[2], lach.[2], par., sumb., upa.[11]

am.[16]: chin.

emotions, from

lach., phos.

exertion, from least

alum., merc.[2], olnd.[2], sep., sumb.

fainting, with[2]

crot-t., SULPH.

headache, during[16]

agar.

leucorrhoea, with[2]

lach., lyc., sulph.

lying down am.

nux-v.[2, 11], thuj.[11]

menses, before

alum., ferr.[8], glon.[8], iod., kali-c.[15], lach.[8], sang.[8], sulph.[8]

during
nat-p.

mental exertion, from

lach.[2], olnd.

motion, from

helon.[1, 7], nux-v.[11], sep.[2, 7]

nausea, with[2]

merc.[2, 7], nux-v., sang.

palpitation, with

calc.[2, 7, 15], iod.[2], KALI-C., lach.[15], sep.[15], sul-i.[1']

perspiration, with

acet-ac., am-m., ant-c., aran-ix.[10, 14], aur., bell., camph.[1', 7], carb-v., chin.[7], cob.[2, 7], CON.[2, 7], hep., hipp.[7], ign.[2, 7], ipom.[2], jab.[6], kali-bi., kali-i.[7], kres.[14], lach., lyss.[7], nux-v.[6], op., ox-ac.[2, 7], petr.[15, 16], PSOR.[2, 7], sep., SUL-AC.[1, 7], sulph., ter.[2, 7], TUB., valer.[6], xan.

face and hands[16]

calc.

and anxiety
ang., kali-bi.

without[7]
LACH.

pregnancy, during[2, 7]

glon.[6], sulph., verat.

room, in[11]

helon.

running[1']

sul-i.

sleep, before[2, 7]

carb-v.

during
cham., nat-m., **phos.,** ran-b.[11], sil.,
zinc.

preventing the[2, 7]

psor., puls.

sexual excess, after[2]

dig.

sitting, on[16]

sep.

stool am., after[11]

agar.

upwards

alum., alumn., ars., ars-h.[2], asaf.,
calc., carb-an., carb-v., chin.,
cinnb., **ferr.,** ferr-ar., **GLON.,**
graph., indg., iris, kali-bi., **kali-c.,**
laur., **lyc.,** mag-m., mang., nat-s.,
nit-ac., **phos.,** plb., psor., **SEP.,**
spong., **sulph., sumb.,** tarent.,
valer.

from back[2, 7]

sumb.

from the hips

alumn.

vomiting, after[11]

tab.

walking am.[11]

fago.

walking in open air

caust., tarax.[11]

warm water were poured over one,
as if

ARS., bry., ph-ac., phos., **PSOR.,**
puls., rhus-t., SEP.

dashed over one

calc., cann-s., nat-m., phos.,
puls., rhus-t., sep.

water

when an idea occurs vividly

phos.

weakness, with[2]

phos.

after fl. of h.

dig.[12], **SEP.**[2, 7], **SULPH.**[2], **xan.**[7]

HEAT, sensation of

acet-ac.[1'], achy.[14], agar., agn.,
allox.[9], **alum., alumn.**[2], am-c.,
anh.[9, 10], ant-t., **APIS**, aran-ix.[10],
arg-n., ars., ars-i., asaf., **asar.**[2, 3, 6],
aur., aur-i., aur-m., bar-c., bov.,
bry., **calc., calc-i., CALC-S.,**
camph., CANN-S., canth., caps.,
carb-an.[3], caust., chel., chin., cina,
cob-n.[9], **COC-C.,** cocc., **COFF.,**
colch., com., **croc.,** cycl., cyt-l.[14],
dros., euph., **FL-AC.,** flor-p.[10],
graph., hed.[10], hell., hist.[10, 14],
hyos.[5], hypoth.[14], ign., **IOD., ip.,**
kali-c., **kali-i.,** kali-n., **KALI-S.,**
kreos., **lach., laur., LIL-T., LYC.,**
lyss.[10], mag-c., **mag-m.,** mand.[9],
mang., meph.[3, 6], **merc.,** nat-c.,
NAT-M., NAT-S., nit-ac.[3, 16],
nux-m., nux-v., oci-s.[9], ph-ac.,
phos., plat., psor., ptel. PULS.,
ran-b., rauw.[9], rheum, rhod.,
rhus-t., **sabad., sabin.,** samb.,
sars., **SEC., seneg.,** sep.[3], **spong.,**
staph., **SUL-AC., SUL-I., SULPH.,**
tab.[3, 6], teucr., thuj., **tub.**[1], valer.,
verat., zinc.

evening, in bed

bry., fl-ac.[1']

night
bar-c.[16], cham., con.[16], fl-ac.[1'],
nat-m., **phos.,** puls.[6, 16], rhus-t.[16],
sil., zinc.

alternating with sensation of cold[14]

hist.

ascending[9]

cob-n.

beer, after[7]

bell.

eating, after[1']

cycl.

eating warm food

carb-v., ferr., kali-c., lach.,
mag-c., PHOS., PULS., sep.,
sul-ac.

coughing, on[16]

squil., sep.

exertion, on

alum., squil.

hand has lain, where[16]

hyos.

nausea, with[7]

chel.

motion, at least[16]

squil.

rest agg.[14]

achy.

single parts, in[3]

apis, bor., par., ph-ac.

talking, on[16]

squil.

waking, on

BAR-C., fl-ac., graph., nat-m.,
sil., zinc.

walking, on[16]

samb.

bloodvessels, in

agar., am-m.[1'], ARS., aur.,
benz-ac.[7], bry., calc., hyos., med.,
nat-m., nit-ac., op., RHUS-T.,
sulph., syph.[1', 3, 7], verat.

vital, lack of

aesc., agar., allox.[9, 14], alum.,
alum-p.[1'], ALUMN.[1], am-br.[6],
am-c., am-m.[1], anac.[7], ang.[4, 6],
anh.[9, 10, 14], ant-c., ARAN.,
aran-ix.[9, 10, 14], arg-m., arg-n.,
arist-cl.[9, 10], ARS., ars-h.[2], ars-i.,
asar., aur., aur-s.[1'], BAR-C.,
bar-m., bar-s.[1'], bor., brom., bufo[1],
buth-a.[9, 10], cact., cadm-s., CALC.,
CALC-AR., calc-f., CALC-P.,
calc-s., calc-sil.[1'], calen.[7],
CAMPH., caps.[1], CARB-AN.,
carb-v., carbn-s., caul., CAUST.,
chel., chin., chlor.[2], chloram.[14],
chlorpr.[14], cic.[14], cimic., cinnb.,
CIST., cob-n.[10], cocc., colch.[6],
con., CROT-C., cupr-a.[2], cycl.,
cyt-l.[9, 10], dicha.[10, 14], dig., DULC.,
elaps, esp-g.[10, 13], eucal.[2],
euph.[4, 6, 16], FERR., ferr-ar.,
ferr-p.[1'], GRAPH., guaj., hed.[14],
HELO., HEP., hir.[14], hydr-ac.[4, 6],
ip., KALI-AR., KALI-BI., kali-br.[2],
KALI-C., KALI-P., kalm., kreos.,
lac-ac., lac-d., lach., lat-m.[9, 14],

laur.[1], LED., lyc., lycps.[2], mag-c.,
mag-m., MAG-P., mag-s.[10],
mang., med., merc., mez., mosch.,
naja, nat-ar., nat-c., nat-m.,
nat-p., nat-sil.[1'], nep.[10], NIT-AC.,
nux-m., NUX-V., ol-j., penic.[13, 14]
perh.[14], petr., PH-AC., PHOS.,
plb., PSOR., PYROG., ran-b.,
rhod., RHUS-T., rumx., sabad.,
sarcol-ac.[14], saroth.[10, 14], sars.,
senec., sep., SIL., spig., stann.,
staph., stront-c., sul-ac., sulph.,
sumb., tarent., thal.[14], ther., thuj.,
tub., v-a-b.[13, 14], verat.[1', 12],
vip-a.[14], x-ray[9], zinc., zinc-p.[1']

afternoon after siesta[16]

con.

and warmth agg.[7]

agar., ALUM., ant-c., APIS,
arg-n., ars-i., aur., bar-c., bor.,
BRY., CAMPH., CARB-AN.,
carb-v., CARBN-S., caust., cocc.,
dig., dros., dulc., GRAPH., guaj.,
ip., kali-s., lach., laur., LED.,
LYC., merc., MEZ., nat-c., nat-m.,
nat-s., ph-ac., phos., PULS.,
sabad., spig. staph., sulph., thuj.,
zinc.

climacteric period, during[7]

chin.

exercise, during

plb., sil.

nausea, with[9]

arist-cl.

walking, after

gins.

warm covering does not am.

asar.

HEATED, becoming

acon., am-c., **ANT-C., arg-n., arn.,
bell.,** bor.[3], **brom., BRY.,** calc.[3],
calc-s., calc-sil.[1]', **camph.,** caps.,
carb-v., coff., **cycl., dig.,** dros.,
dulc.[1]', **ferr.,** fl-ac.[3], gels.[1]', **glon.,
graph.**[7, 10], hep., ign., **IOD.,** ip.,
kali-ar.[1]', **KALI-C., KALI-S.,** lach.[3],
lyc.[1', 3], merc., mez., **nat-m.,** nux-m.,
nux-v., olnd., **op., phos., PULS.,
ran-b., sep., SIL.,** staph., **thuj.,
zinc.**

old drunkards

bar-c.

HEAVINESS externally

acon., **AESC.,** agar., agn., aloe,
alum., alum-p.[1]', alum-sil.[1]', am-c.,
ambr., ammc.[4], anac., ang.[3], ant-c.,
an-t., arg-n.[3], arn., **ars., ars-i.,** asaf.,
asar., aur., aur-ar.[1]', **bar-c.,** bar-m.,
bar-s.[1]', **BELL.,** berb.[4], bor., bov.,
BRY., cact., calc., camph., cann-i.,
cann-s., canth., caps., carb-ac.,
carb-an.[4], **carb-v., carbn-s.,** caust.,
cham., chel., **chin.,** cic., cimic.[3],
cina[4], clem., cocc., coff., colch.,
coloc., **CON.,** croc., crot-h., crot-t.,
cupr., cur., dig., dulc., euph., euphr.,
ferr., ferr-ar.[1]', **GELS.,** graph., grat.[4],
hell., hep., ign., iod., **ip.,** kali-c.,

kali-m.[1]', kali-n., kali-s., **kreos.,**
lach.[4], laur., **led.,** lyc., m-arct.[4],
m-aust.[4], mag-c., mag-m., **meli.,**
meny., **merc., mez.,** mosch., mur-ac.,
nat-c., nat-m., nat-sil.[1]', nit-ac.,
nux-m., **NUX-V.,** ol-an.[4], **onos.,** op.,
par., **petr.,** ph-ac., **PHOS.,** pic-ac.,
plat., plb., **psor., PULS.,** ran-b.,
rheum, **rhod., RHUS-T., ruta,**
sabad., sabin., samb., sars., sec.,
SEP., sil., SPIG., spong., squil.,
STANN., staph., stram., stront-c.,
sul-ac., sul-i.[1]', **SULPH.,** teucr.[3],
ther.[4], **thuj.,** valer., **verat.,** verb.,
viol-o., **zinc., zinc-p.**[1]'

internally

ACON., agar., agn., **ALOE,** alum.,
am-c., am-m., ambr., anac., ang.[3],
ant-t., arg-n., arn., ars., ars-s-f.[1]',
asaf., asar., aur., **bar-c.,** bar-m.,
bell., BISM., bor., bov., bry., calad.,
CALC., calc-sil.[1]', camph., **cann-i.,**
cann-s., canth., carb-ac., **carb-an.,
carb-v.,** carbn-s., caust., cham.,
CHEL., chin., cic., clem., **cocc.,**
coff., colch., **coloc., con., croc.,
cupr., dig.,** dros., dulc.[1], euphr.,
ferr., ferr-ar.[1]', **GELS., graph., hell.,**
hep., hyos., ign., iod., ip.[1], **iris,**
kali-bi.[3], **kali-c.,** kali-m.[1]', kali-n.,
kreos., **lach., laur., lob., lyc., mag-c.,
mag-m.,** mang., **meny., merc.,** mez.,
mosch., **mur-ac.,** nat-c., **NAT-M.,**
nat-sil.[1]', nit-ac., **nux-m., NUX-V.,
olnd., onos., op.,** par., **PETR.,** ph-ac.,
PHOS., plat., **plb., prun.,** psor.[3],
PULS., ran-b., ran-s., rheum, rhod.,
RHUS-T., ruta, **sabad., sabin.,**
samb., **sang.,** sars., sec., sel.,
senec., seneg., SEP., SIL., spig.,
spong., squil., **STANN., staph.,**
stram., stront-c., sul-ac., sul-i.[1]',
SULPH., tarax., thuj., valer., verat.,
verb., viol-o., viol-t., zinc.,
zinc-p.[1]'

morning[16]
kali-c., lyc., nat-c., zinc.

night[16]
mag-c.

menses, during[16]

kali-c.

sleep, after[16]

rheum

storm, before and during[16]

sil.

walking in open air, on[16]

nit-ac.

bones, of[3]

sulph.

muscles, of[9, 10]

mand.

high see ascending–high

HODGKIN'S disease, lymphogranulo-matosis[8]

acon.[8, 12], acon-l.[8, 12], **ars.**[8, 12], **ars-i.,**
bar-i., buni-o.[14], **calc-f.**[8, 9, 12], ferr-pic.,
iod., kali-m.[8, 12], nat-m.[8, 12], phos.,
saroth.[14], scroph-n., syph.[1', 7]

HUNGER agg.[6]*

anac., ars-i.[1'], chel., cina, graph.,
iod., kali-c., lyc., olnd., phos., sil.,
staph.

ailments from

alum., aur., **cact.,** calc-f.[10, 14], canth
caust., CROT-H.[1], ferr., GRAPH.,
hell., IOD., KALI-C., olnd., phos.,
plat., ⌐sor., rhus-t., SIL., spig.,
stann., SULPH., valer., verat.,
zinc.

HYPERTENSION[7]

acon.[6], adon.[6], **adren.**[6, 7], agar.[6],
aml-ns.[6], anh.[14], ant-ar., aran.[10, 14],
aran-ix.[10], arg-n., arn.[7, 10], ars., asar.[6],
aster.[14], **aur.**[6-8, 10], aur-br., aur-i.[6, 7],
aur-m., aur-m-n., **bar-c.**[6, 7, 10],
bar-m.[6, 8], cal-ren., calc., calc-f.[6],
calc-p., caust., chin-s., chlor.[11],
chloram.[14], chlorpr.[14], coff.[6, 7, 11],
convo-s.[9], cortico.[9, 10], cortiso.[14],
cupr., cupr-a., cupr-ar., cyna.[14],
cyt-l.[9, 10, 14], dig., ergot.[14], esp-g.[14],
fl-ac.[6], gels.[11], glon.[6-8, 10], **grat.,** ign.,
iod.[6, 7, 10], iris[6], kali-c., kali-m., kali-p.,
kali-sal., kres.[10, 13, 14], lach.[7, 10],
lat-m.[9, 14], lyc., mag-c., mand.[14],
methys.[14], naja[10], nit-ac., nux-v.[6, 7],
onop.[14], ph-ac., phos., pic-ac.,
pitu.[9, 14], **plb.**[6, 10], plb-i.[6, 7], psor.,
pulm-a.[13], puls., rad-br., reser.[14],
rauw.[9, 10, 14], rhust.[15], sang., **sec.**[6, 7, 10],
sep., sil., squil.[6], **stront-c.**[6, 7], **stront-i.**[6],
sulph., **sumb.,** tab., thal.[14], thlas.,
thuj., valer.[6], vanad., **VERAT.,**
verat-v.[7, 8], **visc.**[6-8, 10, 14]

HYPOTENSION[10]

acon., adlu.[14], agar., aran., chlorpr.[14],
cortico.[14], cur.[7], gels.[8], halo.[14], hist.[9],
lach., lat-m.[9, 14], levo.[14], lyc.[1'],
meph.[14], naja, nat-f.[9], rad-br.,
rauw.[9, 14], reser.[14], rib-ac.[14], staph.,
sulfa.[14], thiop.[14], thymol.[9], v-a-b.[13, 14],
verat.

INDOLENCE and luxury, ailments from[7]

carb-v., helon., nux-v.

INDURATIONS

ambr., **ant-c.**[3], **anthraci., apis**[2, 3],
arg-m., arg-n., arn., **ars.,** ars-i.,
ars-s-f.[1'], asaf., **aur.,** aur-ar.[1'],
aur-i.[1'], **aur-m., AUR-M-N.**[2],
aur-s.[1'], **BAD.,** bar-c., bar-i.[1'],
bar-m.[4], **BELL.,** bov.[4], **bry., calc.,**
CALC-F., calc-i.[1'], camph.,
cann-i.[2], cann-s., caps.,
CARB-AN., CARB-V., carbn-s.,
caust., cham., chel., **CHIN.,** cina,
cist.[3, 6], **CLEM.,** cocc.[4], coloc.,
CON., cupr., cycl., dulc., ferr.,
ferr-ar., fl-ac.[3, 6], **graph., hep.,**
hydrc.[2], hyos., ign., **iod.,** kali-c.,
kali-chl., kali-i., kali-m.[1', 3],
LACH., lap-a.[6], led., **lyc.,** mag-c.,
MAG-M., mang.[1', 3], **merc.,**
merc-i-r.[3], mez., nat-c., nux-v.,
op., **petr.**[4], **PHOS., phyt.**[3], **plb.,**
plb-i.[8], **psor., puls.,** ran-b.[3, 6],
ran-s., rhod., **RHUS-T.,** sec., **SEL.,**
SEP., SIL., spig., spong., squil.[4],
STAPH., stram., sul-i.[3], **sulph.,**
syph.[7], tarent.[3], thuj., valer.,
verat.

painful[16]

bell.

pressure, from[1']

sulph.

glands, of

aethi-a.[6], agar., agn., **alum.,**
alumn.[1', 8], am-c., **am-m.**[3, 6],

ambr., ant-c., **anthraci.**[2], **apis**[2],
arg-n.[2], arn., ars., ars-br.[8], ars-i.,
asaf.[2, 3, 6], astac.[2], **aster**[8], **aur.,**
aur-ar.[1'], aur-i.[1'], **aur-m.,**
aur-m-n.[2], aur-s.[1'], **BAD., bar-c.,**
bar-i.[1', 8], **BAR-M.,** bar-s.[1], **BELL.,**
berb-a.[8], bov., **BROM., bry.,**
bufo[3], **CALC.,** calc-chl.[8],
CALC-F., calc-i.[6], **calc-s.**[1', 2],
calc-sil.[1'] camph., cann-s., canth.,
caps., **CARB-AN., carb-v.,**
carbn-s., caust., cham., **chin.,**
cinnb.[2], cist., **CLEM.,** cocc.,
coloc., **CON.,** cupr., cycl., **dig.,**
dulc., ferr., **ferr-i., graph.,**
hecla[2, 8], hep., hydr.[1'], hyos., ign.,
IOD., kali-c., **kali-chl., kali-i.,**
kali-m.[1'], kali-n.[2], kali-sil.[1'],
lap-a.[6, 8], **lyc., mag-m.,** mang.,
merc., **merc-aur.**[6], **merc-c.**[2],
merc-d.[3, 6], **merc-i-f.**[2, 6, 8],
merc-i-r.[3, 6, 8], merc-sul.[2], nat-ar.,
nat-c., nat-m.[3, 6], nat-sil.[1'], nit-ac.,
nux-v., oper.[8], petr., phos.,
PHYT., plb., **psor., puls.,** raph.[4],
rhod., **rhus-t., sars.,** sep., **sil.,**
spig., **SPONG.,** squil., staph.,
SUL-I.[1', 3, 6], **SULPH.,** syph.[7],
thuj., thyr.[8], trif-r.[8], tub.[6], verat.,
viol-t.[2]

injuries, after

CON.

knotty like ropes

aeth.[3], **BAR-M.,** berb.[3], **calc.,**
cist., con., **dulc.,** hep., **iod.,** lyc.,
nit-ac.[3], rhus-t., **sil.,** sul-i.[1', 3],
tub.

nodes under the skin, like

bry., **calc.,** caust., mag-c., nit-ac.

sensation of small foreign bodies

cocain.

muscles, of

alum., **anthraci., bad.,** bar-c., **bry.,**
CALC-F.[1], carb-an., carb-v., **caust.,**
con., dulc., hep., hyos., iod., kali-c.,
kali-chl., kali-m.[1]', kali-sil.[1]', lach.,
lyc., nat.-c., nux-v., ph-ac., puls.,
ran-b., rhod., rhus-t., sars., sep.,
sil., **spong.,** sul-i.[1]', sulph., **thuj.**

INFLAMMATION externally

acon., agar., **agn.[4],** alum.[7], **alumn.[1]',**
am-c., ambr., ant-c., **apis[2, 3],** arn.,
ARS., ars-i., asaf., asar., aur.
aur-ar.[1]', bar-c., **BELL.,** bor.[1] (non:
brom.), bov., **bry., cact., calc.,**
calc-i.[1]', calc-sil.[1]', camph., cann-s.,
canth., caps., carb-an., carb-v.,
caust., **cham.,** chel., chin., chin-s.[4],
cina[4], clem., cocc., coff., colch.[4],
coloc., **con.,** cortiso.[9], croc.[4],
crot-h., crot-t.[4], cupr., cupr-a.[4], dig.,
dulc., **ECHI.,** euph., **euphr., ferr.,**
ferr-ar.[1]', **FERR-P.[2], fl-ac., gels.[2],**
gran.[4], graph., **gunp.[7],** hell., **hep.,**
hyos., ign., iod., ip., **kali-ar.,**
kali-c., kali-m.[1]', kali-n., kreos.,
LACH., lact.[4], led., **lyc., m-arct.[4],**
mag-c., mag-m., mang., **merc.,**
merc-d.[4], mez., mur-ac., myris.[3],
nat-ar., nat-c., nat-m., nat-sil[1]',
nit-ac., nux-v., op., **petr.,** ph-ac.,
phos., plb., **PULS.,** ran-b., **rhus-t.,**
sabad., sabin., samb., sars., sep.,
SIL., spig., spong., squil.[2], stann.,
STAPH., stram., sul-ac., sul-i.[3],
sulph.[2, 3, 4], tarax., teucr., thuj.,
valer., verat., **VERAT-V.[2],** zinc.

internally

ACON., agar., aloe[3], alum., ang.[3]
ant-c., ant-t., **apis,** arg-m.,
arg-n.[3], arn., **ARS.,** ars-i.,
ars-s-f.[1]', **arum-t.,** asaf., **aur.,**
aur-ar.[1]', aur-i.[1]', aur-s.[1]', bar-c.,
bar-i.[1]', **BELL.,** bell-p.[9], **berb.,**
bism., **BRY., cact.,** calad., calc.,
calc-sil.[1]', camph., **cann-s.,**
CANTH., caps., carb-ac., carb-v.,
cham., chin., cic., cina, clem.,
coc-c., cocc., coff., colch., coloc.,
con., cortiso.[9], crot-h., **cub.,**
cupr., dig., dros., dulc., **ECHI.,**
equis., euph., **ferr.,** ferr-ar.[1]',
FERR-P.[2], GELS., graph., guaj.,
ham., hell., hep., hydr-ac.[6], **hyos.,**
ign., **IOD.,** ip., **kali-ar., kali-c.,**
kali-chl., kali-i., kali-n., LACH.,
laur., lil-t., **lyc.,** mag-m., mang.,
MERC., MERC-C.[3], mez., nat-ar.,
nat-c., nat-m., nat-s.[6], nit-ac.,
nux-m.[2], **NUX-V.,** op., par.,
pareir., petr., ph-ac., **PHOS.,**
phyt., **PLB.,** podo.[6], **PULS.,** ran-b.,
ran-s., rheum, rhus-t., ruta,
sabad., sabin., samb., sang.,
sang-n., **SEC.,** senec., seneg., sep.,
sil., spig., spong., **squil.,** stann.,
stram., stront-c., sul-ac., sul-i.[1]',
sulph., tab.[6], tarent.[6], **TER.,** thuj.,
uva, **verat., verat-v.[6],** vip.[6]

blood vessels, of

acon., **ant-t.,**   **ARN., ARS.,**
ars-i., **BAR-C.,** calc., cham., **cupr.,**
ham., kali-c., kreos., lach., lyc.,
puls., sil., spig., **SULPH.,** thuj.,
zinc.

arteriitis[8]
ars., calc.[2], echi., hist.[14], **kali-i.,**
lach., **nat-i.,** sec., sulfa.[14]

phlebitis, milk leg

ACON.[3, 8], agar.[8], all-c., ant-c.,
ant-t.[2, 3, 12], apis, arist-cl.[10, 14],
arn., ars., bell., both.[7], BRY.,
bufo, CALC., calc-ar.[6], calc-f.[6],
carb-v.[3, 6, 10], carbn-s., cham.,
chin., chlorpr.[14], crot-h., ferr-p.[2],
graph., ham., hecla[14], hir.[14], hep.,
iod., kali-c., kali-m.[6], kreos.,
LACH., led., lyc., lycps., mag-c.[10],
mag-f.[14], merc., merc-cy.[12],
merc-i-r.[10]. nat-s., nux-v., phos.[8],
puls., rhod., RHUS-T., ruta[8],
sep., sil., spig., stront-br.[12],
stront-c.[8, 12], sulfa.[14], sulph.,
thiop.[14], thuj.[3, 4], verat.,
VIP.[3, 6-8, 10, 12], vip-a.[14], zinc.

injuries, after[6]

rhus-t.

bones, of; osteitis

acon., ang.[3, 6], ars., ars-i., asaf.,
aur., aur-ar.[1'], aur-i.[1', 7, 8], aur-m.,
aur-s.[1'], bell., bry., calc., calc-f.[3, 6],
calc-sil.[1'], chin., clem., coloc.,
con., conch.[7, 8, 11, 12], cupr., dig.,
euph., FL-AC., guaj., hecla[2, 7, 8],
hep., iod., kali-i.[7, 8, 11], kreos.,
lac-ac., lach., lyc., mag-m., mang.,
MERC., merc-c.[3], merc-sul.[7],
MEZ., nat-c., nat-sil.[1'], nit-ac.,
PH-AC., phos., phyt.[2], plb., psor.,
PULS., rhus-t., sep., SIL., spig.,
STAPH., still.[7, 8], stront-c.[7, 8],
sulph., symph.[2], thuj., verat.,

osteomyelitis[7, 8]

achy.[14], acon., arg-m.[14], bell.[6],
chin-s., conch.[11], des-ac.[14], gunp.,
ph-ac.[12], phos., sil.[6]

periosteum, of; periostitis

acon.[2, 3, 7], ant-c., apis, aran.[8],
ars., asaf., aur., aur-ac.[1'], aur-m.,
bell.[1, 7], calc.[1', 3, 8], calc-p.[3, 6],
calc-sil.[10], chin., clem.[8], colch.[8],
con.[3, 7, 8], conch.[11], ferr-i.[2, 7, 8, 12],
ferr-p.[2, 7], FL-AC., graph.[8], guaj.[8],
hecla[2, 7, 8, 12], hep.[3], iod.[8, 10],
kali-bi.[3, 7, 8], kali-l., lach.[3], led.,
mang., merc., merc-c., MEZ.,
nat-sal.[12], nit-ac., PH-AC.,
phyt.[2, 7, 8, 10], plat-m.[8], psor.,
puls., rhod.[8], rhus-t., RUTA[1, 7],
SABIN.[3], sars.[8], sep.[3], sil., staph.,
still.[7, 8, 10, 12], sulph.[3], symph.[2, 7, 8],
tell.[3]

bursae, of; bursitis[2]

ant-c., apis, ars., bell., bell-p.[7],
graph., hep., iod., lycpr.[7], puls.,
ruta[7, 12], SIL., stict., sulph.

cartilages, of; chondritis, perichon-
dritis

asaf[1], ARG-M., bell.[8, 12], cham[8, 12],
cimic.[8, 12], lob-s.[12], nat-m., olnd.[8, 12],
plb.[8, 12], Ruta[8, 12]

cellulitis[8]

apis[3, 8], arn., ars.[3, 8], bapt., bell.[3],
crot-h., graph[3], hep.[3], lach., mang.,
merc-i-r., myris.[3], rhus-t[1', 3, 8],
sil.[3, 8, 12], sul-i[3], sulph[3], vesp

chronic appendicitis[6]

bell-p.[14], but-ac.[14], coloc.,
iris-t.[6, 8], kali-c.[14], merc-d., plb.,
pyrog.[7], sil., sul-i.[6, 10], sulph.,
tub-k.[10]

hepatitis

adlu.[14], **arn., aur.**[2], **bell.**[2], cael.[14],
calc-f.[10, 14], **card-m., corn.,**
crot-h., flor-p.[10], **iod.**[6], kali-c.[6, 14],
lach., LYC., mag-m., mand.[10],
nat-c., **nat-m., NAT-S., nit-ac.,**
nux-v., phos., phyt.[2], **podo.**[2],
psor., ptel.[2], ran-s., sel., **sil.**[2],
stann.[10, 14], **sulph.,** vip-a.[14]

ovaries, of[2]

ars., bry., chin., cod., coloc.,
con.[8], graph.[8], **guaj.,** ign., **iod.**[2, 8],
lach.[2, 8], **lil-t., lyc.,** nux-v., **pall.**[2, 8],
ph-ac., **plat.**[2, 8], pyrog.[7], rhus-t.,
sabal[8], sabin., sep.[8], staph.,
thuj.[8]

prostatitis[8]

alum., anac.[14], arg-m.[14], **aur.**[6, 8],
bar-c., brach., calad., carbn-s.,
caust.[2, 8], cic.[14], clem., **con.,**
ferr-pic., graph., hep., hydrc.,
iod.[6, 8], **kali-bi.**[2], kali-c.[14], **lyc.**[6, 8],
merc., merc-c., nit-ac., nux-v.[2, 8],
phyt., **puls.,** pyrog.[7], sabad.,
sabal, sel., senec.[2], **sep.**[8, 10], sil.,
solid., **staph.**[2, 8], sulph., **thuj.,**
trib.

sinusitis[6, 8]

ant-c.[8, 10], ars-i., aur.[8], **calc.**[2, 3, 6, 8],
calc-f.[8, 10], calc-s.[7], cinnb.[6, 10],
eucal.[8], fl-ac.[10], hecla[14], **hep.**[6, 8, 10],
hydr., kali-bi., kali-c.[8, 10],
kali-i.[2, 6, 8], kali-s.[7], lyc.[3, 6],
mag-c.[10], mag-f.[10], mag-m.[10],
med.[10], **merc.,** nat-m.[3, 6],
nit-ac.[3, 6, 10], penic.[14], **phos.,**
puls.[3, 6], pyrog.[7], spig.[8],
SIL.[2, 3, 6, 8, 10], stann.[10, 14],
stict.[8, 10], **sulph.**[6, 8, 10], teucr.,
thuj.[8]

tonsillitis

alum.[6], **alumn., BAR-C.,**
bar-i.[6, 10], **bar-m.,** bar-s.[1'],
brom.[3, 10], calc.[6, 10], calc-i.[6, 10],
calc-p.[7, 8], con.[6], fuc.[6, 8], guaj.[7],
hep., ign.[2, 6], iod.[6, 10], kali-bi.[6],
kali-i.[3, 6], lach., lyc., mag-f.[10, 14],
nat-m.[3, 6], **NIT-AC.**[2, 6], **PSOR.**[1, 7],
sang., sep., **sil., staph.**[2, 6],
sul-i.[3, 6, 10], sulph., teucr.[6],
thuj.[3, 6, 10], **TUB.**[6, 7], v-a-b.[14]

gangrenous

ARS., bell., CANTH., carb-an.,
carb-v., chin., colch., crot-h.,
euph.[16], hep., **iod., kali-n.**[16],
kali-p., LACH., merc., **phos.,**
plb., rhus-t., **SEC., SIL.**

glands, of; adenitis

acon., ail.[8], **alumn., anan.,**
apis[2, 3, 8, 10], arn., ars., ars-i.,
ars-s-f.[1'], **aur.,** aur-ar.[1'], aur-i[1'],
aur-m., aur-s[1'], **bad., bar-c.,**
bar-i.[1', 8, 10], **BAR-M.,** bar-s.[1'], **BELL.,**
berb.[4], **brom.,** bry., bufo, **CALC.,**
calc-f.[10], calc-hp.[10], calc-i.[10],
calc-sil[1', 10], **camph.,** canth.,
caps.[3], **carb-an.,** carb-v., **cham.,**
cist., clem., **con.,** cor-r.[12],
crot-h.[2, 3], dros.[7], dulc., echi.[3],
ferr-ar., fl-ac.[10], **graph.**[3, 4, 8], **hep.,**
hippoz.[2, 12], iod.[8, 10], **iodof.**[8], kali-ar.,
kali-c., kali-i., kali-m.[2], kali-p.,
lach., laur., **lyc.,** m-aust.[4], mag-m.[4],
MERC., merc-c.[11], **merc-i-r.**[8, 10],
nat-s.[3], **nit-ac., nux-v.,** oper.[8], petr.,
ph-ac., **PHOS., phyt.,** plb., **psor.,**
puls., pyrog.[3], raph.[4], rhus-t., samb.,
sanic.[10], sars., scroph-n.[10], sieg.[10],
sil., sil-mar.[8], spig., spong.[1', 10],
squil., staph., still.[10], sul-ac.,
sul-i.[1', 10], **SULPH.,** tarent-c.[3], thuj.,
tub.[10], verat., zinc.

joints, of; arthritis

abrot.[3, 6, 8], **ACON.,** am-be.[6], am-c.[6], am-caust.[6], am-m.[6], am-p.[6], **ang.,** ant-c.[6], **ant-t.**[2, 6], **APIS,** aran.[10, 14], aran-ix.[10], arb.[8, 11, 12], arist-cl.[9], **arn.,** ars.[6], asar.[6], **aur.,** bar-c.[6], **BELL., benz-ac.**[3, 6, 8], berb.[6, 8], **BRY., calc.,** calc-p.[6], caul.[6], **caust.,** cham.[6, 12], chin.[6, 8], chin-s.[6], cimic.[8], clem.[6], **colch.**[6, 8], coloc.[6], conch.[11], cortiso.[9], crot-h.[6], cycl.[6], **dulc.**[1', 3, 6], elat.[8], eup-per.[6], euphr.[10], ferr.[6], **ferr-p.,** fl-ac.[3], form.[3, 6], **form-ac.**[6, 10], **gaul.**[6], gins.[6], gnaph.[8], **guaj.,** hed.[10], hep.[6], hyper., ichth.[12], **iod.,** kali-ar.[1'], kali-bi.[8], **kali-c., kali-i.,** kali-m.[6], **kalm., kreos., lac-ac.,** lach., **LED.,** lil-t.[8], **lith-be.**[6], lith-c., **lyc.,** mand.[10, 14], **mang.,** meny., **merc.,** mez.[6], **nat-m., nat-s.,** nat-sil.[8], nit-ac.[8], ph-ac.[6], phos.[6], **phyt., psor., puls.,** pyrog.[6], rad-br.[6, 8], ran-b.[6], **rhod., rhus-t., ruta,** sabad.[6], sabin., sal-ac.[6, 8], sang.[6], **sars., sep., SIL.,** solid.[8], spong.[6], **stel.**[6, 8], stict.[6], stront-c.[6], sul-i.[10], sul-ter.[8], **sulph.,** syph.[1'], tarax.[6], thuj.[6], tub.[6], ven-m.[14], verat.[6], verat-v., viol-t.[8], visc.[10]

arthritis deformans[6, 8]

abrot.[6], **am-p.,** ant-c., aran.[10], aran-ix.[10], arb.[8], arn.[8], **ars.**[3, 8], aur.[3], **benz-ac.,** cal-ren.[8], **calc.**[6, 8, 10], calc-caust.[6], calc-f.[10], calc-p.[6], caul., **caust.**[3, 6, 8, 10], **chin.**[8], **cimic.**[8], clem.[6], colch., colchin.[8], cupr.[3], euphr.[10], ferr-i.[8], ferr-pic.[8], fl-ac.[10], form-ac.[6, 10], graph.[6], **guaj.**[3, 6, 8], hed.[10], hep.[3, 6], ichth.[6], **iod., kali-br.**[8], **kali-i.,** kalm.[10], lac-ac.[8], **led.,** lith-be.[6], lith-c.[6], lith-sal.[6], lyc., mand.[10], mang.[6], merc.[3], merc-c.[8], nat-br.[8], nat-p.[8], nat-s., nit-ac.[6], onop.[14], **pipe.**[8], **puls.**[3, 8], rad.[8], rad-br.[3, 6, 10], rhod.[6], **sabin.**[3, 6, 8], sal-ac.[8], sars.[6], sep., **sil.**[6], staph.[6], sul-i.[10],

sul-ter.[8], **sulph.**[6, 8, 10], symph.[10], **thuj.**[6], thyr.[8], urt-u.[6], visc.[10]

lymphangitis[6]

aethi-a., all-c., **anthraci.**[6-8], apis[6, 8], arn., **ars.,** ars-i.[6, 8], **bell.**[6, 8], both.[6, 8], **BUFO**[6-8], **buth-a.**[9], carb-v., **chin-ar.,** croth-h.[6, 8], cupr.[7], **echi.**[6, 8], euph., graph., hep., hippoz.[8], iod.[7], **lach.**[6-8], lat-k.[8], **merc.**[6, 8], merc-i-r.[8], mygal.[7, 8], **myris.,** nat-s., **pyrog.**[6, 8], **rhus-t.**[6, 8,], sil., sulph., **tarent-c.**

muscles, of; myositis[8]

arn., bell., bry., ham[1'], hep., kali-i., merc., **mez., rhus-t.**

nerves, of; neuritis

ACON., aesc.[8], **all-c.**[8], **alum-sil.,** anan.[8], **ant-c.,** arg-n.[8], **arn.**[8], **ars., BELL.,** bell-p.[8, 9], ben-d.[8], berb.[8], **cact., carbn-s.**[8], caust., **cedr.**[8, 12], **cic.,** cimic.[8], **coca,** con.[8], ferr-p.[8], **gels., hep., hyper.,** iod., **ip.,** kali-i., **kalm.,** lac-c., **lec., led., merc., nat-m.,** nit-ac.[1'], **nux-v.,** pareir.[8], ph-ac.[8], **PHOS.,** plb-p.[8], **puls., rhus-t.,** sang.[8], **sil., stann.**[8], stront-c.[8], stram., stry.[8], sul**ph., thal.**[8, 12], urt-u.[8], zinc., zinc-p.[8]

serous membranes, of

acon.[1], am-c., **APIS, apoc.**[1], arg-m., **ARS.,** ars-i., asaf., **aur., aur-ar.**[1'], aur-i.[1'], **aur-m.,** aur-s.[1'], bell., **BRY., CALC.,** calc-p., **carb-v.,** colch., ferr., fl-ac., **HELL.,** indg., **iod., kali-c.,** lach., **led., LYC.,** mag-m., **merc., nat-m., ph-ac., phos.,** plat., **psor., puls.,** samb., seneg., **SIL., squil., stram., sulph., ter.,** zinc.

sudden[16]

bell.

synovitis

acon.[8], **am-p.**[8], ant-t.[1z], apis, arn.[8], bell., **benz-ac.**[8], **berb.**[8], bry., calc., calc-f.[8], calc-p.[8], canth.[8], caust., ferr-p., fl-ac.[8], **hep.**[8], iod., kali-c., kali-i., led., lyc., merc., phyt., puls., rhus-t., ruta[8], **sabin.**[8], sep., sil., slag[8], staph.[8], **stel.**[8], stict.[8], sulph., tub.[8], verat-v.

tendency to[16]

camph.

tendons, of; tendinitis

anac.[7], ant-c.[12], **rhod., rhus-t.**

wounds, of[4]

acon., arist-cl.[9], arn., calc-f.[2], calen.[2, 11], **cham., con.**[2], hyper.[1'], kali-bi.[11], lach., led.[1'], mez.[4, 16], nat-m., plb., **puls., rhus-t.**[4, 11], **sul-ac., sulph.,** vip.[11]

IJURIES (including blows, bruises, falls)

absin.[2], acet-ac.[7, 8], **acon.**[2, 3, 4, 7, 8, 12]. **agn.**[2], all-c.[3, 8, 12], aloe.[3], alum.[3, 4], **am-c.**[3, 4], am-m.[3], ang.[3, 6-8, 12], ant-c.[2, 3], apis[12], **arg-m.**[2, 3], arg-n.[3], **ARN., aur-m.**[2], **bad.,** bell.[3, 4], **bell-p.**[1, 7], bor.[3, 4], bry., bufo[3, 7, 8], calc., calc-p.[3], calc-s.[12], **CALEN.**[1'-3, 6-8, 10], **CAMPH.**[7], **CANN-I.**[7] cann-s.[3], canth.,

carb-v., **caust.**[2, 3, 4], cham., chin., chion.[3], chin-s.[4], **cic., CON.,** croc., crot-t.[7, 8], dig.[3], **dros.**[2, 3], **dulc.,** echi.[3, 7, 8], erig.[12], eug.[4], euph.[3], euph-pi.[12], euphr., ferr-p.[12], **form.**[2, 12], gamb.[12], **glon.**[2, 3, 6-8, 12], **ham.**[2, 3, 6-8, 12], hell.[12], **HEP.,** hyos., **HYPER., iod.,** ip.[12], kali-c., kali-i.[3], kali-m.[12], kali-p.[12], kali-s.[12], kalm.[3], kreos., lac-c.[12], lac-d.[12], **lach.,** laur., **led., lith-c.**[2, 3, 12], lyc., mag-c.[7, 8, 12], merc., mez., **mill.**[2, 3, 7, 12], mosch.[2], **naja**[3], nat-c., nat-m., **nat-s., nit-ac.,** nux-m.[3], nux-v., oena.[12], **olnd.**[2, 3], par., pareir.[2], **petr.**[2, 3, 4], ph-ac., **phos.,** phys.[3, 7, 8, 12], **plan.**[2, 12], plat., plb., polyg-h.[2], psor.[12], **PULS.,** pyrog.[3], ran-b.[12], **rhod.**[2, 3], **RHUS-T., ruta,** samb., sec., seneg., sep.[2, 3, 4, 12], **sil.,** spig.[3], **staph.,** stict.[12], stront-c.[3, 7, 8], **SUL-AC.,** sul-i.[1'], **sulph., symph.,** tab.[3], tarent.[3, 12], tell.[12], ter.[12], teucr.[2, 3], urt-u.[12], valer.[3], vario.[12], verat., **verb.**[2, 3, 7, 8], zinc.

lifting
shocks

ailments from[12]

acon., all-c., arn., bell-p., con., dulc., ferr-p., glon., ham., hell., hep., ip., kali-m., kali-p., kali-s., lac-c., lac-d., lach., led., lith-c., mag-c., mill., nat-s., nux-v., oena., paeon., par., ph-ac., phys., plan., psor., ran-b., ruta, sec., sep., sil., staph., stict., sul-ac., sulph., symph., tarent., tell., ter., teucr., urt-u., valer., vario.,

wounds-constitutional effects

concussion[2, 3]

acon., **anac.**, **ARN.**[2, 3, 6], aur.,
BAD.[2], **bell.**[2, 3, 7], bry.[3, 4], **calc.**,
calen.[2], camph., cann-s., caust.,
chin.[2, 3], cic.[2, 3, 6, 8, 12], cina, **cocc.**,
con.[2], cupr., euphr.[2], **glon.**[3],
hell.[2, 12], hyos., **HYPER.**[2, 7], iod.[2],
kali-p.[2], kreos., **lach.**[2], laur., **led.**,
lyc., m-arct.[3], mag-m., **mang.**,
mez., nat-m., **NAT-S.**[2], nux-m.,
nux-v.[2, 3, 6], ph-ac., **puls.**[2-4],
rhus-t.[2, 3], seneg., **sep.**[2, 3, 12], **sil.**,
spig., staph., stry.[6], sul-ac.[2],
sulph.[3], valer., **verat.**, viol-t.

ailments from[6]

am-c., **arn.**, **hyper.**, valer.

am.[3]
hell.

**commotion of the brain, ailments
from**[12] ✱

sul-ac., teucr.

convulsions–c
faintness–injury–c.

dislocation, luxation[3]

acon., agar., **AGN.**[2, 3, 12], alum.,
am-c.[2, 3, 12], **am-m.**, **ambr.**[2, 3],
anac., ang.[2, 3], ant-c., ant-t.,
ARN.[2-4, 7], ars., asar., aur.,
bar-c.[2, 3], **bell.**[2, 3], bov.[2, 3], **bry.**[2-4],
calad., **CALC.**[2, 3], **calc-f.**, calc-p.,
camph., cann-s.[2, 3], caps.[3, 4],
carb-an.[2-4], **carb-v.**[2-4],
carl.[11], caust.[2, 3], cham.,
chel., chin., cina, cocc., **coloc.**,
con.[2-4], croc., cycl., dig., dros.,

dulc., euph., **ferr-s.**[2], **form.**[2, 12],
graph.[2, 3], hell., hep.[2, 3], **IGN.**[2-4],
ip., kali-c., **kali-n.**[2, 3], kreos.[2, 3],
lach.[4], led., **LYC.**[2, 3], m-arct.[4],
m-aust.[12], mag-c.[3, 4], mag-m.,
mang., meny., **merc.**[2-4], mez.[2],
mosch.[2-4], mur-ac., **NAT-C.**[2-4],
NAT-M.[2-4], **nit-ac.**[2, 3], nux-m.,
nux-v.[2, 3], par.[4], **PETR.**[2-4],
ph-ac., **PHOS.**[2-4], plat., plb.,
prun., psor.[3, 12], **PULS.**[2, 3], ran-b.,
rhod.[2, 3], **RHUS-T.**[2-4, 7], **ruta**[2, 3, 12],
sabin.[2, 3], sars., seneg., sep.[2, 3, 4],
sil., **spig.**[2-4], spong., stann.[2, 3],
staph.[2, 3], **stront-c.**, **sulph.**[2-4],
thuj., valer., verat., verb.,
zinc.[2, 3]

ailments from[12]

psor., rheum

extravasations, with

acet-ac.[2], agar.[2, 7], **ARN.**, **bad.**,
bell-p.[7], both.[7], bry., calen.[2, 7],
cham., chin., cic., **con.**, crot-h.[4, 7],
dulc., euphr., ferr., **ham.**[2], **hep.**,
hyper.[7], iod., **lach.**, laur., **led.**[2, 3, 7, 8],
mill.[2], nux-v., par., plb., **puls.**,
rhus-t., **ruta**, sec., staph.[7], **SUL-AC.**,
sul-i.[1], **sulph.**, symph.[7]

operation, disorders from[8] ✱

acet-ac., **acon.**[2, 3, 7, 12], all-c.[12],
apis[8, 12], **arn.**[3, 6-12], **bell-p.**[7-9],
berb.[6, 8], calc-f., calc-p.[12],
calen.[1'-3, 8], camph., carb-v.[1'],
chin.[6], croc.[8, 12], ferr-p.,
hyper.[3, 6, 8, 12], kali-s., led.[1'],
merc.[12], mill., naja, nit-ac.,
nux-v.[6], op.[6], ph-ac.[12], pop.[6],
raph., rhus-t., ruta[1'],
STAPH.[1', 7, 8, 12], **stront-c.**[1', 3, 7, 8],
sul-ac.[12], verat., zinc.[12]

fistulae–operation

weakness-operation

ailments from[12]

acon., all-c., calc-p., ph-ac.,
staph., stront-c., sul-ac., zinc.

stretching, with[1']

staph.

overexertion, strain, from[12]

arn.[2, 7], ars.[2, 12], **CALC.**[2, 12], calc-f.,
carb-an., carb-v., cocc., **con.**[2],
ham.[2], lyc., **mill.**[2], nat-c., ovi-p.,
rhus-t.[2, 12], sanic., sil., ter.

prophylaxis of tetanus[7]

ARN., HYPER., LED., tetox., thuj.

convulsions–tetanic

rupture of bloodvessel[2]

mill.

muscles, of[2]

calen.

tendons, of[7]

rhus-t.

sprains, distorsions[3]

acet-ac.[8], **acon.**[8], agar.,
AGN.[2-4, 8, 12], all-s.[12], **am-c.**[2-4, 6, 12],
am-m.[6, 12], am-p., ambr.,
amgd-p.[12], ang.[3, 4],
ARN.[1'-3, 4, 6-8, 10, 12], ars.[12],
asaf.[2], asar.[6], bar-c., bell.[2-4, 8, 11],
bell-p.[6-8, 10], benz-ac., bov.[3, 6],
bry.[2-4, 6, 7], **CALC.**[2, 3, 4, 7, 8],
calc-f.[8, 12], calc-p.[3, 6], calc-sil.[1'],
calen.[8], cann-s., canth.[4], caps.,
carb-an.[2-4, 6, 8], carb-v.[2-4], carl.[12],
caust.[3, 4, 6], chin.[4], **cic.**[3, 4, 11, 12],
coloc., con., cupr.[4], ferr-p.[1', 2, 12],
ferr-s.[2], form.[8], graph.[3, 4, 6],
guaj., hep., hyos.[3, 4], **hyper.**[8],
ign.[2-4], kali-i., **kali-n.**, kreos.[3],
led.[3, 6, 7], lith-c., **LYC.**[2-4, 6, 12],
m-aust.[3, 4], mag-c.[6], **merc.**,
mez.[3, 6], **MILL.**[2, 7, 8, 12], mosch.,
NAT-C.[2-4, 6], **NAT-M.**[2-4, 6],
nit-ac.[2-4, 6], **nux-v.**[2-4, 6, 8],
onos., **PETR.**[2-4, 6, 8, 12],
PHOS.[1'-4, 6, 12], plat., polyg-h.[2],
polyg-pe.[12], **prun.**[6, 12], psor.[12],
puls.[2-4, 6], rad., rhod.[3, 6, 8, 12],
RHUS-T.[1'-3, 6-8, 10, 12],
RUTA[1'-4, 6-8, 10, 12], sabin.,
sep.[2-4, 6], sil.[3, 6, 12], sol-n.[4],
spig.[3, 4], stann., staph.[3, 6], stram.,
stront-c.[2, 3, 6-8, 12], **sulph.**[2-4, 6],
sumb.[11], **symph.**[2, 8, 10, 12],
tarent.[11], thuj., zinc.

ailments from[12]

agn., kali-m., kreos., lach., petr.,
phos., polyg-h., prun., psor.,
rhod., rhus-v., ruta, seneg.,
stront-c., sul-ac., sulph.

traumatic fever[3]

acon.[2, 3, 7, 8, 12], **apis.**[3, 7],
ARN.[2, 3, 7, 8, 12], **ars.**[7, 8, 12], bry.,
cact.[12], **calen.**[2, 7], carb-v., **chin.**[7, 8, 12],

coff.[2, 7], croc., euphr., hep., iod.[7], lach.[3, 7, 8, 12], **lyss.**[7], merc.[3, 7], nat-c., nit-ac., ph-ac., phos., **puls., rhus-t., staph.**, sul-ac., **sulph.**[1', 3]

bones, of; fractures✱

acon.[7], ang.[3, 6], **arn.**[1', 3, 4, 6-8], asaf.[2], bell-p.[9, 10], calc., **calc-f.**[2, 3, 6], calc-p., **calen**[2, 3, 4, 6, 7], **CARB-AC.**[2], con.[3], cortico.[9], cortiso.[9], croc.[3], **eup-per.**[3, 12], ferr.[3, 6], hep.[3], iod.[3, 6], kali-i.[3, 6], lyc.[2], nit-ac.[2], **petr.**[3], **ph-ac.**[3, 4, 6], phos.[3, 4], **puls.**[3, 4], rhus-t.[1', 3, 4], **RUTA, sil.**[2, 3, 4, 6, 7, 12], staph.[3, 4], stront-c.[7], **sul-ac.,** sulph.[2, 3, 6], **symph.,** valer.[3]

shock–injury

ailments from[12]

hecla, ruta, symph.

compound fracture[3]

ang., **ARN.**[2, 3, 7, 8], **calc., calen.**[3, 6-8], con., crot-h.[2], hep., hyper.[12], iod., **lach.**[2], petr., ph-ac., phos., puls., rhus-t., **RUTA,** sil., staph., symph.

slow repair of broken bones

asaf., **CALC.,** calc-f.[3, 7], **CALC-P.,** calen.[7, 8], des-ac.[14], **ferr.**[1, 7], fl-ac.[1'], iod.[7, 8], lyc., mang.[7, 8], merc., **mez.**[1, 7], nit-ac., **ph-ac.,** phos., puls., **RUTA**[1, 7], sep., **sil.,** staph., sulph., **SYMPH.**[1, 7], **thyr.**[7, 8, 12]

children, in[7]

calc., calc-f., calc-p., sil.

glands, of

arn., aster.[8], cann-s.[3], cic., **CON., dulc.,** hep., **iod.,** kali-c.[3], kalm.[2], merc., **petr.**[2, 3, 4], **phos.,** puls., rhus-t., **sil., sul-ac., sulph.**[3, 4]

muscles, of[3]

arn.[1', 3], calc.[1'], nat-c., nat-m., phos., **RHUS-T.**[1', 3]

nerves with great pain, of

bell-p.[7-9], **cur.**[2], glon.[3, 6], **HYPER.,** led.[1'], mag-p.[2], meny.[2, 12], **phos.,** tarent.[2], ther.[2], xan.[12]

ailments from[12]

hyper., meny., xan.

periosteum, of

calc.[1'], **ruta,** symph.[12]

ailments from[12]

symph.

soft parts, of

ARN., bell-p.[7], cham., **CON.,** dulc., euphr., ham.[7], hyper.[7], lach., **nat-c.**[4], nat-m.[4], phos.[4], **puls., rhus-t.**[4, 7], samb., **sul-ac.,** sulph., **symph.**[7]

stump neuralgia[2, 6, 7]

all-c., am-m., arn.[2, 6], **hyper.**[2, 7], kalm.[2, 6], ph-ac.[2, 6], symph.

pain-amputation

tendons, of

anac., calen.[7], rhus-t.[7], ruta[1']

INTOXICATION, after

abies-c.[11], absin.[11], acet-ac.[11], acon., aether[11], agar., agn.[11], **am-m.**, aml-ns.[11], amyg.[11], arg-m., ars.[11], atro.[11], bart.[11], bell., bov., **bry.**, camph.[11], cann-s.[11], **caps.**[3, 11], carb-an.[11], **carb-v.**, chel.[11], chin., cic.[11], cinch.[11], coca[11] **cocc., coff.**, con.[3, 11], conin.[11], cori-r.[11], dat-m.[11], eucal.[11], fagu.[11], ferr.[11], **gels.**[3, 11], grat.[11], hyos.[11], ign.[11], ip., kali-bi.[11], kali-c., kali-i.[11], kali-n., kiss.[11], kreos., lach.[3], lact.[11] **laur.**, led.[11, 12], lol.[11], merc.[11], mez.[11], mill.[11], morph.[11], nabal.[11], naja[11], nat-m., nux-m., **NUX-V., OP.,** ph-ac., phel.[11], pip-m.[11], **puls.**, ran-b.[3], rheum, rhod.[11], sabad.[11], samb., sec.[11], **spong.**, squil., **stram.**, tab.[11], tax.[11], ter.[11], teucr., thea.[11], til.[11], tus-fr.[11], valer., verat.[11], vip.[11], zinc.[3, 11]

index: *alcohol*

IODINE, after abuse of[6]

ant-c., ant-t.[2], **ars.**[2, 4, 6, 12], bell., camph., chin., chin-s.[2], coff., **conv.,** **hep.,** lycps., merc.[2], **op., phos.**[2, 4, 6], **sec.,** spong.[2], sulph.[4, 6]

IRON, after abuse of

ars., calc-p.[6], **chin.**[2, 3, 6, 8], chin-ar.[6], cupr.[3, 6], **hep.**[2, 3, 6, 8], iod.[2], ip.[2, 3], merc.[2], nat-m.[6], **puls., sulph.,** thea[3], verat.[3], **zinc.**

IRRITABILITY, excessive physical

absin., acon., agar., alum.[12], **ambr.,** anac., ant-c., ant-t.[1], **APIS, arg-n.**[8], **ARN., ars., asaf., ASAR., AUR.,** aur-ar.[1'], **aur-m.**[2], bar-c., bar-m.[2], **BELL., bell-p.**[8], **berb.**[12], bor., bov., bry., **calad.**[12], calc.[3], camph., cann-i., **CANTH.,** carb-ac.[12], **carb-v.**[3, 12], carbn-s., caust., **cham., CHIN.,** chin-ar.[8], **chin-s.,** chlol.[2], cina[3], cob.[8], **coc-c.**[12], **coca**[2] **cocc., COFF., coll.**[12], con.[3], croc., cupr., dig.[3], **dulc.**[12], ery-a.[2], **ferr.,** ferr-ar.[1'], ferr-i.[11] **gels.,** graph., gua.[8], hell., hep., hyos., **hyper.**[8], **ign.,** indg.[2], kali-c.[3, 8], kali-p.[8], kreos., **lach.,** laur., **lil-t., lyc.**[3, 12], mag-c., mag-m., mang., **MED.,** meny.[3], **MERC.,** mez., **morph.**[12], mosch., naja[8], nat-ar., nat-c., **nat-m.,** nat-p., nat-sil.[1'], **NIT-AC.,** nux-m.[3], **NUX-V.,** ox-ac.[8], par., ped.[12], petr., **ph-ac., phos., phys.**[8], **pic-ac.**[8], plat., podo.[2], **puls.,** ran-b.[8], rhus-t., **rhus-v.**[12], **rumx.**[12], sabin., sars.[3], sec., sel., sep., **SIL.,** spig., spong.[2, 3], squil., **STAPH.,** stram., stry-p.[8], sulph., **TARENT., tell.**[8], **TEUCR.,** ther.[8], tub.[8], **valer., verat., vib.**[2], **zinc.**[8], zinc-val.[8], ziz.[2]

sexual excesses, from[8]

agar., kali-p., nat-m.

when too much medicine has prod-
uced an over-sensitive state and
remedies fail to act

ph-ac., **TEUCR.**

medicaments

lack of

acon.[3], agn., **alum.**, alum-p.[1'],
am-c., am-m.[3], **ambr.**, **anac.**,
ang.[3], ant-c., ant-t., arn., **ars.**,
asaf., asar.[3], bar-c., bell.[3],
bism., bor.[3], brom., bry., **CALC.**,
CALC-I., **camph.**, cann-s., canth.[3],
CAPS., **carb-an.**, **CARB-V.**, caust.,
cham.[3], chel.[3], chin.[3], cic., clem.[3],
cocc., colch., coloc., **CON.**, croc.,
cupr., dig.[3], **dulc.**, euph., ferr.,
ferr-i.[1'], **GELS.**, graph., **guaj.**, **HELL.**,
hep.[3], hyos.[3], ign.[3], **iod.**, **ip.**, **kali-br.**[1]
(not : kali-bi.), kali-c., kali-s.[1'], lach.,
LAUR., led., **lyc.**, mag-c., mag-m.,
merc.[3], mez., **mosch.**, mur-ac.,
nat-c.[3], nat-m.[3], **nit-ac.**[3], nux-m.,
nux-v.[3], **OLND.**, **OP.**, petr., **PH-AC.**,
phos., plb., **PSOR.**, puls.[3], **rhod.**,
rhus-t., sec., seneg., **sep.**, sil.[3],
spong., stann., staph.[3], **stram.**,
stront-c., **sulph.**, **TEUCR.**[7], thuj.,
valer., verat.[4, 6], verb., **zinc.**

anaesthesia
analgesia
painlessness

reaction

ITCHING of **glanas**

am-c., **anac.**, ant-c., canth.,
carb-an., carb-v., **caust.**, cocc..
CON., **kali-c.**, mag-c., merc.,
nit-ac.[16], **phos.**, ran-s., rheum,
rhus-t., sabin., sep., **sil.**, **spong.**,
sulph.[3]

affected parts, of[16]

dig.

bones, of[16]

verat.

internal[16]

phos.

ITCHING and **TICKLING** internally[3]

acon., agar., alum., am-c., am-m.,
AMBR., anac., ang., ant-t., apis, arn.,
asar., bar-c., bell., bor., bov., brom.,
bry., calc., caps., carb-v., caust., cham.,
chin., cic., cina, cocc., colch., **con.**,
croc., dig., euph., **ferr.**, fl-ac., graph.,
hep., ign. **IOD.**, ip., **kali-bi.**, kali-c.,
lach., **laur.**, led., mag-c., mag-m.,
meny., merc., mosch., nat-c., nit-ac.,
nux-m., **NUX-V.**, olnd., petr., ph-ac.,
PHOS., plb., puls., rhod., rhus-t., ruta,
sabad., sabin., sang., seneg., sep.,
sil., spig., spong., squil., **stann.**,
sulph., tarax., teucr., thuj. verat.,
zinc.

JAR, stepping **agg.**

acon., aloe[3], alum., alum-p.[1'],
alum-sil.[1'], am-c., ambr., **anac.**,
ang.[3], **ant-c.**, arg-m., **arg-n.**,

ARN., ars., **asar.**, bapt.³,
bar-c., **BELL.**, berb.³, ⁷, ⁸, bor.,
BRY., cact., calad., **calc.**, calc-p¹',
calc-sil.¹', camph., canth., carb-ac.³,
carbn-s., **caust.**, cham., chel., **chin.**,
CIC., cina³, **cocc.**, coff., **CON.**,
crot-h.⁸, dros., dulc., euphr., **ferr.**,
ferr-ar., ferr-p.¹', form.³, glon.,
graph., ham., hell., hep.,
ign., kali-c., **kali-i.**, kali-n.,
kali-sil.¹', **lac-c.**⁶, ⁷, **LACH., led.**,
lil-t., lyc., mag-c., **mag-m.**, meny.,
merc., nat-ar., **nat-c., nat-m.**,
nat-p., nat-s.³, nat-sil¹', **NIT-AC.**,
nux-m., **nux-v., onos.**, par., petr.,
ph-ac., phos., plat., plb., podo.³,
puls., rhod., **RHUS-T.**, ruta, **sabad.**,
sabin., **sanic.**, seneg., **sep., SIL.**,
spig., spong., stann., staph., **sulph.**,
tab.³, tarax.³, **THER., thuj.**, valer.⁶,
verb., viol-t.

am.

caps., gels.³, hell.³, nit-ac.³

JERKING internally

acon., agar., ambr., anac., ang.³,
aran-ix.¹⁰, arn., ars.,**bell.**, bov., bry.,
calad., **CALC., CANN-I., cann-s.**¹,
caust., cic., clem., coca, colch.,
con., croc., dig., dulc., **GLON.**,
kreos., **lyc.**, mag-c., mang., mez.,
mur-ac., nat.-c., nat-m., **nux-m.**,
nux-v., petr., phos., **PLAT., PULS.**,
ran-s., rhod., rhus-t., ruta, samb.,
sep., **sil., SPIG., spong., STANN.**,
stront-c., sul-ac., sulph.³, teucr.,
thuj., **valer.**

shocks, electric-like

twitching

bones, in³

chin., sil.

convulsions, as in

acon., agar., **alum.**, am-c.⁴, am-m.⁴,
AMBR., ant-c., ant-t.⁴, arg-m., arn.,
ars., asaf.⁴, bar-c.⁴, bar-m.⁴, bell.,
bry., **calc.**, camph., cann-s., canth.⁴,
caps., carb-v., **CAUST., cham.**,
chin., chin-s.⁴, chlol.⁷, **cic.**, cina⁴,
cocc.⁴, coff.⁴, colch.⁴, coloc.,
crot-h.⁴, **cupr.**, cupr-a.⁴, cupr-c.⁴,
dig., dros., dulc., graph.⁴, hep.,
hyos., ign., ip., kali-c., kali-chl.⁴,
kreos.⁴, lach., lact.⁴, laur., led.⁴,
lil-t., lob.⁴, lyc., m-arct.⁴, mag-c.,
mag-m.⁴, mang.⁴, **meny, merc.**,
mez., mosch.⁴, mur-ac., nat-c.,
NAT-M., nat-s.⁴, nit-ac., nux-v., op.,
petr., ph-ac.⁴, phel.⁴, **phos.**, plat.,
PLB., puls.⁴, **ran-b.**, ran-s.⁴, rat.⁴,
rhod., rhus-t.⁴, sabad., **sec.**, sep.,
sil., sol-n.⁴, squil., staph., **stram.**,
stront-c., sul-ac., **sulph.**, tarent.¹',
teucr.⁴, thuj., valer.⁴, verat., viol-t.,
vip.⁴, **zinc.**

night¹⁶
staph.

joints, in³

alum., bell., bry., bufo, **coloc.**,
graph., nat-m., puls., sil., spig.³, ⁶,
spong., **sul-ac.**, sulph.³, ⁶, **verat.**

muscles, of

acon, aesc., **agar.**, alum.,
alum-p.¹', alum-sil.¹', am-c.,
ambr.⁶, **anac.**, ant-c., **ant-t., apis**,
aran-ix.¹⁰, **arg-m., arg-n.**, arn.,
ars., **asaf.**¹, asar., **bar-c.**, bar-s.¹',
bell., berb.⁴, bor.³, **bry.**, bufo¹',
cadm-s., calc., calc-f.¹⁰, ¹⁴,
CALC-P., cann-i., caps.,
carbn-s., caust.⁴, ⁶, cham.,
chin., **chion., CIC., cimic.**,
clem.⁴, cocc., **colch.**, coloc.³, ⁴,
con., croc., cupr., cyt-l.¹⁰, dulc.,
eucal.⁶, euph., euphr., **ferr.**,

ferr-ar., **gels., glon., graph.,**
hist.[9, 10, 14], **HYOS.,** hyper.[1'],
ign.[4, 6], ind.[14], iod.[6], ip., kali-i.,
kali-n.[4], kali-p.[1'], kali-s., **lach.,**
lil-t., lyc.[3, 6], lyss.[10], mag-c.,
mag-m.[1'], **meny, merc.,** merc-c.,
MEZ., mosch., **nat-c.,** nat-f.[10],
nat-m., nit-ac., **nux-m., nux-v.,**
olnd., **op.,** petr., ph-ac., **phos.,**
phyt.[1'], **plat., plb., puls.,**
ran-b.[4], rat.[3], **rhus-t.,** ruta,
sabad., sabin., sal-ac.[6], sec.[4, 6],
SEP., sil., **spig., stann.,** staph.,
STRAM., stront-c., SUL-AC.,
sul-i.[1'], **SULPH.,** tab.[3], tarax.[14],
tarent., ter., teucr.[4], **valer.,**
viol-t., **visc., ZINC.,** zinc-i.[3],
ZINC-P.[1']

paralyzed parts, of

arg-n., merc., **nux-v.,** phos.,
sec.[1'], stram.[1'], **stry.**

side lain on, in

cimic.

sleep, on going to

acon., **agai.,** all-s.[2], **aloe²,**
alum., arg-m., **ARS.,** bell.[3],
cob., **colch¹,** hyper., **ign.,**
iodof.[2], **KALI-C.,** kali-cy.[7],
nit-ac.[3], nux-v.[1'], op.[3], phys.,
puls.[16], ran-b., **sel.,** sep.[3], sil.,
stront-c., stry., sul-ac., **sulph.,**
tub.[1', 7], **zinc.**

shocks, electric-like sleep

during

agar., aloe, **alum.,** ambr.,
anac., ant-t., arg-m., **ars., bell.,**
bry., calc.[4], carb-v.[3], cast.,
cham., cimic., cob., colch.[1],
con., cor-r., **cupr.,** cupr-ar.[6],
daph., dig.[3], dulc., hep.,
ign., ip., **kali-c.,** lyc., merc.,
nat-c., **nat-m.,** nat-s., nit-ac.,
nux-v.[1', 6, 7], op., phos., puls.,
ran-s., rheum, rhus-t., sel., sep.,
sil., stann., staph., stront-c.,
sul-ac., **sulph.,** thuj., tub.[1', 7],
viol-t., zinc.

KNEE in[7]

bar-c., lach., nux-v.

out[7]

calc., nux-v., sulph.

KNEELING, ailments on

calc.[3], **cocc.,** mag-c., puls.[3], sep.,
spig.[3], tarent.[3]

am.[3]
euph.

KNOTTED sensation internally

ambr., ant-t., arn., **ars.,** asaf.[3], bell.[3],
bry., carb-an., carb-v.[6], cham., cic.,
cina³, con., cupr., gels., graph.[3],
hydr.[3], hydr-ac., ign.[8], kali-p.[6, 6],
kreos., **LACH.,** lob.[3], mag-m.,
mag-p.[3, 6], **merc-i-r.,** nux-v., petr.,
phyt., puls., **rhus-t., sabad.,** sec., sep.,
SPIG., staph., stict., **SULPH.,** valer.[3],
zinc.[3, 6]

ball

LABOR agg., manual[3]

am-m., bov., ferr., kali-c., **lach.,**
mag-c., merc., **NAT-M.**[3, 6], nit-ac.,
phos., **sil., verat.**

LASSITUDE

abies-n.[2], **ACON., aesc.,** aeth.,
agar.[1], ail., **alet.**[2], **aloe**[2], **ALUM.,**
alumn.[1'], **ALUM-P.**[1'], alum-sil.[1'],
AM-C., am-m.[2], **ambr., aml-ns.**[2],
ammc.[2], anac.[2], ang.[2], anh.[9], ant-c.,
ant-t., APIS, apoc., **ARAN.,**
aran-ix.[10], arg-m., arg-n.[2], **arn.**[2],
ars., ars-h.[2], **ars-i.,** ars-met.[2],
ars-s-f.[1'], arum-d.[2], arum-m.[2],
arum-t.[2], asaf., asar., asc-t.[2],
aspar.[2], astac.[2], aster., atro.[2],
aur., aur-m-n., bar-c., bar-i.[1'],
bar-m., bar-s.[1'], **bapt., bell.,** bell-p.[7],
benz-ac., berb., bism., **bol-la.**[2], bor.,
bov., brach.[2], bry., cact.,
cadm-met.[9], cain.[7], **CALAD.,**
CALC., calc-ar.[1', 2], calc-i.[1']
CALC-P.[2], calc-s.[2], calc-sil.[1'],
calen.[2], **camph.,** cann-s., canth.,
caps., carb-ac., carb-v., CARBN-S.,
card-m.[2], **casc., caust.,** cedr.[2],
cham., **chel.,** chen-v.[2], **CHIN.,**
chin-ar.[2], **chin-s.,** chlf.[2], chlol.[2, 7],
chr-ac.[2], **cic.,** cina, cinnb.[2], cist.[2],
cob-n.[9, 14], coc-c.[2], **coca**[2], **cocc.,**
coff., **colch., coloc., CON.,** conv.[7],
cop., croc., **CROT-C.,** crot-t.[2],
CUPR., cupr-ar[2], cupr-s.[2], cyn-d.[14],
daph.[2], dicha.[14], **dig.,** dios.[2], **dulc.**[2],
ery-a.[2], eucal., eup-pur.[2], euph.[2],
euphr., **FERR.,** ferr-ar., ferr-p.,
fl-ac[2], **form.,** gamb.[2], **GELS.,**
GRAPH., grat.[1', 2], guaj., **guar.**[2],
halo.[14], **ham.**[2], harp.[14], **hell.**[2],
hep., hippoz.[2], **hydr., hydrc.**[2], hyos.,
ign., iod., ip., **kali-bi.**[2, 3], **kali-br.**[2],
kali-c., kali-m.[1', 2], kali-n., **kali-p.,**
kali-sil.[1'], lac-ac.[2], **lac-d.**[1', 2, 7],
LACH., laur., led., **lept.**[2], levo.[14],
lob., luf-o.[14], **lyc., lyss.**[2], mag-c.,
mag-m., manc.[2], **mang., med.**[2],
meny., **merc.,** methys.[14], **mez.,**

mosch., **mur-ac.,** myric.[2], naja[14],
nat-ar., **nat-c., nat-m., nat-p.,**
nat-s.[2], **nat-sil.**[1'], nep.[13, 14], nit-ac.,
nuph.[2], **nux-m., NUX-V.,** ol-an.[2],
olnd., onop.[14], **op., ox-ac.,** oxyt.,
pall.[2], petr., **PH-AC.,** phel.[2], **phos.,**
phyt., **PIC-AC.,** plat., **plb., psor.,**
ptel.[2], puls., **ran-b., raph.**[2], **rat.**[2],
rhod., **rhust-t., rhus-v.**[2], rib-ac.[14],
RUTA, sabad., sabin., **SANG.,**
sarr.[2], sec., sel., **senec.**[1', 2], **seneg.,**
sep., **SIL.,** spig., **spong., stann.,**
staph., **stram.,** stront-c., **SUL-AC.,**
sul-i.[1'], sulfa.[14], sulfonam.[14], **sulph.**
sumb., tab.[2], tarax., **TARENT.,**
tell.[2], **ter.**[2], **teucr.,** ther., thiop.[14],
thuj., **tub.**[2], uran-n.[2], **ust.**[2], vac.[2],
valer., verat., viol-t., x-ray[9], **ZINC.,**
ZINC-P.[1'], zing.[2]

weakness

daytime[2]

am-m., asc-t., **calc.,** calc-f., cob-n.[9],
ferr., kali-bi., senec.

morning
am-c., ant-c., **calad.**[2], **kali-m.**[2],
lyc., **mag-m.**[2], nat-c., nat-p.,
nux-v., staph.[2], **sulph.**[2], sumb.

and afternoon[2]

bry.

bed, in[4]

acon., alum., **ambr.**[2, 4], **aur., bell.,**
bor., **bry., carb-v.**[2, 4], **caust.,**
cham.[2], clem., con., crot-t., dros.,
hell. iod., kali-c., **lach.,** mag-c.,
mag-s., mang., nat-m., **op.,**
petr.[2, 4], phos., plb., **puls.,** ran-s.,
sep., sil., spig., **squil.,** thuj.,
verat., zinc.[2, 4]

rising, on[4]

dig., **ferr.**[2], kreos., **nux-v.**[2], **osm.**[2], petr., ph-ac., plb., **sep.**[2], sil., stann., vib.[2]

am.[4]
acon., mag-c.

forenoon
alum., ran-b.

noon[2]
cic.

afternoon
arg-n., **calc-s.**[2], **card-m.**[2], gels., hyos.[16], lil-t.[7], lyc., petr.[16], thuj.

siesta, after[16]

kali-c.

16 h[14]
trios.

evening
am-c., ars., calc-sil.[1'], carb-v., **CAUST.**, **graph.**, **ign.**[2], **myrt-c.**[2], naja, nat-m., pall.[2], sang.[7], spig., sulfonam.[14], thuj.

night[1']
calc-sil.

2 h[14]
trios.

and morning[2]

nat-s.

Addison's disease, in[2]

calc.

air agg., in open[2]

petr.

alternating with activity

aloe, aur.

coldness, objective or subjective[2]

spig.

chilliness, with[2]

cimic., corn.

coition, after

agar.[2, 4, 6, 15], **CALC.**, con.[4], graph.[4], led.[4], lyc.[4], nat-m.[4], **phos.**[6], plb.[4], sep.[4], staph.[4], tax.[4], **ziz.**[2]

conversation, from

sil.

eating, after

act-sp.[2], ant-c.[2], bar-c.[2, 16], bov.[2], calc-p.[2], **carb-an.**[2], **card-m.**[2], chin.[2], lach.[2], lyc., lyss.[2], mur-ac., **nat-m.**[2], nux-m.[2], ol-an.[7], **PH-AC.**, **rhus-t.**[2], sel., sep.[16]

emissions, from seminal[2]

bar-c.[4], ery-a., ham.

lie down before dinner, must

mez.

if he does not eat frequently[2]

sulph.

menses, before

alum.[4, 6], **bell.**[2, 6], calc., **lyc.**,
nux-m.[4, 6]

during[4]
alum.[4, 6], **am-c.**[2], bell.[6], bor.[2, 4],
bov., calc-p.[2], carb-an.[4, 6], cast.,
caust.[2, 4], ign., iod.[2, 4], **kali-c.**[2, 4],
kali-n., lyc., **mag-c.**, mag-m.,
nit-ac.[2], **nux-m.**[2], **petr.**[2, 4], phel.,
phos., thuj.[2]

after[2, 4]
berb., nux-v., thuj.[2]

mental exertion, from[2]

AUR., podo., **puls.**

motion, on

phos.

am.[16]: nat-c.

pregnancy, during[2]

calc-p.

restlessness, with[2]

dios., tell.

sexual excesses, after[6]

agn.

sitting, on

merc.[2], phos.

---

sleep, after

ant-t.[2], kali-c.[16], **PULS.**[2], sil.

spring, in[2]

apis, **bry.**, **gels.**

stool, before[2]

mez.

during[2]
bor., ip.

after
ip.[2], **lyc.**[2], mag-m.

stormy weather

psor., **sang., tub.**

talking, after

alum., dor.[2]

waking, on[4]

acon., alum., ambr., **arg-m.**[2], aur.,
bell., bor., **bry., carb-v.,** card-m.[2],
caust., chin.[2], clem., crot-t., dios.[2],
dros., hell., hyper.[2], kreos., lac-ac.[2],
lach., mang., **op.,** petr., **ph-ac.**[2, 4],
phos., plb., **podo.**[2], **ptel.**[2], puls.,
ran-s., sep., sil., spig., **squil., stann.,**
thuj., verat., xan.[2], zinc.

walking in open air am.

alum., **am-c.,** graph.[16]

warm room, in

iod.

weather, during warm

nat-p.

wet[2]
   SANG.

LEAD, chronic effects of

alum., alum-sil.[12], **alumn.,** ant-c.[2],
ars., **bell.,** carbn-s.[8], **CAUST.,** chin.,
cocc.[2, 6], **coloc.**[6, 8, 12], crot-t.[6], cupr.[6],
gels.[6], hep.[2, 10], iod.[8, 10], kali-br.[8],
kali-i.[6, 8], kreos.[2], lyc.[2], mang.[6],
merc.[8], **nat-s.**[6], nux-v., **op.,** petr.[2, 8],
pipe.[12], **plat.,** plb.[3, 10], sul-ac., **sulph.,**
zinc.[2]

paralysis-poisoning

LEAN people

acet-ac.[12], alum.[3, 5-7], **AMBR.,**
arg-m.[1', 3, 6, 14], **arg-n.,** ars.[12], ars-i.[7],
bar-c.[3, 6], beryl.[9], bry., cadm-met.[9],
calc-f.[9], **CALC-P.,** caust., chin.[12],
coff.[7, 12], cupr.[7], ferr.[3, 6], fl-ac.[7],
flor-p.[14], graph.[5, 12], ign., **iod.,** ip.[3, 6],
kreos.[3, 6, 12], lach., **lyc.,** mag-c.[3, 5, 6],
mang.[3, 6], merc.[12], nat-c.[6], nat-m.[5, 12],
nit-ac., nux-m.[3, 6], **nux-v.,** perh.[14],
petr.[1', 3, 6, 12], ph-ac.[7], **phos.,** plb.[12],
saroth.[14], **SEC.,** sep., **sil.,** stann.[12],
SULPH., tub., v-a-b.[14], verat.[12]

LEANING against anything **agg.**[3]

arg-m., arn., bell., cann-s.,
canth., cimic., coloc.[6], con.,
cycl., graph., **hell.,** hep., mag-m.,
nit-ac., phos., plat., samb., sil.,
stann., staph.[3, 6], sulph., ther.,
thuj.

after[3]
   coloc.

am.[3]
   bell., **carb-v.,** dros., **FERR.,**
   kali-c., mang., merc., **nat-m.,**
   nux-v., rhod., rhus-t., sabad., sabin.,
   seneg., spig., staph.

backward agg.[3]

nit-ac., staph.

desire for[11]

gymne., op., tub.[7]

hard am.[3]

bell., **rhus-t.**

pressure

sharp edge agg., a[3]

agar.[3, 6], caust., chin-s., lyc.,
ran-b., ruta, **samb.**[3, 6], stann.,
valer.

am.[3]
   nat-c., stann.

sideward agg.[3]

meny.

LEUCORRHEA am.[3]

arist-cl.[9], cimic., lach., puls.

mucous secretions

LEUKAEMIA

acet-ac., acon.[2], **aran.**[2, 8], ars., **ars-i.**[8], bar-i.[8], benzol.[8], bry.[8], **calc., calc-p.,** carb-v., **carbn-s.,** cean.[8], **chin.,** chin-s.[8], con.[8], cortiso.[9], crot-h., ferr-ar.[10], **ferr-pic.**[8], ip., **kali-p.,** merc.[8], **NAT-AR., nat-m., nat-p.,** NAT-S., nux-v., op.[11], phos.[8], **pic-ac.,** sulfa.[14], sulph., thuj., tub.[7], **x-ray**[9, 14]

LIE DOWN, desire to[11]

abrot., absin., acon., adlu.[14], aether, alet.[1'], alum-p.[1'], **alumn.,** aur-ar.[1'], aur-s.[1'], bar-s.[1'], bell., caj., carbn-o., cench.[1'], chlor., cocc., coloc., dor., dros., ferr., ferr-m., gels., grat., ham., hell., hipp., hydr., iber., kali-m.[1'], **kali-sil.**[1'], lach., lyc., manc., merc., merc-i-f., mez., nat-c., nat-sil.[1'], nux-v., op., ox-ac., paull., phos., polyp-p., **rhus-t.,** sal-n., sang., sel., sumb., tab., tarent., thea, wildb., zinc., zinc-p.[1']

inclination to

ACON., ALUM., am-c., ambr., amor-r.[14], **anac., ant-c.,** ant-t., **apis, ARAN.,** arn., **ARS.,** ars-s-f.[1'], asar., **aur., bapt., bar-c.,** bar-m., bell.[1], bism., bor., bry., buni-o.[14], **CALAD., calc.,** calc-s.[2], cann-s.[3, 4], canth., **caps., carb-an., carb-v., CARBN-S.,** casc., **caust., CHAM., chel.,** chin., chin-ar., **chlol.**[3], cic.[4], cina, clem.[4], **cocc.,** coff., colch.[1', 3], **con.,** croc., crot-h.[4], crot-t.[4], cupr., **cycl.,** daph.[4], dig., dros., dulc., euonin.[4], **FERR.,** ferr-ar.[1'], ferr-p., **form.**[3, 16], gels., gran.[4], **graph.,** grat.[4], **guaj.,** hell.[4], hep.[4, 16], hipp., hyos.[4, 16], iber.[14], **ign.,** ip., **KALI-AR., kali-bi., kali-br.**[3], **KALI-C.**[1, 7], **kali-n.**[3, 4, 6], kali-s., **lach.,** laur.[4], led., lil-t.[3], **lyc.,** m-arct.[4], mag-c.,

mag-m., mang.[16], merc., merc-c.[3], mez.[3], mosch.[2], mur-ac., nat-ar., nat-c., **nat-m.,** nat-p., nat-s.[3, 4], nit-ac.[1], nux-m.[3, 4], **NUX-V.,** olnd.[3, 4], op., ox-ac.[4, 6], par.[4], **petr., ph-ac., phos., phyt., pic-ac.,** plan.[3], plb.[4], **psor.**[1', 6], **puls.,** ran-b., raph.[4], **rhus-t.,** ruta, sabad., sabin.[4], **SEL.,** senec.[6], **seneg.**[2], **sep., SIL., spong., stann.,** staph., **stram.,** stront-c., sulfonam.[14], **sulph., sumb.,** tarax., **tarent.,** teucr., thea[4], ther.[4], thuj., verat., vip.[4], visc.[9], **zinc., zing.**[2]

abdomen in pregnancy, on[7]

podo.

but agg. thereby[3]

alum.

eating, after

ant-c.[3, 16], caust.[3], chel.[16], **chin.**[3, 16], clem.[16], **lach.,** nat-m.[3, 16], nit-ac.[16], **sel.**

will not lie down, sits up in bed

kali-br.

LIFTING, straining of muscles and tendons, from

acet-ac.[7], **acon.**[7], **agn.**[2, 7, 12], alum., alum-sil.[1'], alumn.[2], **ambr.,** arist-cl.[9], **ARN.,** ars.[3], bar-c., bell.[7], **bell.-p.**[7], **bor., bov.**[2], **bry., CALC.,**

calc-f.[7, 9], calc-p.[12], **calc-s.,**
calc-sil.[1'], calen.[7], **CARB-AN.,**
carb-v., carbn-s., caust., chin., **cocc.,**
coloc., **CON.,** croc., cur., **dulc.**[1, 7],
ferr., ferr-p., **form.**[2, 7, 12], **GRAPH.,**
hyper.[1', 7], **ign.**[3], iod., **kali-c.,**
kali-m.[1'], kali-sil.[1'], **kalm.**[2], lach.,
lyc., mag-c.[4], merc., **mill.,** mur-ac.,
nat-c. nat-m., nit-ac., nux-v., olnd.,
ph-ac., phos., plat., podo.[2, 12],
prun.[12], psor.[12], rhod., **RHUS-T.,**
RUTA[1, 7], **sec.,** sep., **SIL.,** spig.,
stann., staph., stront-c.[7], sul-ac.,
sulph., thuj., valer.

ailments from[12]

agn., alum., calc., calc-p.,
carb-an., carb-v., graph., lyc.,
mill., ph-ac., phos., podo., prun.,
psor., rhus-t., ruta, sec., sep.

arms, of[12]

rhus-t., sul-ac.

reaching high[12]

sulph.

tendency to strain o.s. in lifting[6]

arn., bry., **calc.,** carb-v., con.,
graph., lyc., **nat-c.**[6, 7], nat-m.[7],
psor.[7], **rhus-t., SIL.**[6, 7], **symph.**[7]

LIGHT agg.[3]

achy.[14], **acon.**[3, 8], agar., aqn., alum.,
am-c., am-m., anac., anh.[10, 14],
ant-c., arg-n.[3, 7], arn., **ars.,** asar.,
bar-c., BELL.[3, 7, 8], bor., bry.,
buth-a.[10], **CALC.**[3, 8], camph.,
carb-an., caust., cham., **chin.,**
cic., cina, clem., coca[8], cocc.,

coff., **colch.**[3, 8, 14], **CON.**[3, 8], **croc.,**
culx.[1'], cupr., dig., **dros., EUPHR.,**
glon.[3, 12], **GRAPH.**[3, 8], hell., **hep.,**
hyos., **ign.**[3, 8], kali-c., kali-n., lach.,
laur., levo.[14], **lyc., lyss.**[8], mag-c.,
mag-m., mang., **merc.,** mez.,
mim-p.[14], mur-ac., **nat-c.,** nat-m.,
nat-s., nit-ac., nux-m., **nux-v.**[3, 7, 8],
op.[7], petr., **ph-ac., PHOS.**[3, 8], plat.,
puls., rhod., **rhus-t.,** ruta, samb.,
sang.[3], sars., sel., seneg., **SEP., sil.,**
spig.[3, 8], stann., staph., **stram.**[3, 8],
sul-ac., **sulph.,** tarax., thuj., valer.,
verat., zinc.

ailments from bright[12]

glon.

snow

am.[2, 3]

am-m., anac., ars., bar-c., **calc.,**
carb-an.[2, 3, 6], **carb-v.**[2, 3, 6], **caust.,**
coff.[3], **plat.**[2, 3, 6], **staph.,**
stram.[2, 3, 6, 8], **STRONT-C.**[2, 3, 6],
valer.

artificial l. agg.[3]

agn., am-m., anac., **apis, bar-c.**[3, 6],
bell.[3, 6], bor., **CALC-C.**[3, 6], carb-an.,
caust., chin-s., cina, **CON.**[3, 6],
croc.[3, 6], **DROS., GLON.**[3, 6],
graph.[3, 6], **hep.**[3, 6], **ign.,** kali-c., laur.,
LYC., manc., mang., **MERC.**[3, 6],
mez., nat-c., nat-m., **nat-s.,** nit-ac.,
nux-m., petr., **ph-ac., PHOS.**[3, 6],
plat., **PULS.,** ruta[3, 6], sars., seneg.,
sep.[3, 6], **sil.**[3, 6], staph., stram.[3, 6],
sulph.

daylight agg.[3]

acon., am-m., **ant-c.,** bell., **calc.,**
CON., dros., EUPHR.[3, 6], GRAPH.,
hell., **HEP.,** hyos., mag-c., mang.,
merc., nit-ac., **NUX-V.,** petr.,
ph-ac., **PHOS.,** rhod., samb., sang.,
sars., **sep., SIL., stram.,** sulph., thuj.

fire agg., of[3]

ant-c., bry., **euph., glon.,** mag-m.,
merc., puls., **zinc.**

sunlight agg.[3]

acon., agar., anh.[9, 10], **ant-c.**[3, 6],
ars., asar., bar-c.[3, 6], bell.[3, 10],
bry., **CALC.**[3, 6], camph., **chin.**[3, 6],
con.[3, 6], **euphr.**[3, 6], **GLON.,**
GRAPH.[3, 6], **ign.**[3, 6], lach.,
mag-m., merc-c., **nat-c.**[3, 6],
nux-v.[3, 6], **PH-AC.**[3, 6], phos.[3, 6],
puls.[3, 6], sang.[6], sel., seneg., sil.[6],
stann., stram., **sulph.**[3, 6], valer.,
verat., zinc.

sun

am.[2, 3]
anac., con., **plat., stram.,**
STRONT-C., thuj.[3]

LIGHTNESS, sensation of[16]

mez.

LIGHTNING, ailments from[12]

crot-h., morph., phos.

weather–storm

LOSS of blood[6] *

abrot., arn., carb-an., **chin.**[1, 6],
chin-ar., **ferr.**[1, 6], ferr-pic.[12], ham.,
helon., hydr., ip.[12], **nat-m.,**
ph-ac.[1, 6], phos., sep.[1], **staph.**[1]

fluids, of *

abrot.[3], acon.[3], agar., alet.[6],
alum., anac., ant-c., ant-t.,
arg-m., arn., **ars.,** ars-i., **aven.**[6],
bell., bism.[3], bor., bov.,
brom.[3], bry., bufo[3], **calad.,**
CALC., CALC-P., cann-s., canth.,
caps., carb-ac.[3], **carb-an.,**
CARB-V., carbn-s., caust., cham.,
CHIN., chin-ar., CHIN-S., cimic.[3],
cina, coff., **con.,** crot-h., **cupr.**[3, 6],
dig., dulc., **ferr.,** ferr-ar., **GRAPH.,**
ham.[3, 6, 8], helon.[3, 6], hep., ign.,
iod., ip., **kali-c., kali-p.,** lach.[3],
led., lyc., mag-m., **merc.,** mez.,
mosch., nat-c., nat-m., **nat-p.,**
nit-ac., nux-m.[1], **nux-v.,** petr.,
PH-AC., phos., plat.[3], plb., psor.[8],
PULS., ran-b., rhod., rhus-t., ruta,
sabad., samb., sec., **SEL., SEP.,**
sil., spig., **squil.,** stann., **STAPH.,**
stram.[3], sul-ac.[7], **sulph.,** thuj.,
valer., verat., zinc.

emissions

nursing

ailments from[12]

calc., carb-an., chin., nat-m.,
ph-ac., phos., sel., sil.

LYING agg.

abies-n., **acon.,** aesc.[3, 6], **agar.,**
agn.[3], alum., alum-p.[1], **alumn.**[2],
am-c., **am-m., ambr.,** anac.,
ang.[2, 3], ant-c., **ant-t., APIS,**
apoc., aral., aran.[3], **arg-m.,** arn.,
ARS., ars-i., ars-s-f.[1], arum-t.[8],
asaf., asar., **AUR.,** aur-ar.[1], **aur-i.**[1],
aur-s.[1], **bapt.,** bar-c.[2, 3], **bell.,**
bism., bor., bov., **bry.,** cact., calad.,
calc., calc-p., camph., cann-i.,
cann-s., canth., **CAPS.,** carb-an.,
carb-v., carbn-s., caust., cench.[7, 8],
CHAM., chel., chin., cic., cina,
clem., cocc., coff., colch., **coloc.,**

CON., croc., crot-h.[3], crot-t., cupr., **cycl.**, dig., dios., **DROS., dulc., EUPH., euphr., FERR.**, ferr-ar., ferr-i., ferr-p., fl-ac., gels., **glon.**, gnaph.[7], graph., grin., guaj., **hell.**, hep., **HYOS.**, iber.[8], ign., iod., ip., kali-bi., **kali-br., KALI-C.**, kali-i., kali-m.[1'], **kali-n.**, kali-s.[1'], **kalm.**[3, 6], kreos., **lach.**, lact., laur., led., lil-t.[3], **LYC.**, mag-c., **mag-m.**, mang., **MENY.**, meph.[3], merc., mez., **mosch., mur-ac.**, murx., naja, nat-ar., **nat-c.**, nat-m., **NAT-S.**, nit-ac., nux-m., **nux-v.**, olnd., **op.**, ox-ac.[3], par., petr., **ph-ac.**, phel., **PHOS., PLAT.**, plb., prot.[14], **PULS.**, **ran-b.**, ran-s.[3], raph., rheum, **rhod.**, **RHUS-T., RUMX., ruta, sabad.**, sabin., sal-ac., **SAMB., SANG.**, sars., sec., sel., seneg., **sep.**, **sil.**[2, 3, 6, 8], spig., spong., squil., stann., staph., stict., stram., **stront-c.**, sul-ac., sul-i.[1'], **sulph.**, **TARAX.**, tarent.[3], teucr., thuj., **trif-r.**[8], **valer.**, verat., **verb.**, viol-o., **viol-t.**, x-ray[8], zinc., **zing.**

am.

acon., agar., agn., alum., alum-sil.[1'], alumn.[2], am-c., **AM-M.**, ambr., anac., ang.[2, 3], anh.[8, 10], ant-c., ant-t., arg-m., **arn.**, ars., asaf.[3], **ASAR.**, aur.[3], **bar-c.**, bar-i.[1'], **BELL.**, bell-p.[8], bor., bov.[3], brom.[8], **BRY.**, calad., **CALC.**, calc-i.[1'], **calc-p.**, calc-sil.[1'], camph., cann-s., **canth.**, caps., carb-ac., **carb-an., carb-v.**, carbn-s., **caust.**, cham.[2, 3], chel., chin., cic., cimic., cina, clem., **coc-c.**[2], cocc., coff., **colch.**, coloc., con., conv., croc., cupr., cycl.[3, 6], dicha.[10], dig., dios., dros., dulc., equis.[8], euph., euphr.[3], **FERR.**, fl-ac.[3], form.[3], gels.[3], **glon.**, **graph.**, guaj., hell., hep., hyos., **ign.**, iod., ip., kali-c., kali-n., kalm., kreos., lach., laur., **led.**, lyc., mag-c., mag-m., mag-s.[4], **MANG.**, merc., merc-c.[3], methys.[14], mez., mur-ac., nat-c., **NAT-M.**, nat-sil.[1'], **nit-ac.**, nux-m., **NUX-V.**, olnd., onos.[8], op., par., petr., ph-ac., phos.,

PIC-AC., plat.[3, 6], plb., **psor.**, pulx.[8], **puls.**[3, 8], rad-br.[8], ran-b., rheum, rhod.[3], rhus-t., ruta, sabad., sabin., samb.[3], **sang.**[3], sars., sec., sel., seneg., sep., sieg.[10], **sil.**[2, 3], **spig.**, spong., **SQUIL., stann.**[2, 3, 6, 8], **staph.**[2, 3, 6], **stram.**[2, 3], stroph-s.[14], stry.[8], sul-ac.[2, 3], **sulph.**, sym-r.[8], tarax.[3], teucr.[2, 3], thuj.[2, 3], valer.[3], **verat.**[2, 3, 4, 6], verb.[3], zinc.[2, 3, 16]

after l. agg.

acon., agar., agn., alum., **am-c.**, am-m., **AMBR.**, ant-c., ant-t., **arg-m.**, arn., **ARS., asaf.**, asar., **AUR.**, bar-c., bell., bism., bor., bov., bry., calad., calc., canth., **caps.**, carb-an., carb-v., caust., **cham.**, chel., chin., **clem.**, cocc., coff., colch., coloc., **con.**, croc., cupr., **cycl.**, dros., **DULC., euph.**, **euphr., ferr.**, graph., guaj., hell., hep., **hyos.**, ign., ip., **kali-c.**, kali-m.[1'], kali-n., lach., laur., led., **LYC., mag-c., mag-m.**, mang., **meny.**, merc., mez., mosch., mur-ac., nat-ar., nat-c., nit-ac., nux-m., nux-v., olnd., op., par., petr., ph-ac., phos., **PLAT.**, plb., **PULS.**, ran-b., ran-s., rhod., **RHUS-T.**, ruta, **sabad.**, sabin., **SAMB.**, sars., sel., seneg., **sep.**, sil., spig., stann., staph., **STRONT-C.**, sul-ac., **sulph.**, **tarax.**, teucr., thuj., valer., verat., verb., viol-o., viol-t., zinc.

am.

acon., agar., agn., am-m., ambr., anac., ant-c., ant-t., arg-m., arn., **ARS.**, asaf., aur., bar-c., **bell.**, bov., **BRY.**, caj., calad., **CALC.**, calc-f., camph., cann-s., **canth.**, caps., carb-an., **carb-v.**, carbn-s., caust., chel., chin., cic., **cina**, cocc., coff., colch., coloc., con., **croc.**, crot-h., cupr., dig., dios., dros., dulc., euphr., **fl-ac., graph.**, guaj., hell., **hep.**, hyos., ign., **iod.**, ip., kali-c., kali-n., kreos., **lach.**,

laur., led., lyc., mag-c., mag-m.,
meli., **merc.**, nat-c., **NAT-M.,
NIT-AC.**, nux-m., **NUX-V., olnd.,**
pall., par., petr., ph-ac., phos.,
PULS., ran-b., rheum, rhod.,
rhus-t., sabin., samb., sars., sec.,
sel., **sep.**, sil., sin-n., **spig.**, spong.,
SQUIL., stann., **staph., stram.,**
sul-ac., sul-i.[1]', **sulph.**, tarax.,
thuj., valer., verat., verb.

abdomen agg., on[3]

ambr.

am.
acet-ac., adlu.[14], aloe, am-c.,
ambr., ant-t.[8], ars., bar-c., **BELL.,**
bell-p.[3], bry., calc., calc-p.[3, 7],
chel., chion.[3], **cina, coloc.**, crot-t.,
cupr.[3, 6], **elaps, eup-per.**[3, 6], ind.[3],
lach., lept.[3, 7], mag-c., **MED.**[3, 7, 8],
nit-ac., par.[3, 7], pareir.[3], **phos.,**
phyt., plb., **podo.**[3, 7, 8], psil.[14],
psor.[3], rhus-t., rib-ac.[14], sel., sep.,
stann., stram.[3], **tab.**[8], thyr.[3]

pregnancy, in[15]

podo.

back agg., on

acet-ac., acon., agar.[3], aloe,
alum., alum-p.[1]', alum-sil.[1]',
alumn.[2], am-c., **am-m.**, ang.[2, 3],
arg-m., arg-n.[3, 6], arn., **ars.,**
ars-s-f.[1]', aur-m., bar-c., bar-i.[1]',
bell., bor., bry., bufo, calc., canth.,
carb-v.[16], **caust., cham.**, chin.,
cimic.[3, 6], cina, clem., **colch.**[2, 3],
coloc., cupr., cycl.[3], dulc.,
eup-per., euph., hyper., **IGN.**[2-4],
iod., kali-c., **kali-n.**[2, 3, 6], kreos.[3, 6],
lach., lob.[3], mag-m.[2, 3], mag-p.[3, 6],
merc., merc-i-f.[3], nat-c., nat-m.,
nat-s., NUX-V., op., par., **PHOS.,**
plat., **plb.**[3], **puls.**[2-4, 8], ran-b.,
rhus-t., rib-ac.[14], sang.[3, 6], **sep.,
sil., spig.**, sponq., stront-c.,
sul-i., **sulph.**, thuj.

am.
acon., aeth., am-c., **AM-M., anac.,**
ang.[2, 3], **apis**, arn., bar-c., bell.,
bor., **BRY., cact.**[1], calad., **CALC.,**
calc-sil.[1]', **camph.**[7], **canth.,**
carb-an., caust., chin., cimic.,
cina, clem., **colch.**, con., conv.,
crot-h.[3, 6], cycl.[3, 6], **dig.**[3, 6, 8], ferr.,
grat., hell., **ign.**, ip., **kali-c., kalm.,**
kreos., lach., **lyc.**, mag-m.[3], merc.,
MERC-C., mosch., nat-c., **nat-m.,
nat-s.**, nux-v., ox-ac., par., **phos.,**
plat., **PULS.**, ran-b., **RHUS-T.,**
sabad., sabin.[3, 6], **sang.**, senec.,
seneg., sep., sil., spig., **spong.,
stann.**, sulph., sym-r.[8], tell.[14],
thuj., verat., viol-t.

unable to turn from the back

cic., elaps

bed agg., in

acon., **agar.**, agn.[1], aloe, alum.,
am-c., am-m., **AMBR.**, anac.,
ang.[3], ant-c., **ant-t., arg-m.**, arn.,
ars., ars-i., asaf., asar., **aur.,**
aur-i.[1]', aur-s.[1]', bar-c., bar-i.[1]',
bell., bism., **bor.**, bov., **bry.,**
bufo[3], calad., calc., calc-i.[1]',
camph., cann-s., canth., caps.,
carb-an., carb-v., caust., cham.,
chel., chin., cic., cina, **clem.,**
cocc., coff., colch., **coloc.**, con.,
croc., cycl., dig., dios., **dros.,**
dulc., **euph.**, euphr., **FERR.,
FERR-I.**, ferr-p.[1]', fl-ac.[3], graph.,
guaj., hell., hep., hyos., ign., **IOD.,
kali-c.**, kali-i., kali-m.[1]', kali-n.,
kali-p., kali-s., **kalm.**, kreos.,
LACH., laur., **led., lil-t., lith-c.,
LYC.**, mag-c., mag-m.[3], **mang.,**
meny., **MERC.**, merc-c.[3],
merc-i-f., mez., mosch., mur-ac.,
nat-c., **nat-m.**, nit-ac., nux-m.,
nux-v., olnd., op., **ox-ac.**, par.,
petr., **ph-ac., PHOS.**, phyt., **plat.,**

plb., **PULS.,** ran-b., rheum, **rhod.,
rhus-t., RUMX.,** ruta, sabad.,
sabin., samb., **SANG., sars.,** sec.,
sel., seneg., **SEP., SIL., spig.,**
spong., squil., stann., staph.,
stict., stram., **stront-c.,** sul-ac.,
sul-i.[1'], **SULPH.,** tarax., **tell.,**
teucr., thuj., valer., **verat.,** verb.,
viol-o., viol-t., **zinc.,** zinc-p.[1']

am.
acon., agar., **am-m.,** ambr., anac.,
ang.[3], ant-c., ant-t., arg-m., arn.,
ars., asar., aur., aur-ar.[1'], **bar-c.,**
bell., bov., **BRY.,** calad., calc.,
calc-sil.[1'], camph., cann-s., **canth.,**
caps., carb-an., carb-v., **caust.,**
cham., chel., chin., **CIC.,** cina,
clem., **coc-c., COCC.,** coff., colch.,
coloc., **con.,** croc., cupr., dig.,
dulc., ferr., graph., guaj., hell.,
HEP., hyos., ign., iod., ip., kali-c.,
kali-n., kreos., **lach.,** laur., led.,
lyc., mag-c., mag-m.[3], merc.,
mez., mur-ac., nat-c., **nat-m.,**
nit-ac., nux-m., **NUX-V.,** olnd.,
par., petr., ph-ac., phos., puls.,
ran-b., rheum, rhod., **rhus-t.,**
sabad., sabin., samb., sars., sec.,
sel., sep., **sil.,** spig., spong.,
SQUIL., STANN., staph., stram.,
stront-c., sul-ac., sulfonam.[14],
sulph., tarax., thuj., valer., verat.,
verb., viol-t.

doubled up agg.[3]

hyos., lyc., spong., teucr., valer.

am.[2, 3, 6]
bell.[3], cham.[3], cocc.[3], **colch.,
COLOC.,** mag-m.[3, 6], mag-p.[3, 6],
merc-c.[3], plat.[3], **puls., rheum,**
rhus-t.[6], staph.[3], stram.[3], **sulph.**[2],
verat.[3]

down, immediatly after[1']

cench., ferr-i.

face am., on the [3, 6]

led., **psor.,**

half reclining posture am.[3]

acon., gels., sang.

hand knee position am.[3]

con., eup-per., euph., **lach.,** med.,
pareir., sep., tarent.

hard bed agg., on a[6]

arn., bapt., bar-c., graph., kali-c.,
lach., puls., **rhus-t.,** sil.

am.[3, 6]
acon.[3], bell., mag-m.[3], nat-m.[3],
rhus-t.[3], **sep.**[3]

head high am., with[8]

petr., puls., spig., spong.[6]

head low agg., with[2, 3]

ant-t., apis[3], **arg-m.**[3], arn.,
ARS.[2, 3, 8], bell.[3], cact.', **cann-s.,**
caps., carb-v.[3], **chin., clem.,
colch.,** con.[3], gels.[3], glon.[1'], **hep.,
KALI-N., lach., nux-v., petr.,**
phos., **PULS.,** sang.[3], **spig.,**
spong.[3], stront-c., **sulph.**

am.[3]
apis, **arn.**[2, 3, 8], bell., calc.[3, 6],
caust.[3, 6], cycl., lach., laur.[3],
nat-m.[3, 6], sang.[3], **spong.**[2, 3, 8],
tab., **verat., verat-v.**[7]

knee chest position am.[3]

sep.

knee elbow position am.[3]

con.[3, 6], eup-per., euph.[3, 6], **lyc.**[3, 6], med., pareir., petr., sep.

legs drawn up am.[6]

bell., cocc., coloc., **mag-p.**, stram., verat.

moist ground or floor agg., on a[3]

ars., calc., calc-p.[3, 6], caust., **dulc.**[3, 6], rhus-t.[3, 6], sil., sulph.[3, 6]

side agg., on

ACON., am-c., am-m., **ANAC.,** ang.[2, 3], **arg-n.,** arn., ars.[16], aur., bar-c., bell., bor., **BRY., calad., CALC.,** canth., **CARB-AN.,** caust., chin., **cina,** clem., colch., **con., ferr., ign., ip., KALI-C.,** kali-n.[16], kreos., lach., lil-t.[1', 3], **LYC.,** mag-m.[2, 3], **merc., merc-c.,** mosch., nat-c.[2, 3], nat-m., **nat-s.,** nux-v., **par., ph-ac., phos.,** plat., **puls.,** ran-b., **RHUS-T.,** sabad., **seneg.,** sep., **sil.,** spig., spong., **STANN., sulph., thuj.,** verat., viol-t.

am.
  acon., alum., am-c., am-m., ang.[2, 3], arn., ars., bar-c., bell., bor., bry., calc-p., canth., caust., cham., chin., cina, clem., **COCC.,** colch., **coloc.**[2, 3], cupr., dulc., euph., ign., iod., kali-c., **kali-n.**[2, 3], lach., mag-m.[2, 3], merc.[2, 3], nat-c.[2, 3], nat-m., **NUX-V.,** par., **phos.,** plat., puls.[2, 3], ran-b., rhus-t., **sep., sil.**[2, 3], spig., spong., stront-c., sulph., thuj.

left s. agg.

acon., ail., **am-c.**[2, 3, 6], anac., ang.[2, 3], ant-t., apis[3], **arg-n.,** arn., **bar-c.,** bell., brom.[6], bry., **cact.,** calad.[8], calc.[2, 3], canth., carb-an., chin., coc-c.[8], **colch.,** con., cycl.[3], dig.[3], eup-per., glon.[3], hydroph.[14], iber.[3, 8], ind.[3], ip., kali-ar., kali-c., kalm., kreos., lil-t.[3], lyc., mag-m., magn-gr.[8], merc., **naja, nat-c., nat-m.,** nat-p., **nat-s.,** op., **par.,** petr., **PHOS.,** plat., **ptel.**[3, 8], **PULS.,** rhus-t., rumx.[3], seneg., **sep.,** sil., **spig.**[2, 3, 8], **stann.**[2, 3], **sulph.,** tab., **thuj.,** tub.[3], vib.[3], visc.[8], zinc-i.[3]

am.[2]
  acon., **am-m.,** anac., arg-n.[3, 6], **bor.,** bry., calc., carb-an., **caust.,** cina, clem., con., ign.[8], ip., kali-c., lach., lyc., **mag-m.,** merc., mur-ac.[8], nat-c., nat-m.[8], **nux-v.,** puls., ran-b., seneg., spig., **spong.,** stann., sulph., thuj.

pain goes to side on which he is not lying[3]

arn., **bry.,** calc-ar., cupr., cur., fl-ac., graph., **ign.,** kali-c., kali-bi., merc., ph-ac., puls., **rhus-t.,** sil.

lain on[3]

arn., **ars., bry.,** calc., cimic., graph., **kali-c.,** merc., mosch., **nat-m., ph-ac.,** phos., phys., **PULS.,** sep., sil.

painful s. agg.

acon., agar., am-c., am-m.,
ambr., anac., ang.[2, 3], **ant-c.**,
arg-m., arn., **ars.**, ars-i., **bapt.**,
BAR-C., bell., bry., **CALAD.**,
calc., calc-f., cann-s., caps.,
carb-an., carb-v., caust., **chin.**,
cina, clem., croc., cupr.,
CYCL.[3, 16], dios., **dros., graph.**,
guaj., **HEP.**, hyos., ign., **IOD.**,
kali-c., kali-i., kali-m.[1', 2],
kali-n., **LACH.**[2, 3, 6], **laur.**[3], led.,
lyc., mag-c., MAG-M.[2, 3],
mang., **merc.**, mez., **mosch.**,
mur-ac., nat-m., **nit-ac.**,
NUX-M., nux-v., olnd., **par.**,
petr., **ph-ac., phos.**, plat., puls.,
pyrog.[3, 6], ran-b., ran-s., **rheum,**
rhod., **rhus-t., rumx., RUTA,**
sabad., sabin., samb., sars.,
sel., sep., **SIL., spong.**, staph.,
stram., sulph.[2, 3], tarax.,
tell.[3, 8], teucr., thiop.[14], thuj.,
valer., verat., verb., vib.[8]

am.

am-c.[8, 15], ambr., arn., bell.,
bor.[8], **BRY., calc.**, cann-s.,
carb-v., caust., **cham.**, chel.[3],
coloc., cupr-a.[8], esp-g.[13], fl-ac.[3],
ign., kali-c., lyc., mag-p.[3, 6],
nux-v., plb.[3, 6], **puls.**, rhus-t.,
sec.[3], **sep.**, stram., sul-ac.[8],
sulph., viol-o., viol-t.

painless s. agg.

ambr., arg-m., arn., bell., **BRY.,**
calc., cann-s., carb-v., **caust.,**
CHAM., chel., chin.[3, 16],
COLOC., con.[3], cupr., **FL-AC.**[3],
graph.[3], hyper., **ign., kali-c.,**
lyc., merc-i-r., naja, nat-c.[1],
nat-m.[3], nat-s.[3], nux-v., phos.,
plan., ptel.[8], **PULS., rhus-t.,**
SEC.[3], **sep.**, stann., sul-ac.,
ter.[3], viol-o., viol-t.

am.

acon., agar., am-c., am-m.,
ambr., anac., ang.[2], ant-c.,
arg-m., arn., ars., **bapt., bar-c.,**
bell., bry., **calad.**, calc.[2], calc-f.,
cann-s., caps., carb-an.,
carb-v., caust., chin., cina,
clem., croc., cupr., dios., dros.,
graph., guaj., **hep.**, hyos., ign.,
iod., kali-c., kali-m.[1'], kali-n.,
lach., led., lyc., mag-c.,
mag-m.[2], mang., merc., mez.,
mosch., mur-ac., naja[14], nat-m.,
nit-ac., **nux-m., nux-v.**, olnd.,
par., petr., ph-ac., **phos.**[2], plat.,
puls., ran-b., ran-s., rheum,
rhod., rhus-t., **ruta,** sabad.,
sabin., samb., sars., sel., sep.,
sil., spong., staph., stram.,
sulph.[2], tarax., teucr.[2], thuj.,
valer., verat., verb.

part on which he is lying, agg.[3]

aloe, am-c., ars., **arn.**, bar-c., **bry.**,
calc., caust., **chin., graph.**, hep.,
hyper., mag-m., merc., mosch.,
nat-s., nit-ac., ph-ac., **PULS.**,
rhus-t., sep., sil., thuj.

right s. agg.

acon., **alum., am-c., am-m.,**
anac., bad.[3], bell.[3], benz-ac.,
bor., bry., bufo, calc.[2, 3, 16],
cann-i.[8], carb-an., caust.[1],
cimic.[14], cina, clem., con.,
hydr.[3], ip., iris[3], **kali-c.**, kali-i.,
kali-m.[1'], kreos., lach.[2, 3], lyc.,
lycps.[3, 6], mag-c.[3'], **mag-m.,**
MERC., mur-ac., nat-c.[?, 3],
nux-v., phos., prun-s., psor.,
puls.[2, 3], ran-b., **rhus-t.**[3, 8],
rumx.[3, 6], sang.[3'], scroph-n.[8],
sec.[3], seneg., spig.[2, 3], **spong.,**
stann.[2, 3, 8], sul-ac., sulph.,
thuj.

am.$^{2, 3}$
  acon., am-c., anac., ang.,
  ant-t.^{8}, arn., **bar-c.,** bar-m.^{3},
  bell., brom.^{3}, **bry.**$^{2, 3, 6}$, cact.^{3},
  calc., canth., **carb-an.,** chin.,
  colch., con., crot-h.^{3}, ip.,
  kali-c., kreos.^{3}, **lyc.,**
  mang.$^{3, 6}$, merc., **nat-c.,**
  nat-m.$^{2, 3, 8}$, **par., PHOS.**$^{2, 3, 8}$,
  plat., ptel.$^{3, 6}$, **PULS.,** seneg.,
  sep., sil., spig.$^{2, 3, 6}$, **stann.,**
  sulph.$^{2, 3, x}$, tab.^{x}, **thuj.**

with head high^8

  ars., cact., **spig.,** spong.

stretched out l. agg.^{3}

  cham., colch., coloc., plat., puls.,
  rheum, rhus-t., staph.

MAGNETISM am.

  acon., bar-c., **bell., calc.,** calc-p., chin.,
  con., **CUPR.,** graph., ign., iod., nat-c.,
  nux-v., PHOS., sabin., sep., **sil.,**
  sulph., teucr., viol-o.

hand-laying

MANY SYMPTOMS^3

  agar., **tub.**

contradictory

MASTURBATION, onanism, from∗

  abrot.^{8}, agar., agn.$^{3, 8}$, aloe^{12},
  alum., **ambr.,** anac., anan.^{11}, ant-c..

apis$^{8, 12}$, **arg-m.,** arg-n.$^{7, 12}$, ars.,
aur.^{3}, aven.^{6}, bar-c.$^{3, 6}$, bell.^{2},
bell-p.$^{7, 8, 12}$, bov., **bufo,** calad.,
CALC., calc-p.$^{3, 6, 8, 12}$, calc-s.,
calc-sil.$^{1'}$, cann-i.^{6}, cann-s.^{3}, **carb-v.,**
carc.^{7}, **caust.**$^{5, 7}$, **CHIN.,** cina^3, cob.^{12},
COCC., coff.$^{5, 7}$, **CON., dig.,**
dios.$^{3, 6, 8, 12}$, dulc.^{3}, ferr., **GELS.,**
graph.^{8}, grat.$^{7, 8, 12}$, **hyos.,** ign.^{3}, **iod.,**
kali-br.$^{3, 6, 8, 12}$, kali-c., **kali-p.,**
lach.$^{3, 12}$, **lyc., mag-p.**^{1}, med.^{12}, **merc.,**
merc-c.^{1}, mosch., nat-c., **nat-m.,**
NAT-P., nux-m., **nux-v.,** op.^{11}, **ORIG.,**
petr., **PH-AC., phos., pic-ac.**$^{3, 6, 8}$,
plat.$^{3, 8, 12}$, plb., **puls., sal-n.**$^{8, 12}$,
sars.^{12}, **SEL., SEP.,** sil., **spig.,** squil.,
stann.$^{3, 12}$, **STAPH.,** stict.$^{3, 6}$, still.^{8},
stram.$^{3, 6}$, **SULPH.,** tab.$^{8, 12}$, **thuj.**$^{3, 8}$,
trib.^{8}, ust.$^{3, 8}$, zinc.$^{8, 12}$, zinc-o.^{8}

MEASLES, after

  acon.^{3}, am-c.^{3}, ant-c., **ant-t.**^{3},
  arg-m.^{2}, **ars.**$^{2-4}$, **bell.,** bry., **calc.**^{2},
  CAMPH., CARB-V., carbn-s.,
  caust.^{2}, cham., chin., cina^3, coff.$^{3, 6}$,
  cupr-a.^{3}, **dros.**$^{2, 3}$, **dulc.**$^{2, 4}$, euphr.^{2},
  hell.^{3}, **hyos.,** ign., iod.^{4}, **ip.**^{7},
  kali-c.$^{3, 6}$, **kali-m.**$^{2, 6}$, lob.^{7}, **MORB.**^{7},
  mosch., nux-m.^{2}, nux-v., oxyd.^{7},
  phos.^{4}, **PULS., rhus-t., sep.**$^{2, 3}$,
  stict.^{2}, stram.^{2}, **sulph.,** zinc.^{3}

exanthema repelled$^{3, 4}$

  bry.^{3}, **phos., puls.,** rhus-t.

MEDICAMENTS, abuse of^7

  aloe^8, ars.^{3}, bapt., camph.$^{3, 6}$,
  carb-v., cham.$^{3, 4, 6}$, coff.^{4}, hep.^{3},
  hydr.$^{3, 8}$, kali-i.^{3}, **lob.**^{7}, mag-s.^{9},
  nat-m.^{3}, nit-ac.^{3}, **NUX-V.**$^{2-4, 6-8, 12}$,
  puls.$^{3, 6}$, **sulph.**^{3}, teucr.$^{2, 8, 12}$,
  thuj.^{12}

arsenical poisoning

china
iodine

iron, abuse

mercury, abuse

narcotics
paralysis-poisoning

purgatives
quinine, abuse

sulphur, abuse

vegetable[8]
   camph., **nux-v.**

addiction

   buth-a.[9], tab.[12]

Vol. I: *morphinism*

narcotics-desire

oversensitive to[5, 7]

   acon., arn., asar.[3], cham.[3, 5, 7],
   chin.[3], coff., **ign.**[3], lyc., nit-ac.[1'],
   NUX-V.[1', 3, 5, 7], **PULS.**[3, 5, 7], sep.[5],
   sil.[5], **SULPH.**, teucr.[3, 12], **valer.**[3]

   high potencies, to[1']

      ars-i., caust.[5], hep.[5], lyc.[5],
      NIT-AC.[1', 4, 5, 7], nux-v.[1', 5],
      sep.[5]

quick reaction[1']

   bell., cupr., nux-v., zinc.

reaction, lack-remedies

MENSES, before

   alum., alum-p.[1'], **am-c.**, am-m.,
   arg-n., arist-cl.[9, 10, 14], asaf., asar.,
   bar-c., bar-i.[1'], bar-m., bar-s.[1'],
   bell., berb.[4], bor., **BOV.**, brom.[3],
   bry., **CALC.**, **CALC-P.**, calc-sil.[1'],
   canth., carb-an., **carb-v.**, carbn-s.,
   caul.[3, 6], **caust.**[1, 7], cham., chin.,
   cimic.[3, 14], cina, cocc., coff., **coloc.**[3],
   con., croc., **CUPR.**, dig.[3], dulc.,
   ferr.[1], ferr-i., foll.[14], gels., graph.,
   hep., **hyos.**, ign., iod., ip., **kali-c.**,
   kali-m.[1'], kali-n., **kreos.**, **LACH.**,
   LYC., mag-c.[1, 7], mag-f.[9, 10, 14],
   mag-m., mag-s.[9, 10], **mang.**, **merc.**,
   mez., mosch., mur-ac., nat-c.,
   NAT-M., **nat-p.**, nit-ac.[3, 4], nux-m.,
   nux-v., ol-an.[4], petr., **ph-ac.**, **phos.**,
   plat., psor.[3, 6], **PULS.**, rhus-t., rob.[7],
   ruta, sabad., sars., **SEP.**, sil., spig.,
   spong., stann., staph., **sul-ac.**,
   SULPH., thuj.[7], valer., **VERAT.**,
   vib., vip-a.[14], **ZINC.**, zinc-p.[1']

at beginning of

   acon., arg-n.[3], asar., bell., bry.,
   cact., **CALC-P.**, **caust.**, **cham.**,
   cimic.[3], cocc., coff., graph.,
   HYOS., ign., iod., ip., **KALI-C.**,
   LACH.[3, 8], lac-c.[7], **lyc.**, mag-c.,
   mag-m., mag-p.[3, 6], merc., mosch.,
   nat-m., nit-ac., **phos.**, **plat.**, plb.[3],
   puls., ruta, sars., **sep.**, **sil.**, staph.,
   zinc.[3]

   am.[6]
      lach., mag-p., plb., zinc.

during

acon., agar., aloe, alum., alum-p.$^{1'}$,
AM-C., am-m., ambr., **ant-c.,**
ARG-N., ars., ars-i., ars-s-f.$^{1'}$,
asar., aur.^{3}, bar-c., bar-i.$^{1'}$,
bar-m., bars-s.$^{1'}$, bell., berb.^{4},
bor., **BOV.,** bry., **bufo,** but-ac.^{14},
calc.^{1}, calc-p., calc-sil.$^{1'}$, cann-s.,
canth., caps., carb-an., carb-v.,
CARBN-S., cast.$^{3,\ 4,\ 6}$, caust.,
CHAM., chel., chin., chin-s.^{4},
cimic., cocc., coff., con., croc.,
crot-h., crot-t.^{4}, cupr., ferr.,
ferr-i., ferr-p., gels., gran.^{4},
GRAPH., ham.$^{3,\ 8}$, hep. **HYOS.,**
ign., iod., **KALI-C.,** kali-i.^{4},
kali-m.$^{1'}$, kali-n., **kreos.,** lach.,
laur., **lyc., MAG-C., mag-m.,**
mag-s.$^{4,\ 9,\ 10}$, merc., mosch.,
mur-ac., nat-c., **nat-m.,** nat-p.,
nat-s.$^{3,\ 4}$, nicc.^{4}, nit-ac., **nux-m.**^{1},
NUX-V., oena., ol-an.$^{3,\ 4,\ 6}$, op.,
petr., ph-ac., phel.^{4}, **phos.,** plat.,
prun.^{4}, psor.$^{3,\ 6}$, **PULS.,** rat.^{4,}
rhod., rhus-t., sabin., sars., sec.,
sel., **SEP., sil.,** spong., stann.,
staph.$^{3,\ 4}$, stram., stront-c., sul-ac.,
SULPH., thea, thyr.^{14}, **verat.,**
vib., vinc.^{4}, **ZINC., ZINC-P.**$^{1'}$

àm.

all-s.^{3}, alum., am-c.^{8}, apis, aran.,
arg-n.^{3}, arist-cl.$^{9,\ 10,\ 14}$, bell.,
calc., calc-f.$_t$ cimic., cortiso.$^{9,\ 14}$,
cycl., dicha.$^{10,\ 14}$, ferr-p.^{3}, foll.^{14},
gels.^{3}, ign.^{3}, iod.^{3}, kali-bi., **kali-c.,**
kali-p., lac-c., **LACH.,** lycps.^{2},
mand.^{14}, **mosch.,** phenob.$^{13,\ 14}$,
phos., plb.^{6}, puls., rhus-t., senec.,
sep., **stann.,** sulph., ust., verat.,
vip-a.^{14}, **zinc.**

retarded^2

lach.

after

alum., alum-p.$^{1'}$, am-c.,
arist-cl.$^{9,\ 10,\ 14}$, ars.^{4}, berb.^{4}, **BOR.,**
bov., bry., calc., calc-sil.$^{1'}$,
canth., carb-an., carb-v.,
carbn-s., chel., chin., **cocc.**^{6}, **con.,**
cupr., **ferr.,** ferr-i., **GRAPH.,** iod.
kali-c., KREOS., LACH., lil-t.,
lyc., mag-c., merc., **nat-m.,**
nat-p., **NUX-V., nit-ac.,** ph-ac.^{1},
phos., plat., puls., rhus-t., ruta,
sabin., **SEP.,** sil., **stram.,** sul-ac.,
sulph., tarent.^{6}, verat., **zinc.,**
zinc-p.$^{1'}$

am.$^{3,\ 6}$

aran.., arist-cl.^{9}, calc., cimic.,
lycps.^{3}, thyr.^{14}, **zinc-p.**$^{1'}$

MERCURY, abuse of*

acon.^{3}, agn.^{3}, alumn.^{7}, anan.^{7}, ang.$^{3,\ 6,\ 8}$,
ant-c., ant-t.^{8}, **arg-m.,** arn.^{3}, ars.$^{3,\ 6}$,
asaf., AUR., aur-m.$^{1'}$, aur-s.$^{1'}$, **bell.,**
bor.^{7}, bry.$^?$, calad.$^{2,\ 3}$, **calc.,** camph.$^{2,\ 3}$,
CARB-V., caust.$^{3,\ 8}$, **chel., chin.,** cic.,
cina^3, **clem.,** cocc.$^{1',\ 3,\ 16}$, coff.^{3}, **colch.,**
con., **cupr.,** dig.$^{3,\ 7}$, dulc., **euph.,**
euphr.^{3}, ferr.$^{2,\ 3}$, fl-ac.$^{3,\ 6,\ 8}$, graph.,
guaj., HEP., hydr.$^{3,\ 6,\ 7}$, **iod.,** iris^6,
kali-bi., **kali-chl.**$^{2,\ 3,\ 6,\ 12}$, **KALI-I.,**
LACH., laur.^{3}, **led., lyc.**$^{3,\ 4,\ 16}$, merc.^{2},
merc-i-r.^{12}, **mez., mur-ac., nat-m.**$^{3,\ 7}$,
NAT-S., NIT-AC., nux-v.^{3}, op.$^{2,\ 3,\ 8}$,
ph-ac., PHYT., plat.^{3}, plat-m.$^{8,\ 12}$,
podo., **puls.,** rheum, rhod., rhus-t.^{3},
sabad.^{3}, **sars.,** sel., sep., **sil.,** spong.,
STAPH., still.$^{2,\ 3,\ 6}$, stram., stront-c.,
sul-i.$^{1'}$, **SULPH.,** thuj., valer., verat.^{3},
viol-t., zinc.

paralysis-poisoning

METASTASIS

ABROT., agar.[1',7], apis[3], **ant-c.**[1',3,6], **ars.**[1',3,6], asaf.[6], cact.[6], calc.[3], **carb-v.**, **caul.**[6], **cimic.**[6,7], colch., **crot-t.**[6], **cupr.**, dig.[6], **dulc.**[6], graph.[6], hep.[3], kali-bi.[6], **kalm.**[6], kreos.[3], lac-c., **lach.**[3,6], lith-c.[6], lyc.[3], mag-c.[10], merc.[3], mez.[6], **nat-m.**[6], nat-p.[15], **nux-v.**[6], **plat.**[6], **puls.**, sang., **senec.**[6], **sep.**[3,6], sil.[3], sulph., zinc.[6]

MINING, ill effects of[8]

card-m., nat-ar., sulph.[1']

stone-cutters

moistening affected part am. see bathing–affectet am.

MOON agg., **full** (Kent's Rep.1897) ✶

alum., **apis**[7], arn.[3,6], **ARS.**[3,7], bar-c.[7], **bell.**[3,7], brom.[3], bry.[7], **calc.**, calc-p.[7], canth.[7], caust.[3,6,7], **cina**[3], **croc.**[3,6], cupr.[7], cycl., fl-ac.[3], gels.[7], **graph.**, hep.[7], ign.[7], kali-bi.[6,7], kali-n., **lach.**[2], led.[7], **LYC.**[3,7], **merc.**[7], nat-c., nat-m., nit-ac.[7], nux-v[7], ph-ac., **PHOS.**[3,7], psor.[3,7], **PULS.**[7], **rhus-t.**[7], sabad., sang.[7], **sep., sil.**, sol-m.[7], sol-t-ae.[7], spong., sul-i.[7], **sulph.**, teucr., thuj.[7], thuj.[7], verat-v.[7]

convulsions–moon

decreasing m. agg.

alum.[15], **apis**[7], ars.[7], bry.[7], **calc.**[7], clem.[3], **daph.**[2-4], **dulc.**, gels.[7], kali-bi.[7], kali-c.[7], **lach.**[7], **lyc.**[3,7], **merc.**[7], merc-i-r.[7], **nat-m.**[7], nux-v.[7], ph-ac.[7], phel.[2,3], **PHOS.**[7], phyt.[7], plat.[7], **PULS.**[7], **RHUS-T.**[7], **SEP.**[3,7],

sil.[7], sul-i.[7], **SULPH.**[3,7], **tab.**[7], thuj.[7], tub.[7], verat.[7]

new m. agg. ✶

agar.[7], alum., am-c., **apis**[7], arg-n.[7], arn.[3,6,7], **ARS.**[3,7], ars-i.[7], bell.[7], **bry.**[7], bufo, calc., calc-p.[7], canth.[7], caust., chin.[7], **cina**[3], clem., croc.[3,6], cupr., daph., graph.[7], hep.[7], kali-bi.[6,7], **lach.**[7], lyc., merc.[7], merc-c.[7], merc-i-f.[7], nat-m.[7], **NUX-V.**[3,7], **PHOS.**[7], phyt.[7], **PULS.**[7], **RHUS-T.**[3,7], sabad., **sep.**, sil., **SULPH.**[7], thuj.[3,7]

chorea–moon

convulsions–moon

increasing m. agg.

alum.[3,6,7], apis[7], arn., **ARS.**[3,7], arum-t.[7], bell.[7], **bry.**[3,7], **CALC.**[7], calc-p.[7], caust.[7], chin.[2], cimic.[7], clem., cupr.[3,7], graph.[7], ign.[7], kali-bi.[7], kali-c.[7], **lach.**[7], **lyc.**[3,7], **med.**[7], merc-i-f.[7], **nat-m.**[3,7], nit-ac.[7], **nux-v.**[7], phel.[2,3,7], **PHOS.**[7], **PULS.**[7], rhus-t.[7], sang.[7], **SEP.**[7], **sil.**[7], staph.[3], sul-i.[7], **SULPH.**[7], **thuj.**[3,4,6,7]

MOONLIGHT agg.

ant-c., bell., calc.[3,6], ovi-p.[7], sep.[3], **sulph.**[3], thuj.

morphinism

MOTION agg.

abrot., achy.[14], **acon.**, adlu.[14], aesc.[8], **agar., agav-t.**[14], **agn.**, aloe,

aml-ns.⁸, anac., **ang.**²⁺ ³, ange-s.¹⁴,
anh.⁸⁺ ¹⁰⁺ ¹⁴, ant-c., ant-t., **apis**, apoc.,
aq-mar.¹⁴, arg-m.²⁺ ³, arg-n.⁷, **arn.**,
ars., ars-h., **ars-i.**, **asaf.**, **asar.**,
aspar., aster.¹⁴, **aur.**, aur-ar.¹′,
aur-i.¹′, aur-s.¹′, **bapt.**, **bar-c.**,
bar-i.¹′, bar-s.¹′, **BELL.**, **berb.**,
beryl¹⁴, **BISM.**, bor., bov.,
BRY., bufo, **but-ac.**⁸, **cact.**,
cadm-met.¹⁰⁺ ¹⁴, cadm-s., **calad.**,
calc., calc-ar.⁸, **calc-p.**, **calc-s.**,
calc-sil.¹′, **camph.**, cann-i., **cann-s.**,
canth., **caps.**, **carb-an.**, **carb-v.**,
carbn-s., card-m., **caust.**, cean.⁸,
cham., **CHEL.**, **CHIN.**, chin-ar.,
chion., cic., **cimic.**, **cimx.**, cina,
cinnb., clem., coc-c., **COCC.**, **coff.**,
coff-t.⁷, **COLCH.**, **COLOC.**, **con.**,
cortico.⁹, **croc.**, **crot-h.**, crot-t.,
cupr., cupr-ar., cur.⁷, **cycl.**²⁺ ³,
des-ac.¹⁴, **dig.**, dros., dulc.²⁺ ³, elaps³,
eup-per., euph., equis.⁸, **ferr.**, ferr-i.,
ferr-p.¹′⁺ ³⁺ ⁸, **fl-ac.**, foll.¹⁴, form.,
gels., get.⁸, **glon.**, **graph.**, **GUAJ.**,
guat.¹⁴, hed.⁹, **hell.**, helon.⁸, **hep.**,
hip-ac.⁹⁺ ¹⁴, hist.¹⁰⁺ ¹⁴, hoit.¹⁴, hyos.,
iber.⁸, ign., **iod.**, **ip.**, **iris**, jac.,
jug-c.⁸, jug-r.⁷, **kali-bi.**, **kali-c.**²⁺ ³⁺ ⁶,
kali-m.¹′⁺ ⁸, **kali-n.**, kali-p., kali-sil.¹′,
kalm., **kreos.**²⁺ ³, lac-c.¹′⁺ ⁸, **lac-d.**¹′⁺ ⁷,
lach., lat-m.¹⁴, laur., **LED.**, lina.⁸,
lob.⁸, lyc.²⁺ ³, lycpr.⁸, lycps., mag-c.,
mag-m., **mag-p.**, **mang.**, med.¹,
meli., meny., meph.⁴, **MERC.**,
merc-c., mez., mim-p.¹⁴, mosch.,
mur-ac.²⁺ ³, naja³⁺ ¹⁴, **nat-ar.**,
nat-c.²⁺ ³⁺ ⁴⁺ ¹⁶, **nat-m.**, **nat-p.**, **nat-s.**,
nat-sil.¹′, nit-ac., nux-m., **NUX-V.**,
ol-an., olnd., onop.¹⁴, **onos.**, op.,
osm., ovi-p.⁷, **ox-ac.**, pall., par.,
paro.¹⁴, penic.¹³⁺ ¹⁴, **petr.**, ph-ac.,
phos., **phyt.**, pic-ac.⁸, plan.¹²,
plat., **plb.**, psil.¹⁴, **psor.**, ptel.,
puls., puls-n.⁸, pulx.⁸, pyrog.³,
RAN-B., ran-s., **rheum**, rhod.²⁺ ³,
rhus-t.²⁺ ³, rumx., ruta²⁺ ³⁺ ⁸, sabad.,
SABIN., samb., sal-ac.⁶, **sang.**,
sanic., sarcol-ac.⁹⁺ ¹⁴, **sars.**²⁺ ³, **sec.**,
sel., senec., seneg., **sep.**, sieg.¹⁰,
SIL., **spig.**, spong., **squil.**, **stann.**,
staph., still.⁸, stram., stront-c.,
stroph-s.⁹⁺ ¹⁴, stry.⁸, sul-ac., sul-i.¹′,

SULPH., syph.⁷, tab.³⁺ ⁸, tarax.,
tarent.³⁺ ⁶⁺ ⁸, teucr., thea⁸, **ther.**,
thuj., thymol.⁸, tril., trios.¹⁴, tub.³⁺ ⁷,
valer.²⁺ ³, **verat.**, verb., vib.³,
viol-o., viol-t., **visc.**, x-ray¹⁴, **zinc.**,
zinc-p.¹, zinc-val.³

am.

abrot.⁸, **acon.**, aesc.³⁺ ⁸, **agar.**,
agn.³, **aloe**, **alum.**, alumn.², **am-c.**,
am-m., ambr., **anac.**, **ang.**²⁺ ³,
ant-c.²⁺ ³, ant-t., apis⁶, aran-ix.¹⁰⁺ ¹⁴,
arg-m., **arg-n.**, arist-cl.¹⁰⁺ ¹⁴, arn.,
ars., ars-s-f.¹′, asaf., asar., **atro,**
AUR., **AUR-M.**, aur-m-n., bar-c.,
bar-m., bell.²⁺ ³⁺ ⁶⁺ ⁸, bell-p.⁸⁺ ¹⁰⁺ ¹⁴,
benz-ac., **bism.**, bor., bov., **brom.**,
bry.²⁺³, cact.⁶, calc., calc-p., cann-s.³,
canth., **CAPS.**, carb-ac., carb-an.,
carb-v., **caust.**, cham., chel.³, chin.,
chin-ar., cic., **cina**, coc-c.²⁺ ⁸,
coca, **cocc.**, **coloc.**, **com.**, **CON.**,
cupr., **CYCL.**, dig.³, **dios.**, **dros.**,
DULC., erig.¹⁰, **EUPH.**, euphr.,
FERR., ferr-ar., ferr-p., **fl-ac.**³⁺ ⁶⁻⁸,
gamb., gᵊls., glon.³, graph.³, guaj.,
hed.¹⁰⁺ ¹′, **hell.**³, **helon.**³⁺ ⁸, hep., hom.⁸,
hyos., ign., **indg.**, **iod.**³, iris⁸,
kali-br.⁶, **kali-c.**, **kali-i.**, **kali-n.**,
kali-p., **KALI-S.**, **kreos.**, lach., laur.,
led.³, **lil-t.**, lith-c., lith-lac.⁸, lob.,
LYC., **mag-c.**, **mag-m.**, magn-gr.⁸,
mand.⁹, mang., **meny.**, **med.**,
merc.²⁺ ³, **merc-c.**, **merc-i-f.**, mez.²⁺ ³,
mosch., mur-ac., nat-c., nat-m.²⁺ ³,
nat-s., nit-ac., nux-m., olnd., op.,
par., parth.⁸, petr., **ph-ac.**, phel.⁴,
phos.²⁺ ³, pip-m.⁸, **plat.**, plb.²⁺ ³,
pneu.¹⁴, **PULS.**, **PYROG.**, rad-br.⁸,
raja-s.¹⁴, **rat.**, **RHOD.**, **RHUS-T.**,
ruta, **SABAD.**, sabin.²⁺ ³, **SAMB.**,
sars.²⁺ ³, sel., seneg., **sep.**, sel.²⁺ ³,
spig., spong.²⁺ ³, **stann.**, staph.²⁺ ³,
stel.⁸, **stront-c.**, sul-ac., **SULPH.**,
syph.⁸, **TARAX.**, **TARENT.**, teucr.,
thala.¹⁴, thiop.¹⁴, thuj., **tub.**,
VALER., ven-m.¹⁴, verat., **verb.**,
vib., viol-o.³, **viol-t.**, visc.¹⁴, xero.⁸,
zinc., zinc-p.¹′

affected part agg., of

acon., **AESC.,** agar., am-c., anac.,
ang.[3], **ant-t., ARN., ars.,** asaf.,
asar., bar-c., **bell., BRY.,** bufo[3],
camph., **cann-s., caps.,** caust.,
CHAM., chel., **chin.,** cic., cimic.,
clem., **cocc.,** coff., **COLCH.,**
coloc., com., con., croc., cupr.,
dig., ferr-ar., form., **gels., glon.,**
guaj., hep., ign., iod., kali-bi.[3],
kali-c., **kalm.,** lach., **LED.,** mag-c.,
mang., meny., **merc., mez.,** nat-c.,
nat-m., nux-m., nux-v., olnd.,
petr., **phos.,** phyt., plat., plan.[12],
puls., ran-b., rheum, RHUS-T.,
rhod., rumx., ruta, sabad., **sabin.,**
samb., **sang., sars.,** sel., sep.,
sil., SPIG., stann., staph., **sulph.,**
thuj., zinc.

am.
abrot., acon., **agar.,** agn., am-m.,
ang.[3], apis[3], arn., **ars.,** ars-i.,
asaf., asar., **aur.,** bell.[3], calc.,
CAPS., cham., **chin.,** cina, **con.,**
croc., **DULC., euph., FERR.,**
hyos.[3], **kali-bi.,** kali-c., lith-c.[3],
lyc., mag-c., **mag-m.,** meny.,
mosch., mur-ac., nat-c., **ph-ac.,**
PULS., rhod., RHUS-T., sabad.,
samb., **sep.,** squil., stann.,
stront-c., **SULPH., tarax.,** thuj.,
valer., verb., viol-t.

after m. agg.

AGAR., am-c., anac., arn., **ARS.,**
aspar., calad., camph., **CANN-S.,**
carb-v., caust., **cocc.,** coff., **croc.,**
dros., hydr.[3], **hyos.,** iod., **kali-c.,**
laur., merc., **nit-ac.,** nux-v., olnd.,
phos., plb., **PULS., RHUS-T., ruta,**
sabin., sep., spig., **SPONG.,**
STANN., staph., **stram.,** sul-ac.,
VALER., zinc.

aversion to

abrot.[7], **ACON.,** agar.[11], alco.[11],
aloe[1,11], alum., alum-p.[1'], alum-sil.[1'],
am-c., ambr., anac., ant-c., ant-t.,
arn., **ARS.,** ars-s-f.[1'], asar., atro.[11],
bapt.[3,11], **bar-c., BELL.,** bol-la.[11],
bor., **BRY.,** cadm-s., **CALAD.,**
CALC., CALC-S., cann-i.[11], canth.,
caps., carb-an., carb-v., carbn-s.,
caust., cham., **chel., chin.,**
chin-ar., cina, coc-c.[11], **cocc.,** coff.,
colch.[1'], **con.,** croc., cupr., **cycl.,**
dig., dios.[11], dros., dulc., eryt-j.[11],
ferr., ferr-i., **gels.,** gins.[11], **graph.,**
GUAJ., ham.[11], hell.[4], hydr-ac.[11],
hyos., hyper.[2], **ign.,** iod.[4], ip.,
kali-ar., **kali-bi., kali-c.,** kali-p.,
kali-sil.[1'], **LACH.,** led., lob.[11], **lyc.,**
mag-c., mag-m., merc., **mez.,**
mur-ac., myric.[11], **nat-ar.,** nat-c.,
nat-m., nit-ac., nux-m.[11], **NUX-V.,**
oena.[11], op., peti.[11], petr., **ph-ac.,**
phos., phys.[11], psor., ptel.[11], puls.,
RUTA, sang., sapin.[11], sep., **SIL.,**
stann., stront-c., **SULPH.,** tarax.,
tarent.[11], teucr., **thuj.,** zinc.,
zinc-p.[1']

at beginning of m. agg.

agar., am-c.[7], ant-t., asar., bry.[3],
cact., calc., **CAPS., carb-v., caust.,**
chin., cina, cocc., **CON.,** cupr.,
dig.[16], dros., **EUPH., FERR.,** fl-ac.,
graph., hecla[14], hed[19], **kali-p.,**
lach., led., **LYC.,** mag-c., mand.[14],
med.[7], nit-ac., petr., **ph-ac., phos.,**
plat., plb., **psor., PULS.,** rhod.,
RHUS-T., ruta, **sabad.,** sabin.,
samb., sanic.[3,7], sars., sep.[1'], **sil.,**
stront-c.[8], **ther.,** thuj., tub.[7], valer.,
verat., **zinc.,** zinc-p.[1']

walking – beginning

continued m. am.

agar., **am-m., ambr.,** anac.[3],
aran-ix.[10], bell-p.[10], bry., **cact.,**
CAPS., carb-v., caust., chin., **cina,**
cob.[3], com., **CON., cycl., dros.,**
EUPH., FERR., FL-AC.[3], gels.,
graph.[3], hecla[14], hed.[10], ind., iod.[10],
iris, kali-c., **lyc.,** mag-c.[10],
mand.[10, 14], med.[1'], plat., plb., **ptel.,**
PULS., rauw.[14], **rhod., RHUS-T.,**
ruta, **sabad.,** sabin., **SAMB.,** sep.,
sil., SYPH.[7], tarax., thuj., **valer.,**
verat., zinc.[3]

desire for[3]

acon., agar., alum.[3, 4], am-c., **ambr.,**
arg-m., arg-n., **arn.**[3, 4], ars.,
ars-i.[1'], asar., aur., aur-ar.[1'], **bell.**[3, 4],
bell-p.[10, 14], bism., bor., bry.[3, 4],
calc.[3, 4], con., canth., cench.[1'],
CHAM.[3, 4], **CHIN.**[3, 4], coff., coloc.,
con., **cupr.,** euphr., **FERR.**[3, 4],
ferr-ar.[1'], ferr-i.[1'], hyos., ign., iod.,
ip., kali-i.[1'], kreos., lyc.[3, 4, 11],
macro.[11], mag-c., mag-m., mang.,
merc.[3, 4], mosch., mur-ac., nat-c.,
nit-ac., nux-m., nux-v., op., petr.[11],
ph-ac., phos., puls., ran-b., rhod.,
RHUS-T., ruta, samb., sec., sep.,
sil., squil.[3, 4], stann., staph.,
stront-c., sul-i.[1'], sulph.[1', 3], **teucr.**
tub.[1'], valer., verat.

open air agg., in[3]

bell., bry., **calc.,** cocc., colch.,
led., nux-v.

am.[3]
dios., **iod.,** kali-i., **lil-t.,** mag-c.,
mag-m., **PULS.**

rapid m. am.[3]

ars., aur-m., **bry., ferr.**[1'], fl-ac., sep.,
sil., stann., sulph.

slow m. agg.[3]

sep.

am.[3]
agar.[3, 8], alum., ambr.[3, 8], asaf.[1'],
aur., bell., calc.[15], coloc.,
FERR.[1', 3, 6-8, 15], ferr-a.[8], ferr-ar.[1'],
ferr-p.[1'], glon., kali-bi., **kali-p.,**
mag-m., plat.[8], **PULS.**[1', 3, 7, 15],
stann.[8], **sulph.**[15], sumb.,
SYPH.[3, 7, 15], tarent., zinc.[8]

violent m. agg.[3]

acon., arn., ars., bry., calc.,
camph., lyc., mag-c., nux-v.,
rhus-t., ruta, sep., sil., sul-ac.,
sulph.

am.[3]
aesc.[3, 6], **ARS., BROM.,** dulc.,
phys., **SEP.**[3, 6], sil., **sul-ac.**[3, 6]

MOUNTAIN sickness[7]

acon.[2, 8], ars.[6-8, 12], aur., bell.,
CALC., carb-v., caust.,
COCA[2, 6-8, 12], con., conv., cupr.,
gels., kola[6], **lach.,** lyc., nat-m.,
olnd., puls., spig., verat.[12]

ascending–high

am. in mountains

prot.[14], **syph.**[7, 8]

climbing m., ailments from[12]

ars.

MUCOUS SECRETIONS increased

acet-ac., acon., agar., agn.[4],
ALL-C., alum., alum-sil.[1'], am-c.,
am-m., ambr., **ammc.,** ang.[3, 4],
ant-c., ant-t., aphis[4], **arg-m., arg-n.,**
arn., **ars.,** ars-i., arum-m.[4], asaf.[4],
asar., aur., aur-s.[1'], **bar-c., bar-m.,**
bell., benz-ac., bism., bond.[11], **bor.,**
bov., bry., **CALC.,** calc-s.[3],
calc-sil.[1'], camph., **cann-s.,** canth.,
caps., carb-an., **CARB-V., carbn-s.,**
caust., cham., chel., **chin.,** chlor.[11],
chr-ac.[11], cina, cinnb.[11], **coc-c.,**
cocc., coff., colch., coloc., **con.,**
cop., croc., cupr., dig., dros.,
DULC., euph., **euphr., ferr.,** ferr-i.,
graph., grat.[4], guaj., hell., **hep.,**
HYDR., hyos., ign., **IOD., ip., iris**[3],
jab.[3], kali-ar., **KALI-BI., kali-c.,**
kali-chl.[4], **kali-i.,** kali-m.[1'], kali-n.,
kali-sil.[1'], kreos., **LACH.,** lact.[4],
laur., **LYC.,** m-arct.[4], m-aust.[4],
mag-c., mag-m., mec.[11], med.[3, 7],
MERC., mez., mur-ac.[4, 11], myric.[2],
nat-ar., **nat-c., nat-m., nat-s.**[3, 4],
nicc.[4], **nit-ac., nux-m., NUX-V.,**
olnd.[1], op.[3], **par., PETR.,** ph-ac.,
phel.[4], **PHOS.,** plat., plb., podo.,
PULS., ran-b., raph.[4], rat.[4], rheum,
rhod., **rhus-t., rumx.,** ruta, sabad.,
sabin., **samb.,** sars., sec., sel.,
seneg., sep., sil., sin-n.[2], spig.,
spong.[3, 4], **squil., stann.,** staph.,
stroph-h.[3], sul-ac., sul-i.[1'], **SULPH.,**
TAB., tax.[11], teucr., thal.[11], thuj.,
tong.[4], valer., verat., zinc.

am.[3]

apis, arg-m., arist-cl.[9, 10], ars.,
bry.[3, 6], calc., camph., cimic.[3, 6],
cupr.[3, 6], dulc.[6], graph.[6], ip.,
kali-bi.[6], **LACH.**[1', 3, 6, 8], lyc.,
mosch.[6, 8], nux-v.[3, 6], ph-ac., psor.,

puls.[3, 6, 10], rhus-t., senec.[6], sep.[3, 6],
sil., squil., stann.[8], stict., stram.,
SULPH.[3, 6], thuj.[6], verat., **zinc.**[3, 6, 8]

leucorrhea

acrid[4]

aesc.[7], all-s.[3], **alum., am-c.**[1', 4, 7],
am-m., anac., ant-c., arum-t.[1', 3],
ars.[1', 3, 4], ars-i.[3], **bor.,** bov., **brom.**[3],
calc., cann-s., canth., carb-an.,
carb-v.[1', 4], **caust.**[3], **cham.**[3, 4], chin.,
con., euph., **ferr.,** fl-ac.[1', 7], **graph.**[3],
hep.[3, 4], **ign., iod.**[3, 4], kali-c.,
kali-i.[3, 4], **kreos.**[1', 3, 4, 7], **lach.,**
lyc.[3, 4], m-arct., mag-c., **mag-m.,**
mang., **merc.**[3, 4], merc-c.[3], **mez.,**
mur-ac., **nat-m.**[2, 4], **nit-ac.**[2-4], **nux-v.,**
ph-ac., **phos.**[3, 4], prun., **puls.,**
rhus-t.[3], **ran-b.,** ruta, sang.[1'], **sep.**[3, 4],
sil.[3, 4], spig., squil., sul-ac.,
sulph.[1', 3, 4], thuj.

albuminoid[3, 4]

alum.[3], am-m., berb.[3], bor., bov.[4],
coc-c.[3], graph.[1'], grat.[1'], jatr.[4],
kali-m.[2], mez., **NAT-M.**[3], pall.[3],
petr., plat., sep.[3], stann.[3]

bitter taste[8]

aloe, cocc., **kali-bi.,** nat-m., nux-v.,
puls.

bland[6]

alumn.[1'], arg-n., cycl., euphr.[3],
hep.[3], kali-i.[3], kali-m.[3], kali-s.,
merc.[0, 0], **PULS.**[1'-3, 6, 7], sil.[3],
sulph.[3]

bloody[4]

acon.[3, 4, 6], ail.[3], aloe[3], alum.[3, 4],
alum-sil.[1'], am-c., am-m., aphis,

arg-n.[3, 6, 7], arn.[3, 6], ars.[1', 3, 4],
ars-s-f.[1'], asar., bar-c.[3, 4], bar-m.[1'],
bell.[1', 3, 4], bor., brom.[3], bry.[3],
calc-s.[1', 2], canth.[3, 4, 6], caps.,
carb-an.[6], carb-v.[1', 3, 4], caust.[3, 4],
chin.[3, 4], cocc.[3, 4], cop., crot-h.[3, 6],
daph., dros.[3], euon., ferr.[3, 4], form.[6],
graph., ham.[1', 2], hep., iod.[3, 4],
kali-ar.[1'], kali-c., kali-chl., kali-n.,
kreos.[1', 3], lach.[3, 4, 6], led., lyc.[3, 4],
mag-c., mag-m., mang.[6], merc.[3, 4, 6],
mez., mur-ac.[3], murx., nat-m.[3, 4],
nit-ac.[1', 3, 6], nux-m., nux-v.[3, 4], op.,
par., petr., phos.[3, 4, 6], puls.[1', 3, 4],
sabin.[3, 4], sang.[3], sep.[3, 4], sil.[3, 4, 6],
sul-ac.[1', 3, 4], sul-i.[1'], sulph.[3, 4],
ter.[2, 6], thuj.[3, 4], verat.[3, 4], vip.,
zinc.[3, 4, 6], zinc-p.[1']

bluish[3, 4]

ambr., ars., cupr.[3], cupr-a.[4], lach.[6]

brownish[3, 4]

am-m.[4], ambr.[3], ars., **bell.**, bism.[4],
bor., carb-v., grat.[4], nit-ac., sulph.

burning[6]

acon., aesc., **ail.**[3, 6], all-c.[3, 6], alum.[4],
alum-p.[1'], am-c.[4, 6, 7], am-m.[4],
ars.[1', 3, 4, 6], ars-i.[6, 7], ars-s-f.[1'],
arum-t., bad., brom.[3, 6], calad.[4],
calc.[3, 4], canth., caps., carb-ac.,
carb-an.[4, 6], carb-v., cast.[4], chin.[4, 6],
chlor., cina[4], **con.**[4], crot-h., fl-ac.[1', 6],
gels.[3, 6], graph., guaj., hep., hydr.,
iod.[6], kali-c., **kali-i.**[3, 4, 6], kreos.[3, 6],
lach., lyc.[6], mag-s.[4], **merc.**[3, 6],
merc-c.[3], mez.[4], mur-ac., nat-m.,
nit-ac.[6, 7], petr., phos., phyt.,
puls.[3, 4], ran-s., **sabad.**[3, 6], sang.,
sep., sil., sin-n.[3], sul-ac.[4, 6],
sulph.[3, 4, 6, 7]

cold[1']

verat.

corrosive[3]

ALUM., am-c.[1', 3, 7], **am-m.**, ant-c.[4],
ARS.[1'-4, 6], ars-i.[7], **ars-s-f.**[1'], arum-t[1']
bor., **bov.**, carb-v., **CAUST.**,
cham.[3, 4], **con.**[4], ferr.[3, 4], **HYDR.**,
ign., **iod.**[6], ip.[4], kali-ar.[1'], **kali-bi.**,
kali-i.[2, 3, 6], **kreos.**[1', 3], **lach.**[3, 4], lyc.[6],
MERC.[3, 4, 6], mez., nat-m.[3, 4, 6],
NIT-AC.[1', 3], **nux-v.**, phos.[3, 4], **puls.**,
rhus-t., ruta, sep.[3, 6], **SIL.**[3, 4, 6],
staph., sul-ac.[1', 3], **sulph.**[1', 3, 4, 7],
thuj.

flocculent[3]

agar., ambr., kali-bi., kali-c.,
kreos., mag-c., merc., phos.,
sabad., sep., sil., sulph., thuj.

frothy[4]

aphis, ars., ferr., **NAT-M.**[2], op.,
sec., sul-ac.

gelatinous[3, 4]

aloe[2, 3], arg-m., **arg-n.**[3], bell.[3], berb.,
caust.[3], chin-s.[4], cocc.[1'], **colch.**[3],
coloc.[3], dig.[3], **hell.**, **kali-bi.**[1', 3],
laur., podo.[3], **rhus-t.**, sabin.[3], sel.,
sep.[3]

gray[3, 4]

ambr., **anac.**, **arg-m.**[1', 3, 4], ars.,
carb-an., caust., chin., cop.[4],
kali-m.[6], kreos., lach., **lyc.**[3],
mag-m., merc., sep., **sil.**, thuj.

greenish[3, 4]

acon.[3], **ars.**, asaf.[4], aur.[4], bor.[4, 6],
carb-v., caust.[4], cham.[3], colch.[4],
con.[3], **dros.**, ferr., hyos.[4], ip.[3],
kali-bi.[3, 4, 7], kali-c.[4], **kali-i.**[1'-3],
kali-s.[1', 2], kreos., lach.[4], led., **lyc.**,
m-aust.[4], **mag-c.**, mang.[4], med.[3, 7],
merc., murx.[4], nat-c., nat-m.[4],
nat-s.[1', 3], nit-ac.[4], nux-v.[4], **par.**[4],
phos., **PULS.**[1', 3, 4, 6], rhus-t.,
sabad.[4], sec.[3], **sep.**, sil.[4], **stann.**,
sul-ac.[3], **sulph.**, thuj., **verat.**[3]

hard[3]

agar., bry., con., **KALI-BI.**, mosch.,
nat-c., **phos.**, **sep.**, **sil.**, stict.[6],
sulph., **thuj.**

honey-like[1']

ars-i.

hot[3]

acon., **ars.**, **bell.**, bor., euphr., **iod.**,
kreos., op., **puls.**, sabin., **sulph.**

lumpy[4]

calc-s.[2], **hep.**[2], kali-c., kreos., phos.,
sabad., sabin., sin-n.[2], stann.

metallic taste[4]

calc., cupr., ip., nux-v., rhus-t.

milky[4]

calc.[3, 4], carb-v., con., ferr.,
kali-m.[1', 3], kali-p.[3], lyc., nat-s.[3],
ph-ac.[3], phos., **puls.**[3, 4], sabin.,
sep.[3, 4], **sil.**, sul-ac.

musty smell[3]

bor.[3, 4], **carb-v.**[3, 4], **coloc.**, crot-h.,
merc., nux-v., **phos.**, **puls.**, **rhus-t.**,
stann.

offensive, fetid[6]

ail., arg-n., arn., arum-t.[3],
ars.[1'-3, 4, 6], **ars-s-f.**[1'], **asaf.**[1', 6],
aur-s.[1'], bals-p., **BAPT.**[1'-3, 6], bell.[4],
calc.[3, 4], calc-f., calc-sil.[1'], caps.[4],
carb-ac., carb-an., **carb-v.**[1'-3, 6],
chel.[4], chin., chlor., cist.[1'], con.[4],
cop., crot-h., cupr.[4], cur.[7], echi.,
ferr.[4], fl-ac.[1', 6, 7], **graph.**[1', 2, 4, 6],
guaj.[1', 2, 6], helon., hep.[1', 3, 4, 6],
kali-ar.[1'], kali-bi., kali-br.[6], kali-i.,
kali-p.[1'], kali-perm., kali-s.,
KREOS.[1', 2, 4, 6], **LACH.**[2, 3, 6],
lyc., mag-c.[4, 10], **merc.**[2, 4, 6],
mur-ac.[4, 6], **NAT-C.**[1', 3, 4],
NIT-AC.[1'-3, 4, 6], **nux-v.**[4], petr.,
psor.[1', 3, 6, 7], **puls.**[1', 4], **pyrog.**[1', 3, 6],
rob.[2], **sabin.**[4], sang., sec.[3], **sep.**[3, 4, 6],
sil.[4, 6], stann.[4], **sulph.**[1', 3, 4], ther.,
tril.[2], vip.

purulent[3]

aur., **CALC.**, **CON.**, cop.[4], **graph.**,
ign.[4], lyc.[6], **merc.**[3, 4, 6], nat-c.[6], **puls.**,
sep.[4], **sil.**, **sulph.**[7]

ropy, tenacious[*]

acon., agn., **alum.**[4, 6], alum-p.[1'],
am-m., anac., **ant-c.**, ant-s-aur.[11],
ant-t.[3, 4], arg-m.[1', 3, 6], arg-n.[3], **ars.**,
asaf., bar-a.[6], bar-c.[4, 6], bar-m.[6],
bell., **bor.**[3, 6], **bov.**[2-4], bry.[3, 4, 6],
calc.[3, 4], cann-s.[4], canth.[4, 6], carb-an.,
carb-v.[4, 6], carbn-s.[1'], caust.[1', 3, 4, 6],
cham., chin., **chin-s.**, cist.,
coc-c.[1', 3, 6, 15], cocc., colch., con.,
croc.[3], culx.[1'], dulc.[4, 6], euphr.,
form.[6], graph.[1', 3, 4, 6], hep.,
hydr.[1'-3, 6, 15], iod., **KALI-BI.**[1'-3, 6, 7, 15],

kali-c.³, ⁴, ⁶, **kali-m.**¹', ³, kali-s.¹',
lach.³, ⁴, ⁶, lact., lap-a.³, laur., lob.,
lyc.³, m-arct., m-aust., **mag-c.,**
mag-m., **merc.**³, ⁴, **mez.**³, ⁴, myrt-c.³,
nat-c., nat-m.³, nux-v., ol-an., osm.³,
par., ph-ac., phos.³, ⁴ phyt.³, ⁶,
plat., plb.⁴, ⁶, puls.¹', ³, ⁴, **ran-b.,**
raph., rhus-t., sabad., sabin., **samb.,**
scroph-n., **seneg.,** sep., sin-n.²,
spig., spong., squil., **STANN.**³, ⁴,
staph., sul-ac.³, **sulph.,** sumb.¹²,
tab., thuj.⁶, tong., ust.³, verat.³, ⁴,
zinc.

salty taste⁴

alum., **ambr., ars., bar-c.,** calc.,
chin., dros., fl-ac.⁷, **graph., iod.⁶,**
kali-i.⁶, lyc.⁴, ⁶, mag-c., mag-m.,
merc., nat-m.⁶, **nat-c.,** nux-v., **petr.,**
phos., puls., samb., **sep., sil.,** stann.,
staph., sulph., zinc.

sour taste⁴

calc., graph., **hep.**¹', ², ⁴, kali-c.,
kali-n., lam., mag-m., merc., nat-c.,
nat-p.⁷, nit-ac.⁷, nux-v., **plb.,** sep.,
sulph.⁴, ⁷, tarax.

suppressed

abrot.⁷, ⁸, agar.¹¹, **ant-c.²,** arist-cl.¹⁴,
ars.¹', asaf.⁶, ⁸, **ASAR.,** aur-m.⁸,
bar-c.⁸, bell.¹', **bry.**³, ⁸, ¹², bufo¹',
calc.¹', carb-v.¹', cupr.¹', ⁸, **dulc.**³, ⁶,
graph.¹', ⁸, **lach.**³, ⁶, ⁸, led.¹², **lob.⁸,**
med.⁸, merc.⁶, ⁸, mill.⁶, **mosch.²,**
nux-v.³, ⁶, plb.⁶, **psor.⁸, puls.**³, ⁶, ⁷,
sanic.⁸, senec.⁶, **sil.**¹', ³, ⁸,
STRAM.², ³, ⁶, ⁸,¹¹, **sulph.**¹', ³, ⁶, ⁸,
verat.³, viol-o.¹², zinc.⁶⁻⁸

sweetish taste⁴

asar., **calc.**¹', cham.¹¹, lach.⁴, ¹¹, •
mag-c., merc-c., phos.¹', stann.¹'

thick, slimy⁴

acon., agar., **alum.,** alum-sil.¹',
am-m., ant-c., arg-m.¹', ³, ⁴, **arg-n.⁶,**
ars.³, ⁴, ars-i.¹', ars-s-f.¹', **aur-s.**¹',
bals-p.⁶, **bar-c.,** berb., bor.³, ⁴, ⁶,
calc.³, ⁴, calc-s.¹', ³, carb-an.,
carb-v.³, ⁴, carbn-s.¹', cast., caust.¹',
chin.³, cist.¹', coc-c.¹', con.³, ⁴, cop.,
croc.³, cycl.⁶, graph., helon.³, **hep.⁶,**
hydr.¹', ³, ⁶, iod., ip., **kali-bi.**¹', ³
kali-br.⁶, **kali-i.**¹', ⁴, **kali-m.**¹', ²,
kali-s.¹', ⁶, kali-sil.¹', kreos., lac-ac.⁶,
lam., lith-c.⁶, lyc.³, ⁴, m-arct.,
mag-c.³, **mag-m.,** mag-s., mang.⁶,
merc.¹', ³, ⁶, merc-d.³, mur-ac.,
murx., **nat-c.**⁴, ⁶, nat-m.¹', ³, ⁴,
nat-s.¹', nat-sil.¹', nicc., nit-ac.,
ol-an., op., par.³, ⁴, phos.³,
PULS.¹'⁻⁴, ⁶, ruta, sabad., samb.,
sars., scroph-n., sec., sel., seneg.,
sil.¹', ³, ⁴, staph., **sulph.**¹', ³, ⁴, tong.,
tub.⁷, zinc., zing.

thin⁴

ambr., ant-t., **ars.**¹', ⁶, **ars-s-f.**¹',
asaf.⁶, asar., **bell.**¹', ⁴, bor., bov.,
calc., canth., caps., **carb-v.**¹', ⁴,
caust., colch., **con.,** ferr., **fl-ac.**¹', ⁶,
gels.⁶, **graph.,** kali-i.², ⁴, kali-n.,
kali-s.¹', laur., lyc., **mag-c.,** mez.,
mur-ac.⁶, nat-m.⁴, ⁶, **NIT-AC.**¹', ², ⁶,
nux-v., ol-an., **puls.**¹, ⁴, rhus-t.,
seneg., **sil.⁶,** stann., staph.,
sul-ac.¹', ⁴, ter.⁴, ⁶, thuj.⁶

transparent⁴

aesc.⁷, alum., cast., crot-h., ferr-m.,
fl-ac.⁷, graph., kali-i., mag-s., mang.,
NAT-M.², ⁴, phos., puls., sabad.,
sep., sil., stann., sul-ac.

urinous odor³

benz-ac., canth., **coloc.,** nat-m.,
nit-ac., ol-an., sec., urt-u.

vicarious[3]

bry., con., dig., ferr., ham., **lach.,**
lycps., mill., nux-v., **PHOS., puls.,**
sec., senec., **sep.,** sulph.

watery[4]

acon.[6], aesc.[7], **agar.,** alum., **am-c.,**
am-m., ambr., ant-c., arg-m.,
ars.[3, 4, 6], **asaf.**[1', 3], asar., bell.,
bov., brom.[6], calc., cann-s.,
carb-an., carb-v., cast., **caust.**[3],
cham.[3, 4], **chin.,** chlor[6], clem., coff.,
con., crot-h.[3], cupr.[3], elat.[2], fl-ac.[1'],
gamb.[3], **gels.**[2], **graph.**[3, 4], grat.[3],
guaj., ign., iod., iris[3], kali-i.[3, 4, 6],
kali-n., **kali-s.**[1'], kreos.[1', 4], **lach.,**
m-arct., mag-c., mag-m., meny.,
merc.[3, 4], **mez.,** murx., **mur-ac.,**
NAT-M.[1', 2, 6], nat-s.[3], nicc., **nux-v.,**
par., phos.[3, 4], **plb., podo.**[3], puls.[1', 4],
ran-b., rhus-t.[3, 4], sabin.[3], sec.[3],
seneg., **sep., sil., squil.,** stann.,
staph., sul-ac., **sulph.,** thuj.,
verat.[1', 3]

white[4]

bell.[1'], ferr., graph., grat., hell.,
kali-m.[1', 2, 6] kali-n., kreos., lyc.,
m-arct., mag-c., **merc.,**
NAT-M.[1', 2, 4], nat-s.[1'], nux-v.,
ol-an., **phos.,** prun., **puls.,** raph.,
rat., sabin., **sep.**[1', 4], **sil.,** sul-ac.,
tab.

yellow[4]

acon., agar.[2], agn., **alum.,** alum-p.[1'],
alum-sil.[1'], alumn.[1'], am-c., am-m.,
ambr., anac., ang., **ant-c.,** arg-m.[1', 4],
arg-n.[6, 7], **ars.,** ars-i.', **ars-s-f.**[1'],
aur., aur-ar.[1'], **aur-i.**[1'], **aur-s.**[1'],
bar-c., bar-i.[1'], bar-s.[1'], **bell., berb.,**
bov., **bry., calc.,** calc-s.[1'], calc-sil.[1'],
cann-s., canth., caps., **carb-an.**[3, 4],

carb-v., cast., caust., cench.[1'],
cham., cic., cist.[1'], clem., con.,
cor-r., croc., cycl.[6], **daph., dros.,**
dulc., **eug.,** form.[6], gran., **graph.,**
hep., hydr.[1', 3, 6], **iod.,** kali-ar.[1'],
kali-bi.[3, 7], **kali-c., kali-m.**[1', 2], kali-n.,
kali-s.[1'-3, 6], kali-sil.[1'], **kreos.,**
lac-ac.[6], lach., **lyc.,** mag-c., mag-m.,
mag-s., mang., merc., merc-i-f.[3],
mez., mur-ac., nat-ar.[11], **nat-c.,**
nat-m., nat-p.[2], nat-s.[2, 3], **nat-sil.**[1'],
nit-ac., nux-v., ol-j.[3], ph-ac., **phos.,**
prun., **puls.**[1', 4, 6], rhus-t., ruta,
sabad., sabin., sec., **sel.,** seneg.,
sep., sil.[1', 4], **spig., stann.,** staph.,
sul-ac.[1, 4], **sul-i.**[1'], **sulph.,** sumb.[3, 12],
thuj., verat., viol-t., zinc-p.[1']

yellowish-green[1']

ars-i.[1', 3], **calc-sil.,** kali-bi.[7],
mang.[3, 6], **merc.**[1', 3], nat-s.[1'],
NIT-AC.[1', 2], **PULS.**[1'-3], sulph.

MUSHROOMS POISONING[7, 8]

absin., agar.[2, 8], ars.[7], atro., **bell.,**
camph., pyrog.

MYATROPHY, progressive spinal[8]

ars., carbn-s.[8, 12], hyper., kali-hp.,
PHOS.[2, 8, 12], phys.[8, 12], **plb.**[1', 2, 8, 12],
sec.

MYXEDEMA[14]

ars.[2, 7], cortico., dor.[12], penic., sulfa.,
thyr.[7, 8, 12]

NARCOTICS agg.

acet-ac.[8, 12], acon., agar., am-c.[3],
apom.[8], ars., aur., **aven.**[6, 8], **BELL.,**
bry., calc., **camph.**[6, 8], cann-i.[8],
canth., carb-v., caust., **CHAM.,**
chin., cic.[3, 6], cimic.[8], **COFF.,** colch.,
croc., cupr., **dig.,** dulc., euph., **ferr.,**
graph., hep., **hyos.,** ign., **ip.,**
kali-perm.[6], **LACH.,** lob.[7], **lyc.,**
macro.[8], mag-s.[9], merc., mosch.,
mur-ac.[3, 6, 8], nat-c., nat-m.,
nat-p.[3, 6, 7], nit-ac., nux-m.,
NUX-V., op., ox-ac.[7], oxyg.[12],
passi.[6], ph-ac., phenob.[14], phos.,
plat., plb., **puls.,** rhus-t., seneg.,
sep., staph., sulph., thuj.[8], **valer.,**
verat., zinc.

ailments from[12]

ip., oxyg., verat.

desire for[11]

buth-a.[9], op., tab.

Vol. I: *morphinism*

NECROSIS bones

ang.[6, 8], aran.[6], **arg-m.**[6, 8], **ARS.,** asaf.,
aur.[3, 6], aur-i.[8], **aur-m.**[2, 8], bac.[12], bell.,
both.[11, 12], **calc.**[2, 6, 8], **calc-f.**[2, 6, 8],
calc-i.[3, 6], calc-hp.[6, 8], calc-p.[6, 8],
calc-sil.[8], caps.[6], carb-ac., carb-an.[6],
chin.[6, 8], **cist.**[6], con., euph.,
FL-AC.[1, 2, 6-8], graph.[6, 8], hecla[6, 8],
hep.[1, 6, 8], **iod.**[3, 6, 8], kali-bi.[6, 8], kali-c.[6],
kali-i.[6, 8], kreos., lach.[6, 8], lap-a.[6], lyc.[6],
mang.[1], med.[8], **merc., merc-c.,**
mez.[1, 6, 8], **nat-sil-f.**[8], **nit-ac.**[3, 6, 8],
ph-ac., **phos.,** plat.[6], plat-m.[8], plb.,
psor.[6], puls.[3], rad-br.[3], **sabin.,** sal-ac.[2],
sec., sil., staph.[8], stront-c.[6], sul-ac.[8, 12],

sulph., symph.[8], syph.[8], teucr.[6], thea[8],
ther., thuj., **tub.**[6, 8], vitr.[8]

caries
softening

NOISES am.[1']

apoc., aur-ar., calad.[2], calc.[3], graph.[3],
hell.[3], kali-ar., mag-p., med., puls.[3],
pyrog., stram.[3], tarent.

Vol. I: *sensitive – noise*

NUMBNESS externally

abrot., absin., acet-ac.[11], **acon.,**
acon-f.[11, 12], aesc.[3, 6], ail., agar.,
aloe[3, 6], alum., alum-p.[1'],
alum-sil.[1', 8], alumn.[1'], am-c.,
am-m., **ambr., ANAC.,** ang.[3, 4],
anh.[9], ant-c., **ant-t., apis,** aran.[6],
aran-ix.[J], **arg-m.**[1'-3, 6], **arg-n.,** arn.,
ars., ars-i., asaf., asar., aur., **bapt.,**
bar-c., bar-m., **bell., BERB.,** bism.,
bov., brom., bry., bufo, cact., caj.,
calc., **calc-p.**[8], calc-sil.[1'], camph.,
cann-i., cann-s., canth., caps.[3],
carb-ac., **carb-an., carb-v.,**
CARBN-S., caust., cedr., **cham.,**
chel., chin., chlor., **cic.,** cimic.,
cinnb., cob-n.[9], coca, **cocain.**[8],
COCC., cod.[8, 11, 12], coff.[3], colch.,
coloc., **CON.,** conin.[12], croc.,
crot-c., crot-h., crot-t.[4], cupr., cur.,
cycl.[3, 4], dig., dios., dulc., euph.[3],
euphr., elaps, ferr., fl-ac., form.[6],
gast.[11], **gels., glon., gnaph.,**
GRAPH., guaj.[2, 3, 4], **hell.,**
helo.[8, 12], hep.[3], hydr-ac., **HYOS.,**
hyper., ign., iod., ip., irid.[8, 12],
iris, kali-ar.[1'], kali-bi.[3], kali-br.,
KALI-C., kali-fcy., kali-n., kali-p.,
kalm., keroso.[11], kreos.[3], lach.,
lath.[6], laur., **led.,** lepi.[11], **LYC.,**
mag-m., mag-s.[9], **mand.**[10],

mang.[3, 6], **merc., mez.**[3, 4, 6],
mosch., mur-ac.[3], naja[3],
nat-m.[2, 3, 4], nit-ac.[3], **nux-m.,**
nux-v., OLND., onos., **OP., ox-ac.,**
oxyt., par., petr., **PH-AC., PHOS.,**
phys., phyt.[6], **pic-ac., plat., PLB.,**
puls., raph.[8, 11, 12], rheum[3, 4],
rhod., **rhus-t.,** samb.[3, 6], sang.[3],
SEC., sep., sil., spig., spong.,
stann.[3, 8], staph., **STRAM.,**
stront-c.[3, 6], sul-ac.[3], sulph., tab.,
tanac.[11], tang.[11], teucr.[3, 4], thal.[8],
thea, thuj.[3, 4, 6], thymol.[9], **urt-u.,**
valer., verat., verat-v., verb.,
vip.[11], **zinc.,** zinc-p.[1']

night[16].
    sil.

on waking[16]

    mez.

alternating with
    hypersensitiveness[3]

plat.

bruised part, in the

arn.

climacteric period, during

cimic.

epilepsy, before

bufo

feels neither heat nor cold[3']

berb.

left half of body

caust.[1], mez.[16], xan.[12]

right half of body[3]

ars., lyc.[16]

whole body

acon.[11], apis[11], arg-n., asc-t.[11],
bar-m.[1], bell.[11], caj.[11], caps.[16],
cedr., chel.[16], crot-c.[11], gels.[11],
gymno.[11], kali-bi.[11], **KALI-BR.,**
kreos.[11], lyss., merc.[11], nitro-o.[11],
nux-v.[16], **OLND.**[1], **ox-ac.,**
pic-ac.[11], tarent.[11], tab.[11]

glands, in

anac., asaf., bell., cocc., con., lyc.,
plat., puls., rhus-t., sep., sil., spong.

internally

acon., aloe[3], alum.[3], am-c., ambr.,
ang.[3], ant-c.[3], **ant-t.**[3], arg-n.[3], **ars.,**
asaf., asar.[3], aur.[3], bar-c., **bell.,**
bism.[3], bor.[3], **bov., bry.**[3], bufo[3],
calad.[3], calc., camph.[3], cann-s.[3],
CANTH.[3], caps.[3], carb-an., carb-v.[3],
carbn-s., caust., cham., chel.[3], chin.,
cic.[3], cina, cocc.[3], coff., colch.,
coloc.[3], con., croc.[3], crot-t., cupr.,
dig., dulc.[3], euph.[3], ferr., **GELS.,**
glon.[3], graph., **hell.**[3], hep. [3], **hyos.,**
ign., iod.[3], ip.[3], **kali-br.,** kali-c.,
kali-n.[3], kreos.[3], lach.[3], laur., lyc.,
mag-c., mag-m., mang.[3], meny.[3],
merc., merc-c.[3], mez.[0], mosch.[3],
mur-ac., nat-c.[3], nat-m., nit-ac.,
nux-m., **NUX-V.**[3], olnd., **op.,** par.[3],
petr., ph-ac.[3], phos., **PLAT.,** plb.,
podo.[3], puls., ran-b., ran-s.[3], rheum,
rhod.[3], rhus-t.[3], ruta[3], sabad.[3],
sabin.[3], sars., sec.[3], seneg., sep.[3],
sil., **spig.,** spong.[3], squil.[3], stann.,

staph.[3], stram., stront-c., sul-ac.[3],
sulph.[3], tarax.[3], teucr.[3], thuj., valer.,
verat., verb.[3], viol-o.[3], zinc.[3]

lower half of body, of[3]

spong.

pains, after[3]

acon., agar., graph., mez., plat.

from[3]
cham., **coloc.,** kalm., plat., puls.,
rhus-t.

parts, lain on

ambr., am-c., **arn.**[3], ars., **bar-c.,**
bufo[3], **calc.,** calc-sil.[1]', carb-an.[3],
carb-v., carbn-s., chin.[3, 15], cop.,
graph., ign., kali-c., **lach.,** mag-c.[3],
nat-m., pall.[7], **phos., PULS.,**
RHUS-T., sep.[7], sil., sumb., zinc.

single parts, in

acon., agar., alum., alum-p.[1]',
alum-sil.[1]', am-c., am-m., **ambr.,**
anac., ang.[3], anh.[9], ant-c., **ant-t.,**
aran-ix.[9], **arg-n.,** arg-n., arn., ars.,
ars-i., asaf., asar., aur., aur-ar.[1]',
aur-i.[1]', aur-s.[1]', **bar-c.,** bar-s.[1]',
bell., bor., bov., bry., cadm-s.[1', 7],
calc., calc-i.[1]', **calc-p.,** calc-sil.[1]',
camph., cann-s., canth., caps.,
CARB-AN., carb-v., CARBN-S.,
caust., **cham.,** chel., **chin.,** cic., cina,
COCC., colch., **coloc.,** con., **CROC.,**
dig., dros., dulc., euph., euphr.,
ferr., ferr-ar.[1]', ferr-p., **GRAPH.,**
guaj., hep., hyos., **ign.,** iod., ip.,
kali-ar., **KALI-C., kali-fcy.,**
kali-m.[1]', **kali-n.**[1], kali-p., kali-s.[1]',
kreos., laur., led., **LYC.,** mag-c.,
mag-m., mang., **MERC.,** mez.,
mosch., **mur-ac.,** nat-c., **nat-m.,**

nat-p., nit-ac., **nux-v.,** olnd., op.,
par., petr., ph-ac.[7], **phos.,** plat., plb.,
PULS., rheum, rhod., RHUS-T.,
sabad., sabin., samb., **sars., sec.,**
sep., SIL., spig., spong., squil.,
stann., staph., **stram.,** sul-ac.,
sul-i.[1]', **sulph.,** teucr., thuj., valer.,
verat., zinc., ZINC-P.[1]'

spots, in

cadm-s.[7], caust.[7], **lyc., plat.**

suffering parts, of

acon., alum., alum-sil.[1]', **agar.**[3],
ambr., **anac.,** ang.[3], ant-t., aran.[3],
arn., **ars.,** ars-i., **asaf.,** aur., aur-ar.[1]',
aur-i.[1]', bell., bor., bov., bry., calc.,
calc-sil.[1]', cann-s., carb-an., carb-v.,
caust., **CHAM.,** chel., chin., cic.,
cina, **cocc.,** coff., colch., coloc.,
CON., croc., cupr., cycl., dig., dulc.,
elaps, euphr., ferr., ferr-ar., ferr-p.,
gnaph., graph., hell., hep., hyos.,
ign., iod., kali-c., **kali-n.**[1], **KALM.**[3],
kreos., **lyc.,** mag-m., mang.[3], merc.,
mez., mur-ac., nat-m., nux-m.,
nux-v., **olnd.,** petr., ph-ac., phos.,
PLAT., PLB., PULS., rheum, rhod.,
rhus-t., ruta, samb., sec., sep., sil.,
spong., stann., staph., stram.,
stront-c., sul-ac., sul-i.[1]', sulph.,
thuj., verat., verb., viol-o., zinc.

bruised parts

arn.

unilateral[3]

ars., caust., chel., **COCC.,** nat-m.,
phos., puls.

upper half of body, of

bar-c.

NURSING, suckling agg.[3, 13]*

abrot.[6], acon., agn., ant-t.[13], ars.[3],
bell., **bor.**[3, 6, 13], **BRY.**[3, 6, 13],
CALC.[3, 6, 13], **calc-p.**[3, 6, 13], carb-an.,
carb-v.[3, 6, 13], cast-eq.[13], caust.[13],
cham., chel., **chin.**[3, 6, 13], chin-ar.[6],
chion.[12], cina, **cocc.**[2], con., crot-h.[2],
crot-t.[13], **dulc.**, ferr., graph., ign.,
iod., ip., **kali-c.**[3, 6, 13], lac-c.[13],
lach., lyc., **merc.**, mill.[13], nat-c.,
nat-m., **nit-ac.**[13], nux-v., olnd.[3, 6, 13],
ph-ac.[3, 6, 7, 13], phel.[3, 6, 13], phos.,
PHYT.[3, 6, 13], **PULS.**[3, 6, 13], rheum,
rhus-t., samb., sec., sel.[3], **SEP.**[3, 6, 13],
SIL., spig., squil.[3], stann., **staph.**[3, 6],
stram., **sulph.**[3, 6, 13], zinc.[3, 6, 13]

loss – fluids

trembling–nursing

weakness – lactation

NURSLINGS[13]

acon., aeth., ant-c., ant-t., **arn.**, **ars.**,
bell., **BOR.**, **BRY.**, **CALC.**, **calc-p.**,
camph., carb-v., **CHAM.**, chin., cina,
coloc., crot-t., dulc., ferr., graph.,
hep., ign., **ip.**, kali-bi.[3], kali-c., lach.,
lyc., **mag-c.**, **merc.**, nat-c., nat-m.,
NAT-P., nux-v., **OP.**, ph-ac., phos.,
podo., psor., **PULS.**, rheum, **rhus-t.**,
samb., sec., **sil.**, stann., staph., stram.,
verat., **sulph.**, zinc.

OBESITY

acon.[3], adon.[6], agar., ail.[12], alco.[11],
all-s.[7, 8], **am-br.**[2, 8, 12], **am-c.**[3, 6–8, 12, 16],
am-m., ambr., **ang.**[2, 3], **ant-c.**,
ant-t.[2, 3], apis[3], aran-ix.[10],
arist-cl.[9, 10, 14], arn.[2, 3], **ars.**[2, 5, 8],

asaf.[1], **aur.**, bac.[12], bar-c., **bell.**[2, 3],
blatta[6, 8, 12], bor., brom.[3, 11], bry.,
bufo[3], calad.[6], **CALC.**, calc-a.[6],
calc-ar., calc-caust.[6], **calo.**[8].
camph., canth., **CAPS.**, carb-v.[3, 8],
caust.[3], cham.[2, 3], chin., chlorpr.[12],
cic.[3], cimic.[10, 14], clem.[2, 3], **coc-c.**[2],
coca[12], cocc., coloc.[2, 3, 8], con.,
cortiso.[14], **croc.**[2, 3, 8, 12],
crot-h.[4, 6], **cupr.**, cyna.[14], dig.[2, 3],
elaps[7, 8], euph., euphr.[2], **FERR.**,
fuc.[6, 8, 10, 12], **GRAPH.**, guaj.,
hell.[2, 3], **hura**[7], **hyos.**[2, 3], iod., ip.,
kali-bi., kali-br.[8, 12], **kali-c.**, **lac-d.**,
lach., laur., lith-c.[12], lob.[8], **lyc.**,
lycpr.[12], mag-c., mag-p.[12], mang.[8],
med.[7], merc., merc-d.[6], mur-ac.,
nat-ar.[11], nat-c., **nat-m.**[5, 16], nux-m.,
nux-v.[5], olnd., op., **phos.**[3, 8, 12],
PHYT.[2, 3, 6, 8, 10, 12], plat., plb., **puls.**,
rauw.[9], rheum[2], rhus-t.[3], sabad.,
sabal[8, 12], sars., sel.[3], seneg., sep.,
sil., spig., spong., stram.[2, 3],
stront-c.[3], **sulph.**, thuj.,
thyr.[8, 11, 12, 14], tus-fr.[7, 8, 11, 12],
valer.[3], verat., viol-o.[2, 3]

weakness–reaction

body fat, but **legs thin**

am-m., ant-c.[3]

children. in

ant-c.[2, 8], **bad.**[2], bar-c.[6, 8],
CALC.[1-3, 7, 8, 12], **caps.**[1, 8], **ferr.**[8],
kali-bi.[2, 8, 12], sacch.[8, 12], seneg.[12]

climacteric period, during

calc-ar.[12], **GRAPH.**[6, 7], sep.[6]

old people, in

am-c.[7], **AUR.**[7], bar-c.[6], fl-ac.[7],
KALI-C.[1, 7], op.[7], sec.[7]

young people, in

ant-c.[2, 4, 6, 7], calc.[4], calc-a.[6], lach.[6]

OLD AGE, premature

agn.[1, 7], alco.[11], alum.[6], **ambr.,**
arg-m.[14], arg-n.[7], **bar-c.,** berb.[1'],
bufo, carb-v.[1'], chin-s.[1], coca[11],
con.[3, 6, 10], cortico.[14], **cupr.**[1'],
des-ac.[14], esp-g.[14], **fl-ac.**[3, 6, 7, 12],
kali-c., kres.[14], lyc., mag-f.[10],
nux-v.[1'], op.[11], prot.[14], psor.[6],
reser.[14], sars.[1'], **SEL.,** sep.[1'], staph.[6],
stram.[7, 12], sulph.[6], **vip.**[7, 11, 12]

old people*

acet-ac.[7, 12], **acon.,** agar., **agn.**[7],
all-s.[7], aloe, **alum.**[3, 7, 8, 12], alumn.,
am-c., am-m.[7], **AMBR., ammc.,**
anac., ant-c., ant-t., apis[12], **arg-n.**[7],
arn.[3, 6], **ars.,** ars-s-f.[1'], **AUR.,** bapt.[12],
BAR-C., bar-m.[8], **bry.**[1, 7], calc.[3, 7],
calc-p., camph., cann-i.[7], caps.[8],
carb-an., carb-v., caust., cham.[7, 12],
chin.[3, 12], chin-s.[4, 6], cic., cit-v.[8],
COCA, cocc.[3], **colch., con.,** crot-h.[8],
cupr.[1'], dig.[7], **fl-ac.,** gamb.[7], gins.[3],
graph.[7, 12], **hydr.**[2, 3, 7, 8, 12], hyos.[3],
iod., irid.[7, 12], **iris**[7], kali-ar.[7], kali-bi.[7],
KALI-C., kreos.[3, 12], **LACH.**[3, 7, 12],
LYC., mag-f.[14], merc.[5, 7],
mill.[2, 7, 8, 12], nat-c.[7], **nat-m.,** nat-s.[12],
nit-ac., nux-m.[8, 12], nux-v.[3], **OP.,**
orch.[7, 12], **ov.**[7, 8], perh.[14], ph-ac.[3],
phos.[3, 7, 8], puls.[7], rhus-t.[3], ruta[3, 7],
sabad., sanic.[3], sarcol-ac.[14], sars.[3],
SEC., SEL., seneg., sep.[7], **sil.**[5, 7],
sul-ac., **sulph.**[1, 7], sumb.[3], syph.[3],

ter.[6, 12], **TEUCR.**[1, 7], thiosin.[7], thuj.[7],
tub.[3], **verat.**[3, 7, 8, 12], zinc.[7]

senile decay[8]

agn., **arg-n.,** ars., **bar-c.,** cann-i.,
con., fl-ac., iod., **lyc., ov.,** phos.,
thiosin.

onanism see masturbation

ORGASM of BLOOD

ACON., aloe, alum., alum-p.[1'],
alum-sil.[1'], alumn., **am-c., am-m.,**
ambr., aml-ns., ant-c., ant-t.,
anthraco.[2], arg-m., **ARG-N., arn.,**
ars.[3, 16], **ars-i., asar.**[1], **AUR.,** aur-ar.[1'],
aur-i.[1'], aur-s.[1'], bar-c., bar-s.[1'],
BELL., berb., bor.[2, 3], **bov., bry.,**
CALC., calc-ar., calc-i.[1'], calc-s.,
cann-i., cann-s., carb-an., **carb-v.,**
CARBN-S., caust., cench.[1'], **cham.,**
chin., cina, cocc., coff., **con.,** corn.[3],
croc., cupr., dig., dulc., erig.[10],
FERR., ferr-ar., **ferr-i.,** ferr-p., **gels.,**
GLON., graph., guaj., **hep.,** hyos.,
ign., **iod.,** jab.[3], kali-bi.[3], kali-br.[3],
kali-c., kali-p., kali-s., kali-sil.[1'],
kiss., **KREOS., LACH.,** lil-t., **LYC.,**
mag-c.[3], mag-m., mang., **meli.,**
merc., merl., **mill.**[1'], mosch., nat-c.,
nat-m., nat-p., nit-ac., **nux-m.,**
nux-v., op., ox-ac.[1'], **petr.,**
PH-AC.[2, 3], **PHOS.,** plb., rhod.,
puls., rhus-t., sabad., sabin., **samb.,**
sang., **sars., sel.**[3], **seneg., sep., sil.,**
SPONG., stann., staph., **STRAM.,**
stront-c.[3], **sul-ac.**[3], sul-i.[1'], **SULPH.,**
tab., tell., ter.[3], **thuj.,** ust.[3], valer.[3],
verat.

heat—flushes

morning in sleep

ang.

after restless sleep

calc.

on waking

calc.[16], graph., kali-c.[16], lyc., nux-v.

rising am.

nux-v.

evening
arn., **asar.**[1], **caust.**, dig., kali-c.[16], lyc., **merc.**[2], petr., phos., rhus-t., sars.[2], thuj.

after lying down

ign., samb., sars.[16], sil.

during sexual excitement

clem.

sitting am.

thuj.

night
am-c., arg-n., **calc.**, **carb-an.**, **carb-v.**, hep., ign., mag-c., **merc.**, mur-ac., **nat-c.**, nat-m., **phos.**, **puls.**, ran-b., raph.[2], senn.[7], **sep.**, **sil.**, **sulph.**

heat–flushes–night

Vol. III: *sleeplessness– climacteric period*

bed, drives him out of

iod.

beer, after

sulph.

anxiety with[2]

acon., aloe, am-m., **bar-c.**, chel.

ascending stairs. on[16]

thuj.

burning in hands, with[2]

SULPH.

skin, of[2]

sang.

coition, after

am-c., **sep.**

disagreeable news, from

lach.

eating am.

alum., chin,

warm food, while

mag-c.

emotions, after

acon., apis, **aur., bell.,** bry., calc.,
CHAM., coff., colch., **coloc., con.,**
cupr., **HYOS., IGN.,** kali-c., **kali-p.,**
lach., lyc., mag-c., nat-m., **nat-p.,**
nit-ac., nux-v., op., **petr., ph-ac.,**
phos., plat., **PULS.,** sep., **staph.,**
stram., teucr., thuj., verat.

everything were moving in body,
as if

croc.

faintness, with[7]

petr.

falling asleep, on

petr., sep.[16]

lying on left side

bar-c.

menses, before

alum., cupr., merc.

during
calc., merl.

motion, on[16]

nat-m.

motion or speaking agg.

iod., nat-c., thuj.[16]

nervousness, from

ambr., **bell.,** calc., ferr., kali-n.,
merc., nit-ac., ph-ac., phos., sep.

palpitation, with[16]

kali-c., phos., sul-i.[1']

restlessness, with[2]

aloe, ph-ac.

sensual impressions, from

phos.

sitting, while

mag-m.

smoking tobacco, on[16]

phos.

vertigo, during

nat-c.

vexation, after

acon., **CHAM.,** coloc., ign., merc.,
petr., SEP., staph.

vomiting, after[16]

verat.

walk, after a long

arg-n.

walking, after

arg-n., berb., **petr.**[2], sul-i.[1']

am.
mag-m.

wine. after[16]

sil.

OVULATION, at

foll.[14]

PAIN, ailments from[12]

cham., scut.

sensitiveness–pain

Vol. I: *sensitive – pain*

morning[16]
sil.

evening[16]
ars.

night[16]
con., kali-c.

in sleep[4]

alum., aur., bell., kali-n., lach., lyc., **merc.**, mosch., **nit-ac.**, vip.

appear gradually

acon., bry., calc-sil.[8], carbn-o., caust., chin.[8], con., ign., lact., lob., rad-br.[8], sars., sul-ac., tell.[8]

and disappear gradually

acon., **arg-n.**[2, 6, 8], arn., ars., bar-c., bufo, cact.[3], cast.[3], chel.[3], coloc.[3], crot-h., epiph.[3], euphr.[3], form.[3], **gels.**[3, 6], glon., **ign.**[3], jab., kali-bi.[6], **kalm.**, **lach.**[3, 6], lol.[3], mez., **nat-m.**, op., **phos.**, pic-ac., **PLAT.**, psor., **puls.**[3, 6], sabin., **SANG.**[3, 6], sars., sel.[3], sep.[3], **spig.**, **STANN.**, staph., stront-c., **sul-ac.**, sulph., **SYPH.**[1', 6-8], verb.

suddenly

arg-m., **arg-n.**[2], bell.[3], caust., ign.[3, 8], **puls.**, rhus-t.[3], rad.[3], **sul-ac.**

appear suddenly

acon.[3, 6], agar., am-c.[3, 6], anh.[9], **arg-m.**, ars.[6], aster., atro.[6], bar-a.[3, 6], **BELL.**, berb., camph., canth.[3, 6], carb-ac.[3, 6], caust.[6], cimic., cob-n.[10], **coloc.**[3, 6], croc., **crot-h.**[3, 6], **cupr.**[3, 6], cupr-ar.[6], daph.[7], **dios.**[6], eup-per.[3], ferr., form.[3, 6], **glon.**[3, 6], kali-bi[3, 6], lyc., mag-c.[3, 6], mag-p.[3, 6], med.[7], mez., morph., **nat-s.**[3, 6], **NIT-AC.**, **nux-v.**[6], ox-ac.[3, 6], phys., plb.[3, 6], **podo.**[3, 6], **puls.**, ran-b.[3, 6], **sabin.**, sep., sil.[6], spig.[3], stann.[3, 6], stry-p.[6], sul-ac.[3, 6], **tab.**, **tarent.**[3, 6], thala.[14], thuj.[3, 6], **valer.**, **verb.**[6], vip.[3, 6], zinc.[6], zinc-val.[6]

and disappear gradually

asaf., **bell.**[3], buni-o.[14], calc., coloc.[3], fl-ac., **hyper.**[3], ign.[6], **lach.**[3], **med.**[3], **puls.**, rad.[3], rad-br.[3], ran-s., sabin.[1], sep.[1], sul-ac.[8]

suddenly

arg-n., asaf., aster., BELL.,
bor.[3], cact.[8], canth.,
carb-ac.[3, 6, 8], carbn-s.,
cham.[7], coff.[7], crot-h.[3], cupr.[3],
dios.[3], eup-per.[8], eup-pur.,
fl-ac., ictod.[8], ign., KALI-BI.,
kalm., lyc., mag-p., merc-c.,
nat-f.[10], NIT-AC., nux-m.[3],
ovi-p.[3, 7], oxyt.[3], petr.[7, 8],
phyt., puls.[8], rhus-t.[3, 8], sabin.,
spig., stry.[8], thal.[14], thuj.[3],
tub.[8,] valer.[3]

disappear suddenly[3]

arum-t.[2], BELL.[2, 3, 6], carb-ac.[2, 6],
caust., cimic.[2], dios.[6], mag-p.[6], puls.,
sul-ac., stry-p.[6], sulph., thuj.[6]

direction of pain backward[3]

bar-c., bell., bry., chel., con.,
crot-t., cupr., gels., kali-bi.,
kali-c., kali-i., lil-t., merc.,
nat-m., par., phos., phyt., prun.,
puls., sep., spig., SULPH.

crosswise[3]

acon., ambr., anac., arg-m., bell.,
berb., bov., bry., calc., canth.,
caust., cham., chel., chin., cocc.,
ferr., hell., kali-bi., kali-c.,
kali-m., lac-c.[3, 6], laur., lyc.,
mang.[6], merc., mur-ac., phos.,
rhus-t., seneg., sep., sil., spig.,
stront-c., sul-ac., sulph., tarax.
valer., verat., zinc.

downward[3]

acon., agar., agn., aloe[3], alum.,
alumn.[2], ant-t., apis[7], arn., asaf.[6],
aur., bar-c., bell., benz-ac.[3, 6],

berb., bor.[8], bry., cact.[8], canth.,
caps., carb-v., caust., chel., chin.,
cic., cina, coff., FERR., goss.[11],
graph., hyper., kali-c.,
kalm.[1', 3, 6-8], lach., led.[7], LYC.,
merc., mez.[1'], nat-c., nat-m.,
nux-v., ph-ac., puls., rheum[2, 7],
rhod., rhus-t., sanic.[8], sars.,
sel.[2, 3], seneg., sep., sil., sulph.,
verat., verb., zinc.

forward[3]

berb., bry., carb-v., gels., lac-c.,
sabin., sang., sep., sil., SPIG.

inward[3]

alum., arg-n., ARN.[3, 6], bell.,
bov., calc., cann-s., CANTH.[3, 6],
carb.-v., caust., chin., cina, con.,
hyos., ign., laur., meny., merc.,
mez., petr., phel., phyt.[6], plb.[3, 6],
ran-b.[3, 6], rhus-t., sabin.[3, 6], sep.,
spig., spong., squil., stann.,
staph., sul-ac., sulph., valer.,
verb.

left side, on[11]

penz-ac., brom., chel., cinnb.,
crot-c., crot-h., daph., ind., kalm.
lepi., lil-t., lycps., merc.,
merc-i-f., oena., ol-j., op., ox-ac.,
phys., pic-ac., plan., puls-n.

outward[3]

alum.[3, 6], am-m., anh.[9, 14], arg-m.,
arg-n.[3, 6], arn., ASAF.[1', 3, 6], bell.,
berb., bry., calc., canth., carb-v.,
chel.[3, 6], chin.[3, 6], cimic.[3], cocc.,
CON.[3, 6], dros., dulc., hyos.,
kali-c.[3], kali-bi., kali-m., kalm.,
led.[1'], lith-c., lyc.[1', 3], mang.,
merc.[3, 6], mez., mur-ac., nat-c.,
nit-ac., phel.[6], phos., phyt.[3, 6],
plat., plb., prun.[3], ran-b.[3, 6],

rhod., rhus-t., sabad., sabin.,
sep.[3], sil.[3, 6], spig.[3, 6], spong.[3, 6],
stann.[3, 6], stann-i.[6], staph.,
SULPH.[3, 6], tarax., **valer.**[3, 6],
viol-t., zinc.

radiating[3]

agar.[3, 6], apis[6], arg-n.[3, 6], ars.[3, 6],
bapt., berb., caust., cham., cimic.,
coloc., cupr.[3, 6], **dios.**[3, 6], hyper.,
kali-bi., kali-c.[3, 6], kalm., lil-t.[6],
mag-m., mag-p., **merc.**, mez.,
nux-v., phyt., plat., plb., sec.,
sil., spig.[3, 6], xan.

right side, on[11]

arist-m., brach., bry., cedr., oena.,
pic-ac., sulph., tarent., wye., yuc.

upward[3]

acon., aloe, alum-sil.[1'], anac.,
arn., ars., **asaf.**[3, 6], aur., **BELL.**,
calc., canth., caust., cham., chin.,
cimic., colch., con., croc.,
cupr.[3, 6], dulc., eup-pur.[3, 6],
euphr., gels., **glon.**, hyper.[6],
IGN., kali-bi., kalm.[1', 3], kreos.,
LACH.[1', 3], **led.**[1', 3, 6, 8], mag-c.,
mang., meny., naja, nat-c.,
nat-m., nit-ac., nux-v., op.,
PHOS., puls., rhus-t., sabad.,
samb., **SANG., SEP., SIL.**, spong.,
stront-c., stroph-h., sulph., thuj.,
valer., zinc.

amputation, after

acon.[7], **all-c.**[2, 7], am-m.[2, 7], arn.[2],
asaf., bell.[7], cupr.[7], hell.[7], **hyper.**[7],
ign.[7], kalm.[2], **ph-ac.**[2, 7], rauw.[10],
spig.[7], **staph.**[7], symph.[2, 7], verat.[7]

bones, of

abies-n., acon., **agar.**, agn.,
all-c.[11], alum.[4], am-c., am-m.,
ambr.[4], anac., ang.[3, 4, 8, 12],
ant-c.[3, 4], aran.[2], **arg-m.**, arn.,
ars., ars-i., **ASAF., aur.**, aur-ar.[1'],
aur-i.[1'], aur-m.[1', 8], aur-s.[1'],
bar-c., bar-i.[1'], bar-s.[1'], bell.,
berb.[1], bism., bry., **calc., calc-p.**,
calc-s., camph.[4], cann-s., canth.,
caps., carb-an., carb-v., carbn-s.,
cast-eq.[8], caust., **cham.**, chel.,
chin., chin-m.[2, 12], chin-s., cic.,
cinnb., cinnm.[2, 12], clem., cob-n.[14],
cocc., colch., coloc., **con.**,
conch.[11], crot-c.[8, 11], **crot-h.**[4, 8, 11],
cupr., cycl., **daph.**[4], dig., dios.,
dros., dulc., **EUP-PER.**, euph.,
ferr., ferr-ar.[1], **fl-ac., gels.**[3], glon.,
graph., guaj., halo.[14], hell., **hep.**,
hom.[12], ictod.[4], ign., iod., **IP.**,
kali-bi., kali-c., **kali-i.**[2, 8, 11],
kali-s., kreos., lach., led., **lyc.**,
lyss., m-arct.[4], mag-c., mag-m.,
mang., mang-m.[12], **MERC.**,
merc-c.[8], merc-i-f., **mez., mur-ac.**[4],
nat-c., nat-m., **nat-s.**[2], nat-sil.[1'],
NIT-AC., nux-m.[3, 4], nux-v.[4],
oci-s.[9], ol-an.[3], olnd., op., petr.,
PH-AC., phos., phyt.[1', 3, 8], plb.,
PULS., pyrog.[1', 3], ran-s., raph.[11],
rhod., rhus-t., RUTA, sabad.,
sabin., sacch.[11], samb., sarr.[11, 12],
sars., sec., **sep., sil.**, sol-t-ae.[11],
spig., spong., **staph.**, still.,
stront-c., sul-i.[1'], sulph., **symph.**[8],
syph.[8], teucr., ther., thuj., valer.,
verat., viol-t., vitr.[8], wildb.[12],
zinc.

morning[16]
sil.

night
asaf.[1], **AUR.**, caust., **cham.**,
cinnb., **fl-ac.**, guare.[11], hep.[8],
iod.[8], **KALI-I.**, kalm., **mang.**,
MERC., merc-i-f., mez., **NIT-AC.**,
ph-ac., phyt., rhod.[8], **sars.**, sil.[1'],
staph.[1'], still.[8], syph.[8], thuj.,
verat.

long, in[8]

cinnb., eup-per., staph., stront-c., syph.

weather, change of[3]

am-c.

blood vessels, of[6]

ham., zinc.

cancerous affections, in[8]

acon.[7], **apis**, anthraci., **ars.**, aster., bry., bufo[7], calc., **calc-a.**[8, 12], calc-o-t., calc-ox., carb-an.[1'], carc., cedr., cinnm., **cit-ac.**[2], coloc.[2], **con.**, cund., echi.[7, 8], **euph., hydr.**, mag-p., merc.[1'], morph., op., ph-ac.[7, 8], sil.

cartilages, of[8, 12]

arg-m., lob-s.[12], ruta

chill, during[16]

ars., petr.

eructation am.[7]

jal.

glands, of

acon., all-s.[11], **alum.**, am-c., ambr., ant-c., ant-t., apis[3], **ARN.**, ars., **ars-i.**, arund.[2, 11], asaf.[3], **aur.**, aur-ar.[1'], aur-i.[1'], aur-s.[1'] **BELL.**, berb.[4], bor.[4], **bry.**, calc., calen.[4], **cann-s.**, canth. **carb-an., carb-v., carbn-s., caust.**, cham., chin., cic.,

clem., **coloc.**, con., cor-r.[4], dulc., graph., ham.[3, 6], hell., hep., ign., **iod.**, kali-c., kali-s., lach.[3, 6], **LYC.**, m-arct.[4], mag-c., mag-m.[4], **MERC.**, murx.[4], **nat-m., nit-ac.**, nux-v., petr., **ph-ac., PHOS., puls.**, rheum, rhus-t., sel., sep., sil., **spig.**, spong., squil., stann., staph., stram., **sul-ac.**, sul-i.[1'], **sulph.**, **THUJ.**, verat.

half sleep, during[16]

nit-ac.

joints, of[1]

acon., **acon-c.**[11], aesc., agar., agar-ph.[11], all-c., **alum.**, anh.[9], **apis., apoc., apoc-a.**[11], aran., **ARG-M., ARN., ars., ars-i.**, asaf., asc-t., aster., aur., bar-c., bar-m.[3], **bell.**, berb.[3], **bol-la., BRY.**, caj., **calc., CALC-P.**, calc-s., cann-i., **caps.**, carb-ac., carb-an., **carbn-s.**, casc.[2], **caus.t.**, cedr., **cham., chin.**, chin-ar., **cimx**, cinnb., cist., **cit-v.**[2], **cocc.**, colch., **coloc.**, con., cop., croc., crot-t., cycl., daph., dig., dios., **dulc., ferr., ferr-ar.**, ferr-i., **ferr-p.**, gels., **guaj.**, harp.[14], hell., hist.[9], hydr., hydrc., ign., **iod.**, ip. iris, jac-c., jatr., **kali-bi., kali-c.**, kali-n., kali-p., **kalm., lac-ac., lac-c., LED., lyc.**, lyss., mag-f.[14], mand.[9, 14], **mang.**, merc., mez., morph., **nat-ar.**, nat-f.[14], nat-m., **nat-s.**, nit-ac., **NUX-V.**, ol-an., par., **ph-ac., phos., phyt., PLB., PULS.**, ran-s., raph., **rheum, rhod., RHUS-T., ruta**, sabad., **sabin., sang.**, sel., senec., **sil.**, sol-n., sol-t-ae., **staph.**, stroph-s.[14], sul-ac., **sulph.**, syph.[1'], ter., thala.[14], thuj., tub-r.[14], verat-v.

muscles, of[8, 12]

achy.[14], **acon.**, agav-t.[14], alet.[12], am-caust.[11], **ant-t., arn.**[6, 8], ars.[8],

aster.[14], bell.[8], bell-p.[8, 9, 12],
brach.[11], **bry.**[6, 8, 12], carbn-s.[8],
caust.[6, 8, 12], **cimic., colch.**[6, 8, 12],
dulc.[6, 8, 12], eryt-j.[11], ferr-p.[6],
form.[11], **gels.**[6, 8, 12], harp.[14], hist.[9],
ign.[6], lat-m.[9], led.[8], lyc.[11], **macro.**,
mag-s.[9, 14], mand.[9, 14], merc.[8],
merc-c.[11], morph.[8], nat-f.[9, 14],
nat-m.[6, 11], op.[11], **phyt.**[6], plb.[11],
puls.[6], **ran-b.**[8], rham-cath.[8],
rauw.[9], **rhus-t.**[6, 8], **ruta**[8], sal-ac.[8],
sil.[6], staph.[6], stram.[8], stroph-s.[14],
stry.[8, 11], sulfa.[14], tab.[11], tarax.[14],
thal.[6, 14], thuj.[11], valer.[8],
verat.[6, 8, 11], **verat-v.**, zinc.[11]

hot bathing am.[9]

lat-m.

motion agg.[9]

bell-p.

stretching, on[9]

mag-s.

paralyzed parts, of

agar., arn., **ars.**, bell., cadm-f.[1'],
calc., **caust.**, cina[1], **cocc.**, crot-t.,
kali-n. lat-m., nux-v., phos., **plb.**,
rhus-t., sil., sulph.

paralysis–painful

parts, of affected[16]

con. dig.

injured long ago[7]

glon.

lain on, in[16]

caust., hep., kali-c., phos., sep., sil.

lying–pain

recently lain on

PULS.

uncovered, of[16]

bell.

periosteum

AM-C.[7], ant-c., **ARN.**[7], **ASAF.**,
aur., **AUR-M.**[7], bell., bry., camph.,
cann-s.[7], **cham.**, chin., colch.,[1, 7]
coloc., cycl., graph., guare.[7], hell.,
ign., kali-c.[7], **KALI-I.**[7], **kalm.**, led.,
mang., merc., merc-c.[7], **mez.**,
mur-ac.[7, 16], **nit-ac.**[7], **PH-AC., phyt.**,
puls.[1, 7], rhod., rhus-t., **RUTA**[1, 7],
sabad., sabin., **sil.**, spig., **staph.**[1, 7],
symph.[12], syph.[1', 7]

small spots, in

agar.[3], **alum.**[3], am-c.[3], am-m.[3],
ambr.[3], apis[3], arg-m.[3], arg-n.[3], arn.[3],
ars.[3], asaf.[3], bell.[3], **berb.**[3], bry.[3],
bufo[3], calc.[3], **calc-p.**[3, 7], cann-s.[3],
canth.[3], carb-v.[3], caust.[3], cham.[3],
chel.[3], **cist.**[3], coff.[8], **colch.**[3, 6], con.[3],
croc.[3], cupr.[3], dios.[3, 6], ferr.[3], fl-ac.,
gels.[3], glon.[3], graph.[3], hep.[3], hist.[9],
ign., iod.[3], **KALI-BI., LACH.**[3], led.[3],
lil-t., lith-c., lyc.[3], mag-c.[3], mag-m.[3],
mag-p., meny.[3], merc.[3], mosch.[3],
nat-m.[3], nit-ac.[3], nux-m., ol-an.[3, 6],
ol-j.[3], **onos.**, ox-ac., petr.[3], ph-ac.[3],
phos.[3], psor., puls.[3], ran-b., ran-s.[3],
rhod.[3, 6, 11], rhus-t.[3], rhus-v.[11],

sabin.³, samb.³, sars.³, sel.³, **sep.³,**
sil.³, spig.¹⁶, squil.³, sul-ac.³,
SULPH.³, thuj., verat.³, zinc.³

tendons, in³

am-m., arn., benz-ac., berb., **bry.²,**
caust., colch., coloc., harp.¹⁴, iod.,
kali-bi., kalm., mag-f.¹⁴, prun.,
RHUS-T.²,³, ruta¹'⁻³, sabin., thuj.,
zinc.

benumbing

acon., agar., agn., am-c., anac.,
ant-c., ant-t., arg-m., arn., asaf.,
asar., aur., bell., bov., bry., **calc.,**
cann-s., carb-an., carb-v.³, **CHAM.,**
chin., cic., **cina,** cocc., con., croc.,
cupr., cycl., dros., dulc., euph.,
euphr., **gnaph.⁷, graph.,** hell., hep.,
hyos., ign., **iris,** kali-n., laur., led.,
mag-c., mag-m., mang., meny.,
mez., mosch., mur-ac., nat-c.,
nat-m., nux-m., nux-v.³, **OLND.,**
op., par., ph-ac., phos., **PLAT.,**
puls., rheum, rhus-t., ruta, **SABAD.,**
sabin., **samb.,** seneg., sep., stann.,
staph., sul-ac., sulph., tarax., valer.,
verat., VERB., zinc.

right side. in¹⁶

ars.

biting

acon., agar., agn., aloe¹¹, alum.,
am-c., **ambr.,** ang.³, ant-c., ant-t.,
arg-m., arn., ars., asar., aur.,
bar-m.⁴, bell., **berb.⁴, bov.⁴,** bry.,
calad., calc., camph., cann-s.,
canth., caps., carb-an., **CARB-V.,**
caust., cham., chel.⁴, **chin., clem.,**
cocc., colch., coloc., con., croc.,
dros., dulc., euon.¹¹, **euph., euphr.,**
graph., grat.⁴, **hell.,** hep., hyos.,
ign., iod., **ip., kali-c.,** kali-m.¹',

kali-n., **kreos.,** lach., lact.⁴, lam.⁴,
laur., led., lyc., m-arct.⁴, m-aust.⁴,
mag-c., mang.⁴, **merc., mez.,**
mosch., mur-ac., nat-c., nat-m.,
nicc.⁴, **nit-ac.,** nux-m., **NUX-V.,**
ol-an.⁴, olnd., op., paeon., par.,
petr., **PETROS.,** ph-ac., phos.,
plat.⁴, **prun., puls.,** ran-b., **RAN-S.,**
rheum, rhod., **rhus-t., ruta,** sabad.,
sabin., sars., sel., seneg., **sep.,** sil.,
spig., **spong.⁴,** squil., stann., **staph.,**
stram., stront-c., sul-ac., **SULPH.,**
teucr., thuj., valer., verat., viol-t.,
voes.¹¹, **ZINC., ZINC-P.¹'**

boring

acon., **agar.,** aloe, alum.,
alum-p.¹', alum-sil.¹', am-c.,
am-m., anac., ang.³, ant-c., ant-t.,
apis, **arg-m., ARG-N.,** arn., ars.,
asaf., AUR., aur-ar.¹', **aur-s.¹',**
bar-c., bar-s.¹', **BELL., BISM.,**
bor., bov., **calc.,** calc-sil.¹',
cann-i., canth., caps., carb-an.,
carb-v., carbn-s., **caust.,** chin.,
cimic., **cina,** clem., coc-c., cocc.,
colch., coloc., con., cupr., cycl.,
dig., dios., dros., **dulc.,** euph.,
euphr., **hell., hep.,** ign., ip.,
kali-c., kali-n., kreos., **lach.,**
laur., led., lyc., m-arct.³, mag-c.,
mag-m., mang., meny., **merc.,**
merc-i-f.¹¹, **mez.,** mur-ac., **nat-c.,**
nat-m., nat-sil.¹', nit-ac., nux-m.,
nux-v., olnd., par., petr., **ph-ac.,**
phos., plan.³,, plat., **plb., PULS.,**
ran-b., **RAN-S., rhod.,** rhus-t,
ruta, sabad., sabin., sel., **seneg.,**
sep., **sil., SPIG.,** spong., stann.,
staph., stram., stront-c., **sulph.,**
tarax., thuj., valer., **zinc.,**
zinc-p.¹'

inward
alum., bell., calc., cocc., **kali-c.,**
mang., zinc.

outward
ant-c., asaf., bell., **bism.**, bov.,
calc., dros., **dulc.**, ip., puls.,
sep., **spig.**, spong., **staph.**

bones
agar., anac.[4], ang.[3, 4], aran., **asaf.**,
AUR., bar-c., bell., brom., **calc.**,
carb-an., clem., dulc., hell., hep.,
kali-c.[4], kali-i.[3], lach., **lyc.**, mang.,
MERC., mez., nat-c., nat-m.,
nit-s-d.[11], ph-ac., phos., **puls.**,
ran-s.[4], rhod., rhus-t., sabad.,
sabin., **sep., sil., spig.**, staph.,
sulph., **thuj.**

glands
bell., lyc.[3, 4], puls., sabad., sabin.[4]

small spots, in[11]

fl-ac.

broken, as if bones

agar.[1'], am-c.[1'], **ang.**[2, 3], arg-m.[11],
arn.[1', 3], ars.[1'], **aur., BELL.**[3], bor.[3],
bov.[3], **bry.**, calc.[3], calc-p.[3],,
caust.[3], **cham.**[2, 3], **chel.**[2, 3], cina[3],
coc-c.[2], **COCC.**[2, 3], cupr., **dros.**[2, 3],
EUP-PER[1', 3, 7], graph.[3], guaj.[3],
hep., hyos.[3], **IGN.**[2, 3], kreos.[3],
lyc.[3], lyss.[2], m-arct.[3], mag-m.[2, 3],
merc.[2, 3, 7], mez.[3], mosch.[3],
nat-m., nux-v.[1', 3], par.[3], ph-ac.[3],
PHOS.[2, 3], puls., rhus-t[1', 3], **ruta**,
samb.[2, 3], sep., **sil.**[11], sulph.[3],
symph.[2], **tarant.**[11], ther., **thuj.**[2],
valer.[3], **verat., vip.**, zinc.[3]

ioints, in[3]

bov., calc., carb-an.[3, 11], caust.,
dros., hep., merc., mez., par.[2, 3, 11],
sep.

part on which he was lying, in[11]

mosch.

bruised see sore

burning externally

acet-ac.[11], achy.[14], **acon.**,
acon-f.[12], **agar.**, all-c.[6], aloe,
alum., **alum-p.**[1'], **alum-sil.**[1'],
am-c., **am-m.**, ambr., anac.,
ang.[3, 11], ant-c., ant-t., **anthraci.**,
APIS, arg-m., **arn., ARS.**,
ars-i., **ARS-S-F.**[1'], **ARUM-T.**,
asaf., asar., atro.[11], aur.[4],
aur-ar.[1'], **aur-m.**[1'], **bapt.**,
bar-c., bar-m., bar-s.[1'], **bell.**,
berb., bism., **bor.**, bov.,
brom.[11], **BRY.**, **bufo**, buni-o.[14],
calad., calc., calc-ar.[1'], calc-i.[1'],
calc-p., camph., cann-s.,
canth., caps., carb-ac.[3, 11],
carb-an., **CARB-V.**, carbn-o.[11],
CARBN-S., CAUST., cham.,
chel., chin., chin-s.[4, 11], cic.,
cimic., cina, **clem.**, coc-c.,
cocc., coff., colch., **coloc.**,
com.[6], **con.**, convo-d.[11], cop.[11],
corn., croc., crot-c.[11], crot-h.,
crot-t., culx.[1'], cupr., **cycl.**,
dig., **dros., dulc.**, eucal.[7],
euon.[4], euph., euph-l.[11],
EUPHR., fago.[11], **ferr.**,
fl-ac.[1', 3, 6], **gels.**[2], **graph.**, **grat.**,
guaj., hell., helon., hep.,
hist.[9, 10, 14], **hyos.**[3, 4], **ign.**, iod.,
ip., **IRIS**, juni.[11], kali-ar.,
kali-bi., kali-br.[11], **kali-c.**,
kali-m.[1'], kali-n., kali-s.,
kali-sula.[11], **kreos.**, lac-ac.[6],
lach., lachn.[11], lap-a.[6], lat-m.[9],
laur., led., lil-t.[11], lob., **lyc.**,
m-arct.[3, 4], m-aust.[3, 4], mag-c.,
mag-m., mag-s.[4], **manc.**,
mand.[10], mang., meny., **MERC.**,
merc-c., merc-sul.[2], merl.[11],
mez., mosch., **mur-ac., nat-ar.**,
nat-c., NAT-M., nat-s.[4],
nat-sil.[1'], nicc.[4], **nit-ac.**, nux-m.,
NUX-V., ol-an.[4], **olnd., op.**,

ox-ac.[1'], paeon., par., petr.,
PH-AC., phel.[4], **PHOS.**, phyt.,
pic-ac.[6], plat., plb., **prun., psor.,
puls., ran-b.**[2, 4, 11], ran-s.,
raph.[4], **RAT.**, rauw.[9], **rheum,**
rhod., **RHUS-T.**, rhus-v.[11],
rumx., ruta, **sabad.**, sabin.,
sal-ac., samb., sang.[4, 6], sars.,
SEC., sel., seneg., **SEP., SIL.,**
sol-n.[11], spig., spong., squil.,
STANN., staph., stram.,
stront-c., sul-ac., sul-i.[1'],
SULPH., tab.[4], **tarax.,
tarent.**[1', 2, 11], tarent-c.[6], teucr.,
thuj., til.[11], trib.[11], valer.,
verat., **viol-o.**[4], viol-t.,
vip.[3, 6, 1], wies.[11], **zinc.,**
zinc-p.[1']

left upper part of body

kreos.

heat am.[3, 7]

alum., **ARS., caps.**, carb-v.,
lyc.

right side of body[8]

phos.

internally

abies-c., acet-ac., achy.[14],
ACON., acon-f., aesc.[3, 6], **agar.,**
aloe[6], **alum.**, alumn., **am-br.,**
am-c., **am-m.**, ambr., amor-r.[14],
ang.[3], ant-c., ant-t., **apis,** arg-m.,
arg-n., arn., ARS., ars-i.,
ARS-S-F.[1'], **ARUM-T.**, asaf.,
asar., **aur.**, aur-i.[1'], **bapt., bar-c.,**
bar-m., **BELL., BERB.**, bism.,
bor., bov., brom.[3, 6], **BRY., bufo,**
calad., **calc., calc-p.**, calc-sil.[1'],
camph., **CANN-I.**, cann-s.,
CANTH., caps., carb-ac.,

carb-an., **carb-v., CARBN-S.,
caust.**, cedr., cham., **chel., chin.,
cic.**, cina, **clem.**, cocc., coff.,
colch., coloc., **com., con.**, crot-t.,
cund., **cupr.**, dig., **dios.**, dol.,
dros., dulc., equis., eucal.[6],
eup-pur., **euph.**, euphr., **fl-ac.,**
form.[6], **gamb., GRAPH.**, hell.,
hep., hist.[14], hydr., hyos., ign.,
iod., ip., **iris**, kali-ar., **KALI-BI.,**
kali-c., **kali-i.**, kali-n., kali-s.,
kalm.[6], **kreos.**, lac-ac.[6], **lach.,
laur.**, led., **lil-t.**, lith-c., **lob., lyc.,**
m-arct.[3], m-aust.[3], mag-c.,
mag-m., mang., **MERC.,
MERC-C., merc-i-f., MEZ.,**
mosch., mur-ac., **nat-ar., nat-c.,
nat-m., NIT-AC.**, nux-m.,
NUX-V., oena.[6], ol-j.[6], **op.**, osm.,
ox-ac., par., petr., ph-ac., **PHOS.,**
phyt., plat., plb., **PRUN., psor.,
PULS.**, pyrog.[6], **ran-b.**, ran-s.,
rat., **rhod., RHUS-T.**, rob., **rumx.,**
ruta, **SABAD.**, sabin., **SANG.,**
sang-n., **sars., SEC.**, seneg.,
SEP., sil., sin-n., **SPIG., SPONG.,
stann.**, staph., stram., stront-c.,
sul-ac., **SULPH.**, tab.[3], tarax.,
tarent.[1'], **tell., ter., thuj.**, uran.,
ust., uva, **verat.**, verat-v.,
viol-o., viol-t., wye., **ZINC.,
ZINC-P.**[1']

with external coldness[3]

ars., verat.

as from burning

agar., aloe, alum., ambr., **apis,
arum-t., bapt., bar-c.**, bell.,
berb., bry., cann-s., caust., chin.,
coloc., ferr., hyos., **ign., IRIS,**
kali-c., **lil-t., mag-m.**, merc.,
mez., mur-ac., nat-c., **nux-v.**, op.,
osm., par., phos., **phyt., plat.,
puls., ran-s.**, sabad., sang., **sep.,**
still., sul-ac., tarent., thuj., verat.

as from glowing coals[16]

ars., carb-v.

as from hot coals[16]

sabad.

blood-vessels, in

agar., **ARS.**, **aur.**, brom.[3], **bry.**,
calc., carb-v.[3], chin.[3], com.[3],
hyos., med., nat-m., nit-ac., **op.**,
phos.[3], plb.[3], **RHUS-T.**, sec.[3],
sulph., syph.[3], verat., xan.[3]

night[16]
ARS.

bones, in

ang.[3], ant-t.[4], arn.[4], ars., **asaf.**,
aur., bell.[11], bry., **carb-v.**,
caust., chel.[3], coloc.[3], con.,
dros.[3], **euph.**, fl-ac.[8], form.,
hep., ign., kali-i.[3, 8], **lach.**, lyc.,
mang., merc., **MEZ.**, nat-c.,
nit-ac., par., **ph-ac.**, phos.,
puls., **rhus-t.**, **ruta**, sabin., **sep.**,
sil., staph., **sulph.**, tarent.[2],
thuj., **ZINC.**

night
mez.[2], ph-ac., phos.[11]

menses, during

carb-v.

cold parts, in[3]

sec., verat.

glands, in

alum., ant-c., arn., **ARS.**, **bell.**,
brom., bry., calc., **cann-s.**,
carb-v., caust., cic., clem., cocc.,
con., graph., **hep.**, **ign.**, kali-c.,
laur., merc., mez., nat-m., nux-v.,
phos., phyt., plat., **PULS.**,
rheum[3, 4], rhus-t., **sep.**, **sil.**,
staph., sul-ac., sulph., ter.[4],
teucr., **zinc.**

joints, in[3]

abrot.[3, 11], anac.[14], ant-t.[3, 11],
arg-n., berb., carb-v., caust.,
cimic., guare.[11], hist.[14], ign.[4],
kali-n., lyc., nit-ac.[3, 4, 11], plat.
rhus-t., sabin.[1'], sulph.,
thuj.[3, 11], zinc.

spots[2]
mang.

parts grasped with the hand

bry., **CAUST.**

on which he lies at night[11]

sulph.

spots, in[11]

agar.[3, 11], ambr., apis, atha.,
carb-v., chin., coloc., glon.[3], ign.,
lim., lyc., mand.[14], nat-s., plat.,
raph. sang.[3], **SULPH.**[3, 11], viol-o,

constricting, externally

acon., acon-c.[11], agar., alum.,
alum-sil.[1'], **am-c.**, ambr.,
AML-NS.[3,] anac., ang.[3], ant-c.[3],

apis³, arg-m., **arg-n.**, arn., ars.³,
asaf.³, **asar.³, aur.³**, bar-c., **bell.,**
bism.³, bor.³, brom.³, bry.,
cadm-s.³, calad., **calc.**, camph.,
cann-s., **canth.³, ⁴**, caps.³,
carb-an.³, **carb-v.**, caust., cham.,
chel., **chin.³**, cic., **cina**, coc-c.³,
cocc., coff.³, colch., coloc.,
CON.³, ⁴, croc., crot-h.³, cupr.³,
cycl., **dig.**, dros., dulc., euphr.,
ferr.³, gamb.¹¹, gels.³, glon.³,
graph., guaj.³, hell.³, hep.³,
hist.⁹, ¹⁰, hydr-ac.³, hyos., **IGN.⁴**,
iod., kali-c., **kali-n.**, kreos.,
lach.³, laur.³, led., lob.³, lyc.,
mag-c.³, mag-m.³, ⁴, manc.³,
mang., meny., merc., mez.,
mosch., mur-ac.³, nat-c.,
nat-m.³, ⁴, nit-ac., NUX-M.³,
nux-v., oena.³, olnd., **op.³**, par.³,
petr., ph-ac., **phos.**, phys.³,
PLAT., PLB³, pneu.¹⁴, **PULS.**,
ran-b., ran-s.³, rheum³, rhod.,
rhus-t., ruta, sabad., sabin.³, sars.³,
sec.³, sel.³, sep., sil., spig.,
spong.³, squil., **stann.³**, staph.³,
stram.³, stront-c., **sul-ac.³**, sulph.,
sumb., tab.³, teucr., thuj., valer.,
verat., verb., viol-o.³, viol-t.,
zinc.

constriction

internally

acon., agar.³, agn., **alum.³**,
am-c.³, am-m., **AMBR.**, anac.,
ang.³, ant-c.³, ant-t., arg-m., arn.,
ars., asaf., asar., aur., bar-c.,
bell., bism., bor., bov.³, bry.,
bufo³, cact.¹, ³, calad.³, **calc.**,
camph., cann-s.³, canth., caps.,
carb-an., **carb-v.**, caust.³, cham.,
chel., chin., cic.³, cina, clem.³,
cocc., coff.³, **colch., coloc.**, con.,
croc., cupr.³, cycl., dig., dros.,
dulc., euph.³, ferr., graph.,
guaj.³, hell.³, hep.³, hyos., **IGN.**,
iod., ip.³, **kali-c.**, kali-n.³, lach.,
laur.³, led., lyc., mag-c., mag-m.³,

mang.³, meny., merc., **mez.,**
mosch.³, mur-ac., nat-c.³, nat-m.,
nit-ac.³, nux-m.³, nux-v., olnd.,
op.³, par.³, petr., **PH-AC.**, phos.,
PLAT., PLB.³, puls., ran-s.,
rheum, rhod., rhus-t., ruta³,
sabad.³, sabin., samb.³, sars.,
sec.³, sel., seneg., sep., sil.,
spig.³, spong., squil., stann.,
staph., stram., stront-c., sul-ac.,
sulph., tab.³, tarax.³, **teucr.**, thuj.,
valer., verat., verb.³, viol-t.³,
zinc.

bones, in

alum., am-m.³, anac.³, **apis⁸**,
aur.³, carb-ac.⁸, chin.³, cocc.³,
con.³, gels.³, **graph.³**, hep.⁸,
kreos.³, lyc.³, merc.³, nat-m.³,
NIT-AC.³, ⁸, nux-v.³, petr.³,
phos.³, **PULS.³**, rhod.³, **rhus-t.³**,
ruta³, sabad.³, sep.³, sil.³,
stront-c.³, **SULPH.³, ⁸**, valer.³,
zinc.³

glands, in

acon.³, ⁴, alum.³, ⁴, am-c., anac.,
arn.³, ⁴, bell., **bor.³, ⁴, calc.,**
carb-v., caust., chin., cocc.³, ⁴,
con.³, ⁴, ign., iod., kali-c., lyc.,
mang.³, ⁴, nat-c., **nit-ac.³, ⁴**,
nux-v., ph-ac., phos.³, ⁴, **plat.,**
plb.³, ⁴, **puls., rhus-t.³, ⁴**, sabad.,
sep., sil., spong., sul-ac.³, ⁴,
sulph.³, ⁴

joints, in³

acon., am-m., **ANAC., AUR.,**
calc., carb-an., chin., coloc.,
ferr., **GRAPH.**, kreos., lyc.,
meny., **NAT-M., NIT-AC.,**
nux-m., nux-v., **petr.**, pyrus¹¹,
ruta, sil., spig., squil., stann.,
stront-c., sulph., zinc.

orifices, of; sphincter spasm[3]

alum., ars., **bell.**, calc., carb-v.,
chel., cocc., colch., con., dig.,
dulc., ferr., graph., hep., hyos.,
ign., iod., ip., lyc., mez., nat-m.,
nux-v., phos., plat., plb., rhod.,
sabad., sars., sep., staph., stram.,
sulph., tarax, thuj., verat.

cramping in joints[3]

acon., am-m., **anac., ANG.,** arn.,
ars., aur., bar-c., **bell.,** bov., **bry.,**
CALC., camph., cann-s., canth.,
carb-an., caust., cham., chel.,
chin., cic., cocc., colch., coloc.,
con., cupr., dulc., euph., hep.,
hist.[14], hyos., ign., kali-c., kali-n.,
kreos., lach., laur., led., lyc.,
m-arct., mez., nux-v., olnd., op.,
par., petr., ph-ac.[2], phos., **PLAT.,**
plb., rhus-t., sarcol-ac.[14], **sec.,**
sel., spig., spong., staph., stram.,
sulph., tab., verat., verb.,

muscles, in[3]

acon., agar., alum., am-c., am-m.,
ambr., **ANAC.**[2, 3], **ANG.,** arg-m.,
arn., ars., asaf., asar.[3, 14], aur.,
bar-c., **BELL.**[1', 3], bism, bov.,
bry., bufo, **CALC., CAMPH.**[2, 3],
cann-s., caps., carb-an., carb-v.,
carbn-s.[11], **caust.**[2, 3], cham., chin.,
cic., cimic., **CINA,** clem.,
cocc.[2, 3], colch., **COLOC.**[2, 3], **con.,**
conin.[11], croc., **CUPR.**[2, 3], **cupr-a.**[2],
cyt-l.[14], dig., dios.[2], dros., **dulc.,**
euph., euphr., ferr., **gels.**[2],
graph.[2, 3], hell., hep., hist.[14],
hyos., **ign.**[2, 3], iod., ip., **kali-br.**[2],
kali-c., kali-n., kreos., lach.,
lat-m.[9], **LYC.,** mag-c., **mag-m.,**
mag-p., mang., meny., **MERC.,**
mez., morph.[11], mosch., **mur-ac.,**

nat-c., nat-f.[14], nat-m., **nit-ac.,**
nux-m., **nux-v.**[2, 3], olnd., **op.**[2, 3],
petr., ph-ac., phos., phyt.[1', 3],
PLAT., plb.[2, 3, 11], puls., ran-b.,
rhod., **rhus-t.,** ruta, sabad., samb.,
sang., sarcol-ac.[14], sec., **SEP., sil.,**
spig., spong., squil., **stann.,**
staph., stram., stront-c., sul-ac.,
sulph., tab.[2, 3], **thuj., valer.,**
VERAT., verb., viol-o., viol-t.,
zinc.[2, 3]

crushed, as if

anh.[9], apis[11], **canth.**[11], ran-b.[3],
verb.[3]

cutting, externally

acon., **alum.,** alum-p.[1'],
alum-sil.[1'], **alumn.**[2], ambr.,
anac., ang.[2, 3, 4], ant-c.,
arg-m., arn., ars-s-f[1'], asaf.,
asar., aur., aur-ar.[1'], aur-s.[1'],
BELL., berb.[3], bism., bor.,
brom., bry., **calad.**[2], **CALC.,**
calc-i.[1'], **CALC-SIL.**[1'], camph.,
cann-s., canth., carbn-s., caust.,
chin., chin-s.[4], cimic., cina[3],
clem., colch., **coloc., CON.,**
conv., dig., **DROS.,** dulc., euph.,
graph., hell., hep., hyos., **ign.,**
kali-c., **kali-m.**[1'], kali-s., led.,
lyc., mag-c.[1'], mag-m., mang.,
meny., **merc.,** mez., mosch.,
mur-ac., NAT-C., nat-m.,
nat-sil.[1'], nit-ac., **nux-v.,** olnd.,
osm., ox-ac.[1'], oxyt., par., **PETR.,**
ph-ac., phos., plat., puls., ran-b.,
rheum[2], rhod., **rhus-t.,** ruta,
sabad., **samb.,** sang.[1'], sars.,
seneg., **sep., sil.,** spig., stann.,
staph., stram., **stront-c.**[2], **sul-ac.,**
sul-il.[1'], **sulph.,** teucr., thuj.,
verat., **viol-t.,** zinc., **ZINC-P.**[1']

internally

abies-n., acon., aesc., aeth.,
agar., agn., all-c., alum., am-c.,
am-m., ambr., anac., **ang.**[3],
ant-c., ant-t., arg-m., arg-n.,
arn., ars., asaf., asar., aur., bar-c.,
bar-m., **BELL., berb.**, bism., bor.,
bov., bry., **calad., CALC.**, calc-p.,
camph., cann-i., cann-s.,
CANTH., caps., carb-an., carb-v.,
caust., cham., **chel., chin.**, cic.,
cina, clem., coc-c., cocc., coff.,
colch., **coll., COLOC., CON.**,
conv., croc., crot-h., crot-t.,
cub., cupr., cycl., dig., **DIOS.**,
dros., **dulc., elat., equis.**, ferr.,
gamb., gels., graph., guaj., hell.,
hep., hydr., **HYOS.**, ign., iod.,
ip., iris, **KALI-C.**, kali-chl.,
kali-n., kali-s., lach., laur., led.,
LYC., m-arct.[3], m-aust.[3], mag-c.,
mag-m., mang., meny., **MERC.**,
merc-c., mez., mosch., **mur-ac.**,
nat-c., **NAT-M.**, nit-ac., nux-m.,
NUX-V., op., **par., petr.**, ph-ac.,
phos., plat., plb., **PULS.**, ran-b.,
ran-s., **rheum**, rhod., rhus-t.,
ruta, sabad., sabin., samb., sars.,
sel., seneg., **sep., SIL., spig.**,
spong., squil., **stann., staph.**,
stront-c., sul-ac., **SULPH.**, teucr.,
thuj., valer., **VERAT.**, verb., **vib.**,
viol-t., **ZINC.**, zing.

blood-vessels, in[3]

calc.

bones, in long

anac.[2, 4], aur-m.[3], calc., dig.[2, 4],
kali-bi.[3], kali-m.[3], osm., sabad.

glands, in

arg-m., **bell.**, calc., con., graph.,
ign., **lyc.**, nat-c., ph-ac., **sep.**,
sil., staph., sulph.

around glands[16]

con.

joints, in[2, 11]

cadm-s., guare., hyos.[4, 11],
sabad.[4, 11], vesp.[11]

digging up (burrowing, rooting
sensation)

acon., agar., alum., alum-p.[1'],
alum-sil.[1'], am-c., **am-m.**, ambr.,
anac., ang.[3], ant-c., ant-t., arg-m.,
arg-n., **arn.**, ars., **asaf.**, asar.,
aur., bar-c., bar-m., **bell.**, bism.,
bor., **bov., bry.**, calc., cann-s.,
canth., caps., carb-an., **carb-v.**,
caust., cham., chel., chin., **cina**,
clem., cocc., colch., **coloc.**, con.,
croc., dig., dros., **DULC.**, euph.,
ferr., graph., guare.[11], hell., hep.,
ign., **kali-bi., kali-c.**, kali-n.,
kreos., laur., led., lyc., m-arct.[3],
m-aust.[3], mag-c., mag-m., mang.,
merc., mez., mur-ac., **nat-c.**,
nat-m., nux-m., nux-v., olnd.,
petr., ph-ac., **phos., plat.**, puls.,
rheum, **RHOD., rhus-t., ruta**,
sabad., sabin., samb., seneg.,
sep., sil., **SPIG.**, spong., squil.,
stann., staph., stront-c., sul-ac.,
sulph., thuj., valer., zinc.

bones, in

aran., arg-m.[11], asaf., **aur.**[8], calc.,
carb-ac.[8], **carb-an., cocc.**, dulc.,

kali-i.[8], **mang.**, merc.[8], rhod.,
ruta, sep., spig., symph.[8], thuj.

night[16]
   mang.

glands, in

acon., am-m., arn., asaf., bell.,
bov., bry., calc., **dulc.**, kali-c.,
nat-c., phos., plat., **rhod.**, rhus-t.,
ruta, sep., spig., stann.

joints, in

bell.[11], colch.[3]

drawing

acon., adon.[6], agar.[4], aloe,
alum.[4], am-c., ambr.[4], anac.,
ang.[4], ant-t.[4], aphis[4], aran-ix.[10],
arg-m., arn.[3, 4], ars.[3, 4], asar.[4],
aur-m.[1'], bar-a.[11], bar-c.,
bell.[1', 3, 4], bor.[4], **bry., calad.**[3],
calc.[4, 6], calc-p.[1'], calen.[4],
camph., cann-s.[4], canth.[4],
caps.[4], carb-ac.[6], carb-an.[4],
CARB-V., card-m.[1'], **caul.**,
caust., **cham.**[3, 4, 6], **CHEL.**,
chin.[1', 3, 4], chin-ar., chin-s.[4],
cic.[4], cimic.[1', 3], cist.[4], clem.,
coc-c., cocc.[4], colch., **COLOC.**,
con.[3], **crot-t.**, cycl.[1', 4], dig.,
digin.[11], **dros.**[3], **dulc.**[3, 4, 6],
esp-g.[13], euon., euph.[3], euphr.[3],
eupi., ferr-ar., **gamb.**, goss.,
GRAPH., guaj.[1'], guare.,
hell.[3], hep.[3, 4], hist.[10], hydrc.,
hyos.[4], ip.[4], kali-bi., kali-c.,
kreos., lach., lact., lam.[4],
laur.[3], led.[1], lup.[4], lyc.,
m-arct.[4], mag-c.[10], mag-m.[1', 4],
mang., med.[1'], merc., merc-c.[4],
mez., **mosch.**[3, 4], mur-ac.[3, 4],
nat-c.[3, 4], **NIT-AC.**, nux-m.[4],
nux-v., ol-an., olnd.[4], petr.[4],
ph-ac.[4, 6], phos., phyt.[1'], plat.,
PLB.[1', 3, 4], **puls.**, ran-s.[4], raph.,

rhod., **RHUS-T.**[1', 3, 4], ruta[3],
sabad.[4], sabin.[4], samb.[4],
sars.[4, 16], sec., sep., **sil.**[3, 6, 16],
stann., staph., stram.[4], sul-ac.[4],
sulph., tab., ter.[4], thuj., tub.[1'],
VALER., verat.[4], verb.[3],
viol-o.[4], **zinc.**[1', 3, 6], zinc-o.[4]

left side night[16]

lyc.

right side[16]

sep.

morning, after rising

graph.

after waking

coloc.

evening,
   coc-c., raph.

20 h
   rhus-t.

22 h
   bry.

night,
   coc-c.

alternating with heart symptoms

acon.

backward as by a cord[3]

crot-t., par., plb.

chill, during[16]

lyc.

cold, as from a[16]

plat.

cramplike[16]

plat.

eating, after[16]

camph.

increasing and decreasing
rapidly[16]

nit-ac.

menses, during

phos.

motion, on

calc., cycl.

paralytic

coc-c., staph.[16]

rest, during[1']

tub.

rheumatic

am-c.[16], carb-v., chel., sul-ac.

rising, after

coloc.

sitting, while

samb., **VALER**

upwards

ol-an.

walking, agg.

calc., coca
am.
rhus-t.[16], tub.[1']

weather agg., bad

rhod.

wrong position, from[16]

staph.

extending to fingers

apis

toes

apis

bones, in[3]

acon.[4], agar.[3, 4], agn., anac.[4],
ang.[4], ant-t., asaf.[4, 8], atha.[4],
aur.[3, 4], **bar-c.**[4], bry.[3, 4], calc-f.,
cann-s., canth., **carb-v.**[4],
caust.[4], cham.[3, 11], **chin.**[3, 4, 11, 16],
cocc.[3, 11], colch., crot-h.[4], cupr.[4].
cycl., gels.[3, 11], graph.[16], hell.,

ign.[4], indg.[4], ip., kali-bi.,
kali-c.[3, 4], kreos.[4], led., **lyc.[4]**,
m-arct.[4], mang.[4], meny.[4],
merc.[3, 4, 11] nat-m., nit-ac.[8],
nux-m., olnd., par.[3, 4], petr.[16],
ph-ac.[4], plb.[4], puls., rhod.[3, 4],
sabad., **SABIN.**[3, 4], samb.[3, 4],
seneg.[3, 4], sil., spig., stann.[4],
staph.[3, 4], sulph., ter.[4], teucr.,
thuj.[4], valer., verat., zinc.[16],
zinc-o.[4]

thread, as from a

bry.

threads

glands, in[3]

agn., alum.[4], **bell.**, bov., calc.,
cann-s., cham., **chin.**, cycl.,
guaj.[11], **ign.**[3, 4], merc.[4], mez.,
nit-ac., phos.[3, 11, 16], **puls.**[3, 4],
seneg., sil.[3, 4], sulph., thuj.

joints, in[3]

acon.[2, 3], agn., am-c.[4], ang.,
ant-c., ant-s-aur.[11], **ant-t.**[3, 11],
arg-m.[3, 11], asaf., asar., bar-c.,
bell., **bry.**[11], calc.[4], cann-s.,
canth., caps., **carl.**[11], **caul.**,
cham.[3, 11], chel., chin., cina,
cist.[4, 11], clem.[11], coc-c., cocc.,
colch., cupr., cycl., graph.[4], hep.[4],
hyos.[3, 4, 11], ign., kali-c.[4], led.,
lyc.[4, 11], **m-aust.**, meny., merc.,
mez.[3, 4, 11], nat-c., nat-m.[11],
nat-s.[11], nit-ac.[4, 11], nit-s-d.[11],
nux-m.[2], nux-v., olnd., par.,
phos.[11], plat.[3, 4], plb., puls.[3, 4],
rheum, **rhod.**[3, 4, 11], rhus-t.,
sabad.[3, 4], sabin.[3, 4], sec.[3, 4, 11],
seneg., sep.[4], spig., spong.,
STAPH.[3, 4], tarax., teucr., valer.,
verat., viol-o.

muscles, in[3]

acon., agn., alum., ambr., anac.,
ang., **ANT-C.**, **ANT-T.**, apis,
arg-m., arn., asaf., asar., aur.,
bar-c., **BELL.**, berb., bism., bov.,
bry., calc., **camph.**, cann-s.,
canth., **caps.**, carb-ac., **carb-v.**,
caust., **CHAM.**, **chel.**, chin.[1, 3],
cic., **cina, clem.**, **COCC.**, coff.,
colch., croc., cupr., **CYCL.**, dig.,
dros., dulc., euph., ferr.,
GRAPH., hell., hep., hydr.[11],
hyos., **ign.**, ip., kali-bi., kali-c.,
kali-n., led., **lyc.**, **meny.**, merc.,
mez., morph.[11], **mosch.**, nat-m.,
nit-ac., **nux-m.**, nux-v., olnd.,
par., petr., ph-ac., phos., **PLAT.**,
plb., **PULS.**, ran-b., ran-s.,
raph.[11], **RHOD.**, **rhus-t.**, ruta,
sabad., sabin., samb., sec., sep.,
sil., spig., spong., **squil.**, staph.,
stram., sul-ac., **sulph.**, tarax.,
teucr., thuj., VALER., verat.,
verb., viol-o., viol-t., **zinc.**

tendons, in[3]

am-m.[1'], kali-bi., nat-m., rhus-t.,
thuj.

gnawing

agn.[6], alum-sil.[1'], **ars.**, bar-s.[1'],
caust., lach.[6], **MERC.**, mez.[6],
nat-m.[6], sil., staph., sulph.

externally

acon., agar., **AGN.**, alum.,
alumn.[2], am-c., ambr., arg-m.,
arn., aur., **bar-c.**, bar-m., bell.,
bry., calad., calc., calc-p.[11],
canth., caps., cham., **crot-t.**,
cycl., dig., **dros.**, dulc., euph.,
ferr., gamb.[11], **glon.**, graph., hell.,
hyos., ign., **kali-c.**, kreos., laur.,

led., lyc., mag-c., mag-m., mang., **meny.**, merc., mez., mur-ac., nat-c., nux-v., olnd., op., **par.**, **ph-ac., phos., PLAT.**, plb., **puls., RAN-S.**, rheum, rhod., rhus-t., **ruta,** samb., sep., sil., spig., **SPONG.**, stann., **STAPH.**, stront-c., sulph., **tarax.**, thuj., verat., zinc.

internally

agar., alum., am-m., arg-m., arg-n.[3], **ars.**, bar-c., **bell.**, calad., **calc.**, cann-s., canth.[1], carb-an.[3], **carb-v., CAUST.**, chel., cocc., **coloc., con., cupr.,** dig., dros., dulc., **gamb., glon.**[3], hep., iod., kali-bi., kali-c., kali-i.[3], **kreos.,** lach., **lyc.**, merc., mez., nat-m.[3, 6], nux-v., olnd., ph-ac., phos., **plat.**, psor.[3], **PULS.**, ran-b.[3, 6], **ran-s,,** rhod., **RUTA**, seneg., **SEP.**, sil., stann., staph.[6], stront-c.[6], sulph., teucr., verat.

bones, in

am-m., arg-m., **aur.**[8], **BELL.**, brom., canth., carb-ac.[8], **con.**[1], **dros.,** graph., kali-bi.[3], kali-i., lyc., **mang.**, merc.[8], nat-s.[3, 11], **ph-ac.**, phos., plb.[11], puls., rhod.[3], **ruta,** samb., **staph.**, stront-c., sulph.[3, 6], symph.[8]

glands, in

bar-c., cham., mez., ph-ac., **plat.**, ran-s., **spong.**, staph.

joints, in

am-c., aur-m.[1'], canth., colch., **dros.**[2, 3, 11], dulc., graph., mag-c., mang., phos., **RAN-S.**, stront-c., zinc.

growing pains[3]

acon.[11], agar.[1', 3] bell., calc-p.[1', 3, 8], **ferr-a.**[3, 6], **guaj.**[3, 6, 8, 12], mang.[3, 8], ol-an., **PH-AC.**[2, 3, 6, 8], phos.[3, 6], sil.[7]

legs, in the

bell., **calc-p.**[7], cimic., **eup-per.**, **GUAJ.**, kali-p.[7], m-aust.[7], mag-p.[7], mang.[7], **PH-AC.**

intolerable[16]

ars., **cham.**, nux-v.

sensitiveness–pain

Vol. I: *sensitive–pain*

jerking externally

acon., agar., agn., **alum.**, alum-p.[1'], alum-sil.[1'], **alumn.**[2], ambr., anac., ang.[3], ant-c., ant-t., arg-m., **arn.**, ars., **ASAF.**, asar., **aur.**, bar-c., **bar-m.,** bar-s.[1'], **bell.**, bism., bor., bov., **bry., CALC.**, calc-a.[6], calc-i.[1'], calc-sil.[1'], camph., **cann-s.**[2, 6], canth., caps., carb-v., **carbn-s., CAUST.**, cham., **chin.**, cic., cimic.[1'], **cina, clem.**, cocc., coff., colch., coloc., con.[3], croc.[3, 6], cupr.[6, 16], cycl.[3], dig.[3], dros.[3], dulc.[3], **graph.**[2, 3, 6], hell.[3], hep.[3], hyos.[3], **IGN.**[2, 3, 6], iod., kali-bi.[3], kali-c., kali-m.[1'], kali-s., kreos., lach., laur., led., **lyc.**, mag-c., **mag-p.**, mang., **MENY., merc.**, mez., mosch., mur-ac., **nat-c., NAT-M., nit-ac.**, nux-m.[2], **NUX-V.**, olnd., op., par., **petr., petros.**[2], ph-ac., phos., phyt., plat., plb.,

PULS., **ran-b.**, ran-s., rheum, rhod., **RHUS-T.**, ruta, sabad., sabin., sec., **sep.**, **sil.**, spig., spong., **squil.**, **stann.**, staph., stront-c., sul-ac., sul-i.[1'], sulph., **TARAX.**, teucr., thuj., **VALER.**, verat., verb., viol-t., zinc.

affected parts, of

arn.[16], **merc.**

on rising from bed[16]

mag-c.

internally

acon., agar., aloe, am-m., ambr., anac., ang.[3], arn., ars., **BELL.**, bor., bry., **calc.**, cann-s., carb-v., caust., cham., **CHIN.**, clem., cocc., colch., con., croc., graph., **IGN.**, **KALI-C.**, lyc., mang., meny., **merc.**, mez., nat-m., **NIT-AC.**, nux-v., petr., ph-ac., plat., plb., **PULS.**, ran-b., ran-s., rhus-t., **sep.**, **SIL.**, **spig.**, **stann.**, stront-c., sul-ac., **SULPH.**, teucr., **THUJ.**, **valer.**

bones, in

anac.[4], **ASAF.**, aur., bell., **calc.**, caust., **chin.**, clem., colch., lyc., mang.[3], merc., **nat-m.**, nux-v., ol-an.[3], petr., phos., **puls.**, rhod., rhus-t., sep., sil., sul-ac.[4], **SULPH.**, **symph.**[2], **valer.**

glands, in

arn., asaf., aur., bell., bry., **calc.**, caps., caust., chin., **clem.**, graph., lyc., meny., merc., nat-c., **nat-m.**, nit-ac., nux-v., petr., **puls.**, rhus-t., sep., sil., sulph.

right side, of[16]

cupr.

paralytic

acon., agar., agn., alum., alum-sil.[1'], am-c., am-m., ambr., ang.[3], ant-c., arg-m., arg-n.[3], ars., ars-i., asaf., asar., **aur.**, bar-c., **BELL.**, **bism.**, bov., **bry.**, calc., cann-s., canth., caps.[4], carb-v., caust., **cham.**, chel., **chin.**, **CINA**, **COCC.**, coff., **COLCH.**, coloc., con., croc., crot-h., **CYCL.**, dig., dros., **dulc.**, eug.[4], euph., euphr., **ferr.**, ferr-ar., ferr-m.[4], gels.[3], graph., grat.[3], hell., hep., hyos., ign., iod., kali-c., kali-n., kali-p., kreos., lach.[4], **laur.**, led., lyc., m-arct.[4], mag-c., mag-m., mang., meny., meph.[4], merc., **mez.**, mosch., mur-ac., nat-c., **nat-m.**, **NUX-V.**, olnd., par., petr., ph-ac., phos., plat., plb., puls., ran-s., raph.[11], rheum[4], rhod., **rhus-t.**, ruta, sabad., **SABIN.**, sars., sel., seneg., sep., **sil.**, spig., stann., **staph.**, stram., stront-c., sul-ac., sulph., teucr., thuj., valer., **verat.**, verb., zinc.

bones, in

AUR., bell., chin., **cocc.**, **crot-h.**[4], cycl., dig., **lach.**[4], led., mez., nat-m., nux-v., petr., phos.[3], puls., rhus-t., sabin., **sil.**, staph., verat., zinc.

joints, in[3]

acon., agn., am-c., ambr., anac., arg-m., arn.[3, 4], ars., asar., **AUR.**, bell., bism., **bov.**, calc., **CAPS.**[2, 3, 4], **carb-v.**, caust.,

cham., **chin.**, cina, cocc., colch.,
coloc., con., **croc.**, dig., **dros.**,
EUPH.[3, 4], ferr., graph., hell., ign.,
kali-c., kali-n., laur.[4], **led.**[2, 3, 4],
lyc., mag-m., meny., merc., **mez.**,
nat-c., nat-m., nux-v., **par.**, petr.,
ph-ac., phos.[3, 4], **plb.**[2, 3], **puls.**[3, 4],
rhus-t.[3, 4], ruta, sabad., **sabin.**[3, 4],
samb., sars., **seneg.**, sep., stann.,
STAPH.[3, 4], stram., stront-c.,
sulph., **VALER.**, verat., verb.,
zinc.

pinching

agar., alum., alum-sil.[1'], **am-c.**[2],
ambr., anac., **ARN.**, **ars.**, ars-i.,
asar., bar-c.[11], **BELL.**, bov., bry.,
calc., calc-i.[1'], cann-s., canth.,
caps., carb-an., carb-v., caust.,
cham., **chel.**[2], **chin.**[2], cina, clem.,
cocc., **colch.**, coloc., con., croc.,
dros., dulc., **euph.**, **gamb.**[11],
graph.[2], guaj., hell., hep., **hyos.**[2],
ign., iod., kali-c., kali-i.[11],
kali-m[1'], kali-n., kreos., **laur.**, lyc.,
mag-m., mang., meny., **merc.**,
mez., mur-ac., **nat-c.**, nat-m.,
nit-ac., nux-m.[1], **NUX-V.**, op.,
par., petr., **phos.**, **plat.**, **puls.**,
ran-b., ran-s., **rheum**, rhod.,
rhus-t., ruta, **sabad.**, sabin., sars.,
seneg., sep., sil., spig., **spong.**,
stann., staph., stront-c., **sulph.**,
teucr., thuj., tub.[1'], valer., verat.,
verb., zinc.

right side, of

sep.

externally

acon., anac., ang.[3], ant-c., arg-m.,
arn., bell., bry., **calc.**, cann-s.,
caps., carb-v., caust., chel., chin.,
cina, **clem.**, cocc., con., croc.,
dig., dros., dulc., euph., euphr.,
hyos., **ip.**, kali-c., kreos., led.,

mang., **MENY.**, **mur-ac.**, nat-c.,
nit-ac., nux-v., olnd., **osm.**, par.,
ph-ac., phos., **RHOD.**, **rhus-t.**,
ruta, **SABAD.**, sabin., samb.,
sars., sil., **spig.**, **SPONG.**,
STANN., staph., sul-ac., **sulph.**,
thuj., verat., **VERB.**, viol-t., zinc.

internally

acon., **agar.**, agn., alum., **am-c.**,
am-m., anac., ang.[3], ant-c., ant-t.,
arg-m., arn., ars., ars-i., asaf.,
asar., aur., bar-c., **bell.**, bism.,
bor., bov., **bry.**, **CALC.**, camph.,
cann-s., **canth.**, caps.[1], carb-an.,
carb-v., caust., cham., **CHEL.**,
chin., cic., **cina**, coc-c., **COCC.**,
coff., **colch.**, **COLOC.**, com.,
con.[3], croc., cupr., cycl., dig.,
dros., **dulc.**, euph., euphr., **gamb.**,
GRAPH., guaj., **hell.**, hep., hyos.,
IGN., iod., **ip.**, **kali-c.**, kreos.,
LYC., mag-c., mag-m., mang.,
meny., **merc.**, mez., mosch.,
mur-ac., **nat-c.**, **nat-m.**, nit-ac.,
nux-m., nux-v., olnd., **par.**, **petr.**,
ph-ac., **phos.**, plat., **plb.**, **puls.**,
ran-b., ran-s., rheum, **rhod.**,
rhus-t., **ruta**, **sabad.**, sabin.,
samb., sars., seneg., **sep.**, sil.,
spig., spong., squil., **stann.**,
staph., stront-c., sul-ac., **sulph.**,
tarax., teucr., **thuj.**, valer.,
verat., **VERB.**, viol-t., **zinc.**

bones, in

bell., calc., cina, ign., mez.,
nux-m.[11], osm., petr., **ph-ac.**,
plat., **VERB.**

glands, in

bry., **calc.**, m-arct.[4], meny.,
mur-ac., prun.[4], **rhod.**, rhus-t.,
sabad., stann., sulph., verat.

muscles, in[4]

bruc., **cann-s.**, lyc.,. m-aust., sulph.[4, 11]

spots, in[11]

caust., daph., lyc.

pressing, externally

abrot., **acon., aesc., AGAR.,** agn., aloe, alum., **alum-p.**[1'], **alum-sil.**[1'], **am-m.,** ambr., **ammc., anac.,** ang.[3], ant-c., **ant-t., APOC.,** arg-m., arn., ars., ars-i., **ARS-S-F.**[1'], **asaf.,** asar., **aspar., aur.,** aur-i.[1'], aur-m.[1'], **aur-s.**[1'], **bapt.,** bar-c., bar-i.[1'], bar-m., bar-s[1]., **bell.,** berb.[4], bism., bor., bov., **bry., calad., calc.,** calc-i.[1'], **calc-p.,** calc-sil.[1'], calen.[4], **camph., CANN-I., cann-s.,** canth., caps., **carb-ac.,** carb-an., **carb-v.**[3], carbn-s., **CAUST.,** cedr., **cham., chel., chin., CHIN-S.,** cic., **cimic.,** cina, cinnb., clem., cob., coc-c., **cocc.,** coff., **colch., coloc., con.,** crot-t., cupr., **cycl.,** daph.[4], dig., dios., **DROS., dulc.,** elaps, **EUP-PER.,** euph., euphr., **FERR.,** ferr-ar., **gels., glon., graph., guaj., hell.,** hep., **hyos., ign.,** iod., **ip., KALI-BI.,** kali-c., kali-m.[1'], kali-n., kali-p., **kalm., kreos.,** lach., **laur., led., lil-t., lyc.,** mag-c., mag-m., mang., meny., merc., **mez., MOSCH.,** mur-ac., nat-ar., nat-c., **nat-m.,** nat-sil.[1'], **NIT-AC.,** nux-m., **NUX-V.,** olnd., **ox-ac.,** par., pareir., **petr., ph-ac., PHOS.,** phyt., plat., plb., **PODO.,** prun., **psor., PULS.,** ran-b., ran-s., rheum, **RHOD., RHUS-T., RUTA,** sabad., sabin., **samb., sang., sars., sec.,** seneg., **SEP., SIL., SPIG.,** spong., **squil., STANN., STAPH.,** stict., stront-c., sul-ac., **sul-i.**[1'], **SULPH.,** tab., **tarax.,** teucr., thuj.,

ust., valer., **verat.,** verb., vib. viol-o., viol-t., **zinc.,** zinc-p.[1']

internally

acon., aesc., agar., agn., **ail., aloe, alum.,** am-c., am-m., **ambr., anac.,** ang.[3], ant-c., ant-t., arg-m., **ARG-N., ARN., ARS., ars-i., arum-t., ASAF.,** asar., **aur.,** aur-ar.[1'], aur-i.[1'], bar-c., **BELL.,** berb., **bism., bor.,** bov., **BROM.,** bry., cact., calad., **CALC., camph., cann-i.,** cann-s., **CANTH.,** caps., **carb-an., CARB-V.,** carbn-s., **caust., cedr.,** cham., chel., chen-a., **CHIN.,** cic., **CIMIC.,** cina, clem., **coc-c., cocc., cod.,** coff., **colch., COLOC., con.,** cor-r., croc., crot-t., **CUPR.,** cycl., **dig.,** dios., dros., dulc., elaps, euph., euphr., **ferr., gamb., gels., glon.,** goss., **graph.,** guaj., **HAM., hell.,** hep., hydr., **hydr-ac.,** hyos., hyper., **ign.,** iod., ip., iris, kali-bi., **kali-c., kali-i.,** kali-n., **kalm.,** kreos., **LACH., laur.,** led., **lept., LIL-T., lith-c., LYC.,** mag-c., mang., **MENY., merc., merc-c.,** merc-i-f., **mez.,** mosch., mur-ac., murx., naja, nat-ar., nat-c., **NAT-M., nit-ac.,** nux-m., **NUX-V.,** olnd., onos., **OP.,** osm., **ox-ac.,** par., **PETR., ph-ac., PHOS., phys., phyt., pic-ac., plat., plb., podo., prun.,** psor., **PULS., RAN-B.,** ran-s., **rheum, rhod., RHUS-T., rumx., RUTA,** sabad., **sabin.,** samb., **SANG., SANG-N.,** sars., **SEC., SENEG., SEP., SIL., SPIG., SPONG., squil., STANN.,** staph., stict., stram., stront-c., sul-ac., **SULPH.,** tab., **tarax.,** tarent., **ter.,** teucr., thuj., ust., **VALER., VERAT.,** verat-v., verb., vesp., vib., viol-o., viol-t., vip., xan., **ZINC., ZINC-P.**[1']

inward

acon., agar., alum., **ANAC.,**
ant-c., ant-t., asaf., asar., aur.,
bar-c., bell., bism., bor., bry.,
calc., cann-s., carb-an., caust.,
chel., chin., **cocc.,** coff., croc.,
cycl., **dulc., hell.,** hep., ign.,
kali-c., **kreos.,** laur., mez.,
mosch., **nit-ac.,** nux-m., nux-v.,
olnd., ph-ac., **PLAT.,** prun.[7],
ran-s., rheum, rhod., rhus-t.,
ruta, sabad., sabin., sars., sep.,
sil., **spig., STANN., staph.,**
sul-ac., **sulph.,** tarax., teucr.,
thuj., valer., verb., viol-t.,
zinc.

deep inward with instruments

bov., verat.

load, as from a

abies-n., ACON., aesc., agar.,
aloe, alum., am-c., **am-m., ambr.,**
ant-t., aran., arg-m., **arg-n.,** arn.,
ars., asaf., asar., aur., **bar-c.,**
BELL., bism., bor., bov., **BROM.,**
BRY., cact., calad., calc., camph.,
cann-s., carb-an., carb-v., caust.,
cham., **chel.,** chin., cina, cinnb.,
cocc., colch., coloc., **com., con.,**
croc., corn., crot-t., **cupr.,** dig.,
ferr., gels., graph., hell., hep.,
hyos., ign., iod., **IP.,** kali-c.,
kali-chl., kali-n., **kreos.,**
laur., led., **LIL-T.,** lyc.,
mag-c., mag-m., mang., **meli.,**
MENY., merc., mosch., **nat-c.,**
nat-m., nit-ac., nux-m., **NUX-V.,**
olnd., **op., PAR.,** petr., **ph-ac.,**
PHOS., plat., plb., **psor., puls.,**
RAN-B., rheum[1], rhod., **RHUS-T.,**
sabad., sabin., **samb.,** sars., **sec.,**
seneg., **SEP.,** sil., **spig.,** spong.,
squil., stann., staph., **STICT.,**

stront-c., sul-ac., **SULPH.,** thuj.,
valer., **verb.,** viol-o., zinc., zing.

together

acon., aeth.[3], agar., **alum.,** am-m.,
ambr., **anac.,** ang.[3], ant-c., ant-t.,
arg-m., arg-n.[3], **arn., ars.,** asaf.,
ASAR., aur. bar-c., **bell., bov.,**
bry., cact.[3], calc., camph.,
cann-s., canth., caps., carb-an.,
carb-v., caust., cham., chel.,
chin., cic., cimic.[3], cina, **COCC.,**
coff., coloc., con., cupr., dig.,
dros., dulc., euph., ferr., graph.,
guaj., **hell.,** helon.[3], hydr-ac.[3],
hyos., ign., iod., **ip.,** kali-c.,
kali-i.[3], kali-n., laur., led., lil-t.[3],
lyc., mag-c., mag-m., meny.,
merc., mez., **mosch., nat-m.,**
nit-ac., nux-m., **NUX-V.,** olnd.,
op., petr., ph-ac., phos., **PLAT.,**
plb., puls., ran-s., rhod., rhus-t.,
ruta, sabad., sabin., **sars.,** seneg.,
sep., sil., spig., **spong.,** squil.,
stann., staph., stram., stront-c.,
sul-ac., SULPH., tarax., teucr.,
thuj., valer., verat., verb.[1],
viol-t., zinc.

upward[3]

calc-p.

within outward, from

•

acon., aloe, alum., am-c., am-m.,
anac., ang.[3], ant-c., ant-t.[3],
arg-m., arg-n.[3], arn., ars.[3],
ASAF., asar., **aur.,** bar-c., **bell.,**
berb., bism., bor., bov.[3], **BRY.,**
calc., camph., cann-s., canth.,
caps., carb-an.[3], carb-v., caust.,
cham.[3], chel., chin., **CIMIC.,**
cina, clem., cocc., coff.[3], colch.,
coloc., con., **cor-r.,** croc., cupr.,
dig., **dros.,** dulc., euph., **ferr.,**
graph., guaj., ham.[3], hell., hep.,
hyos.[3], **ign.,** iod.[3], ip., iris[3],

kali-c., **kali-i.,** kali-n., kreos.,
lach., laur., led., **lith-c.,** lyc.,
mag-c.[3], mag-m., mang., meli.,
meny., **merc., merc-c., mez.,**
mosch.[3], **mur-ac.,** nat-c., **nat-m.,**
nit-ac., nux-m., **nux-v., olnd.,** op.,
par., petr., ph-ac., **phos.,** plat.,
plb.[3], **prun., PULS.,** ran-b., ran-s.,
rheum, rhod., **rhus-t.,** ruta,
sabad., **sabin.,** samb., sars.[3],
seneg., **sep., sil., spig., spong.,**
squil., stann., staph., stront-c.,
sul-ac., **SULPH.,** tarax., **teucr.,**
thuj., usn.[3]**, VALER.**[1]**,** verat.[3],
verb., viol-t., zinc.

bones, in

   alum., am-m.[4], anac., ang.[3, 4],
anis.[4], **arg-m.,** arn.[4], ars., asaf.,
aur., **bell., bism.,** bry., cann-i.,
cann-s.[4], canth., carb-v.[4],
carbn-s., cham., chel.[4], cocc.,
colch., **coloc.,** con., **cupr.,**
cycl., daph.[4]**,** dros., graph.,
guaj., hell., hep., ign., kali-bi.[3],
kali-c., kali-n., **led.**[4]**,** m-arct.[4],
m-aust.[4], mang-o.[11], merc.,
mez., nux-m., nux-v.[4], **olnd.,**
petr.[16], phos., plat., puls., rhod.,
rhus-t., ruta, sabin., sil.,
spong., stann., **staph.,** teucr.[4],
thuj., valer., verat., viol-t.,
zinc.

on going to sleep[16]

   graph.

sticking

   anac.[3], mez., ruta[3], staph.

tearing

   arg-m., bell., cham., coloc.,
thuj.

glands, in

   alum.[4], arg-m., ars., asar., aur.,
bell., calc., carb-v., caust.,
chin., cina, cocc., con.[4], cycl.,
hyos., ign., kali-c., **lyc.,**
m-arct.[4], mag-m.[4], mang.,
meny., **MERC.,** mur-ac.,
nat-m.[4], nit-ac.[4], osm., par.,
ph-ac., puls., rheum, rhust-t.,
sabin., **spong.,** stann., **staph.,**
stram., **sulph.,** teucr.[3], verat.,
zinc.

  inward

   aur., **calc.,** cocc., cycl., rheum,
staph., zinc.

  outward

   arg-m., cina, ign., lyc., mang.,
meny., **merc.,** par., puls.,
rhus-t., **spong.,** sulph., teucr.[3]

joints, in[3]

   agn., alum.[1', 3, 4, 11]**,** anac.,
arg-m., asaf., asar., bar-c.,
bell., calc.[3, 4], camph., carb-an.,
caust., cham., chel., chin.,
clem., colch., coloc.[11], dulc.,
graph., hep., hyos., ign., iod.,
kali-c.[2, 3, 4]**, led.**[3, 11]**,** lyc.[4],
meny., merc., mez., mosch.,
nat-s.[11],, nit-ac.[3, 4], nit-s-d.[11],
nux-v., petr., rhust-t., sabad.,
sabin., sep., sil., spong., stann.,
staph., stront-c., sulph., tarax.,
thuj., viol-o., viol-t., zinc.

sticking[3]

   ph-ac., sars., staph., zinc.

tearing

agn.[3], anac., ang.[3], arg-m.[3],
arn., asaf., bell., bism., carb-v.,
caust., cham., chin [3], coloc.[3],
graph.[3], guaj.[3], hyos., kali-c.[3],
led., lyc., mez.[3], ph-ac.[3], ruta,
sabad.[3], sars.[3], sep.[3], spong.,
stann., staph.[3], zinc.[3]

muscles, in

agar., agn., am-m., **anac.,** ang.[3],
arg-m., arn., **asaf., asar.,** aur.,
bell., bism., **bry.,** calc., camph.,
cann-s., **caps., carb-an.,** caust.,
chel., chin., cina, clem., cocc.,
con., **cupr., CYCL.,** dig., dros.,
euph., euphr., graph., hell., hep.,
ign., kali-n., **led.,** lyc., mag-c.,
mag-m., mang., meny., merc.,
mez., **mosch.,** mur-ac., nat-c.,
nat-m., nitro-o.[11], **NUX-M.,**
nux-v., **olnd.,** petr., **ph-ac.,**
phos., plat., plb., puls., ran-b.,
ran-s., rheum, rhod.[3], rhus-t.,
RUTA, sabad., sabin., samb.,
sil., spig., spong., **stann.,**
staph., stront-c., **sul-ac.,** sulph.,
tarax., teucr., thuj., **valer.,**
verat., VERB., viol-t., zinc.

sticking

am-m.[3], anac., arg-m.[3], arn.[3],
asaf., bar-c.[3], bell., calc.,
chin.[3], colch.[3], coloc., cycl.,
dios.[3], dros., euph., **ign.,**
kali-c.[3], mez.[3], **mur-ac.,** olnd.,
phos.[3], plat., rhus-t.[3], ruta[3],
sabad[3]., sars., sep., spong.[3],
stann.[3], staph.[3], sul-ac., tarax.[3],
thuj., verb.[3], viol-t.[3], **zinc.[3]**

tearing

agar., anac., **ang.[3],** arg-m.,
arn., asaf., asar., aur.,

bell., bism., calc., **camph.,**
cann-s., carb-v., chin., colch.,
cupr., cycl., hyos., led., meny.,
petr., ph-ac., ruta, sars., sep.,
spig., spong., stann., sulph.,
zinc.

twitching[16]

petr.

parts lain on, in[16]

kali-c.

spots, in[11]

bar-a., sul-ac.

upward[3]

calc-p.

radiating

agar.[6], apis[6], **arg-n.,** ars.[6], berb.,
cupr.[6], dios., kali-c.[6], lil-t.[6],
mag-m.[3], **mag-p.,** plb.[3], spig.[6], **tell.**

scraped, as if

acon., aesc., alumn., **arg-n.,** arn.,
asaf., **asar.[2], bell., BROM.,** bry.,
carbn-s., cham., **chin., coc-c.,**
coloc., **con.,** crot-t., dig., **DROS.,**
kali-bi., kali-chl., lach., led.,
lepi.[11], lyc., mez., **NUX-V.,** osm.,
par., ph-ac., **phos.,** phyt., **PULS.,**
rhus-t., rumx., sabad., sel.,
seneg., spig., **stann., SULPH.,**
tell., **VERAT.**

bones, in[2, 3]

asaf., berb.[2], bry.[3], **CHIN.,**

coloc.[3], nat-m.[3], **PH-AC.**, puls., **RHUS-T., sabad.**[2, 3, 11], spig., thuj.[3]

long, in

bry., **sabad.**

periosteum, of ⮞

asaf., **CHIN.**, coloc., **PH-AC.**, puls., **RHUS-T., sabad.**, spig.

sore, bruised

acon., adon.[6], **aesc.**, agar.[1], agn., aloe, **alum., alum-p.**[1'], alum-sil.[1'], alumn., **am-c.**, am-m.[3], ammc., anac.[3], **ang.**[2, 3], ant-c., ant-t., apis, **ARG-M.**, arg-n.[6], **ARN., ars.**[6], ars-i.[1'], arum-t., **asar., aur.**[2, 3], aur-ar.[1'], **bad., bapt.,** bar-a.[11], bar-c., bar-i.[1'], bar-m., **bell.**[3], bell-p.[6, 9, 14], berb., bor., bov., **brom.**[2], **bry.**, calc., calc-sil.[1'], calen., **camph.**[2, 11], cann-s.[3], **canth.**, caps.[3, 6], (not [1]: carb-ac.), carb-an., carb-v., carbn-o.[11], **carbn-s., caust.**, cedr., cent.[11], cerv.[11], cham., chel., **CHIN.**[2, 3, 6], chlor., **CIC., CIMIC., CINA**, cinnb.[1'], clem., cob., cob-n.[9], **COCC.**[2], colch.[6], coloc., con., cot.[11], **croc.**[2], crot-h., crot-t., culx.[1'], cund.[11], cupr., cycl., dig., **DROS.,** dulc., echi.[3, 6], elaps, eucal.[3, 6], **EUP-PER.**[2, 3, 11], euph., eupi., fago., **FERR.**[2], ferr-ar., ferr-p., form.[11], gamb., **GELS.**[9, 3, 6], glon.[3], goss., graph.[1', 3], grat., guare.[11], **HAM.**, hedeo.[11], **hell.**[2], helon.[3, 6], hep., hip-ac.[9], hipp., hist.[9], hyos., **hyper.**[2, 3], **hydrc.**[2], iber.[11], ign., ind.[11], iod., ip., juni.[11], kali-c., kali-i.[3, 6], kali-m.[1', 3], kali-n., kalm., kreos.[3, 4, 6], lach., lap-a.[3],

lec., **led.**, lil-t., **lith-c.**, lyc., lyss.[2, 11], **mag-c.**[2, 11], mag-m., mag-p.[1'], mag-s., **mang., med.,** merc., **merc-i-f.**[2], merc-i-r., mez.[3], mit.[11], morph.[11], mosch., **myric.**[2], narcin.[11], **nat-ar.**, nat-c., nat-m., nat-n.[3], nat-p.[1], nat-s.[1'], nat-sil.[1'], nicc.[2], nit-ac., **nux-m.**, nux-v., oci-s.[9], ol-an.[3], **olnd.**, onos.[3], ox-ac.[1'], pall.[3, 6], par., paull.[11], petr., **ph-ac.**[2, 3, 6], **phos.**, phys.[11], **phyt.**, pic-ac.[1'], plan.[3], **PLAT.,** plb., plect.[11], prun.[3], ptel.[3, 6], **puls.**, puls-n.[11], **PYROG., ran-b.**, raph., rat.[4], **rhod., RHUS-T.,** rhus-v.[11], **RUTA**, sabad., sabin., sars.[3], sec.[11], sel.[3], seneg., sep., **SIL.**, sin-n.[11], sol-n., sol-t-ae.[11], spig., spong., **stann.**[2], staph.[2, 3, 6], stict.[3], still.[11], stry.[11], **sul-ac.**, sul-i.[1'], sulph., tarax.[3], tarent., tart-ac.[11], tell., ter.[3], teucr., thuj., til.[3], **tub.**, uva[2], **valer.**[2], verat., verb., viol-o., wies., x-ray[9], zinc., zinc-p.[1']

externally

acon., aesc., **agar.**, aloe, **alum.,** am-c., am-m., anac., **ang.**[3], ant-t., apis, **ARG-M., ARN.**, ars., asaf., asar., aur., bad., **BAPT.**, bar-c., **BELL., berb.**, bism.[3], bor.[3, 4], bov., bry., calad., **calc.**, calc-p.[3], camph., cann-s., canth., caps., carb-an., carb-v., carbn-s., **caust.**, cedr., **cham.**, chel., **CHIN.**, cic., **cimic.**[1', 3], **cina, clem., COCC.,** coff., **colch.**, coloc., con., **croc.**, cupr., cycl., **daph.**[4], dig., dros., **dulc., EUP-PER.**, euph., euphr.[3], **ferr.**, fl-ac., form., **gran.**, graph., quaj., **HAM.**, hell., **HEP.**, hyos., **ign.**, iod.[3], ip., kali-bi.[3], kali-c., **kalm., kreos.**, lach., laur., **led., lith-c.**, lyc., m-aust.[3, 4], **mag-c.**, mag-m., **mang.**, med., meny., **merc.**[1], mez., mosch.[3, 4], mur-ac., **nat-c., NAT-M.**, nit-ac.[1], **nux-m., NUX-V.**, olnd.[3, 4], **ox-ac.**, par., petr., **ph-ac., phos., phyt.**, plat.,

plb., podo.[3], **puls., PYROG.,
RAN-B.,** ran-s., rheum, **rhod.,
RHUS-T.,** rhus-v.[4], **RUTA,
sabad., SABIN.,** samb., sars.,
sec.[3], sel.[4], seneg., **sep., SIL.,
spig., SPONG.,** squil., **stann.,**
staph., stict.[3], stram., stront-c.,
sul-ac., **SULPH.,** tab.[3, 4], tarax.,
teucr.[3, 4], thuj., **valer., VERAT.,**
viol-t., **zinc.**

internally

acon., **aesc.,** agar., alum.,
am-c.[1', 3], am-m., ambr., anac.,
ang.[3], ant-c.[3], ant-t.[3], **apis,
arg-m.**[3], arg-n.[3], arn., **ars.,** ars-i.,
asaf., asar.[3], **aur.,** aur-i.[1'], **BAPT.,**
bar-c., bar-m., bell.[3], bell-p.[3],
bism.[3], bor.[3], bov., bry., **calc.**[3],
calc-sil.[1'], **CAMPH.,** cann-i.,
cann-s., canth.[3], caps.[3], carb-ac.,
carb-an., carb-v., carbn-s., caust.,
cham., **CHIN.,** cic.[3], cina, clem.,
cocc., coff., colch.[3], **coloc.,** con.,
croc.[3], **cupr.,** dig.[3], **dros., eup-per.**[3],
euph., euphr., ferr., **GELS.,** glon.,
graph., **hell.,** hep., ign., iod., **ip.,**
kali-c., kreos., lach., **laur.,** led.,
lyc., m-arct.[3], m-aust.[3], mag-c.,
mag-m., **mang.,** meny., merc.,
MERC-C., mez.[3, 4], mosch.,
mur-ac., nat-c., **nat-m.**[3], nit-ac.,
nux-m.[3], **nux-v.,** olnd.[3], **op.,**
petr.[3], ph-ac., phos., phyt., plat.[3],
plb.[3], **PULS., PYROG., RAN-B.,**
ran-s., rhod., rhus-t., rumx., ruta,
sabad.[3], sabin., samb., **sang.**[3],
sars., seneg.[3], sep., **sil.,** spig.,
spong., **STANN.,** staph., stram.,
stront-c., sul-ac., **sulph.,** teucr.[3],
thuj., valer., **verat.,** viol-o.[3],
viol-t., **zinc.**

morning,
aesc., bry., carb-an., chin.[16],
cob.[11], euphr., form., lyc., lyss.[2],
mag-m.[16], nat-c.[16], ox-ac.,
phyt.[11], polyp-p.[11], sarr.[11], tab.,
thuj.

bed, in

anac.[11], grat., rhod., nat-m.,
petr.[16], viol-o.[11]

insufficient sleep, after

mag-m.

rising, on

nat-ar., sulph.[16]

am.[11]
anac., crot-h., viol-o.

after

am-m., mag-c.[16], phos., sulph.

waking, on

aesc., bar-c., calc.[16], crot-h.[11],
thuj., til., zinc.[16]

after
bry.[11], carb.-ac.[1], crot-h.,
sep.[1], sulph.[11]

forenoon[11]
mag-m.[16], mag-s., sars.[16]

afternoon[11]
sang.

evening
agar.[16], am-c., caust.[16], lyc.,
par.[6]

23 h
fago.

lying down, after

mag-m., mag-s.

sitting, on

brom.

night
carb-an.[16], caust.[16], ferr-i., **sil.**

midnight, after

caust.

air am., in open

caust.

chill, during

tarent.

coition, after

SIL.

cramp, after[16]

plat.

exertion, as after great

clem.

headache, during

seneg.

heat, during[16]

agar., mang.

heated walk and rapid cooling,
after

bry., RHUS-T.

march, as after a long

chel.

menses, during

nat-c., petr.[16], sep.[16]

motion, on

aesc.[z, 11], **arn.**[2], bapt., bov.[11],
bry., chel., **hep.**[2], lach.,
merc-c.[11], phyt., plb., staph.[16]

am.
ars-h.[2], caust., **pyrog., rhus-t.,
tub.**

bed, in

sol-t-ae.

parts affected with cramp-like pain

PLAT.

parts lain on

ARN., bapt., caust.[16], graph.[16],
hep., mosch., nux-m., (non[1]:
pyrog.) **PYRUS**[1]**, RUTA, sep.,**
sil.[16], thuj.

pressure, on

alum-sil.[1]', **PLAT.**, plb.

red hard nodules

petr.

rising, on[11]

bar-a.[16], pic-ac., ptel.

am.
grat., mag-c.

siesta, during[11, 16]

graph.

after
bar-c.[16], eug.

sitting, on[11]

agar., am-m., caust.[11, 16]

from[7]

spig.

somnambulism, after[16]

sulph.

spots, in

aloe, **ARN.**, calc-p., carb-ac.[1], colch.[1], **KALI-BI.**, nux-v., **ox-ac.**, petr., plat., **SABAD.**

stool, after

calc.[16], grat.

stooping, after

berb.

stormy weather, in

cham.

touch, on[11]

acon., alum-sil.[1]', ars-s-f.[1]', bov., brach., **bry.**, calc-p., calc-sil.[1]', **caust.**[11, 16], clem., **colch.**, mang.[11, 16], nat-m., nicc., nux-v., **rhus-t., ruta,** sil., spig., stram., stry., thuj.

waking, on

aesc.[2], (non: carb-ac.), hydrc., ptel.[2], spong., sulph., thuj.

after
mag-s., (non: sep.), sulph.[11]

walking, while

staph.

am.
coloc.

working am.

caust.

bones, in

acon., **agar.**, am-m., ang.[3, 4], apis.[3], **ARG-M., asaf.**, aur., bar-c., bov., **bry.**[2, 3, 4, 6], bufo[3], **calc.**, calc-sil.[1]', cann-s., canth.[3, 4], carb-v.[3], chin., **COCC.**,

con., conch.[8], cor-r., crot-h.[2],
cupr., dros.[2, 4], EUP-PER.[2, 3, 6, 8, 11],
graph., HEP., ign., IP., jab.[2],
kali-bi., kreos.[2], lac-d.[7], lach.[3],
led., lith-c., lyss.[2, 8], m-aust.[4],
mag-c., mang., meph.[4], merc.[2, 3, 4],
mez., nat-m., nit-ac.[2, 3], nux-m.[11],
nux-v., par., petr., ph-ac.[1], phos.,
phyt.[8], puls., rhus-t.[2-4, 8], RUTA,
sabad., sabin.[4], sarr.[2], sep., sil.,
spig., staph.[4], sulph.[2], syph.[1'],
teucr.[3], ther.[2], thuj.[2], tub.[1'],
valer., verat., zinc.

menses, during[16]

carb-v.

cartilages, in

ARG-M., rhod., rhus-t.

glands, in

alum., ant-c., arg-m., arn., ars.,
bry., calc., carb-an., caust., cic.,
clem.[3, 4], CON., cupr., graph.[1],
hep., ign.[3, 4], iod., kali-c., merc.,
mez., nat-m., nicc.[11], nux-v.[3],
petr.[3], phos., plat., psor., puls.,
rhod., rhus-t., ruta, sep., staph.,
sul-ac., sulph., teucr., zinc.

joints, in[11]

abrot., agar.[3, 11], alumn.[2],
apoc.[3, 11], ARG-M.[2, 3],
ARN.[1', 3, 11], aur.[3], berb.[1'],
calad.[2], carb-an.[3, 11], cham.[2, 3, 11],
chlf., clem., coff.[1'], coloc.[3, 11],
con.[2, 3], crot-h.[2], guaj.[1'], hipp-ac.[9],
hyos.[3, 11], hyper.[2, 11], kali-i.,
lith-c.[2], mang.[4], mez.[2, 3, 11],
mur-ac.[2, 3, 11], nat-p.[2, 11],
nit-ac.[3, 11], petr.[1'], phys., phyt.[1'],
PULS.[3, 11], ran-a.[4, 11], RHUS-T.[2, 3],
sulph.[3], tub.[1'], viol-o.[3]

muscles, in[16]

kali-c., verat.

veins, in[3]

ham., puls.

splinters, sensation of

aesc., AGAR., alum., ANAG.[7],
ARG-N., asaf.[3], bar-c., carb-v., cic.,
colch., coll., dol., fl-ac., HEP.,
kali-c.[3], NIT-AC., petr., plat.,
ran-b., sil., stann.[3], sulph.

*stinging–wounds see wounds–
stinging*

stitching[11]

ACON.[2, 3, 6, 7], aconin., ail.,
alum-p.[1'], alum-sil.[1'], alumn.[2],
am-m.[2], amgd-p., anac.,
apis[1', 3, 6, 11], arg-n.[6], arist-cl.[9],
arn.[2, 3], ars., ars-s-f.[1'], ASAF.[2, 11],
astac., aur-ar.[1'], aur-i.[1'], aur-m.[1'],
aur-s.[1'], bar-c., bar-i.[1'], bar-s.[1'],
bart., BELL.[2, 3], benz-ac.[6], berb.[6],
bor.[3], bov.[2], BRY.[2, 3, 6, 11], bufo[6],
buni-o.[14], CALC.[2, 11], calc-f.[6],
calc-i.[1'], calc-sil.[1'], camph.[3],
cann-i.[6, 11], CANTH.[2, 4, 6],
caust.[2, 3, 11], cham.[3, 11], chel.[2, 11],
CHIN.[2, 3], cina[6], cocc.[2, 3], coff.[1'],
colch.[2, 3], coloc.[3, 6], CON.[2, 6, 11],
culx.[1'], cupr., dig., dros.[2],
esp-g.[13], eucal., ferr-ar.[1'], ferul.,
gamb., gast., graph.[2, 11], hell.[2],
hist.[9, 10], hydr.[6], hydroph.[14],
hyos., hyper.[1', 3], IGN.[2], jac-c.,
kali-ar.[1'], KALI-C.[2, 3, 6, 11, 14],
kali-i.[6], kali-m.[1', 3], kali-n.,
kali-sil.[1'], kreos.[2], lac-c., lach.,
lat-m.[3], laur.[2], led.[6, 11], lyc.,
mag-c.[2, 11], mag-m.[2], manc.,
meny.[2], MERC.[2, 3], merc-c.[1', 6],
merc-i-f., mez., mosch.,

mur-ac.[2, 11], naja, **nat-c.**[2],
nat-m.[2, 11], **nat-sil.**[1'],
NIT-AC.[2, 3, 6, 11], nux-v.[3, 6, 7],
op.[5], **par.**[2], **ph-ac.**[2, 11], **PHOS.**[2, 11],
plat., **plb.**[2], plb-i.[6], pneu.[14],
PULS.[2, 3, 6], pulx.[3], ran-b.[3, 6],
ran-s.[2], rauw.[9], **RHUS-T.**[2, 3, 6, 11],
sabad.[2], **sabin.**[2, 3], sang.[6],
sars.[2, 11], scut., **SEP.**[2], sil.[2, 11],
SPIG.[2, 3, 6], **spong.**[2, 3, 11], squil.[3, 6].
stann.[2], **STAPH.**[2, 3, 6], stict.[6],
stroph-h.[3], stroph-s.[9], sul-ac.[6],
sul-i.[1'], **SULPH.**[2, 3, 6], symph.[3],
tarax.[2], tarent., **THUJ.**[2, 6, 11],
tub.[1'], urt-c., verat., **VERB.**[2],
verin., vip.[6, 11], zinc.[2, 3, 6],
ZINC-P.[1']

left side[11]

aesc., all-c., ant-s-aur., coc-c.,
crot-h., **IGN.**, lach., lepi., merc.,
nicc., **sil.**, sphing., **SQUIL.**,
stann., **sulph.**, sumb., tax., zinc.

right side[11]

bad., carb-an., chel., con., hura,
hyos., kali-bi., mosch., phos.,
plect., sil., sin-n., sol-t-ae.

morning in bed[6]

stann.

night[16]
euphr.

ascending[16]

spig.

crawling[16]

lyc.

one-sided[16]

stann.

parts lain on, in[16]

carb-v.

externally

abrot., **acon.**, **agar.**, agn., **aloe**,
alum., am-c., **am-m.**, ambr.,
anac., ang.[3], ant-c., ant-t., apis,
arg-m., arg-n.[6], **arn.**, ars., ars-i.,
ASAF., asar., aur., **bar-c.**,
bar-m., **BELL.**, benz-ac.[6], **berb.**,
bism., bor., bov., **BRY.**, bufo[6],
calad., **CALC.**, calc-f.[6], **calc-p.**,
camph., **cann-i.**, cann-s., canth.,
caps., carb-ac., carb-an.,
carb-v., **CARBN-S.**, **caust.**,
cedr., cham., **chel.**, **chin.**, chin-ar.,
chin-s.[4], **CIC.**, **cimic.**, cina,
cinnb., **clem.**, **cocc.**, coff.[3, 4],
colch., **coloc.**, **CON.**, croc.,
crot-h., crot-t., cupr., cycl.,
daph.[4], dig., **dios.**, **dros.**, dulc.,
euonir.[4], euph., euphr., **ferr.**,
ferr-ar., ferr-ma.[4], ferr-p.,
fl-ac.[3], form., **gels.**, **graph.**,
guaj., **hell.**, hep., hydr., hyos.,
ign., **indg.**, iod., ip., kali-ar.,
kali-bi., **KALI-C.**, kali-i.[6],
kali-n., **KALI-P.**, **KALI-S.**,
kreos., lach., lact.[4], laur., **LED.**,
lith-c., **lob.**, **LYC.**, m-arct.[4],
m-aust.[4], mag-c., mag-m.,
manc., mang., **med.**, **meny.**,
MERC., merc-c.[4, 6], **mez.**,
mosch., **mur-ac.**, naja, nat-ar.,
nat-c., **nat-h.**, **nat-m.**, **nat-p.**,
nat-s., nicc.[4], **NIT-AC.**, nux-m.,
nux-v., **ol-an.**, olnd., op.[4],
ox-ac., **par.**, petr., **ph-ac.**,
phel.[4], **phos.**, **phyt.**, plat., **plb.**,
plb-i.[6], prun.[4], psor., **PULS.**,
RAN-B., **ran-s.**, **rat.**, rheum,
rhod., **RHUS-T.**, ruta, **sabad.**,
sabin., samb., sang., sars., sel.,
seneg., **sep.**, **sil.**, **SPIG.**, **spong.**,
squil., **stann.**, **STAPH.**, stict.[6],
still., **stram.**, stront-c., sul-ac.,
SULPH., tab.[4], **TARAX.**, teucr.,
THUJ., **valer.**, verat., verb.,

viol-o., **viol-t.**, vip.[4, 6], vip-r.[4],
ZINC.

here and there[3, 6]

BAR-C.[7], sul-ac., zinc.

perspiration, during[7]

cann-s.

rest, during[1']

tub., valer.

vexation, after

rhus-t.

internally

abrot., **acon., aesc., agar.,** agn.,
all-c., aloe, **alum.,** am-c.,
am-m., ambr., ammc., anac.,
ang.[3], ant-c., ant-t., apis,
arg-m., arg-n., arn., **ars.,** ars-i.,
ASAF., asar., aspar., **aur.,**
bar-c., bar-m., **bell., BERB.,**
bism., **BOR.,** bov., **BRY., cact.,**
calad., **calc.,** calc-p., camph.,
CANN-I., CANTH., caps.,
carb-an., carb-v., **CARBN-S.,**
card-m., **caust.,** cham., **CHEL.,**
CHIN., chin-ar., cic., cimic.,
cina, clem., **coc-c.,** cocc., coff.,
colch., coll., **coloc., con., croc.,**
crot-t., cupr., cycl., dig., dios.,
dol.[1], dros., **dulc.,** euph.,
euphr., **ferr., gamb.,** gels.,
glon., graph., **guaj.,** hell., hep.,
hydr., hyos., **IGN.,** iod., ip.,
kali-ar., **kali-bi., KALI-C.,**
kali-i., kali-n., **KALI-S.,** kalm.,
kreos., **LACH.,** laur., **LED.,**
lyc., **mag-c., mag-m.,** mang.,
meny., **MERC., MERC-C.,**

merc-i-r., merc-ns., mez.,
mosch., mur-ac., **naja,** nat-ar.,
nat-c., nat-m., nat-s., NIT-AC.,
nux-m., **nux-v., ol-an.,** olnd.,
op., ox-ac., **par.,** petr., **ph-ac.,**
phel., **PHOS.,** phyt., plan.,
plat., **PLB.,** prun., psor., **PULS.,**
RAN-B., ran-s., rheum, rhod.,
rhus-t., rumx., ruta, **sabad.,**
sabin., samb., sang., **sars.,** sec.,
sel., **seneg., SEP., SIL., SPIG.,**
spong., **SQUIL.,** stann., **staph.,**
stram., stront-c., sul-ac., **sulph.,**
tab., **tarax.,** teucr., **thal.,** 'her.,
thuj., valer., verat., verb.
viol-t., zinc., ziz.

night[16]
euphr.

cold needles like

AGAR.

burning[3]

am-m.[4], ant-c., **apis, ars.,**
bell.[3, 4], **berb.**[3, 11]**, con.,** dig.[4],
dulc., gamb.[11]**, glon.,** ign.[3, 4],
iris, lyc., m-aust.[4], mez.,
nat-s.[4], ph-ac., **phos.,** rat.[4],
rhod.[4], rhus-t., sil., **urt-u.**

externally[4]

acon., alum., **anac.,** arg-m.,
arn., ars., **asaf.,** aur., **bar-c.,**
bell., berb., **bry.,** cann-s., caps.
caust., cina, **cocc.,** con., **dig.,**
hep., hyos., ign., **lach., lyc.,**
m-arct., m-aust., mag-c., meny.,
merc., mez., mur-ac., nat-s.,
nicc., **nux-v., ph-ac.,** phel.,
phos., plat., **puls., ran-b.,**
ran-s., rhus-t., sabad., sel., **sep.,**
sil., spig., **spong.,** squil., **stann.,**
staph., sul-ac., **sulph., thuj.,**
viol-t.

internally

ARS., aur., **mez.**, **ol-an.**, spig.

bones, in[3]

arg-m., euph., zinc.

joints, in[3]

ign.[11], mez., plat., plb., sul-ac., thuj.

muscles, in

acon., **alum.**, am-m., anac., apis, **arg-m.**, arn., **ASAF.**, aur., bar-c., bry., bufo[3], calc., caust., cic., cina, **COCC.**, colch.[3], **dig.**, euph., glon.[3], ign., laur., lyc., mag-c., mang., merc., **MEZ.**, mur-ac., **NUX-V., olnd.**, par., phyt., plat., plb., rhod., **RHUS-T., sabad.**, sabin., samb., sep., spig., stann., **STAPH., SUL-AC.**, tarax., **THUJ.**, viol-t., zinc.

like hot needles

alum.[3], apis[3], **ARS.**, bar-c.[3], **kali-c.**[7], mag-c.[3], naja[3], nit-ac.[3], ol-an., rhus-t.[3], spig.[3], vesp.[3]

drawing[16]

mang.

dull[16]

mang.

downward

ant-c., arn., **asc-t.**, bell., bor., canth., caps., **CARB-V., caust.**, chel., cimic., cina, coloc., dios., dros., **FERR.**, gels., kreos., lyc., mang., mez., nit-ac., nux-v., pall., petr., ph-ac., **phyt., puls., ran-s., RHUS-T.**, sabin., sars., sep., squil., still., **sulph.**, tarax., ust., **valer.**, zinc.

inward

acon., alum., am-m., arg-m., **ARN., asaf.**, bar-c., bell., bov., **bry., calc.**, cann-s., **CANTH.**, caps., carb-v., caust., cina, clem., cocc., coloc., croc., dros., guaj., hyos., **ign.**, ip., **laur.**, mang., meny., mez., nux-v., olnd., par., petr., ph-ac., phos., **phyt., plb., RAN-B.**, rhus-t., **sabin.**, samb., sel., squil., staph., sul-ac., tarax., thuj., verb.

itching[16]

carb-v., euphr., stann.

jerking

ang.[3], arn., **bry., calc.**, carbn-s., caust., **CINA**, cocc., coff., **coloc.**, euph., guaj., **lyc.**, mang., **meny.**, mez., mur-ac., **NUX-V.**, ph-ac., plb., sep., sil., spong., **SQUIL.**, stann., zinc.

outward

alum., am-m., ant-c., **ARG-M.**, arn., **ASAF.**, asar., **bell., bry., calc.**, cann-s., canth., carb-v., caust., cham., **CHEL., CHIN.**, clem., cocc., coff., colch., **CON.**, dros., **dulc.**, hell., hyos.,

kali-c., kali-m.[1'], **lach., laur.,**
lith-c., lob., lyc., mang., meny.,
MERC., mez., mur-ac., **nat-c.,**
nat-m., nit-ac., **ol-an.,** olnd.,
ph-ac., **PHEL.,** phos., phyt.,
PRUN., puls., rhod., **rhus-t.,**
sabad., sabin., sil., SPIG.,
SPONG., STANN., staph.,
stront-c., **SULPH., tarax.,** ther.,
thuj., **VALER.,** verat., verb.,
viol-o., viol-t.

to tips of fingers

lob.

paralytic[16]

sep.

tearing in bones[3]

acon., **ars.,** bell., calc.[11],
camph.[11], chel., merc., mur-ac.,
phos., sabin.[3, 11], thuj.

joints, in[3]

ang., ars., asaf., **asar.,** calc.[11],
camph.[11], carb-v., caust., clem.,
dulc., ferr., merc., mur-ac.,
puls., sabin.[3, 11], stann.,
STAPH., sul-ac., sulph., tarax.,
thuj., verb., zinc.

muscles, in

acon., agn., alum., am-c.,
am-m., ambr., **ANAC.,** ang.[3],
arg-m., **ars.,** asaf., asar., aur.,
bell., bism., bor., **CALC.,**
camph., cann-s., canth., caps.,
caust., chel., **chin.,** cina, clem.,
coloc., con., cycl., dig., dros.,
GUAJ., hell., kali-c., kreos.,
led., **MANG.,** merc., mez.,
mur-ac., nat-m., nux-v., olnd..

ph-ac., phos., **PULS.,** rheum,
rhus-t., ruta, sabin., samb.,
sars., sep., sil., spig., spong.,
squil., staph., sul-ac., tarax.,
THUJ., verb., zinc.

wandering[16]

euphr.

transversely

acon., ambr., anac., arg-n..,
asc-t., atro., BELL., bov., bry.,
calc., canth., caust., cham., **chin.,**
cimic., cocc., cupr., dig., **kali-bi.,**
kali-c., kali-m.[1'], laur., lyc.,
merc., mur-ac., phos., **plb., ran-b.,**
rhod., rhus-t., seneg., **sep., spig.,**
stict., stront-c., sul-ac., **sulph.,**
tarax.

upward

acon., alum., arn., ars., bar-c.,
BELL., bry., calc., canth., carb-v.,
caust. cham., chin., cimic., cina,
coloc., dios., **dros.,** euphr., gels.,
glon., guaj., kali-c., **lach., lith-c.,**
mang., **meny.,** merc., nat-s., petr.,
PHYT., plb., puls., rhus-t., rumx.,
ruta, **SEP., spong., stann.. sulph.,**
tarax., thuj.

bones, in

abrot.[3], acon., aeth.[4], agar., agn.,
am-c., anac., ant-c., arg-m., ars.,
asaf., aur., **BELL.,** berb.[4], **BRY.,**
CALC., canth., carb-v., **CAUST.,**
cedr., chel., **chin.,** cocc., colch.,
CON., daph.[4], **dros.,** dulc., euph.,
euphr.[4], graph., **HELL.,** iod.,
kali-bi.[2], kali-c., kali-n.[4], **kalm.,**
lach., laur.[4], lyc., mag-c.,
mag-m.[4], mang., **MERC.,** mez.,
mur-ac.[4], nat-c.[4], nat-s.[4], nit-ac.,
nit-s-d.[11], nux-v., ol-an.[4], par.,

petr., ph-ac., phel.⁴, phos., **phyt.⁶**,
prun.⁴, **PULS., ran-s.,** raph.⁴, **ruta,**
sabin., samb., **SARS., SEP.,** sil.,
spig., staph., stront-c., **SULPH.,**
tarax.⁴, tax.⁴, **thuj.,** valer., verb.,
viol-t., zinc.

glands, in

acon., agn., alum., **am-m.,** ang.³, ⁴,
apis³, arg-m., arn., **asaf.,** bar-c.,
bar-m., **BELL.,** berb.⁴, bor., **bry.,**
calc., carb-an., caust., chin.,
cocc., con., cupr., cycl., euph.,
euphr.⁴, graph., grat.⁴, hell., hep.,
ign., iod., kali-c., kali-m.¹ʼ, kreos.,
lach., lyc., m-arct.⁴, **MERC., mez.,**
mur-ac., murx.⁴, **nat-c., nat-m.,**
NIT-AC., nux-v.¹, ol-an.⁴, ph-ac.,
phos., plb., **PULS., ran-s.,** raph.⁴,
rheum, **rhus-t.,** sabad., sang.⁴,
sep., sil., spig., **spong.,** stann.,
staph., sul-ac., **sulph.,** thuj.,
verat., zinc.

around glands¹⁶

con.

joints, in³

acon.², ³, ⁴, agar.², ³, **agn.,** aloe¹¹,
alum., am-c., am-m., anac., ang.,
ant-c., ant-t., apis, arg-m., arg-n.,
arist-cl.⁶, **arn.**³, ⁴, ¹¹, ars., **asaf.,**
asar., **bar-c.**³, ¹¹, **bell.,** benz-ac.,
berb., **bov., BRY.**², ³, ⁴, bufo,
CALC.³, ¹¹, calc-f., camph.,
cann-s., canth., caps., carb-an.,
carb-v., carl.¹¹, **caust.**³, ⁴, cham.¹¹,
chel., chin., cina, clem.³, ¹¹, **cocc.,**
colch.², coloc., **con.,** crot-t.,
dros.², ³, ⁴, ¹¹, dulc., euph., euphr.,
ferr., gast.¹¹, **graph.,** guaj.³, ⁴,
HELL.³, ⁴, **hep.**², ³, ⁴, hydr., hyos.,
ign.³, ⁴, indg.¹¹, iod.,
KALI-C.², ³, ⁴, ¹¹, kali-i., **kali-n.,**
kreos.², ³, ⁴, ¹¹, lac-ac.¹¹, laur.,
led.³, ⁴, lyc., mag-c., **mag-m.,**

MANG.³, ⁴, **meny.**³, ⁴, **MERC.,**
merc-c., mez., mosch., mur-ac.,
nat-c.³, ⁴, **nat-m.**³, ¹¹, nit-ac.,
nit-s-d.¹¹, nux-m., nux-v.³, ⁴, olnd.,
par.³, ¹¹, petr., ph-ac., **phos.**³, ¹¹,
plat., plb., plect.¹¹, **puls.,** ran-b.,
rheum, **rhod., RHUS-T.**³, ⁴, ruta,
sabad., **sabin.**³, ⁴, samb., sang.,
sars., sep., **SIL.**³, ⁴, ¹¹, **SPIG.**³, ⁴,
spong., squil., **stann., staph.,**
stict., **stront-c.,** stroph-s.⁹, **sul-ac.,**
sulph.³, ⁴, **TARAX., THUJ.**², ³, ⁴, ¹¹,
valer., verat., verb., viol-t., vip.,
zinc.², ³, ⁴, ¹¹

muscles, in

acon., agar., agn., **alum.,** am-c.,
am-m., ambr., anac., ang.³,
ant-c., ant-t., arg-m., **arn.,** ars.,
ars-i., ASAF., asar., aur.,
bar-c., bar-m., **BELL.,** bism.,
bor., bov., **BRY.,** calad., **CALC.,**
camph., cann-s., canth., caps.,
carb-an., carb-v., **caust.,** cham.,
chel., **chin.,** cic., cina, clem.,
cocc., colch., coloc., **con.,** croc.,
cupr., cycl., dig., dros., dulc.,
euph., euphr., ferr., **graph.,**
guaj., hell., hep., hyos., **ign.,**
iod., **KALI-C., kali-m.**¹ʼ, kali-n.,
kreos., lach., **laur.,** led., lyc.,
mag-c.¹, mag-m., mang., **meny.,**
MERC., merc-c.³, merc-i-r.¹¹,
mez., mosch., **mur-ac., nat-c.,**
nat-m., nit-ac., nux-m., nux-v.,
olnd., **par.,** petr., ph-ac., **phos.,**
plan.¹¹, plat., plb., prun.¹¹,
PULS., ran-b., **ran-s.,** rheum,
rhod., **RHUS-T.,** ruta, **sabad.,**
sabin., samb., sang.³, **sars.,**
sep., sil., **SPIG., spong.,** squil.,
stann., STAPH., stront-c.,
stry.¹¹, sul-ac., **SULPH.,**
TARAX., teucr.³, **THUJ.,**
valer., verat., verb., **viol-t.,**
zinc.

jerking³

ang.

warm in bed, while

carb-v.

tearing externally

ACON., adon.[6], aesc., **agar.**, agn.,
alum., alum-p.[1'], ALUM-SIL.[1'],
alumn.[2], **am-c., am-m., ambr.,
anac.,** ang.[3], ant-c., ant-t., aphis[4],
apis[3], arg-m., **ARN., ars.,** ars-s-f.[1'],
asaf., asar., aur., aur-ar.[1'], aur-i.[1'],
aur-m.[1'], aur-s.[1'], bar-a.[6], bar-c.,
bar-i.[1'], bar-m., bar-s.[1'], **BELL.,
BERB., bism.,** bor., bov., brom.,
bruc.[4], **BRY.,** cact., calad., **calc.,**
calc-caust.[6], calc-i.[1'], calc-p.,
calc-sil.[1'], camph., cann-s., canth.,
caps., carb-an., **carb-v.,
CARBN-S., caust.,** cedr., **cham.,
chel., CHIN.,** chin-ar., chin-s.[4],
cic., **cimic.**[6], cina, cist.[4], clem.,
coc-c.[3, 4], cocc., coff., **COLCH.,
coloc.,** con., croc., **crot-t.**[1], cupr.,
cycl., cyt-l.[10], dig., dros., **dulc.,**
euph., euphr., **ferr., ferr-ar.,**
ferr-m.[4], ferr-p., **gamb., gels.,**
graph., **guaj.,** hell., hep., hera.[4],
hist.[10], hyos., **HYPER.,** ign., **indg.,**
iod., ip., kali-ar., **kali-bi.,
KALI-C., kali-i., kali-n., KALI-P.,
KALI-S.,** kali-sil.[1'], **kalm.**[6], **kreos.,**
lach., lact.[4], lam.[4], laur., **LED.,
LYC.,** lyss., **mag-c.,** mag-m.,
mang., med.[1'], meny., **merc.,**
merc-c.[1'], **mez.,** mosch., mur-ac.,
nat-ar., nat-c., NAT-M., nat-p.,
NAT-S., nat-sil.[1'], nicc., **NIT-AC.,**
nux-m., **nux-v.,** olnd., op.,
ox-ac.[1'], par., petr., ph-ac.,
phos.[1'-3, 4], phyt., plan.[2], plat.,
plb., **PULS.,** ran-b., ran-s., **rat.,**
rheum, **rhod., rhus-t.,** ruta,
sabad., sabin., samb., sang.[1'],
sars., sec., **sel.,** seneg., **SEP., SIL.,
spig.,** spong., squil., stann.,
staph.[1], stram., **stront-c.,** sul-ac.,
sul-i.[1'], **SULPH.,** tarax., teucr.,
thuj., ton.[4], **tub.**[1', 7], **valer.,** verat.,

verb., vinc.[4], viol-o., viol-t.,
ZINC., zinc-o.[4]

internally

acon., aesc., **agar.,** agn., aloe,
alum., am-c., am-m., **ambr.,** anac.,
ang.[3], ant-c., **ant-t.,** apis, **arg-m.,**
arn., ars., ars-i., asaf., asar., **aur.,**
bar-c., **BELL., BERB.,** bism., bor.,
bov., **BRY.,** calad., calc., calc-p.[3],
camph., cann-s., canth., **caps.,**
carb-an., **CARB-V., carbn-s.,**
caust., **cham., chel.,** chin.,
chin-ar., cic., cina, clem., cocc.,
coff., colch., **coloc., CON.,** croc.,
crot-h., cupr., cycl., dig., dios.,
dros., dulc., euph., euphr., ferr.,
gran., graph., guaj., hell., hep.,
hyos., **ign.,** iod., ip., kali-ar.,
kali-bi.[3], kali-c., **kali-n., KALI-S.,
kalm.,** kreos., **lach.,** laur., **LED.,
LYC., mag-c.,** mag-m., mang.,
meny., MERC., mez., mosch.,
mur-ac., nat-ar., nat-c., **nat-m.,**
nit-ac., nux-m., **NUX-V.,** olnd.,
op., par., petr., ph-ac., **phos.,**
plat., plb., **PULS.,** ran-b., ran-s.,
rhod., rhus-t., ruta, sabad., sabin.,
samb., sang., sars., sec., sel.,
seneg., **SEP., SIL., SPIG.,** spong.,
squil., **stann.,** staph., stram.,
stront-c., sul-ac., **SULPH., tarax.,**
teucr[3], thuj., uva, valer., verat.,
verat-v., verb., viol-o., viol-t.,
zinc.

asunder

agar., alum., am-m., anac., arn.,
ars., asar., calc., carb-an., carb-v.,
caust., **COFF.,** colch., con., dig.,
ferr., graph., ign., **mez.,** mur-ac.,
nat-m., **NIT-AC., NUX-V.,** op.,
puls., rhus-t., sabin., sep., spig.,
staph., sul-ac., sulph., **teucr.,**
thuj., zinc.

away

act-sp., coloc., dig., hep., **KALI-BI.**, kreos.[3], led., mosch., nux-v., paeon., petr., phos., **plb.**, **RHUS-T.**, sep., sulph., thlas.[3], thuj., urt-u.[3], uran-n.[3]

downward

acon., agar., agn., alum., anac., ant-c., ant-t., arg-n.[1'], ars., ars-s-f.[1'], asaf., aur., aur-s.[1'], **bar-c.**, bar-i.[1'], bar-m., bar-s.[1'], **BELL.**, bism., **bry.**, calc., canth., **CAPS., carb-v., carbn-s.**, caust., chel., **chin.**, cina, colch., **coloc.**, con., croc., dulc., euphr., **ferr.**, ferr-p., **graph.**, ign., **kali-c.**, kali-m.[1'], kali-n., kali-p., **kali-s.**, kalm.[3], laur., **LYC.**, mag-c., **meny., merc.**, mez., mur-ac., nat-ar., **nat-c.**, nat-m., nit-ac., **nux-v.**, ph-ac., phos., **puls.**, rhod., **RHUS-T.**, sabin., sars., seneg., **sep.**, sil., **spig.**, squil., stann., staph., **SULPH.**, thuj., valer., **verat.**, verb., zinc.

outward

all-c., am-c., bell., bov., **bry.**, **calc.**, cann-s., caust., **cocc.**, cycl., elaps, euph., ip., mang., mez., mur-ac., nat-c., par., ph-ac., **PRUN.**, puls., **rhus-t., sil., spig.**, spong., stram.

rest, during[1']

tub.

upward

acon., alum., **anac.**, ant-c., arn., **ars.**, asaf., aur., **BELL.**, bism., bor., calc., carb-v., caust., chin.,

clem., colch., **con., dulc.**, euphr., mag-c., meny., merc., **nat-ar., nat-c.**, nat-m., **nit-ac., nux-v.**, ph-ac., phos., puls., rhod., rhust-t., samb., sars., **SEP., SIL., SPIG.**, spong., **stront-c.**, sulph., thuj., valer.

bones, in

acon., **agar.**, alum., **am-m.**, anac., ang.[11], **arg-m.**, arn., ars., asaf., **AUR., aur-m.**, aur-s.[1'], **bar-c., bell., berb.**, bism., bor., bov., bry., calc-p., cann-s., canth., **caps., carb-v., caust.**, cham., chel., **CHIN., cina, cocc.**, colch.[8], coloc., con., crot-t., **cupr., cycl.**, dig., **dros.**, dulc., **ferr.**, fl-ac.[8], gamb.[11], graph., hell., hep., ign., iod., kali-bi.[11], **KALI-C., kali-n., kalm.**[2], **LACH.**, lact.[4], laur., **lyc.**, lyss.[2], **mag-c.**, mag-m., mang., meph.[4], **MERC., merc-c., mez.**, mur-ac.[4], nat-c., nat-m., nicc.[4], **nit-ac.**, nit-s-d.[11], nux-v., **ph-ac., phos.**, plb., puls., **RHOD.**, rhus-t., **ruta**, sabad.[4], **sabin.**, samb., sars., sep., **SPIG.**, spong., stann., **staph., stront-c.**, sul-ac., sulph., **tab.**, teucr.[4], **thuj.**, valer., verat., verb., **zinc.**

burning

sabin.

cramp-like

aur., olnd., **verat.**

jerking

ang., **bry.**, **CHIN.**, cupr., mang.

paralytic

bell., **bism.**, chel., chin., **cocc.,**
dig.

pressive

ARG-M., arn., asaf., bism.,
bry., coloc., **CYCL.,** staph.,
teucr.

sticking

bell., cina, mur-ac., sabin.

epiphyses, in[16]

arg-m.

periosteum, in

bry., **mez.,** ph-ac., **rhod.**

glands, in

agn., am-c., **ambr., arn.,** bar-c.,
bar-s.[1'], **bell.,** bov., **bry., calc.,**
cann-s., **caps., carb-an., carb-v.,**
caust., **cham., CHIN.,** cocc., con.,
cycl., **dulc.,** ferr., graph., grat.[4],
ign., **kali-c.,** kali-s., kreos., **lyc.,**
MERC., mez., nat-c., nit-ac.,
nux-v., ol-an.[4], phel.[4], phos.,
PULS., rhod., **rhus-t.,** sel., seneg.,
sep., **sil.,** staph.[1'], **sulph.,** thuj.,
zinc.

joints, in[3]

acon., agar., **agn.,** alum., am-c.,
am-m., **ambr.**[3, 4], anac., ang.,
ant-s-aur.[11], ant-t.[2, 3, 11],
ARG-M., arist-cl.[9], arn.[3, 4], ars.,
ars-i.[1'], asaf., asar., **aur.,** bar-c.,
bell.[2, 3], bism., **bov., bry.,**

cact.[11], **calc.**[2, 3, 4], camph.[2, 3],
canth., carb-an., carb-v., **carl.**[11],
CAUST.[3, 4, 11] cham., chel.,
chin., cic., cina, cist.[2, 4, 11],
clem., cocc., **colch.**[2, 3], con.,
cupr., cycl., dig., dros., dulc.,
euphr., ferr., graph.[3, 4], grat.[11],
guaj.[3, 4], hell., hep., hera.[4],
hyos.[3, 4], ign., iod.[3, 4], **KALI-C.,**
kali-n., kreos., lach.[4], laur.,
mag-m., mang., meny., **MERC.,**
mez., mosch., mur-ac., nat-c.[3, 4],
nat-m., nat-s.[11], nit-ac.[3, 4, 11],
nit-s-d.[11], nux-m., **nux-v.**[3, 4],
olnd., par., petr., **ph-ac.,**
phos.[3, 4], plb., puls., ran-b.,
rheum, rhod.[3, 4], **RHUS-T.,**
ruta, sabad., sabin.[3, 4], samb.,
sars.[3, 4, 11], sec.[3, 4, 11], **sep.**[3, 4],
sil.[3, 4], spig.[2, 3, 4], spong., stann.,
staph., **STRONT-C.**[3, 4], **SULPH.,**
tarax., **teucr.,** thuj.[3, 11], valer.,
verat., verb., viol-o., **ZINC.**

burning, and[3]

carb-v., caust., nat-c., nit-ac.

cramp-like[3]

anac., ars., aur., bov., kali-c.,
OLND., phos., **plat.**

jerking, and[3]

acon., caust., **CHIN.,** cupr.,
laur., mang., olnd., **puls.,**
rhus-t., sulph.

paralytic[3]

bell., carb-v., chel., chin., cocc.,
con., dig., **kali-c.,** meny.,
nat-m., nit-ac., phos., sars.,
stann., **STAPH.**

pressive³

agn., anac., ang., arg-m., arn.,
asaf., bell., bism., **CARB-V.,**
caust., cham., chin., coloc.,
graph., guaj., hyos., kali-c.,
led., lyc., mez., ph-ac., ruta,
sabad., sars., sep., spong.,
stann., staph., zinc.

sticking³

agn., anac.³, bar-c., calc., chin.,
colch., dulc., graph., guaj.³,
hyos., **LED.**³, ¹¹, mag-c., mang.³,
merc., mur-ac., nat-c., nat-m.,
puls., sabin., sep., staph..
thuj.³, **zinc.**

muscles, in

acon., adon.³, aesc.³, agar.,
agn., alum., am-c., **am-m.,**
ambr., anac., ang.³, ant-c.,
ant-t., **arg-m.,** arn., **ars.,** ars-i.,
ars-s-f.¹', **asaf.,** asar., **aur.,**
aur-s.¹', bar-c., bar-i.¹', bar-m.,
bell., bism., bor., bov., **bry.,**
CALC., camph., **canth.,** caps.,
carb-an., CARB-V., CARBN-S.,
CAUST., cham., **chel., chin.,**
cic., cimic.³, **cina,** clem., cocc.,
colch., coloc., con., croc.,
cupr., cycl., dig., dros., **dulc.³,**
euph., ferr., **graph.,** guaj., hell.,
hep., hyos., ign., iod., ip.,
KALI-C., kali-m.¹', **kali-n.¹,**
kali-s., kreos., lach., laur., led.,
LYC., mag-c., mag-m., mang.,
meny., **MERC.,** mez., mosch.,
mur-ac., nat-c., nat-m.,
NIT-AC., nux-v., olnd., par.,
petr., ph-ac., **phos.,** plat., plb.,
puls., ran-b., rheum, **RHOD.,**
rhus-t., **ruta,** sabad., **sabin.,**
samb., sars., sec., sel., seneg.,
SEP., SIL., spig., spong.,
squil., **stann., STAPH.,**
STRONT-C., sul-ac., **SULPH.,**

tarax., **teucr.,** thuj., valer.,
verat., verb., viol-o., viol-t.,
ZINC., ZINC-P.¹'

burning

bell., **carb-v.,** caust., kali-c.,
led., lyc., **nit-ac.,** ruta, sabin.,
tarax., zinc.

cramp-like

ANAC., ang.³, ant-c., arg-m.,
asaf., aur., bism., **calc.,** caust.,
chel., **chin.,** dulc., euph.,
graph., iod., kali-c., mang.,
meny., mosch., **mur-ac.,**
NAT-C., nat-m., nux-v., **petr.,**
ph-ac., phos., **PLAT.,** ran-b.,
ruta, samb., sil., stann.,
stront-c., thuj., valer.

jerking

acon., agar., agn., alum., bell.,
calc., camph., **CHIN.,** cina,
cupr., dig., dulc., guaj., lyc.,
mang., merc., nat-c., ph-ac.,
phos., plat., **PULS.,** rhus-t.,
spig., **staph.,** stront-c., sul-ac.,
sulph.

paralytic

agn., ant-c., asaf., carb-v.,
cham.¹, chin., cic., **cina,** cocc.,
con., dig., graph., **hell.,**
KALI-C., mez., mosch.,nat-m.,
nit-ac., phos., **sabin., sars.,**
seneg., sil., stann., verb.

pressing

acon., ambr., anac., ang.³,
ant-c., arg-m., arn., asar.,
bism., camph., cann-s.,
CARB-V., caust., chin., colch.,

cupr., cycl., dig., euph., guaj.,
kali-c., kali-n., laur., led., lyc.,
ph-ac., ran-b., ruta, sabin.,
sars., sep., spig., **STANN.,**
staph., stront-c., sulph., teucr.,
viol-t., zinc.

sticking

acon., agn., ambr., ang.[3], ant-t.,
arg-m., arn., bar-c., bell., bry.,
camph., cann-s., canth., caps.,
chin., cic., **colch.,** coloc., con.,
dros., dulc., **euph.,** guaj., hyos.,
ign., iod., kali-c., **lyc.,** mag-c.,
mang., merc., mur-ac., nat-m.,
ph-ac., phos., rheum, sars.,
spong., staph., sulph., teucr.,
thuj., **ZINC.**

thread, like a long, evening agg.[7]

all-c.

twinging

acon.[6], **agar.**[6], aloe, alum., **AM-M.,**
ant-c., apis, arg-n.[6], **ars.**[6], aur., bell.,
berb., **bov.,** canth., carb-an., caust.,
cham.[6], **chel.,** **cimic.**[6], cocc., coff.[6],
coloc., **crot-t., dios.,** dros., **ferr.,**
iod., iris[6], **kali-bi.**[6], kali-c., **kali-i.**[6],
kali-m.[1'], **kalm.**[6], lact.[11], **LAUR.,**
lyc., **mag-c.,** mag-m., **mag-p.**[6],
merc., **mez.**[6], **MOSCH.,** mur-ac.,
nat-p., nux-v.[6], ph-ac., phos.,
phys.[11], plan., **PLB.,** plb-i.[6], **prun.,**
puls.[6], **rhus-t.,** sabin., sang.[6], sars.,
seneg., **sep.**[6], sieg.[10], sil., **spig.**[6],
staph., stel.[6], stront-c., sul-ac.,
tab.[6], **valer.**

twisting

agar., alum., am-m., anac., ant-c.,
ant-t., **arg-n.,** arn.[3], ars., asaf.,
bar-c., **bell.,** berb., bor., **bry.,**
calad., calc., **caps.,** canth., cham.,

cina, clem.[3], **coloc.**[3], con., dig.,
dios., dros., dulc., **ign.,** ip., kali-c.,
kali-n., led., **merc.,** mez., nat-c.,
nat-m., nux-m., **nux-v.,** olnd.,
ox-ac., ph-ac., phos., **plat.,** plb.,
podo., ran-b., ran-s., **rhus-t.,** ruta,
sabad., sabin., sars., seneg., sep.,
SIL., staph., sul-ac., sulph., thlas.[3],
thuj., valer., **VERAT.**

ulcerative[2]

alum-sil.[1'], **AM-M., bry., cann-s.,**
caust., cic., cycl., graph., hep.,
ign., iodof., **kali-c.,** kali-m.[1'],
KALI-S.[1'], **LACH., mang., merc.,**
mur-ac., nat-m., nux-v., PHOS.,
PULS., RAN-B., RHUS-T., zinc.

externally

acon., agar., alum., am-c.,
AM-M., ambr., anac., ang.[3],
ant-c., arg-m., arn., ars., aur.,
bar-c., bell., bov., **BRY.,** calc.[4],
camph., cann-s., **canth.,** caps.,
carb-an., carb-v., **caust.,** cedr.,
cham., chin., **cic.,** cocc., colch.,
cycl., dros., dulc., ferr., **graph..**
hep., **ign., kali-c.,** kali-n.,
KALI-S., kreos., lach., laur.,
mag-c., mag-m., **mang.,** merc.,
mur-ac., nat-c., **nat-m.,** nit-ac.,
nux-v., petr., ph-ac., phos., plat.,
PULS., RHUS-T., ruta, sars., **sep.,**
SIL., spig., spong., staph., sul-ac.,
sulph., teucr., thuj. verat., **zinc.**

internally

acon., **am-c., arg-n.,** ars., bell.,
bor., bov., **bry., cann-s.,** canth.,
caps., carb-an., carb-v., carbn-s.,
caust., cham., chel., cocc., **coloc.,**
cupr., dig., **gamb.,** hell., hep.,
kali-c., kreos., **LACH.,** laur.,
mag-c., mag-m., mang., **merc.,**
mur-ac., nit-ac., **nux-v.,** ph-ac.,
phos., **psor., PULS., RAN-B.,**

rhus-t., ruta, sabad., sep., **SIL.,**
spig., stann., staph., stront-c.,
sulph., valer., verat.

bones, in

am-c., am-m., **bry.,** bufo[3], caust.,
cic., graph., ign., mang., nat-m.,
puls., rhus-t.

glands, in

am-c., **am-m.,** aur., bell., bry.,
calc., canth., caust., cham., chin.,
cic., cocc., graph., hep., ign.,
kali-c., merc., mur-ac., nat-c.,
nat-m., nit-ac., petr., **PHOS.,**
puls., rhus-t., ruta, **SIL.,** staph.,
sul-ac., teucr., **zinc.**

undulating

acon., anac., ant-t., arn., asaf.,
chin., cocc., dulc., mez., olnd.,
plat., rhod., sep., spig., sul-ac.[16],
teucr., viol-t.

wandering

acon., adon.[9], aesc., agar.[3, 6],
agav-t.[14], alum-sil.[1'], **am-be.[6],**
am-c., **am-m.,** ambr.[6], aml-ns.[11],
ant-t [3], **apis.**[2, 3, 6, 8], apoc.,
apoc-a.[11, 12], arg-m., **arn.,** ars.,
ars-s-f.[2], arund.[11], asaf., **aur.,**
aur-ar.[1'], bapt.[11], bar-c., **bell.,**
benz-ac., **berb.**[1'-3, 6], berb-a.[6], bry.,
buni-o.[14], calc.[3], calc-caust.[6],
calc-p., camph., caps., **carb-v.,**
carbn-s., **caul.,** caust., cedr.,
cnel., chin., cimic.[3, 6], cina[3], clem.,
COCC.[3], **colch.,** coloc.[11], com.[6],
con.[4, 6], croc., **cupr.**[3, 6], daph.[2, 4, 7],
dios., elat.[11], ery-a.[2], eup-per.[6],
eup-pur., ferr.[3], ferr-p.[1', 6], fl-ac.[11],
form.[6], gels., goss., graph.[3, 11, 16],
hydr.[3, 6], **hyper.[6],** ictod.[2], ign.,
iod., **iris, KALI-BI.,** kali-c.,

kali-fcy., kali-n.[3], **KALI-S., kalm.,**
LAC-C., lach., lact.[4], **LED.,** lil-t.,
lyc.[3, 6], lycps., mag-c.[3, 16],
mag-m.[3], **mag-p.,** magn-gr.[8],
manc., mang., meny.[3], meph.[11],
merc.[3, 11], merc-i-r.[3, 6], mez.[11],
myric.[11], naja[11], nat-m., nat-s.,
nit-s-d.[2, 11], **nux-m.,** nux-v.[6], op.[3],
ox-ac.[6], pall.[3], ph-ac.[3], phos.[3],
phyt., plan.[3, 11], plat., **plb.,**
polyg-h., prun.[3, 6], **PULS.,**
puls-n.[12], pyrog.[6], pyrus[11], rad.[3],
rad-br.[3], **ran-b.,** rat.[3], rhod.,
rhus-t.[3, 6, 11], rhus-v.[11], rumx.[3],
sabad.[6], **sabin.,** sacch.[11], **sal-ac.,**
sang., sars., sec.[3, 4, 6, 11], senec.[6],
sep., sil.[3], **spig.,** spong.[6], stann.[3],
staph.[3], **stel.[1]** (non: still.), sulph.,
syph.[1', 7, 8], tab.[3], tarent., tax.[4],
tell.[11], **thuj.**[3, 6, 11], **tub.,** valer.,
verat.[2, 6], verat-v.[3, 6], zinc.

suddenly[3]

ambr., colch., rad-br.

touch agg.[16]

graph.

joints, in[2]

ang., **ant-t., hyper.,** kali-bi.[1'],
tub.[1']

PAINLESSNESS of complaints usually
painful

ant-c.[3, 7], ant-t.[3], **hell., OP., STRAM.**

analgesia

PARALYSIS agitans

agar.[3, 6, 8], ant-t.[12], aran.[10, 14],
aran-ix.[10, 14], arg-m.[6, 14], **arg-n.**[3],
ars.[6, 8], aur.[6], **aur-s.**[1', 8, 12], aven.[7, 8],
bar-c., bufo, **camph-br.**[6, 8], cann-i.[8],
chlorpr.[14], cimic.[14], cocain.[8],
cocc.[3, 6, 8], **con.**[3, 6, 8, 10], dub.[8],
dub-m.[8], **gels.**, halo.[14], helo., **hyos.**,
hyosin.[8, 12], **kali-br.**, kres.[10],
lath.[6, 8, 12], levo.[14], **lol.**[3, 6, 8, 12], lyc.[12],
mag-p., mang.[6, 8], **MERC.**, nicot.[8],
nux-v.[3], perh.[14], **phos.**,
phys.[2, 3, 6-8, 12], **plb.**, prun.[3], psil.[14],
rauw.[9, 14], reser.[14], **RHUS-T.**, scut.[8],
tab., **tarent.**, thiop.[14], **ZINC.**,
zinc-cy.[8, 12], **zinc-pic.**[6, 8, 12]

alcohol, after abuse of[2]

ant-t., **ars.,** calc., **lach.,** nat-s.,
nux-v., OP., ran-b., sep., **sulph.**

anger, after

nat-m., **nux-v.,** staph.

one-sided[2]

staph.

atrophy, with[2]

cupr., **GRAPH.,** kali-p., **plb., sec.,**
sep.

change of weather from warm to
cold-wet[7]

caust., dulc., rhus-t.

coition, after

phos.

cold, after taking

dulc., rhod.

bathing am.[3]

con.

wind or draft, after[15]

caust.

exertion, after

ars., **caust., gels.,** nux-v., **rhus-t.**

extends from above **downwards**

bar-c., merc., zinc.[3]

upwards

agar., **ars.,** bar-c.[15], **con.,**
hydr-ac., **kali-c.,** karw-h.[14],
lyss.[10, 12], mang., phos.[7], plb.[3],
sulfon.[12]

fright, as if from[16]

nat-m.

gradually appearing

CAUST.

intermittent fever, after

arn.[2], ars.[2], lach.[2], **NAT-M.,** nux-v.[2]

internally

acon., ant-c., arg-n.[3], **ars.**, bar-c., **BELL.**, calc., cann-s., canth., caps., caust., chin., cic., **cocc.**, coloc., **con.**, cycl., dig., **DULC.**, euphr., **gels.**, graph., helo.[3], **HYOS.**, ip., kali-c., lach., **laur.**, lyc., meny., . merc., mur-ac., nat-m., **nux-m., nux-v., op.**, petr., phos., plb., **puls.**, ran-b.[3], rheum, **rhus-t.**, sec., sel.[3], seneg., sep., sil., spig., **STRAM.**, sulph.[3], tab[3], tarent., zinc.[3]

Landry's ascending p.[12]

aconin., con., lyss.

lower half of body, of[1']

alum-p., alum-sil., ars.[11], graph.

lying on a moist ground[15]

rhus-t.

masturbation, from **chin.**[2], stann.

mental shock, from

apis, caust.[15]

mental emotion, after

apis, IGN., nat-m., nux-v., stann.

muscles, extensor

alum., ars., calc., **cocc., crot-h.,** cur.[7], **PLB.**

flexor m.

caust., **nat-m.**

neuralgias, with

abrot.

nicotinism, from[10]

nux-v.

old people, of

bar-c., con., kali-c., OP.[2, 7]

one-sided

acon., acon-c.[11], adren.[7], agar., **alum., alum-p.**[1'], alumn.[2, 8], am-m., ambr.[8], **anac., apis,** arg-m., arg-n., a.n., **ars.,** ars-s-f.[1'], asar., **aur.**[8], bapt., bar-c., bar-m., **bar-s.**[1'], **bell., both.,** bov., cadm-s., caj.[2, 7], calc., carb-v., carbn-o.[11], carbn-s., **CAUST.,** chel., chen-a.[8, 12], chin., chin-s.[4], cob-n.[14], **coc-c., cocc.,** colch., conin.[12], cop., cur.[8], cycl., dig., dulc., **elaps, graph.,** guaj., hell., hep., **hydr-ac.**[2, 8, 12], hyos., ign., irid.[8], **kali-c., kali-i.,** kali-m.[1'], kali-p., **lach.,** laur., led., lyc., merc., mez., **mur-ac.,** nat-c., nat-m., nit-ac., nux-v., olnd., **op.,** ox-ac., perh.[14], petr., **ph-ac., phos.,** phys.[8], pic-ac.[8, 12], plb., podo., rhod., **rhus-t.,** sabin., **sars., sec.**[8], sep., spig., stann., staph., **stram.,** stront-c., stry.[8, 12], **sul-ac.,** syph., tab., tarax., thuj., verat-v.[8], vip.[4, 8], xan.[8, 12], zinc., zinc-p.[1']

left

acon., **all-c.**[2], ambr.[8], **anac., apis,**

arg-n., **arn.**, ars., art-v.^{2}, bapt.,
bar-m., bell., brom., caust., cocc.,
cupr-ar.$^{8,\,12}$, elaps, gels., hydr-ac.,
karw-h.^{14}, lacer.^{11}, **LACH.**, lyc.,
nit-ac., NUX-V., op.^{3}, ox-ac.,
petr., phys.$^{8,\,11,\,12}$, **plb.**$^{2,\,11}$, podo.,
RHUS-T., santin.^{12}, stann., **stram.**,
stront-c.^{3}, sulph., verat-v.^{8}, vip.^{3},
xan.^{8}

right

acon.^{11}, apis, **arn., bell.**, both.^{11},
calc., canth., carbn-s.^{11},
CAUST., chel.^{3}, chen-a.^{8}, colch.,
CROT-C., crot-h., cur.^{8}, **elaps,
graph.**, irid.$^{8,\,12}$, iris-fl.^{12},
iris-foe.^{11}, kali-i., merc-i-r.^{3},
nat-c., nat-m.^{3}, **op.**, phos.,
plb., rhus-t., sang., sil.,
stront-c., sulph., thuj.^{3}, vip.^{4}

anger, after^{15}

staph.

aphasia, with^7

cench.

apoplexy, after

acon.$^{3,\,6}$, **alum.**, anac., apis,
arn., ars.$^{3,\,6}$, **bar-c.**, bell., both.^{10},
cadm-s., caj.^{7}, calc-f.$^{3,\,6}$, calen.^{7},
caust., cocc., con., **crot-c.,
crot-h.**, crot-t.$^{3,\,6}$, **cupr.**, form$^{3,\,6}$,
gels., glon.$^{3,\,6}$, **hyos.**$^{2,\,4}$,
kali-br.$^{3,\,6}$, lach., laur., merc.$^{3,\,6}$,
nux-v., **OP., PHOS., plb.**, sec.,
sep.$^{3,\,4,\,6}$, stann., stram.,
stront-c.$^{3,\,6}$, sulph.$^{3,\,6}$, verat-v.$^{3,\,6}$,
vip.$^{3,\,6}$, zinc.

coldness of the paralyzed part. with

**ars., caust., cocc., dulc., graph.,
nux-v.**, plb., **RHUS-T., zinc.**

convulsions of the well side

apis, **art-v.**, bell., hell., **stram.**

paralyzed side, of

phos., sec.

convulsions, after

ars.^{2}, **bell.**^{2}, **CAUST., CIC.**^{2},
cocc.$^{2,\,3}$, con.^{7}, **CUPR.**$^{2,\,3,\,7}$,
elaps^3, **hyos., ip.**$^{2,\,7}$, laur.^{2},
nux-v.^{2}, **plb.**$^{2,\,4,\,8}$, **sec.**$^{2,\,3,\,8}$, **sil.**^{2},
stann.^{2}, stram.^{2}, sulph.^{2}, **vib.**^{2}

headache, after^{16}

ars.

heat in the paralyzed part, with

alum.$^{1,\,7}$, phos.

hyperesthesia of the well side

plb.

involuntary motion of the paralyzed limb^{16}

arg-n., merc., phos.

mental excitement, after

stann.

shock, after

apis

now here, now there[16]

bell.

numbness of the paralyzed side,
with[2]

apis, cann-i.[7], caust., coc-c.,
rhus-t., staph.[7]

well side, of

cocc.

pain, from

nat-m.

spasms, after

stann.

of the other side[15]

bell., lach., phos., stram.

suppression of eruption, from

caust., dulc., hep., psor., sulph.

twitching of the well side

apis, art-v., bell., stram.

of the paralysed side

apis, arg-n., merc., nux-v.,
phos., sec., stram.. stry.

nettle rash, after disappearance of

cop.

organs, of

absin., acon., agar., agn., alum.,
alum-p.[1'], am-c., am-m., ambr.,
anac., ang.[3], ant-c., ant-t., arn., ars.,
asaf., asar., aur., aur-s.[1'], bar-c.,
bar-s.[1'], BELL., bism., bor., bov.,
bry., calc., camph., cann-s., canth.,
caps., carb-ac., carb-an., carb-v.,
carbn-s., caust., cham., chel., chin.,
cic., cocc., colch., coloc., con.,
croc., cupr., cycl., dig., dros.,
DULC., euphr., gels., graph., hell.,
hep., hydr-ac., HYOS., ign., iod.,
ip., kali-br., kali-c., kali-m.[1'], kreos.,
lach., laur., led., lyc., mag-c.,
mag-m., mang., meny., merc., mez.,
mur-ac., nat-c., nat-m., nit-ac.,
nux-m., nux-v., olnd., op., par.,
petr.[1], ph-ac., phos., plb., PULS.,
rheum, rhod., rhus-t., ruta, sabad.,
sabin., sars., SEC., seneg., sep.,
SIL., spig., spong., squil., stann.,
staph., stram., stront-c., sul-ac.,
sulph., thuj., verat., verb., zinc.,
zinc-p.[1']

painful

agar., alum-sil.[1'], arn., ars., bell.,
cadm-s.[1'], calc., caust., cina, cocc.,
crot-t., kali-n., lat-m., phos., plb.,
sil., sulph.

pain – paralyzed

painless

abies-c., absin., acon., aeth., alum., alum-p.[1'], ambr., **anac.**, ang.[3], **arg-n.**, arn., **ars.**, ars-s-f.[1'], **aur.**, aur-ar.[1'], aur-s.[1'], **bapt., bar-c.**, bar-s.[1'], bell., bov., **bufo**, bry., cadm-s., calc., camph., **CANN-I.**, cann-s.[3], carb-v., **carbn-s., caust.**, cham., chel., chin., chin-s., chlor., cic., **COCC.**, colch., coloc., **CON.**, crot-h., **cupr.**, cur., ferr., **GELS.**, graph., hell., hydr-ac., **hyos.**, ign., ip., kali-c., kalm., karw-h.[14], laur., led., **LYC.**, m-arct.[4], **merc.**, nat-m., nux-m., nux-v., **OLND., op.**, ph-ac., phos., **PLB., puls.**, rhod., **RHUS-T., sec.**, sil., staph., stram., stront-c., sulph., **verat.**, zinc., zinc-p.[1']

paraplegia[12]

anh., arg-n.[3], ars.[3], caul.[2, 12], gels., kali-t., kalm., lath., mang., nux-v.[3], phys., pic-ac., pip-m., rhus-v., stry., thal., thyr., wildb.

parturiton, after[2]

PHOS., RHUS-T.

perspiration, from suppressed

colch., gels.[7], lach.[7], rhus-t.

poliomyelitis[7]

acon.[2, 7, 8], aeth.[8], alum., arg-n., arn.[2, 7], ars., bell.[2, 7, 8], **bung.**[8], **calc.**[8], carb-ac., **caust.**[2, 7, 8], chin-ar., chr-s.[8], cur., dulc., ferr-i., ferr-p., **GELS.**[2, 7, 8], hydr-ac., hydroph.[14], hyos.[2, 7],

kali-i., kali-p.[7, 8], karw-h.[14], kres.[10], lach., lath.[7, 8, 10], merc.[2, 7, 10], nux-v.[2, 7, 8], phos.[7, 8], phys., **plb.**[7, 8], plb-i., rhus-t.[1', 2, 7, 8], sec.[7, 8], stry-p., sulph.[2, 7, 8], verat., verat-v.

paralysis of diaphragm, with

cupr., op., sil.

post-diphtheric

ant-t., apis, arg-m., **arg-n.**[2, 3, 6, 8], arn., **ars.**, aur-m.[8], aven.[8], **bar-c.**[2], botul.[8], camph., carb-ac., **caust., COCC., con.**, crot-h., **diph.**[3, 6, 8, 12], **gels.**, helon.[2], **hyos.**, kali-br., kali-i.[8], kali-p., **lac-c., lach., nat-m.**, nux-v., **phos., phys.**[2, 3, 6], phyt., **plb.**, plb-a.[8], rhod.[8, 12], **rhus-t.**[2, 3, 6, 8], sec., sil., sulph.[2], thuj.[2], zinc.[2]

river bath in summer, from

caust.

sensation of[16]

phos.

senses, of[16]

kali-n.

sexual excesses, from

nat-m., nux-v., PHOS.[2], rhus-t., sil.[3]

single parts

anac., **ars.**, CAUST., dulc., plb.[1', 3]

spastic spinal p.[8, 12]

ben-d., gels., hyper., kres.[10], lachn.,
lath.[10], **nux-v.**, phos.[1'], plect., sec.
reflexes, increased

twitching-paralysed

suppressed eruptions

caust., **dulc.**, hep., **psor., sulph.**

toxic

apis, ars., bapt., crot-h.[2], gels.,
lac-c., **lach.**, mur-ac., rhus-t.

arsenic[2]
chin., ferr., graph., **hep., nux-v.**

lead[8]
alumn., **ars.**[2], cupr.[2, 8], kali-i.,
nux-v., **op.**[2, 8], pipe.[12], **plat.**[2], plb.,
sul-ac.[8, 12]

mercurial[7]
HEP., nit-ac., staph., stram.,
sulph.

typhoid, in

agar., caust.[15], **lach., rhus-t.**

wet, after getting

CAUST., rhus-t.

*paresis–convulsions see convulsions–
paresis*

*parturiton see Vol. I index, Vol II
index, Vol. III*

PERIODICITY

acon., **agar.**[1], aloe[7], **ALUM.**,
alum-sil.[1'], **ALUMN.**[2], am-br.,
ambr.[2, 7], **anac., ant-c.**, ant-t.,
ARG-M., aran., **arn., ARS.**,
ars-met.[8], ars-s-f.[1'], **asar., bar-c.**,
bell., benz-ac.[6], bov., bry., bufo,
cact., calc., calc-sil.[1'], cann-s.,
canth., caps., carb-v., CARBN-S.[2, 7],
carl.[8], **CEDR.**, cent.[7, 11], chel.[6],
CHIN., CHIN-AR., CHIN-S.,
chr-ac.[8], cina, clem., cocc., colch.,
croc., crot-h., cupr., dros., **eucal.**[7],
eup-per.[3, 8], ferr., ferr-ar., **gels.**,
graph., hep.[3], **ign., IP., kali-ar.**,
kali-bi., kali-c.[3], kali-n., lac-d.[1', 7],
lach., lact.[4], lil-t.[6], **lyc., mag-c.**,
mag-s.[10], meny., merc., nat-ar.,
NAT-M., nat-n.[6], **nat-s.**, nicc.[8],
nicc-s.[7], **NIT-AC., nux-v.**, petr.,
phos., plb., prim-o.[8], **puls.**,
ran-s.[4, 6, 8], **rhod., rhus-t.**,
rhus-v.[7, 11], **sabad.**, samb., **sang.**,
sec., senec.[6], **SEP., SIL., spig.**,
stann., staph., sul-ac.[7], **sulph.**,
tarent.[3, 6-8, 11], **tela**[8], thal.[14], **tub.**,
urt-u.[8], valer., **verat.**, vip.[4, 6], zinc.

Vol. I: *absent-minded*

anxiety
confusion
delirium
despair
dullness
ecstasy
fancies
forgetful
indifference

insanity
memory, weakness of

restlessness

sadness
unconsciousness

weeping

Vol. II: *chorea*
convulsions
faintness

menses
moon
seasons
weakness

Vol. III: *sleepiness*

sleeplesness

yawning
abortion

annually

am-c.³, ⁷, **ant-t.³, ARS.¹, ⁷,**
buth-a.⁹, ¹⁴, carb-v.³, ⁸, carc.⁹,
cench., crot-h.³⁻⁴, ⁶, ⁸, echi.³, elaps³,
gels.³, kali-bi.³, **lach.**³⁻⁴, ⁷, ⁸, lyc.³,
naja³, nat-m.³, nicc.³, ⁷, ⁸, psor.³, ⁷,
rhus-r.⁸, **rhus-t.³,** rhus-v.⁷, ¹¹,
sulph.³, ⁸, tarent., thuj., urt-u.³, ⁶⁻⁸,
vip.³, ⁶

same hour, complaints return at

ant-c., **aran.,** ars.³, bov.³, **cact.,**
CEDR.¹, ⁷, cench.⁷, chin.¹',
chin-s.³, ⁴, cina³, cocc.⁴, ign.,
ip.⁶, kali-bi.¹', kali-br.⁷, lyc.³,
nat-m.³, sabad., sel.¹ (not : sil.),
tarent.⁷, tub.⁷

neuralgia every day at

KALI-BI., sulph.¹'

regular intervals, complaints return
at⁷

CARBN-S.

daily³

aran., ars., caps., ip., nux-v., puls.

every other day⁴, ⁶

alum.⁴, ⁶⁻⁸, ¹⁵, ¹⁶, anac.⁶, ars.¹', ³,
calc.⁴, ⁶, ¹⁶, cham.⁶,
chin.³, ⁶, ⁸, ¹⁵, ¹⁶, chin-s.⁴,
crot-h., fl-ac.⁸, **ip.**⁶, ⁷, lyc.¹⁵,
lycps.⁷, nat-c.¹⁶, nat-m.³, ⁶, ¹⁶,
nit-ac.⁸, nux-v.¹⁶, oxyt.⁸,
psor.⁷, puls.¹⁶

morning²
alumn.

evening⁴, ⁷
puls.

third day⁶

anac., aur., chin-s.⁴, kali-ar.¹',
kali-br.⁷

pregnancy, in

lyc.⁷, mag-c.²

fourth day³

ars.¹', ³, ⁴, ⁶, aur.⁶, eup-per.⁶,
kali-br.⁷, lyc., puls., sabad.

seventh day

am-m., ars.¹', ³, ⁶, ars-h.², ⁷,
aur-m.⁶, canth., cedr.⁶, **chin.,**
croc.⁶, eup-per.⁶, gels.³, **iris³, ⁶,**
lac-d.³, ⁶, lyc., nux-m.⁶, phos.³, ⁶,
plan., rhus-t., sabad.⁶, sang.³, ⁶,
sil.³, ⁶, **SULPH.¹, ⁷,** tell.⁷, ¹¹, tub.

tenth day[6]

kali-p., lach.[3, 6], phos.[3]

fourteenth day

am-m., **ARS.**, ars-met.[2, 7, 8], **calc.**,
canth.[7], chel.[6], **chin.**, chin-s.,
con., ign.[6], kali-br.[7], **LACH.,**
nicc.[3, 6, 8], phyt.[6], plan., psor.,
puls., sang.[3], sulph.[3, 6]

twenty-first day

ant-c., ars.[8], ars-met.[8], **aur.,
chin-s., mag-c.**[1'], psor., sulph.,
tarent., tub.

twenty-eighth day

mag-c.[4], nux-m.[1], **NUX-V.**, puls.,
SEP., tub.

forty-second day[3]

mag-m.

PERSPIRATION, agg. during

acon., ant-t., arn., **ARS.**, calc.,
CAUST., CHAM., chin., chin-ar.,
cimx., croc., eup-per., **ferr.**, ferr-ar.,
FORM., ign., **ip.**, lyc., **MERC.**,
nat-ar., nat-c., **nux-v., OP.**, phos.,
puls., **psor., RHUS-T., SEP.**, spong.,
STRAM., SULPH., VERAT.

am.
  acon., aesc., aeth., **ars.**, apis, bapt.,
  bell., **bov., BRY.**, calad., calc.,
  camph., canth., **cham., chin-s.**,
  cimx., **CUPR.**, elat., eup-per.,
  fl-ac.[7], **GELS., graph.**, hep., lach.,
  lyc., nat-c., **NAT-M.**, psor.,
  RHUS-T., samb., sec., **stront-c.**,
  tere-ch.[14], **thuj., verat.**

gives no relief

acon., anac., **ant-c., ant-t.**, apis[1'],
arn., **ARS.**, ars-s-f.[1'], bar-c., bell.,
benz-ac., **calc.**, camph., cann-s.,
carb-v., **CAUST., CHAM.**, chel.,
chin., chin-ar.[6], cimx., cina, cinnb.,
cocc., coff., **colch.**[1], coloc., con.,
croc., **dig.**, dros., dulc., eup-per.,
ferr., ferr-ar., **FORM.**, graph., **hep.**,
hyos., **ign., ip., kali-c.**, kali-n.,
kreos., lach.[3, 6], led., lyc., **mang.**,
MERC., mez., mosch., mur-ac.,
nat-ar., **nat-c.**, nat-m., **nit-ac.**,
NUX-V., OP., par., ph-ac., **phos.**,
plb., psor., **puls., pyrog.**[3], ran-b.,
rhod., **RHUS-T., sabad.**, sabin.,
sal-ac.[3, 6], samb., sel., **SEP.**, spong.,
stann., staph., **STRAM.**, stront-c.,
sul-ac.[3], **SULPH.**, tarax., tarent-c.[3],
thuj., **til., tub.**[3], valer., **VERAT.,
verat-v.**

after p. agg.

acon., ant-t., arn.[2], ars., ars-i.[6],
ars-s-f.[1'], bell., bry., **calc.**, canth.[6],
carb-an.[16], carb-v., cast.[6], cham.,
CHIN., chin-s.[8], cinnb.[1'], **con.**,
ferr.[2], **hep.**[6, 8], ign., iod., ip.,
kali-c., kali-i.[6], lyc., **merc.**,
merc-c.[8], mur-ac.[1', 2], nat-c.,
nat-m., nit-ac.[3, 8], nux-v., op.[8],
petr., **PH-AC., phos., psor.**[6],
puls., samb.[6], sel., **SEP.**, sil.,
spig., **spong.**[2], squil., **stann.**[6],
staph., stram.[8], **sulph.**, tub.[6],
verat.[8]

am.
  acon., aesc., am-m., ambr., ant-t.,
  apis[2], **ars.**, aur.[3, 6], bapt.[3], bar-c.,
  bell., bov., **bry., calad., calc.**[3, 6],
  camph.[2, 3, 6], **canth., CHAM.**,
  chel., **cimx.**[2], clem., cocc., coloc.,
  cupr.[3, 6, 8], elat.[2], ferr-p.[3, 6], **fl-ac.**[2],
  franc.[8], **GELS.**, glon.[3], **graph.**,
  hell., **hep.**, hyos., **iod.**[3, 6], ip.,
  kali-i.[3, 6], kali-n., **lach.**[2], led., lyc.,
  lyss.[2, 10], mag-m., **NAT-M.**,

nit-ac., nux-v., **olnd.**, op., **PSOR.**, puls., ran-b.³, ⁶, rhod., **RHUS-T.**, sabad., sabin., samb., sel., spong., stram., **stront-c.**, sul-ac., **sulph.**, tab.³, tarax., **thuj.**, urt-u.³, ⁶, valer., **verat.**, vip.³, ⁶, vip-a.¹⁴, visc.³, ⁶

acrid

all-s., **caps., CHAM.**, coff.³, **con.**, fl-ac., graph., **hell.**³, iod., ip., **lac-ac.**, lyc., merc., nat-m.³, **nit-ac.**³, ⁶, par., ran-b.³, rhus-t., sil.³, tarax., tarent.³, zinc.³

burning

bloody

anag.², arn., ars.³, ⁶, calc., cann-i.⁶, cann-s.³, cham., chin., clem., cocc.², **CROT-H., cur.**, hell.³, ⁶, **LACH.**, lyc., **nux-m., nux-v.**, petr., phos.³, ⁶

night
cur.

burning

merc., **mez., NAT-C.**, veraᵗ

acrid

clammy, sticky, viscid

absin.¹¹, acet-ac., acon., act-sp.², agar., aloe³, ⁶, aml-ns., anac., ant-c., **ant-t.**, anthraci., anthraco., apis, arn., **ARS.**, ars-s-f.¹′, ben-n.¹¹, both., brom., **bry.**², ³, **calc., CAMPH.**, cann-i., canth., carb-ac.³, ⁶, carb-an., carb-v., carbn-h.¹¹, caust., **cench.**⁷, ¹¹, **CHAM.**, chin., chlor., cimic., cocc., coff., coff-t.¹¹, colch., coloc.³, **corn., crot-c.**, crot-h.,

crot-t., cub.¹¹, cupr., **cupr-ar.**², ¹¹, daph., dig., elat., fago., **FERR., FERR-AR.**, ferr-i., **FERR-P.**, fl-ac., gast.¹¹, glon., guat.⁹, **hell.**, hep., hydr.¹¹, hydr-ac.², ¹¹, hyos., iod., jatr., kali-bi., kali-br., kali-cy.¹¹, kali-n.¹¹, kali-ox.¹¹, lach., lachn., lil-t.³, ⁶, lob.¹¹, **LYC., MERC., merc-c.**, merc-pr-r.¹¹, merc-sul.¹¹, mez., morph., **mosch.**, mur-ac.¹¹, **naja**³, ¹¹, napht.¹¹, nat-m.³, nat-sil.¹′, **nux-v.**, op., ox-ac., **PH-AC.**, phal.¹², **PHOS.**, phys.¹¹, **plb.**, psor., rauw.¹⁴, sec., sol-t.¹¹, **spig., spong.**, stann., stry.¹¹, **sul-ac.**, sul-i.¹′, sulph.¹¹, sumb., tab., tanac.¹¹, tax., ter., trach.¹¹, **tub., VERAT.**, verat-v.³, vip., wies.¹¹, zinc., zinc-m.¹¹, zinc-s.¹¹

morning
mosch.

evening
anthraco., clem., fl-ac., sumb.

night
cupr., fago., hep., **lyc.**², **merc.**²

bed, in²

plb.

climacteric period, at⁷

crot-h., lach., lyc., sul-ac., ter.

falling asleep²

daph.

starting from sleep, with

daph.

cold

acet-ac., **acon.**, act-sp., aeth.,
agar., agar-ph.[11], ail., alco.[11],
aloe[3, 6], **AM-C.**, ambr.[3], **anac.**,
anh.[9], **ant-c.**, **ANT-T.**, **anthraci.**,
apis, aran.[14], **arn.**, **ARS.**, ars-i.,
ars-s-f.[1'], asaf.[3], aur.[3], **aur-m.**,
bar-c., bar-m., bar-s.[1'], bell.,
benz-ac., bol-lu.[11], both., **bry.**,
bufo[1], buth-a.[9], cact.[1'], cadm-s.[1'],
calad., **calc.**, calc-p.[3], calc-s.,
calc-sil.[1'], **CAMPH.**, **cann-i.**[2],
cann-s., canth., caps., **carb-ac.**,
CARB-V., **carbn-s.**, cast.[3], **cench.**[7],
cent.[11], cham., **CHIN.**, **CHIN-AR.**,
chlol.[2], **chlor.**, cimic., **cina**[1], **cist.**,
COCC., coff., coff-t.[11], colch.[1'],
coloc., con.[3], convo-s.[14], corn.,
croc., **crot-c.**, crot-h., cupr.,
cupr-a.[2, 11], **cupr-ar.**[2], **cur.**,
cyt-l.[9, 14], dig., digin.[11], **dros.**,
dulc., **elaps**, esp-g.[13], **euph.**[3],
euphr., **FERR.**, **ferr-ar.**, **ferr-i.**,
ferr-p.[3], frag.[11], gels., **graph.**[3],
hell., **HEP.**, **hydr.**[2], **hydr-ac.**[3, 6],
hyos., hura, **ign.**, iod., **IP.**, jatr.,
kali-ar., kali-bi.[1', 3], **kali-c.**[1', 14],
kali-cy.[11], kali-n., kali-p.[3, 6],
kalm., lac-c.[1] (non: lac-ac.),
lachn., laur., lil-t.[3, 6], **lob.**,
lol.[11], **LYC.**, manc., mang.[3],
med.[1'], **merc.**, **MERC-C.**,
merc-pr-r.[11], **mez.**, morph.,
mur-ac., **naja**[3], narcot.[11], **nat-ar.**,
nat-c., nat-m., nat-p., nit-ac.,
nux-v., op., ox-ac., paeon.[2],
penic.[13], **petr.**, **ph-ac.**[2, 3, 11], **phos.**,
plan., plb., podo., **psor.**, **puls.**,
pyrog., ran-s.[3], **rheum**[2, 3], rhus-t.,
ruta, sabad.[3], sang., **SEC.**, seneg.,
SEP., sil., **spig.**, **spong.**, stann.,
staph., **stram.**, sul-ac., sul-i.[1'],
sulo-ac.[14], **sulph.**, sumb., **tab.**,
ter., tere-ch.[14], thea[11], **ther.**, **thuj.**,
tub., **VERAT.**, **VERAT-V.**, vip.,
vip-a.[14], wye.[11], zinc.

Vol. I: *anxiety-perspiration*

faintness – perspiration

morning
ant-c., canth., chin., esp-g.[13],
euph., ruta

afternoon
GELS., phos., verat-v.

evening
anac., hura, phos.[11]

18 h
psor.

night
am-c., buth-a.[14], chin., coloc.,
croc., cupr., cur., **dig.**, fago., iod.,
lob., mang.[16], op., rhus-t., **SEP.**,
thuj.

am.
nux-v.

cigar, after[.1]

op.

clammy sweats with haemorrhage

CHIN.

chill

corn., cupr.[2], lyss.[2], **VERAT.**[2]

coffee, after[11]

digin.

convulsions, during

camph.[1'], **cupr.**[2], ferr., stram.,
verat.[2]

diarrhoea, in[2]

aeth., ant-t., **ars.**, calc., **camph.,**
cupr., hell., jatr., pic-ac., **sec.,
sil.,** sulph., **tab.,** ter., **verat.**

dysmenorrhoea, in[2]

sars., verat.

eating, while

MERC.

after

digin.[11], sul-ac.

exertion of body, or mind, after the
slightest

act-sp., **calc., HEP., SEP.**

headache, with

GELS.[2], graph., **verat.**[2]

heat, with sensation of internal[14]

anac.

lying, while[11]

thea

menses, during

ars., coff., phos., **sars., sec.,
VERAT.**

motion, on

ant-c., sep.

nausea, with[2]

**calc., ip., lach., PETR., tab.,
verat.,** verat-v.

and vertigo

ail.

over the body, warm sweat on the
palms

dig.

perspiration increases the coldness
of the body

cinnb., cist.

rising from bed, on[11]

bry.

stool, during

merc., sulph., thuj., verat.

sudden attacks of

crot-h.

urination, after

bell.

walking, on[11]

rhus-t.

in cold open air[16]

rhus-t.

vertigo, with[2]

ail., **merc-c.**, ther.

vomiting, with[2]

CAMPH., ip., thea[11], **VERAT., verat-v.**

colliquative

acet-ac., **ANT-T., ars.**, ars-h.[2], camph., **carb-v., CHIN., EUPI.,** iod.[2], jab.[2], **lach.**, lyc., mill., **nit-ac., psor., sec.**

critical

acon.[6], bapt., bell.[6], bry., **canth.**[6], chlor., pneu.[6], **pyrog.**, rhus-t.[6]

hot

ACON., aesc., aml-ns.[3, 6], anac.[3], ant-c.[3], asar.[3], asc-t., aur.[3, 6], **bell.**, bism.[3, 6], bry., calc., calc-sil.[1'], camph.[3], canth.[3], **caps.**[2], **carb-v., CHAM.**, chel., chin., cocc., **coff.**[3, 6], **CON.**, corn., dig., dros.[3], **hell.**[2, 3], **IGN., IP.**, kreos.[3], lach.[3], led.[3], lyc.[3], **merc.**[2], merc-i-r., nat-c., **NUX-V., OP.**, par.[3], penic.[13], **ph-ac.**[2], phos., pip-n.[3], **PSOR.**, puls., **pyrog.**, rauw.[9], **rhus-t.**[2], sabad., sang.[3], **SEP.**, sil.,

stann., staph., **stram., sulph.**, thuj., verat., viol-t.

gives no relief[7]

til.

odor, aromatic

all-c.[3], benz-ac., guare., petr.[3], rhod., sep.[3]

bitter[3]

dig., **verat.**

morning
verat.

blood, like

lyc.

bread, like white[2]

ign.

burnt

BELL.[2, 3], **bry.**[3], mag-c.[3], sulph., thuj.[3]

cadaverous, carrion

ars., art-v., lach.[15], **psor.**[2], thuj.

camphora, like[2, 3, 7]

camph.

cheesy

con.[3], **hep.**, plb., sulph.

drugs, like corresponding

asaf., ben., camph., carbn-h.,
chen-a.[11], iod., ol-an.[11], phos.,
sulph., tab., ter.[11], valer.

eggs, like spoiled

plb.[3], staph., sulpn.

elder-blossoms, like

sep.

fetid

aesc., all-s.[2], aloe[2], am-c.,
am-m.[3], ambr.[2], anac., arn.,
ars.[2, 3], aur-m.[2], **bapt.**[2, 3, 6],
BAR-C.[2, 3, 6], bell.[3], bov.[3, 6],
canth.[2, 3], **carb-ac.**, carb-an.,
carb-v.[3, 6], cimic.[2], coloc.[3], con.,
crot-h.[3, 6], **cycl.**[2, 3], dios.[3], **dulc.**,
eucal.[2], **euphr.**[2, 3], ferr.,
fl-ac.[3, 6], **GRAPH.**[2, 3, 6],
guaj.[2, 3, 6], **HEP.**, **kali-c.**[2, 3, 6],
kali-p.[2, 3, 6], lac-c.[3, 6], lach.[3],
led., lyc., **mag-c.**[2, 3], mag-m.[3, 6],
merc., merc-c.[2],
NIT-AC.[2, 3, 6, 12], **NUX-V.**[2, 3],
petr.[3, 6], **PHOS.**[2, 3], plb.[3], **psor.**,
PULS.[2, 3], pyrog., **rhod.**[2, 3],
rhus-t.[2, 3], rob., **SEL.**[3], **sep.**[1'-3, 6],
SIL.[?, 3, 6, 7], spig.[2, 3],
STAPH.[2, 3, 6], stram.[3, 6],
sulph.[2, 3, 6], tell., thuj., **tub.**,
vario.[2], **verat.**[2, 3], zinc.

coughing, after

hep.

eruptions, with

dulc.

garlic, like

art-v.[2-3', 7, 11], lach.[2], sulph.[7],
thuj.[1']

honey, like

thuj.

leek, like[7]

thuj.

lilac, like[8]

sep.

mice, like[7]

tub.

musk, like

apis, bism.[3], mosch., puls., **sulph.**,
sumb.

musty

arn., **cimx.**, merc.[3], merc-c.[3],
nux-v., **psor.**, **puls.**, **rhus-t.**,
stann., syph.[15], thuj.[3], thyr.[3]

offensive

acon.[3], aloe, all-s., am-c.,
ambr.[3], apis, **ARN., ars.,**
ars-s-f.[1'], art-v., asar.[3], aur-m.,
bapt., bar-c.[3], **BAR-M.,** bar-s.[1'],
bell., bov.[3], bry.[3], calc-sil.[1'],
camph.[3], **canth.**[3], **CARB-AN.,**
carb-v., CARBN-S., caust.[3],
cham.[3], cimic., cimx., cocc.,
coloc.[3], con., cycl., daph., **dulc.,**
euphr., **ferr.,** ferr-ar., **fl-ac.,**
GRAPH., guaj., **HEP.,** hyos.[3],
ign.[3], iod.[3], ip.[3], kali-a.[11],
kali-ar., kali-c., kali-p., **lach.,**
led., **LYC., mag-c.**[1, 7], mand.[9],
med., **MERC., merl.,** mosch.[3],
murx.[1'], nat-m.[3], **NIT-AC.,**
NUX-V., oci-s.[9], oena.[11], **PETR.,**
phos., plb.[3], podo.[1'], **psor.,**
PULS., pyrog., rheum[3], rhod.,
rhus-t., rob., sacch-l.[12], **sel.,**
SEP., SIL., sol-t-ae.[12], spig.,
stann., **staph.,** stram.[3], **SULPH.,**
syph.[1'], tarax., tax.[11], **tell.,**
THUJ., vario.[3, 7], **verat.,**
wies.[12], zinc.[3]

morning
carb-v., dulc., merc-c., nux-v.

afternoon

fl-ac.

night
ars., **CARB-AN.,** carb-v.,
con., cycl., dulc., euphr.,
ferr.[2], graph., **guaj.**[2], **lyc.**[2],
mag-c., **MERC.,** nit-ac.,
nux-v., puls.[16], rhus-t., **sep.**[2],
spig., staph., **tell.,** thuj.

during sleep

cycl.

midnight
mag-c., merl.

cough, after

hep., merl.

exertion, on

nit-ac.

menses, during

stram.

motion, on

eupi., mag-c.

on one side

BAR-C.

onions, like[3]

art-v.[3, 6], bov.[2, 3, 6, 7], **calc.**[16],
lach., kali-p., **lyc.**[2, 3, 6, 7, 16], osm.,
phos., sin-n., tell.

pickled herring, like[7]

vario.

pungent[2]

cop., gast.[11], **ip.,** rhus-t.[3], **sep.**[2, 11],
sulph.[1'], thuj.[1']

putrid

bapt., **CARB-V.,** con., led.,
mag-c.[1, 7], nux-v.[3], **PSOR.,** rhus-t.,
sil.[3], **spig., STAPH.,** stram., verat.

rancid, at night

thuj.

rank

art-v., **bov.**, cop., ferr., goss.,
lac-c.², lach., lyc., sep., tell.

during menses

stram., tell.

rhubarᴅ, like³, ⁷

rheum

sickly

chin., cinch.¹¹, thuj.

smoky

bell.

sour

acon., alco:¹¹, all-s.¹¹, **arn.,
ARS.**, ars-s-f.¹', **asar., bell.², ³,
BRY.**, bufo³, calc., calc-s.,
calc-sil.¹', **carb-v., carbn-s.,
caust., cham.**, chel., chin.³,
cimx., clem.⁷, **COLCH., cupr.²,**
ferr., ferr-ar., ferr-m., **fl-ac.¹,**
gast.¹¹, **graph., HEP.**, hyos.,
ign., **IOD., ip., iris¹**, kali-c.,
kalm.², lac-ac., **lach.²**, led.,
LYC., MAG-C., MERC., nat-m.,
nat-p., NIT-AC., nux-v., pilo.¹¹,
PSOR., puls., **rheum, rhus-t.,**
ruta², samb.², **SEP., SIL.**, spig.³,
staph.³, sul-ac., sul-i.¹', **SULPH.,**
sumb., tarent., tep.¹¹, **thuj.,
VERAT.**, zinc.

morning
bry., carb-v., iod., lyc., nat-m.,
rhus-t., sep.¹⁶, sul-ac., **SULPH.**

forenoon
sulph.

afternoon
fl-ac.

night
arn., ars., asar.², bry.,
carbn-s., **caust.**, cop.¹¹,
graph., HEP., iod., **kali-c.², ¹⁶,**
lyc., mag-c., **MERC.²**, nat-m.,
nit-ac., **phyt.²**, plect.¹¹, **sep.,**
sil.¹⁶, **sulph., thuj.**, zinc.¹⁶

during sleep

bry.

sour-sweet

bry.³, ⁷, **PULS.², ³, ⁷**

spicy

rhod.

sulphur, like
phos., **sulph.¹¹**

sulfuricum acidum, like³'

plb., **staph.**, sulph.

sweetish

apıs, **ars.², calad.**, merc., puls.,
sep.², thuj., **uran-n.²**

urine, like

berb., bov.⁷, **CANTH.,**
card-m.³, caust., coloc., ery-a.,

graph.[3, 7], lyc.[3, 7], nat-m.[3],
NIT-AC., plb.[3], rhus-t.[3], sec.[3],
thyr.[3], urt-u.[3]

horse's

NIT-AC., nux-v.[2]

vinous[3]

sec.

oily

agar., arg-m., arn.[3], **ars.**[2],
aur.[2, 3, 6], **BRY.**, bufo, calc.,
CHIN., fl-ac.[3], lyc.[7], **MAG-C.**,
med.[3], **MERC.**, **nat-m.**[2, 3], nux-v.,
ol-j.[11], petr.[3], plb.[2, 3], **psor.**[2],
rhus-t.[3], **rob., sel., STRAM.**,
sumb., **THUJ.**, thyr.[3]

daytime

bry.

morning
bry., chin.

night
agar.[2], bry., croc., mag-c.[16],
MERC.

periodical at the same hour[16]

ant-c.

single parts, of:

affected parts, on

AMBR., ANT-T., anthraco.[4],
ars., asar.[6], bry., calc.[3, 6],
caust., chin.[6], **cocc., coff.,** fl-ac.,
guaj.[6], hell.[6], kali-c.[3], lyc.[3],
MERC., nat-c., nit-ac., nux-v.,
petr.[6], puls.[6], **RHUS-T., sep.,**

sil., **stann.,** stram., stront-c.,
thuj.[6]

morning
ambr.

all parts except the head

bell.[1, 7], merc., mur-ac.[16], nux-v.,
RHUS-T., SAMB., sec.[2, 7], sep.,
THUJ.[1, 7]

feet[16]

chin., phos.

legs[16]

lyc.

lower limbs[16]

lyc.

thighs[16]

lyc.

back part of body, on[3]

ars., calc., caust., **CHIN.**[2, 3], **dulc.,**
ferr., guaj., lach., led., mang.,
mosch., **mur-ac.,** nat-c., **nux-v.,**
par., petr., **ph-ac., puls.**[2, 3], sabin.,
SEP.[2, 3, 8], **sil.**[2], **stann.,** stram.,
SULPH.[2, 3]

covered parts, on

ACON., BELL., cham., **CHIN.,**
ferr., led., lyc.[3], **nit-ac.,** nux-v
puls., sec., spig., **thuj.**

night
bell., **CHAM., CHIN.,** ferr.,
nit-ac., nux-v., sec., **thuj.**

front of body, on

agar., ambr.³, anac.³, **ARG-M.,**
arn., **asar.³,** bell.²˒³, **bov.²˒³, calc.,**
canth., cina³, **COCC.,** dros.³,
euphr.²˒³, graph., ip.³, kali-n.,
laur.³, merc., merc-c.³, nat-m.³,
nux-v., **PHOS.,** plb.³, rheum³,
rhus-t.², ruta³, sabad.³, sec.³, **SEL.,**
sep.², staph.³

head, only on the

acon., am-m.³, **bell.³, calc.,** cham.,
kali-m.³, phos., **puls.,** rheum³,
sabad., sanic.³, sep., **sil.,** spig.,
stann.

left side, on

ambr.³˒⁶, anac.³˒⁷, **BAR-C., chin.,**
fl-ac., jab.², kali-c.³, phos., **PULS.,**
rhus-t., spig.³, stann.³, sulph.

lain on

.

acon., bry., **bell., CHIN.,**
NIT-AC., nux-v., puls., **sanic.**

one-sided

acon., alum.³˒⁷, **ambr.,** anac.³˒⁷,
ant-t.⁷, arn.⁷, aur-m-n., **bar-c.,**
bell., **bry.,** carb-v.³, **caust.³˒⁷,**
cham., **chin., cocc.²˒³,** fl-ac., ign.³,
jab.⁸, lyc., merc., merl., nux-m.,
NUX-V., PETR., phos., PULS.,
ran-b., rheum³, rhus-t., **sabad.²,**
sabin., **spig.²˒³,** stann.³, stram.,
sulph., THUJ.

lower part of body, on

am-c., am-m., apis, ars., asaf.³,
aur.³, bry.³, calc.³, cinnb., **cocc.²,**
coloc., con.³, **CROC.,** cycl., dros.³,
euph., ferr.², **hyos., iod.²,** kali-n.³,
mang., merc., nit-ac., nux-v.³,
phos.³˒⁶˒⁷˒¹⁵, ran-a.⁸, sanic.⁸,
sep., sil.³, thuj., **zinc.²˒³**

not lain on

ben., thuj.

right side, on

aur-m-n., bell., bry., fl-ac.³, jab.²,
merl., nux-v., **phos., puls.,** ran-b.,
sabin.

uncovered parts, on

bell.⁷, puls., **thuj.**

night, except the head

thuj.

upper part of body, on

acon.³, agar.³, **anac.²˒³, ant-t.²˒³,**
arg-m., arn.³, **ASAR.,** aza.⁸,
bar-c.³, bell.³, berb., **bov.²˒³,**
calc.⁷˒⁸, camph., canth.³, **caps.²,**
carb-v., caust.³, **cham.,** chin.,
cina, coc-c.³, dulc., dig.,
eup-per., euphr.³, fl-ac.,
graph.³, **guaj.²˒³, ign.²,** ip.,
KALI-C., laur., mag-c.³,
mag-m.³, mag-s.⁴, merc-c.³,
mosch.³, mur-ac.³, nat-c.³,
nit-ac., nux-v., **OP., PAR.,**
petr.³, ph-ac.³, phos.³, plb.³,
puls.³, **ran-s.², rheum,** rhus-t.³,
ruta²˒³, sabad.³, **samb.², sars.²,**
sec., sel.³ sep., sil., spig.,

stann.[2], sul-ac., thuj., tub.[3], váler., verat.

before sleep

berb.
.
spots, in[3]

merc., ptel., tell.

salty[3, 7, 14]

nat-m.[3], **sel.**

staining the linen

arn.[2, 3, 7], ars., bar-c., bar-m.,
BELL., benz-ac.[7], **calc.**[2, 3, 7],
carb-an., carl.[7], cham.[3, 7], chin.,
clem.[3, 7], dulc.[3, 7], **graph.**, lac-c.[7],
LACH., **lyc.**[2, 3, 7], mag-c., med.[15],
merc.[1, 7], nux-m.[3], **nux-v.**[2, 3, 7],
rheum, **sel.**[1, 7]

bloody

anag.[7], **arn.**[7] ars.[7], calc.,
cann-i.[7], **cham.**[7], chin.[7],
clem.[1, 7], cocc.[7], crot-h., **cur.**,
dulc.[7], hell.[7], **LACH.**, lyc.[1, 7],
merc.[7], **NUX-M.**, **nux-v.**[7],
phos.[7], **sel.**[7]

night
cur.

blue[7]

indg., iod., kali-i.

brown[15]

iod., nit-ac., sep., wies.[7, 11]

brownish-yellow

ars., **bell.**[1, 7], carb-an., graph.[3],
lac-c.[7], **lach.**[2, 3, 7], mag-c.[3],
sel.[2, 3, 7], thuj.[2, 3, 7]

dark[7]

bell.

difficult to wash off

lac-d.[2, 7], **mag-c.**[1, 7], **merc.**

green

agar.[3], cupr.

red

arn.[1, 7], **calc.**[2, 7], **carb-v.**, cham.[2, 7],
chin.[2, 7], clem.[2, 7], **crot-h.**[3, 7],
dulc.[1, 7], ferr.[7], gast.[2, 7, 11], **LACH.**,
lyc.[2, 7], **NUX-M.**, **nux-v.**[1, 7], thuj.

yellow

ars., **bell.**, ben-n.[11], bry., cadm-s.,
CARB-AN., carl.[11], chin., chin-ar.,
crot-c., **ferr.**, ferr-ar., **GRAPH.**,
guat.[9], hep.[3], **ip.**[1, 7], lac-c.[7], lac-d.,
LACH., **mag-c.**, **MERC.**,
rheum[2, 3, 6, 7, 11], **SEL.**, thuj., tub.,
verat.[2, 3, 7]

white[2, 3]

sel.

stiffening the linen

MERC.[1, 7], nat-m.[3], sel.

suppression of, complaints from *

acon., am-c., anthraci., apis,
arn., **ars., aspar.**[2], atro.[11],
aur-m-n.[2], **BELL.,** bell-p.[8], **BRY.**[1],
cadm-s., **caj.**[2, 12], **CALC.,**
CALC-S., calc-sil.[1'], cann-s.,
carb-v., carbn-s., cary.[11], caust.[3],
CHAM., CHIN., clem., coff.,
COLCH., coloc., cupr., **DULC.,**
eup-per., ferr., ferr-p.[12], **graph.,**
hep., hyos., iod., ip., kali-ar.,
KALI-C.[1], kali-sil.[1'], lach.[3], led.,
lyc., mag-c., **merc.,** mill.[6], nat-c.,
nat-m., nat-s., nit-ac., **NUX-M.**[1],
nux-v., olnd., op., ph-ac., **phos.,**
plat., **plb., PSOR.,** puls., **RHUS-T.,**
sabad., sec., sel., senec.[6], seneg.,
SEP., SIL., spong., squil., staph.,
STRAM., SULPH., teucr., thuj.[3],
verat.[3], verb., viol-o.

paralysis–perspiration

foot, of *

am-c., apis, ars., bad., **BAR-C.,**
bar-m., bar-s.[1'], cham., coch.,
colch., **cupr., form.,** graph., haem.,
kali-c., lyc., merc., nat-c., **nat-m.,**
nit-ac., ol-an.[3, 12], ph-ac., phos.,
plb., psor.[8], **puls.,** rhus-t.,
sal-ac.[12], sanic.[8], sel., **SEP., SIL.,**
sulph. **thuj., ZINC.,** zinc-p.[1']

warm

acon., ant-c., asar., ben., camph.,
carb-v., cham., cocc., dig.[4], dros.,
ign., kali-c., kreos.[4], lach., led.,
nat-m., nux-v., op., phos., puls.[4],
sep., sil.[4], staph., stram., thuj.[4, 16],
verat.[4]

morning[4]
carb-v.

every other morning[4]

ant-c.

evening[4]
anac., puls.

night[4]
staph., thuj.

causing uneasiness

CALC., cham., nux-v., **puls.,**
SEP., sulph.

convulsions with[4]

sil.

epilepsy, after[15]

sil.

sitting, in[4]

asar.

somnolence with[4]

op.

waking, am. on[4]

thuj.

wash off, difficult to

lac-d.[2], **mag-c., merc.,** sep.[15]

PINCHING am.[3]

apis, ars., pip-n.

pressure – hard

PLAYING piano*

anac., calc., cham.[7], kali-c., **nat-c.,**
phos.[1,7], **sep.,** zinc.

weariness – playing

PLETHORA

acon., **aesc.**[1]**, aloe**[1,3,6], alum.,
am-c., am-m.[3], ambr., ant-t.[3], apis[3],
arn., ars., AUR., aur-ar.[1], aur-i.[1],
aur-s.[1], **bar-c.,** bar-i.[1], **BELL.,**
bov., brom.[1], **BRY., CALC.,** canth.,
caps.[3], **carb-an., carb-v., carbn-s.,**
caust., cham., chel., **chin.,** clem.,
cocc., coloc., con., **croc.,** cupr., dig.,
digin.[11], dulc., **ferr.,** ferr-ar.,
ferr-i.[2,11,12], ferr-p., glon.[1,12],
graph., guaj., hep., **HYOS.,** ign.,
iod., ip., **KALI-BI., kali-c.,** kali-n.,
lach., led., **LYC.,** mag-m., **merc.,**
mosch., nat-c., **NAT-M.,** nit-ac.,
nux-v., op., perh.[14], petr., **ph-ac.,**
PHOS., puls., rauw.[14], rhod., **rhus-t.,**
sabin., sacch.[11], sars., sec., sel.,
seneg., **SEP., SIL.,** spig., spong.,
stann., staph., **stram., stront-c.,**
sul-i.[1], **SULPH., thuj.,** tus-fr.[12],
valer., verat., zinc.

plethoric constitution[2]

ACON., aur., **BELL.,** bry.[1], **cact.**[2,7],
calc., **glon., nux-v., op.,** ruta,
seneg., **verat-v.**

portal stasis, pylestasis[2]

aesc., aesc-g.[8], **asaf.,** apoc., **card-m.,**
cimx., ham.[1], **kali-m., NUX-V.,**
SULPH.[2,12]

PLUG externally, sensation of

agar., ang.[3], arn., bufo[3], coloc.[3],
crot-t., hell., hyper.[3], **kali-bi.,** lach.,
plat., ruta

internally

acon., **agar., ALOE,** am-br., am-c.,
ambr., **anac., ant-c.,** apoc.[3,6],
arg-m., arg-n.[3], **arn., asaf.,** aur.,
bar-c., bell. bov., bufo[3], calc.,
caust., cham., chel., cimic.[3],
coc-c., cocc., coff., con., croc.,
dros., ferr., graph., hell., **hep., IGN.,**
iod., **kali-bi.**[3,6], kali-c., kreos.,
lach., led., lith-c.[3], lyc., merc., mez.,
mosch.[3], mur-ac., nat-m., **nux-v.,**
olnd., par., plat., plb., ran-s., rat.[3],
rhod., **ruta,** sabad., sabin., sang.,
sep., spig., **spong.,** staph., sul-ac.[3,4],
sulph., THUJ.

POLYPUS

all-c.[7,8], alum.[3,6], alumn.[12], ambr.,
ant-c., **aur.,** bell., berb.[12], cadm-s.[3,6],
CALC., calc-i.[3,6], **CALC-P., calc-s.,**
carb-an., caust., coc-c.[3], **CON.,**
form.[3,6,8], graph., **hep., kali-bi.**[3,6,8,1?]
kali-i.[3,6,8], kali-m.[6], kali-n.[6,12,]
kali-s.[6,12], lem-m.[8,12], **lyc.,** med.[3,12],
merc., merc-i-r.[6], **mez.,** nat-m., nit-ac.,
petr., ph-ac., **PHOS., psor.**[3,6,8,12],
puls., sang., **sang-n.**[8,12], sep., **sil.,**
STAPH., sul-ac., sulph., **TEUCR.,**
thuj.

POUNDING, foreign hammering side lain on[16]

clem.

PRESSURE agg.

acon., **AGAR.,** alum., alum-sil.[1'], am-br.[1], am-c., am-m., ambr., anac., **ang.**[2, 3], ant-c., **APIS,** aq-mar.[14], **arg-m.,** arg-n.[3], arn., **ars., ars-i.,** asaf., **bapt., BAR-C.,** bar-i.[1'], bar-m., bar-s.[1'], bell., bism., bor., bov., **bry.,** cact., **calad.,** calc., calc-p., camph., **cann-s., canth., caps.,** carb-an., **carb-v.,** carbn-s., card-m., caust., cench.[8], **chel.,** chin., cimic.[14], **CINA,** coc-c., cocc., coloc., cortiso.[14], crot-t., culx.[1'], cupr., dig., dros., dulc., equis.[8], ferr.[3], fl-ac.[3], **guaj.,** hecla[14], hell., **HEP.,** hyos., ign., **IOD.,** ip., **kali-bi., kali-c., kali-i.,** kali-n., kali-p., kali-sil.[1'], **LACH.,** laur., led., **LIL-T., LYC., mag-c.,** mag-m., mang., meny., **merc., MERC-C.,** mez., **mosch.,** mur-ac., nat-ar., nat-c., **nat-m., nat-s., nit-ac.,** nux-m., **nux-v., olnd.,** onos.[8], **op.,** ovi-p.[8], ox-ac., ph-ac., phos., phyt.[3, 8], **plat.,** psor.[3], puls., **ran-b., ran-s.,** rhus-t., **ruta,** sabad., **sabin.,** samb., sars., **sel.,** seneg., sep., **SIL.,** spig., **spong., stann., staph.,** stram., stront-c., sul-ac., sul-i.[1'], sulph., **teucr.,** thal.[14], **ther.**[8], thuj., **valer., verb.,** vib.[3], vip-a.[14], zinc.

am.
abies c., acon., agar., **agn.,** alum., alum-p.[1'], alum-sil.[1'], **alumn.**[2], **am-c., am-m.,** ambr., anac., ant-c, **apis,** arg-m., **arg-n.,** arn., ars., **asaf.,** atra-r.[14], **aur.,** bar-m.[1'], bell., bell-p.[7, 14], bism., **bor.,** bov., **BRY.,** cact., cadm-met.[14], calc., calc-f., camph., **canth., caps.**[8],

carb-ac., **carbn-s.,** cast.[3], caust., **chel., CHIN.,** cina, cinnb., **clem., cocc.**[2, 3], **COLOC., CON.,** croc., crot-t., cupr-a.[8], cupr-ar.[3], dig., dios., **DROS., dulc.,** esp-g.[13], euon.[8], form., **glon., graph.,** guaj., hell., hip-ac.[14], hist.[10, 14], ign., indg.[4, 8], ip., **kali-bi.,** kali-c., **kali-i.,** kali-p., kreos., **lac-d.**[1', 7], **lach.,** laur., led., **LIL-T.,** mag-c., **MAG-M., MAG-P., mang.,** med.[7], **MENY.,** merc., mez., mosch., **mur-ac., NAT-C.,** nat-f.[10, 14], **nat-m.,** nat-p., **nat-s.,** nat-sil.[1'], **nit-ac., nux-m.,** nux-v., olnd., **par., ph-ac.,** phos., pic-ac.[8], **PLB., PULS.,** rad-br.[8], **rhus-t.,** ruta, sabad., sabin., sang., **sep., SIL., spig.,** stann., sul-ac., sulfonam.[14], sulph., thuj., **tril.,** verat., verb., vip-a.[14], zinc.

hard edge am., over a[3]

bell., **chin., COLOC.,** con., ign., **lach.,** samb., sang., stann., zinc.

hard p. agg.[3]

pip-n., spig., tell.

am.[3]
achy.[14], arg-n., arn., coloc., culx.[1'], ign.[1'], mag-m.[14], plb., rauw.[14], sep.[1'], stann.[14]

painless side agg., on

ambr., arn., bell., **BRY.,** calc., cann-s., carb-an., carb-v., **caust., cham.,** coloc., fl-ac.[3], **IGN.,** kali-c., lyc., nux-v., **PULS.,** rhus-t., sep., **stann.,** viol o., **viol-t.**

slight p. agg., hard p. am.[3]

aloe, bell., **cast.**[3], caust., **CHIN.,** culx.[1'], ign., kali-c., lac-c.[1'],

lach.[1', 3, 10], **mag-p., nux-v.,** plb.. sulph.

rubbing – am., gentle

PRICKLING externally

abrot.[3], acon., agar., **ail.,** alum., ant-c., ant-t., **apis**[2, 3, 11], arn.[2], ars.[3, 11], arum-t.[1'], bar-c.[3], bell., bor.[3], brom.[11], bry.[3], calc., cann-i., cann-s., caps., carbn-s., carl.[11], caust., chin.[11], cimic., coloc., con., croc., **crot-c.,** crot-h.[3], delphin.[11], **dros.,** elaps[11], ferr-m.[11], ferr-ma.[4], glon., grat.[4], ham.[3], hep., hydr-ac.[11], hyos.[11], ign.[3], ip.[2], kali-bi.[3], kali-br., kali-p.[3], laur., linu-c.[11], **lob.,** lyc., med., **mez.,** mosch., nat-m.[3], **nit-ac.**[3], **nux-m.,** nux-v.[3], onos., **phos.**[2], **PLAT., RAN-S.,** rhod.[3], rhus-t.[3], ruta, sabad., **sec.,** sep., sil.[3], spira.[11], staph., stram.[11], sul-ac., sulph., symph.[3], tarent.[2, 3], **tep.**[11], thuj.[4], urt-u.[3], verat.[3, 11], verat-v.[3], xan.[2], zinc.

internally

abrot., acon., **ail.,** arum-t.[1'], aur., cann-s., dios., lach., **NIT-AC.,** osm., ph-ac., **phos.,** plat., **ran-b., sabad., sang.,** sec., seneg., verb.[1], viol-o.

PSORA[7]

acon., adlu.[14], aesc., **agar.**[3, 6, 7, 16], alco.[11], aln.[12], alum.[3, 6, 7, 16], alumn.[1'], ambr.[3, 7], am-c.[3, 6, 7, 16], am-m.[3, 6, 7, 16], amyg.[3, 7], anac.[3, 7, 16], ang., anh.[14], **ant-c.**[3, 6, 7, 16], ant-t.[3, 7], apis[3, 7, 16], aran.[14], arg-m.[7, 16], arg-n.[3, 6, 7], arn.[3, 7], ars.[3, 6, 7], **ars-i.**[2, 7], ars-s-f.[1'], asaf.[3, 6, 7], asar.[3, 7], astra-e.[14], aur.[3, 6, 7, 16], aur-m.[3, 7], bac.[12], **bar-c.**[3, 6, 7, 16], bell.[3, 7, 16], berb., berb-a.[14], beryl.[14], bism., bor.[3, 6, 7, 16], bor-ac.[16], bov.[3, 6, 7], bry.[3, 7], bufo, buni-o.[14], **calc.**[2, 3, 6, 7, 16],

calc-ac.[3, 7], calc-f.[14], **calc-p.**[6, 7, 16], calc-s.[3, 7], camph.[3, 7], cann-s.[3, 7], canth.[3, 7], caps.[3, 7], **carb-an.**[3, 6, 7, 16], **carb-v.**[3, 6, 7, 12], caust.[3, 6, 7, 12, 16], cham.[3, 7], chel.[3, 7], chin.[3, 7], cic.[3, 7, 14], cina[3, 7], cinnb.[7], clem.[3, 6, 7, 16], coc-c.[7], coca, cocc.[3, 7], coff., colch.[3, 7, 14], coloc.[3, 6, 7, 16], con.[3, 6, 7, 16], cortiso.[14], croc.[3, 7], **cupr.**[3, 6, 7, 16], cycl.[3, 7], cyna.[14], daph., des-ac.[14], dig.[3, 6, 7], dros., dulc.[3, 6, 7, 16], euph.[3, 6, 7, 16], euph-cy., euph-l., euphr., ferr.[3, 7], ferr-ar.[1'], ferr-ma., ferr-p., fl-ac., flav.[14], galph.[14], graph.[2, 3, 6, 7, 16], guaj.[3, 6, 7, 16], guat.[14], halo.[14], ham., harp.[14], hell., helon., **hep.**[2, 3, 6, 7, 16], hip-ac.[14], hir.[14], hist.[14], hydr., hydr-ac., hyos., hypoth.[14], iber.[14], ign., iod.[3, 6, 7, 16], ip., kali-ar.[1'], kali-bi.[6, 7, 11], **kali-c.**[3, 6, 7, 16], kali-i., kali-n.[3, 6, 7, 16], kali-p., kreos.[2], kres.[14], lac-c., lac-d., lach., laur., led., levo.[14], lil-t., lob., lyc.[3, 6, 7, 16], m-arct., m-aust., **mag-c.**[3, 6, 7, 16], **mag-m.**[3, 6, 7, 16], mag-s.[14], mand.[14], mang.[3, 6, 7, 16], **merc.,** merc-c., mez.[3, 6, 7, 16], mill., mim-p.[14], morph., mosch., mur-ac.[3, 6, 7, 16], murx., **nat-c.**[3, 6, 7, 16], **nat-m.**[3, 6, 7, 16], nicc.[3, 7], **nit-ac.**[3, 6, 7, 16], nux-v., oci-s.[14], okou.[14], **ol-j.**[6, 7, 11], olnd.[6, 7], onop.[14], op., orig., palo.[14], par., paraph.[14], ped.[12], perh.[14], pers.[14], **petr.**[3, 6, 7, 16], ph-ac.[3, 6, 7, 16], phenob.[14], phos.[3, 6, 7, 16], plat.[3, 6, 7, 16], plb.[3, 7], plb-a., plb-m., pneu.[14], podo., prot.[14], **PSOR.**[2, 3, 6, 7, 12], puls., ran-b., rauw.[14], reser.[14], rheum, rhod.[3, 7, 16], rhus-t.[3, 7], rib-ac.[14], rumx., ruta, sabad.[3, 7], sabin., samb., saroth.[14], sarr., sars., sec., sel.[3, 7], seneg.[3, 7, 16], **sil.**[3, 6, 7, 16], spig.[3, 7], spong.[3, 7], squil., stann.[3, 6, 7], staph., stram., stront-c.[3, 7], sul-ac.[3, 6, 7, 16], **SULPH.**[2, 3, 6, 7, 12, 16], tarax., tell.[14], teucr., thala.[14], thiop.[14], thuj., thyr.[14], trif-p., trios.[14], tub., tub-r.[14], ven-m.[14], verat., visc.[14], zinc.

PTOMAINE POISONING, ailments from[12]

ars.[3], pyrog.

PUBERTY ailments in[3, 6]✱

acon.[2, 12], agar.[3], **ant-c.**[3], apoc.[12], aur.[6, 12], bell.[3, 12], **calc.**[2, 6], **calc-p.**[3, 6, 12], caust., cimic.[3], croc., cupr.[6], ferr., **ferr-p., GELS.**[2, 12], **graph.,** guaj.[3], hell.[3], helon., ign.[12], iod., **jug-r.**[3, 6], kali-br.[3], **kali-c., lach.**[3], mag-p.[12], mill.[12], **nat-m., ph-ac., PHOS.,** plat., **PULS.**[3, 4, 6, 12], senec.[3], sep.[12], sil., stram.[12], ther.[4], verat.[12], viol-o.[3]

girls, in[2]

aur.[2, 12], bar-c., bell., calc-p.[1', 2, 12], ferr., fil., hyoth.[14], **LACH., phos., puls.**

PULSATION, externally

acet-ac.[1'], **acon.,** acon-s.[11], **aesc.,** agar., alum., alumn., am-c., am-m., **ambr.,** ammc., anac., ang.[3], **ant-t., arg-m., arg-n.,** arn., **ars.,** ars-i., ars-s-f.[1'], **asaf.,** asar., aster.[3], **bar-c.,** bar-i.[1'], bar-m., bar-s.[1'], bell., benz-ac., berb., bov., brom., bry., bufo[3], **cact.,** calad., **CALC.,** calc-i.[1'], **calc-p., calc-s.,** calc-sil.[1'], cann-s., canth., caps., carb-an., **carb-v., carbn-s., caust.,** cham., chel., chin., chin-ar., chlol., chlor.[11], cina, clem., coc-c., cocc., coff., **coloc., con.,** cop., croc., cupr., dig., dros., dulc., euph.[3], euphr., **FERR.,** ferr-ar., **FERR-I.,** ferr-p., fl-ac., gamb., gast.[11], gels., **GLON., GRAPH.,** guaj., hell., helo., hep., hyos.,

ign., iod., jab.[3], kali-ar., **kali-bi., KALI-C.,** kali-m.[1'], kali-n., kali-p., **KALI-S.,** kali-sil.[1'], kiss., **KREOS., LACH.,** laur., led.[1'], **lil-t., lyc., lyss.,** macro.[11], mag-c., mag-m., manc., mang., med., **MELI., merc.,** mez., mosch., mur-ac., nat-ar., **nat-c., NAT-M., nat-p., nat-s.,** nat-sil.[1'], **nit-ac.,** nitro-o.[11], nux-m., **nux-v., OLND.,** op., par., petr., ph-ac., **phos., phys., phyt., plat.,** plb., polyg-s.[3], **PULS.,** ran-b., rheum, **rhod.,** rhus-t., **rumx., ruta, SABAD.,** sabin., samb., sang., sars., sec., **sel.,** seneg., **sep., sil.,** spig., spong., squil., stann., staph., **still., stram., stront-c.,** stroph-h.[3], sul-ac., sul-i.[1'], **SULPH., tarax.,** teucr., **thuj.,** til., **urt-u.,** verat., **zinc.,** zinc-p.[1']

morning, on waking

bell.

14.30 h pall.

evening
arn., **carb-an.,** caust., nat-m., sep.

during rest

nat-m.

sleep, before going to[16]

sil.

night
am-m., **bry.,** cact., nat-m., **sil.,** sulph.

coughing, from

calc.

half awake, while

    sulph.

midnight
    phys.

    after
        iris, trios.[11]

air am., in open

    aur.

bed. in

    arn., carb-an., caust., nat-m.,
    sep., upa.

coition, after[4]

    nat-c.

cough, during

    calc.

dreams, after[4]

    nit-ac.

eating, after

    arg-n., camph., **clem.**, lyc., **SEL.**

excitement agg.

    ferr, kreos.

exertion, on

    ferr., iod.

after[16]
    anac.

fever, during[11, 16]

    urt-u.[3], zinc.

haemorrhage from anus, after[16]

    kali-c.

headache, during

    lach.

lying, while

    calad., coloc.[16], **glon.**, sel.[3]

    on right side[1']

        arg-n.

menses, before

    cupr., thuj.

motion agg.

    ant-t., **graph., iod.**

am.
    kreos., nat-m.

music agg.

    kreos.

    Vol. I: *music*

plaintive
    kreos.

pregnancy, during

kali-c.

rest, in[11]

kreos.

sitting, while

anac.[16], eupi., phys., **sil.**

sleep, during

aesc.[1'], nat-m., sulph.

speaking in company, while
⊢

carb-v.

standing, while

alům.

starting, on[11]

camph.

touches anything, when body

glon.

tremulous

nat-c.

waking, on

bell.[2], ferr-i., **nat-m.**[2, 4], nit-ac.[4],
sulph.[4]

walking, on

dig., ferr.

in open air, after

ambr.

wandering[3]

puls.

internally

ACON., aesc.[6], aeth., agar., aloe,
ALUM., alum-p.[1'], alum-sil.[1'], am-c.,
am-m., ambr., **aml-ns.**, anac.,
ang.[3, 11], ant-c., **ANT-T.**, apis[3],
arg-m., **arg-n.**, arn., **ars., ars-i.**,
asaf., asar., atro.[6], **aur.**, aur-ar.[1'],
aur-i.[1'], aur-s.[1'], bar-c., bar-i.[1'],
bar-m.[1'], bar-s.[1'], **bell.**, berb.[4], **bor.**,
bov., **BRY.**, **cact.**, calad., **CALC.**,
calc-p., calc-sil.[1'], **camph., CANN-I.**,
cann-s., canth., **caps.**, carb-an.,
carb-v., carbn-s., **caust.**, cedr.,
cench.[1'], **cham.**, chel., chin.,
chin-ar., chin-s.[4], **cic.**, clem.[4, 6, 16],
COCC., coff., colch., **coloc., con.**,
croc., crot-h., crot-t., cycl., **dig.**,
dros., dulc., **FERR.**, ferr-ar.[1'],
FERR-I., ferr-s.[6], gels. **GLON.**,
graph., ham.[6], hell., hep., hyos.,
ign., iod., ip., kali-ar.[1'], kali-bi.[3],
kali-c., kali-i.[3], kali-m.[1'], **kali-n.**,
kreos., lach., **laur.**, led., lil-t.[6], lyc.,
mag-c., mag-m., mang., **MELI.**,
merc., merc-c., mez., mosch., murx.,
nat-c., **nat-m.**, nat-p., **nat-s.**,
nat-sil.[1'], nit-ac., nux-m., **nux-v.**,
ol-an.[4, 6], **olnd.**, op., par., petr.,
ph-ac., **PHOS.**, phys., phyt.[3],
pic-ac., **plan., plat., plb., psor.,
PULS.**, pyrog.[6], ran-b., rheum,
rhod., **rhus-t.**, ruta, **sabad.**, sabin.,
sang., sars., sec., **SEL.**, seneg., **SEP.**,
SIL., spig., **spong.**, stann., **stram.**,
stront-c.[6], sul-ac., sul-i.[1'], **sulph.**,

tab.[6], **thuj.**, verat., verat-v., verb., **zinc.**, zinc-p.[1']

bones, in

asaf., **calc.**, carb-v., lyc., **merc.**, nit-ac., phos., rhod., ruṭa, sabad., sep., sil., **sulph.**, thuj.

glands, in

am-m., arn., asaf., bell., bov., bry., **calc.**, caust., cham., clem., con.[3], **kali-c.**, lach.[4], lyc., **MERC.**, nat-c., nit-ac., **phos.**, rhod., **sabad.**, sep., **sil., sulph.**, thuj.

joints, in[3]

am-m., arg-m., dros., led.[11], **merc.**[3, 11], mez., olnd., ph-ac., rhod., rhus-t., **ruta,** sabad., spig., thuj.

upper part of body[16]

nit-ac.

venous see venous pulsations

PULSE abnormal

ACON., agar., agn., am-c., am-m., ambr., ang.[3], ant-c., **ant-t.**, arg-m., **arg-n., arn., ARS., ARS-I.,** asaf., asar., aur., bar-c., **BELL.,** bism., bor., bov., **bry., CACT.**[3], calad., calc., **camph.,** cann-s., canth., caps., carb-an,, **carb-v., carbn-s.,** caust., cham., chel., **chin.,** chin-s.[3], cic., cina, cocc., colch., coloc., **con.,** croc., **CUPR., DIG.,** dulc., ferr., **gels., glon.,** graph., guaj., hell., **hep., HYOS.,** ign., **IOD.,** ip., kali-c., kali-n., kalm.[3], **KREOS., LACH., laur.,** led., lyc., mang., **meli.**[3], meny., **merc.,** mez., mosch., mur-ac.,

nat-m., nit-ac., nux-m., nux-v., olnd., **OP.,** par., petr., **PH-AC., PHOS.,** plat., plb., puls., ran-b., ran-s., rheum, rhod., **RHUS-T.,** sabad., sabin., samb., sang.[3], **sec.,** seneg., **sep., SIL.,** spig., spong., squil., stann., staph., **STRAM.,** stront-c., sul-ac., **sulph.,** thuj., valer., **VERAT.,** viol-o., viol-t., zinc.

audible

ant-t., **camph.**[3], con.[3], **dig.**[3], hell.[3], iod.[3], kali-c.[3], kreos.[3], merc.[3], op.[3], phos.[3], plb.[3], sep.[3], **SPIG.**[3], sulph.[3], **thuj.**[3]

bounding

acon.[2], aether[11], alco.[11], ars., atro.[11], **bell.**[2, 7], benz-ac., camph., cann-i., canth., chin-s., chlor.[11], colch.[2], corn-f.[11], dulc.[2], eup-per., **eup-pur.**[2], fago.[11], glon , iod., jatr.[11], kali-chl., lil-t., naja, paro-i.[14], plan., raph., trif-p.[11], visc.[11]

ascending stairs, on[16]

petr.

walking, on[16]

petr.

contracted

acet-ac., acon., agar., ant-t., arn., ars., **asaf.,** aster., bell., bism., bor.[3, 16], calc., calth.[11], cann-i., canth., chin.[3], cina, colch., crot-t., cupr.[3], cupr-a.[11], hyos., iod., **kali-bi.,** **kali-br.**[2], kali-s.[11], kiss.[11], lach.[3], laur., merc-cy., morph.[11], nit-ac., op., ox-ac., paeon.[11], petr., phos., plb., russ.[11], **sec.,** spira.[11], squil.[11],

stann., stram.[11], stry.[11], sul-ac.,
tarent.[2], vip.[11], zinc., zinc-m.[11]

hard
spasmodic

thready
wiry

discordant with temperature

lil-t.[8], **PYROG.**[3, 7, 8]

double, dicrotism

acon.[3, 11], agar., aml-ns.[3], amyg.[3],
anan.[2], apis[3], apoc.[3, 11], bell., cycl.,
ferr.[3], gels.[3], glon., iber.[3, 11],
kali-c.[3, 7], phos., pilo.[11], plb., rhod.[3],
stram., zinc.[3], zinc-s.[11].

empty

alco.[11], camph., chin., ferr.[3], **lach.**[2],
petr., **sec.**[2], **verat.**[2]

excited
e

ant-t., anth.[11], cyt-l.[11], dig.[3], iod.,
nux-v., petr., plumbg.[11], sol-t-ae.[11]

febrile

acon., alum., alumn.[11], anthraco.[2, 11],
ars., bell., bov., croc.[2], gins.[11],
lac-ac., merc-c., mez., morph.[11],
plb., sars., sec., **stram., sulph.**[2], .
thuj., vip.[11]

fluttering

apis, **arn., ars.,** cann-i.[1'], carb-ac.[11],
cimic.[1'], coff.[1'], colch., **crot-h.,**
dig.[1'], gels., gins.[11], juni.[11], **kali-bi.,**
kali-n., morph.[11], **NUX-V.,** op.,
ph-ac., **phos.,** ptel.[11], pyrog., sec.[1],

stann., stram., sul-h.[11], thea[11],
verat.[2], zinc., zinc-m.[11]

frequent, accelerated, elevated,
ᴐxalted, fast, innumerable, rapid

abies-n.[8], abrot.[11], acal.[7], **ACON.,**
adon.[8], adren.[7, 8], aesc., **aeth.,**
aether[11], **agar.,** agar-pa.[11],
agar-se.[11], **agn.**[8], **ail.,** alco.[11],
aloe, all-c., alum., alum-p.[1'],
alum-sil.[1'], alumn.[2], am-be.[2],
am-br.[11], am-c., am-m., am-val.[8],
ambr., **aml-ns.**[2, 11], ammc.[2],
amyg.[2, 11], anac., anan.[2], **ang.**[2, 3],
ant-ar.[2, 8, 11], ant-c., ant-m.[2], **ant-t.,**
anthraco.[2, 11], antip.[8], aphis[2, 11],
APIS, apoc.[8], apom.[11], aq-pet.[11],
arg-m., **arg-n., ARN., ARS.,**
aran-ix.[14], **ars-h.**[2], **ARS-I.,**
ars-s-f.[1', 2], arum-d.[2, 11], arum-i.[11],
arum-t.[2], **arund.**[2], **asaf.,** asar.,
asc-c.[2], asc-t.[11], asim.[2, 11], aster.,
atro.[2, 11], **AUR.,** aur-ar.[1'], aur-i.[1'],
aur-m., AUR-S.[1'], aza.[14], **bapt.,**
bar-a.[11], bar-c., bar-i.[1'], bar-m.,
BELL., benz-ac., ben-n.[11], **BERB.,**
beryl.[9], bism., bor., both.[11], bov.,
brom., **BRY.,** bux.[11], **cact.**[8], cain.[11],
caj.[11], calad., calc., calc-ar.[1', 7],
camph., cann-i., cann-s.[3], **canth.,**
carb-ac.[2, 11], **CARB-AN.**[1', 3],
carb-v., carbn-h.[11], carbn-o.[11],
carbn-s.[1'], cary.[11], catal.[11], caust.,
cedr., celt.[11], **cham.,** chel., **chim.**[2],
chin., chin-ar., chin-b.[2], **chin-s.,**
chlol.[2], **chlor.**[2], chloram.[14],
chlorpr.[14], chr-ac.[2], cic.[11, 14],
cimic.[1', 11], **cina,** cinch.[11], cinnb.[11],
clem., coc-c., coca[2, 11], cocc.,
coch.[2], cod.[11], coff., coff-t.[11],
colch., **COLL.,** coloc., **CON.,**
conv.[8], convo-s.[9], cop.[2], corn.[2, 11],
crat.[8], **CROC.**[2, 3], **CROT-C.,**
crot-h.[1], crot-t., cub.[2, 11], cund.[11],
CUPR., cupr-a.[11], cupr-ar.[2],
cupr-n.[11], cupr-s.[2], cur.[7], cycl.,
cyna.[14], cyt-l.[9, 14], daph.[2], dat-m.[11],
DIG., digin.[11], diph.[8], dor.[2, 11],

dubo-m.[11], dulc.[11], **echi.**, equis.[11], erech.[11], erio.[11], ery-a.[11], eucal.[2, 11], euph., fago.[11], fagu.[11], **ferr.**, ferr-i., ferr-m.[11], **FERR-P.,** fl-ac., foll.[14], **form.**[2], gad.[11], gamb.[11], gast.[11], **GELS.**, gins.[11], **GLON.**, gran.[11], grat., guaj., guat.[9], gymno.[11], hall.[11], halo.[14], ham., hed.[14], **hell.**, hep., hipp., hippoz.[2], hist.[9], hoit.[14], hydr-ac.[11], hydrc.[11], **hyos.**, **hyper.**, **iber.**[2, 8, 11, 14], **ign.**, **IOD.**, ip., iris[11], jab.[11], jatr.[11], jug-r.[11], kali-ar.[11], kali-bi., kali-br.[2], kali-c., kali-chl.[8, 11], kali-i., **kali-m.**[2], kali-n., kali-ox.[11], **kali-p.**[2], kalm.[8], keroso.[11], kreos., **lac-c.**[2], **lach.**, lapa.[11], lat-m.[8, 9, 14], **laur.**, **LED.**[2, 3, 8, 11], levo.[14], lil-s.[11], **lil-t.**[8], linu-c.[11], lipp.[11], lob., lyc., **lycps.**, lyss.[2], **mag-c.**[3], **mag-m.**[3], **manc.**, mang., med.[2], **meny.**[3], **MERC.**, merc-c., merc-cy., merc-d.[11], merc-i-f.[11], merc-pr-a.[11], merc-sul.[2], merl.[2], meth-ae-ae.[11], methys.[14], **mez.**, mill., mom-b.[11], **morph.**[8, 11], **mosch.**, **mur-ac.**, mygal.[2, 11], myric.[11], **naja**, narcot.[11], nat-ar., **nat-c.**, nat-f.[9, 14], **NAT-M.**, nat-s., nicc., **nit-ac.**, nit-s-d.[11], nitro-o.[11], **nux-m.**, **NUX-V.**, oena.[11], **ol-j.**[2, 11], olnd., onos., **OP.**, osm., ox-ac., par., penic.[13, 14], petr., **PH-AC.**, phase.[8], phel., **PHOS.**, **phys.**, **phyt.**, pic-ac., pilo.[8, 11], **plat.**, plat-m.[11], **plb.**, plect.[11], podo., prun.[7], **psor.**[2], **ptel.**[2, 11], **puls.**, pyre-p.[11], **PYROG.**, ran-b., **ran-s.**, raph.[11], rham-f.[11], rheum, rhod., rhodi.[11], **RHUS-T.**, **rhus-v.**, ric.[11], **rumx.**[2], rumx-a.[11], **ruta**[3], sabad., sabin.[3], samb., **sang.**, santin.[11], sapin.[11], saroth.[9, 14], sarr.[2, 11], sars., scroph-n.[11], scut.[7], **SEC.**, **sel.**[3], seneg., **sep.**, ser-ang.[8], **SIL.**, sin-n.[11], sol-n.[11], sol-t-ae.[11], solin.[11], **SPIG.**, spig-m.[11], **spong.**, **STANN.**, staph., still.[2], **STRAM.**, **stront-c.**[3], stroph-h.[8], stry.[11], stry-p.[8], sul-ac., sul-h.[11], sulfa.[9], sulo-ac.[14], **SULPH.**, sumb.[11], **tab.**,

tanac.[11], tarax.[11], **TARENT.**[2, 7, 11], tax.[11], **tell.**, tep.[11], ter., **teucr.**[3], thal.[14], thea[8, 11], ther.[11], thiop.[14], thlas.[2], thuj., thymol.[9, 14], **thyr.**[3, 7, 8], til.[11], tox-th.[11], throm.[11], urt-u.[11], vac.[2, 11], **valer.**, vario.[2], **verat.**, **VERAT-V.**, vesp., viol-o.[2], **VIOL-T.**[2, 3, 11], vip.[11], vip-a.[14], visc.[9, 11, 14], wies.[11], xan.[11], **ZINC.**, zinc-m.[11], **ZINC-P.**[1'], zinc-s.[11]

daytime

nat-ar., nat-m.

morning
agar., ail., **ars.**, **ars-met.**[2], asaf., atro.[11], **canth.**, cedr., chin., chin-s.[1] (non: chin-ar.), fago.[11],
• **graph.**, ign., **kali-c.**, merc-c., **mez.**[2], mit.[11], myric.[11], oena.[11], onóp.[14], ox-ac., phos., phys., podo., sang., sulph., sumb.[11], ther.[11], thuj., upa.[11]

slow during the day and in the evening, but[3]

AGAR., alum., **ARS.**, calc., canth., chin., graph., **ign.**[2, 3], **KALI-C.**, lyc., mez., nux-v., phos.

waking, on[11]

alumn.

forenoon
aphis[11], calc., chin., com.[11], lyc.[11], merc-sul.[11], mez., nat-p.[11], oena.[11], op., plan., ptel.[11], trom.[2]

noon[11]
mit., oena., ox-ac.

afternoon
agar.[2], bapt.[2], chel.[11], chin-s.[11],
chr-ac.[2], ferr-i.[11], gels.[11], gins.[11],
kali-chl.[11], kali-n.[16], lyc.,
merc-sul.[11], nat-m.[11], oena.[11],
phos.[11], phys.[11], phyt.[11], podo.[3],
ptel.[11], sumb.[11]

slow in the morning, but[3]

KALI-N., thuj., zinc.

evening
acon., alum-sil.[1'], am-caust.[11],
anth.[11], anthraco.[2], aphis[2],
arg-m., arg-n., ars.[11], arum-i.[11],
aster.[11], atha.[11], bry.,
carb-an., CAUST., chin-s.[11],
cinnb., crot-h., dulc., euph.,
euphr.[11], **ferr.**, gent-l.[11], ham.[11],
hell., hyper.[11], jug-r.[11], **lach.**,
lyc., mez., mill.[11], **mur-ac.**,
murx., **nat-c.**, nat-sil.[1'], **nux-v.**,
oena.[11], olnd., ox-ac.[11], **ph-ac.**,
phos., plan., **puls.**, ran-b.,
rheum[2], sars., sep., **sil., sulph.**,
sumb.[11], teucr.[11], **thuj., tub.**,
upa.[11], **zinc.**

in bed[16]

sul-ac.

slow in the morning, but[3]

arg-m., arn., asar., carb-an.,
caust., chin., **kali-c., KALI-N.**,
lyc., mez., **OLND.**, petr., phos.,
puls., **RAN-B., sars.**, sep.,
SPIG., teucr., **THUJ., ZINC.**

night[11]
alum-sil.[1'], anthraco., arum-i.,
aster., cinnb.[1'], con., nat-sil.[1'],
nux-v., plect., ptel.

slow by day, but[3]

am-c., bor., **bry.**[2, 3], calc.,
carb-an., dulc., hep., kali-n.,
mag-c., **merc.**[2, 3], mur-ac.,
nat-c., nat-m., phos., ran-s.,
sabin., **SEP., sil.**, sulph.

midnight, after

benz-ac., hyper.[11]

chill, during[11]

chin-s., coloc., crot-t., gels., zinc.

convulsions, during[11]

oena., op., stry.

drinking, after[16]

nat-m.

eating, after

arg-n., iod., LYC., mez.[11, 16],
nat-m.[16], **nux-v., phos., puls.**,
rhus-t., **sulph.**

excitement, from[2]

anthraco., bar-m., cain., con.[11],
digox.[11], merc.[11]

faster than the heart-beat

acon., arn., **rhus-t., spig.**

motion agg.

alum-sil.¹', ant-t., **arn.**, **bry.**, **dig.**, digin.¹¹, fl-ac., **gels.**, glon.¹¹, **graph.**, **iod.**, **lycps.**, **NAT-M.**, **nux-v.**, petr., **phos.**, sep., staph., stram.

noticing it, when

arg-n.

rest, during

mag-m.

rising up, on

bry., **dig.**

sitting, while

aspar.¹¹, gins.¹¹, indg.¹¹, **mag-m.**, nat-m.¹¹, oena.¹¹

standing, on¹⁶

nat-m.

stool, after

agar., **CON.**, glon.¹¹

supper, after¹⁶

cupr.

thinking of past troubles

sep.

urine, with copious¹⁶

dig.

vexation, after

acon., arg-n., **CHAM.**, coloc., ign., **nat-m.**, **nux-v.**, **petr.**, **SEP.**, **staph.**

warm applications, from

sulph.

and intermittent

acon., agar., aloe, alum., am-m., ars., **aur.**, bell., benz-ac., bism., cann-i., canth., chin., chin-s., colch., cupr., **dig.**, gels., glon., grat., hyos., ign., kali-chl., lob., merc-c., merc-cy., mez., mur-ac., nat-ar., nit-ac., nux-m., **nux-v.**, olnd., op., ox-ac., phos., phys., plb., sep., stram., **sulph.**, tab., verat-v., zinc.

and small

ACON., aeth., alum., apis, arn., **ARS.**, ars-i.¹, asaf., **aur.**, **aur-m.**, bell., benz-ac., bism., bry., cain.², **camph.**, canth., chin., cocc., colch., coloc., **con.**, crot-t., **dig.**, ferr-m.², fl-ac., gels., glon., grat., **hell.**, hyos., ign., **iod.**, kali-bi., kali-chl., kali-n.¹⁶, **lach.**¹, **LAUR.**, led., lob., lyc., **lycps.**, merc-c., merc-cy., **mur-ac.**, nat-m., nit-ac., **nux-m.**, **NUX-V.**, olnd., op., ox-ac., petr., phos., phyt., pic-ac., puls., ran-s., raph., rhod., rhus-t., samb., **SIL.**, sol-t-ae.¹¹, staph., **STRAM.**, sul-ac., tab., **VERAT.**, zinc.

and irregular[7]

visc.

strong and small

acon., apis, arn., ars., bell., chin.,
crot-t., gels., hyos., merc-c.,
merc-cy., op., raph., stram.

full

acet-ac., **ACON.**, aesc., aether[11],
agar.[2], agar-pa.[11], alco.[11], **all-c.**,
aloe, **ALUM.**[3], alumn.[2], am-m.[8],
aml-ns.[2, 8], **amyg.**[2, 11], anan.[2],
ANT-T., anth.[11], antip.[8], apis,
apoc., aq-pet.[11], **arn.**, ars.,
ars-h.[2, 11], ars-i., ars-met.[2, 11],
arum-d.[2, 11], arum-t.[2], asaf. asar.,
asc-c.[2], asim.[11], atro.[2, 11], **aur.**[3]
bapt., bar-c., bar-i.[1'], bar-m.,
BELL., benz-ac., **BERB.**, bism.,
brom., **BRY., cact.**[8], cain.[2, 11],
caj.[11], **CALC.**[3, 8], camph., **canth.**,
carb-ac.[11], carbn-o.[11], cedr.,
celt.[11], cent.[11], cham., **CHEL.**,
chin., chin-ar.[2], chin-s., chlf.[11],
chr-ac.[2, 11], cimic., coff., colch.,
coloc., con., cor-r., cori-r.[11],
crot-c.[11], crot-h., crot-t., cub.[2, 11],
cupr., cupr-a.[11], cupr-s.[2, 11], cycl.,
cyt-l.[11], daph., dat-f.[11], **DIG.**,
digin.[11], dirc.[11], dor.[11], **dulc.**,
eup-per., eup-pur.[2], fago[8, 11], ferr.,
ferr-p., gast.[11], **GELS.**, gins.[11],
glon., GRAPH.[3], ham., hell., **hep.**,
hydr-ac.[11], **HYOS.**, iber.[2, 11],
ictod.[8], **ign.**[1], iod., jab.[11], jug-r.[11],
juni.[11], kali-bi., **kali-c.**, kali-chl.,
kali-i., kali-m.[1', 2], **KALI-N.**,
kali-ox.[11], kreos.[3, 11], lac-ac.[11],
lach., laur., **led., lil-t.**[8], linu-c.[11],
lipp.[11], lyc., menth.[11], **merc.**,
merc-c., merc-cy., merc-pr-a.[11],
merl.[2], **mez.**, mill., morph.[11],
mosch., mur-ac., myric.[11], **naja**,
nat-m., **nat-n.**[6], nit-ac., nitro-o.[11],
nux-v., ol-an.[11], olnd., onos.[8], **op.**,

ox-ac., par., **petr., ph-ac.,** phel.,
phos., phys.[8, 11], phyt., pilo.[8, 11],
plan , plb., plect.[11], puls.[3, 8],
ran-b., ran-s., raph.[11], rat.[11],
rhus-t., sabad., **sabin.**, samb.,
sang., sarr., sars., scroph-n.[11],
sec.[3], seneg., **sep., sel.**, sin-n.[2, 11],
sium[11], sol-n.[11], **spig.**, spira.[11],
spong., **STRAM.**, stront-c.,
sul-ac., **sulph.**, sumb.[11], **tab.**,
tanac.[11], tarax.[11], tarent., tell.,
tep.[11], thea[11], thuj., til.[11], toxi.[11],
trif-p.[11], trom.[11], valer., **verat.**,
verat-v., vinc.[11], viol-o., vip.[11],
visc.[11], yuc.[11], zinc., zing.[11]

morning
  canth.[2], jac-c.[11], phos., phyt.,
  sep., zinc.

forenoon[11]
  nat-ar., trom.[2], zing.

afternoon
  iod., nat-ar.[11], phyt.[11], zinc.,
  zing.[11]

evening
  acon., anth.[11], anthraco.[2], hell.,
  myric.[11], olnd., ran-b., scut.[11],
  seneg., sulph., thuj., zinc., zing.[2]

night
  com.[11], **merc.**, sep.[2]

hard

ACON., aesc., aether[11],
agar-cps.[11], agar-pa.[11], agro.[11],
alco.[11], **all-c.**, all-s.[2], am-c.,
am-caust.[11], am-m., **aml-ns.**[2],
ammc.[2], **amyg.**[2, 11], anan.[2], ant-c.,
ant-m.[2], **ant-t.**, apis[3], **arn.**, ars.,
ars-h.[2, 11], ars-i., ars-s-f.[2, 11],
arum-d.[2, 11], asaf., asar., aster.,
atro.[11], **bar-c.**, bar-i.[1'], bar-m.,
BELL., benz-ac., BERB., bism.,
brom., **BRY., cact.**, calad.,
calth.[11], camph., **canth.**,
carb-ac.[11], carbn-s.[11], cent.[11],

cham., **CHEL.**, **chin.**, chlor.[11],
cimic., **cina**, clem.[3], cocc., coff.,
colch., coloc., con., cor-r.,
corn.[2, 11], crot-h.[11], **cupr.**, **cupr-a.**[11],
cupr-s.[2, 11], cycl., cyna.[14], daph.,
dig., digin.[11], **dulc.**, **ferr.**, gast.[11],
gels., glon., gran.[11], **GRAPH.**[3],
ham., hell., **hep.**, **HYOS.**,
hyper.[2, 11], iber.[11], **ign.**, indg.[11],
iod., jatr.[11], kali-bi., **kali-c.**,
kali-i., kali-m.[1'], **kali-n.**, **kreos.**,
lach., laur.[3], **led.**, lyc., **lycps.**[2],
merc., merc-c., merc-cy.,
merc-d.[11], **merc-pr-r.**[11], mez.,
morph.[11], **mosch.**, mur-ac.,
nat-c.[11], nat-m., **nit-ac.**, nit-s-d.[11],
nitro-o.[11], **nux-v.**, olnd., op.,
ox-ac., par., petr., ph-ac., phel.,
phos., phyt., plb., plect.[11],
plumbg.[11], puls.[3], ran-b., ran-s.,
rauw.[9], sabin., samb., sang.[2],
sec., seneg., **sep.**, serp.[11], **sil.**,
sin-a.[11], sol-m.[11], sol-t-ae.[11], spig.,
spira.[11], spong., squil., **STRAM.**,
STRONT-C.[2, 3], stroph-s.[9], **stry.**[11],
sul-h.[11], **sulph.**, tab., tanac.[11],
tarent. tep.[11], **ter.**, thuj.[11], til.[11],
uva[11], valer., veıat., verat-v.,
vinc.[11], viol-o., vip.[11], wies.[11],
zinc., zinc-m.[11]

morning
  petr., phyt., zinc.

11 h[11]
  zing.

noon
  ox-ac.

evening
  all-c., **bapt.**, dulc., plb., plumbg.[11],
  ran-b.[2], zing.[2]

climbing, after[9]

rauw.

excitement, with[9]

stroph-s.

exertion, after sudden[9]

rauw.

old people, in[2]

ANT-T.

slow, and[9]

stroph-s.

heavy

crot-c.[11], phos., stram., **verat-v.**[2],
yuc.[11]

night[1]
  com.

imperceptible

ACON., aeth.[15], agar.[11], agn.,
amyg.[2, 11], anil.[11], ant-t., **apis**[3],
arg-n.[2], arn.[3], **ars.**, ars-h.[2],
ars-s-f.[2], bell., benz-ac., **cact.**,
cadm-br.[11], **CAMPH.**[3, 11], cann-i.,
cann-s., **canth.**, carb-ac., **CARB-V.**,
carbn-h.[11], chel., chin., chlor.[11],
cic. cic-m.[11], cit-l.[2, 11], **cocc.**,
COLCH., coloc., con.[2, 3, 16], crot-h.,
CUPR., cupr-ar.[11], cyt-l.[9, 11], digin.[11],
dulc., ferr., gins.[11], gels.[7], guaj.,
hell., **HYDR-AC.**[2, 3, 6, 11], hyos.,
ip., kali-cy.[11], kalm., kreos., lach.,
laur., **led.**[3], mand.[9], **merc.**, merc-c.,
morph.[11], **mosch.**[2, 3], **naja**, nux-v.,
oena.[11], **op.**, ox-ac., petr.[11], ph-ac.,
phos., **phyt.**[2], plb., plat., **podo.**[2],
puls., rhus-t., **sec.**, **SIL.**, stann.,
stram., stry.[11], sul-ac., sulph., tab.,
tax.[11], **VERAT.**, zinc.

imperceptible, almost

ACON., aeth.[15], agar.[16],
agn.[11], am-c., aml-ns.[11],
CAMPH., carbn-o.[11], chin.,
chlor.[11], cic-m.[11], coff-t.[11], crot-h.,
cyt-l.[9], dig., digin.[11], ferr., GELS.,
glon., ham., hell., hydr-ac.[6, 11],
hydrc.[11], ip., kali-bi., lach., laur.,
mand.[9], mang., merc., merc-c.[11],
morph.[11], naja, olnd., op., ox-ac.,
ph-ac., phos., plb., podo., puls.,
rhus-t., ric.[11], seneg., sol-n.[11],
sol-t.[11], spong., stram., tab.,
tere-ch.[14], thea[11], ther., verat.,
vip.[11], zinc.

convulsions, during

nux-v., olnd.

stupor, during

hep.

intermittent

acet-ac., acon., aeth., agar.,
agar-pa.[11], aloe, alum.,
am-c., am-m., amyg.[2], ang.,
ant-t.[3, 11], apis, apoc.[3, 6, 8, 11],
arg-n., arn.[2, 3, 6], ars., ars-h.[2],
ars-i.[1'], ars-s-f.[1''], asaf., atro.[2],
aur., bapt.[3, 6], bell., ben-n.[11],
benz-ac., bism., brom., bry.,
cact.[3, 6, 8], calth.[11], camph.,
cann-i.[11], canth., caps., carb-ac.,
carb-an.[11], carb-v., cedr., CHIN.,
chin-s., chlol.[2], chlor.[11], cic-m.[11],
cimx., cinnb.[11], coff., colch., con.,
conv., crat.[6, 8], crot-h., cupr.,
cupr-ac.[11], daph., DIG., digin.[11],
digox.[11], fago.[11], ferr., ferr-m.[8],
frag.[11], gast.[11], gels., glon., grat.,
hep., hura[11], hydr-ac.[11], hyos.,
iber.[6, 8, 14], ign., iod., jatr.[11],
juni.[11], kali-bi., kali-c., kali-chl.,
kali-i., kali-m.[1'], kali-p., kalm.,

keroso.[11], kreos.[2], lach., lapa.[11],
laur., lil-t., lipp.[11], lob., lycps.,
lyss.[2], mag-p.[3], meny.[3], MERC.,
merc-c.[1], merc-cy.[1], merc-sul.[11],
meth-ae-ae.[11], mez., morph.[11],
mur-ac., murx.[3], naja, nat-ar.,
NAT-M., nit-ac., nit-s-d.[2],
nitro-o.[11], nux-m., nux-v., olnd.,
op., ox-ac., PH-AC., phos.,
phys.[11], phyt., pip-n.[8], plan.[11],
plb., prun-v.[7], ptel.[2, 11], ran-s.[2],
rhus-t., sabin., samb., scut.[11],
SEC., sep., spig., staph.[3], stram.,
stroph-h.[6, 8], stry.[11], sul-ac.,
sulph., tab., tarent.[2], ter.[3, 6, 8],
thea, thuj., trif-p.[11], trom.[2, 11],
verat., VERAT-V.[1, 7], vip.[11], zinc.,
zinc-p.[1']

every other beat[3]

nat-m., ph-ac., spig.[2]

third beat[2]

apis[2, 3], arum-t.[3], ars-h.,
cimic.[3, 7, 14], dig.[3, 8], iber.,
kali-c.[6], mur-ac.[1'-3, 6-8],
nat-m.[2, 3, 6, 7, 15], nit-ac.[3, 6],
phas.[15], sulph., vib.

third or fourth beat[3, 6]

apis[15], cimic.

fourth beat[2, 3]

apis[2], calc-ar.[1', 2, 7, 15],
cimic.[3, 7, 14], dig.[3, 8], iber.,
NIT-AC., nux-v., sulph.[2], tab.[3]

third or fifth beat[2, 6]

crot-h.[6], nit-ac.

fourth or fifth beat[3, 6, 15]

nux-v.

fifth beat[2]

ars-h., **chel., coca**[2, 15], crot-h.[6], dig.[8], nit-ac.[6], **nux-v.**[2, 3]

sixth beat

acon.[3], ars-h.[2], **chel.**[2], dig.[8], **mur-ac.**[8]

seventh beat[8]

dig., **mur-ac.**

tenth beat after exertion or vexation[6]

geis.

tenth to thirtieth beat[2]

agar.[2, 3], **cina**, kali-m., lach.[3]

fortieth to sixtieth beat[2]

agar., ars-h.

dinner, after[16]

nat-m.

menses, before[7]

kali-c.

---

old people, in[7]

tab.

irregular

acetan.[8], **acon.**[1], acon-c.[11], **adon.**[3, 6, 8], **adren.**[7, 8], aeth.[15], **agar.**, agar-pa.[11], agarin.[8], aloe, alum., alum-p.[1'], am-caust.[11], aml-ns., anac.[14], ang., anh.[14], anil.[11], **ANT-C.**, ant-t., antip.[8], apis[1], apoc., arg-m., **arg-n.**, arn., **ARS.**, ars-h.[2], **ars-i.**, ars-s-f.[1'], arum-d.[2, 11], **asaf.**, arar.[14], **aspar.**, **atro.**[2, 11], **aur.**, aur-ar.[1'], **aur-s.**[1'], bapt., bar-a.[11], bar-c.[2], bar-m.[11], bell., bell-p.[9, 14], ben-n.[11], benz-ac., bism., bol-lu.[11], **bry.**, bufo[3], **cact.**, cael.[14], calc., calen.[2], camph., cann-i., cann-s.[3], canth., **caps.**, carb-ac., carb-an., carb-v., carbn-o.[11], caust.[3], cham., chel., **CHIN.**, chin-s., **chlol.**[2], chlor.[11], chlorpr.[14], chr-ac.[11], **cimic.**[14], cimx., cinch.[11], clem.[11], coff., coffin.[8], **colch., con., conv.**[6, 8], convo-s.[9, 14], cor-r., cortico.[14], **crat.**[6, 8], **crot-h.**, cub.[2, 11], cupr., cupr-a.[11], cyt-l.[11, 14], **DIG., digin.**[11], digox.[11], dulc.[11], euph.[11], fago.[11], ferr.[1', 3, 8], ferr-p.[3], form.[11], **gels.**, gins.[11], glon., guare.[11], ham., hed.[14], hell., **hep.**, hir.[14], hist.[14], home.[11], **hydr-ac.**[8, 11], **hyos.**, **iber.**[2, 8, 11, 14], ign., iod., jab.[11], jatr.[11], juni.[11], **kali-bi., kali-c.**, kali-chl., kali-cy.[11], **kali-i.**, kali-m.[1'], kali-n.[11], kali-p., kali-s.[11], **kalm., LACH.**, lachn.[2], laur., **lil-t.**[6, 8], lob., lol.[11], **lycps.**, mag-p.[3], mag-s.[9, 14], manc.[2, 3, 6, 11], mang., meny., meph.[14], **merc.**, **merc-c.**, merc-cy., merc-i-f.[2, 11], merc-sul.[2, 11], mez., morph.[11], **mur-ac.**[3, 6, 8], myric.[2], **naja**, nat-ar., nat-f.[9, 14], **NAT-M.**, nat-n.[6], nat-s.[11], nicc.[11], nit-ac., nit-s-d.[11], nux-m.[3, 6, 8], nux-v., oena.[11], **olnd.**, onop.[14], **op.**, ox-ac.,

penic.[14], **PH-AC., phase.**[8], **phos.,**
phys., **phyt.,** pic-ac.[11], pilo.[8],
pip-n.[3], **plan., plb.,** prun-v.[7],
ptel.[11], puls.[3, 8], pyrog., rauw.[9],
rhus-t., sabad., sabin., sacch.[11],
samb., sang., santin.[11], **saroth.**[8, 9],
SEC., seneg., **sep.,** ser-ang.[8], **sil.,**
sol-n.[11], sol-t-ae.[11], **spig., squil.**[3, 6],
stann.[3], **still., STRAM.,**
stroph-h.[3, 8], stroph-s.[9], stry.[11],
stry-ar.[8], stry-p.[8], sul-ac., sul-h.[11],
sulfa.[14], sulo-ac.[11], **sulph.,**
sumb.[2, 3, 6, 8, 11], **tab.,** tanac.[11],
tarent.[11], tax.[11], thea, thiop.[14],
thuj., trach.[11], trif-p.[11], **tub.**[7],
uva[11], valer., **verat., VERAT-V.,**
vib.[2], vip.[3, 6, 11], vip-a.[14], visc.[9],
wies.[11], xan.[11], yuc.[11], zinc.,
zinc-p.[1']

morning[16]
caust.

exertion, on slight

arg-n., meny., **nat-m.**

lying down, on[11]

lycps., still.

lying on back, while

arg-n.

on left side[2]

nat-m.

stool, after

agar.

and slow

acon., arn., ars., asaf., bell.,

camph., cann-i., chel., chin.,
cimic., colch., **DIG.,** dulc., ham.,
hell., hyos., iod., **KALM.,** laur.,
lob., merc-c., merc-cy., mez.,
naja, nit-ac., nux-v., olnd., op.,
ox-ac., ph-ac., phys., phyt., plb.,
rhus-t., seneg., sul-ac., tab.,
verat., **VERAT-V.,** zinc.

irritable

arg-m., ars., colch., dig., iod.,
kali-bi., meny., ox-ac., stram., tab.

jerking

acon., agar.[3], aml-ns.[2, 3, 11], **arn.**[3],
ars.[3, 11], arum-d.[2, 3, 11], aur., bar-c.,
calad.[2, 3, 11], canth.[3], con.[3], dig.[3],
digin.[11], dulc., fago.[3, 11], gins.[3, 11],
glon.[3, 11], **IBER.**[2, 11], jatr.[3, 11], nat-m.[3],
nat-p.[3], nux-v.[3], plb., thuj.[3]

labored

crot-h.[2], cupr., cupr-a.[11], hydr.[11],
iris, kreos., merc., merc-c.[11],
merc-i-f.[2, 11], mit.[11], morph.[11], op.,
stram.

large[3]

ACON., ant-t., **APIS**[2], **arn.,** asaf.,
asar., atro.[11], bar-c., **BELL.**[2, 3 11],
bism., **bry.**[3, 11], camph.[3, 11], canth.,
cench.[11], **chel.**[3, 11], chin., chin-s.[11],
colch.[2, 3], coloc., **CON.**[2, 3, 11], **cupr.,**
cupr-a.[11], dig., dulc., ferr.[3, 11],
ferr-p., gels., glon., hell., hep.,
HYOS., ign., **IOD.**[2, 3], ip.[2], jatr.[11],
kali-cy.[11], **KALI-N.,** lach., led.,
lycps.[0], manc.[0], merc., mez.,
mosch., mur-ac., nat-m., nat-p.,
nux-v., olnd., op.[3, 11], par., petr.,
ph-ac., phos., plb.[3, 11], ran-b., ran-s.,
sabin., samb., **sep.,** sil., **spig.,**
spira.[11], spong., **STRAM.,** stry.[11],
sul-ac.[11], sulph., syph.[3], **tab.**[2],
verat., **verat-v.,** viol-.

slow

abies-n.[8], acet-ac., achy.[14], **acon.,**
acon-c.[11], acon-f., acon-l.[11],
adon.[8], adren.[8], aesc.[3, 6, 8] aeth.,
aether[11], **agar.,** agar-cps.[11],
agar-pa.[11], agn., **all-c.**[2],
am-caust.[11], aml-ns.[2, 11], **amyg.,**
anan.[2], anh.[9, 14], anil.[11], ant-c.,
ant-t., apis[3], apoc., arn., ars.,
ars-met.[2], ars-s-f.[2], asaf., asc-t.[2],
aspar., atro.[11], bapt., bar-a.[11],
bar-i.[1'], **bell.,** ben-n.[11], benz-ac.,
BERB., both.[11], brom., cact.[8],
cain.[11], **camph., CANN-I.,**
cann-s., canth., caps.,
carb-ac.[2, 11], carbn-o.[11], carbn-s.[1'],
catal.[11], caust., cench.[11], **chel.,**
chin., **chin-s.,** chlor.[2, 11], chr-ac.[11],
cic., cimic., coca[11], coff-t.[11],
colch., coloc., **con.,** croc.[11],
crot-h., cryp.[11], cub.[2, 11], cund.[11],
cupr., cupr-am-s.[11], cur.[7], cyt-l.[11],
daph.[2], dat-f.[11], delphin.[11], **DIG.,**
digin.[11], digox.[11], dubo-m.[11], dulc.,
ery-j.[11], esin.[8], euph-c.[11], eupi.[7, 11],
fago.[11], ferr., ferr-ma.[11], gast.[11],
GELS., gins.[11], glon., grat.[11], ham.,
hell., helo.[8], hep., hippoz.[2],
home.[11], hydr.[3, 11], hydr-ac.,
hyos., ign., iod., iris, jab.[11],
jac-c.[11], jatr.[11], juni.[11], kali-bi.,
kali-br.[2], kali-c., kali-chl.,
kali-cy.[11], kali-m.[1'], kali-n,
kali-s.[11], **KALM.,** kreos., kres.[14],
lach., lachn., lact.[11], lat-k.[11],
lat-m.[8, 9, 11], **laur., lob.,** lon-x.[11],
lup.[8, 11], lycpr.[8], **lycps.,** mag-c.[3],
mag-s.[4, 14], **manc., mang.**[3, 11],
mec.[11], meny., meph.[14], merc.,
merc-c., merc-cy., merc-sul.[2],
meth-ae-ae.[11], mez., **morph.**[8, 11],
mosch., mur-ac., myric.,
myrt-c.[3], **naja,** narcot.[11], nat-ar.[2],
nat-c.[3], **nat-m.**[3], nat-n.[6], nit-ac.,
nit-s-d.[11], nitro.[11], **nux-m.,**
nux-v., oena.[11], ol-an.[11], olnd.,
OP., ox-ac., par., pen.[11], petr.,
ph-ac., phel.[11], phos., phys., phyt.,
pic-ac., pip-n.[3, 8], pitu.[9], plb.,

podo., prop.[11], prun.[11], prun-p.[7],
puls., ran-b.[3], raph.[11], rauw.[9],
rhod., rhus-t., ruta, samb., **sang.,**
sars., **sec.,** **SEP.,** sil., sol-n.[11],
solin.[11], spig., spong., squil.,
STRAM., stroph-s.[9], stry.[11],
sulo-ac.[11], sumb.[11], **tab.,** tanac.[11],
tarent.[2], tax.[11], thea[11], thiop.[14],
thuj., thymol.[9, 14], trif-p.[11], trios.[14],
uva[11], upa.[11], valer., **VERAT.**[1, 7],
VERAT-V.[1, 7], verb.[11], vip.[11],
visc.[9, 11, 14], wies.[11], wye.[11], zinc.,
zing.[2]

daytime

dulc.[2], mur-ac., sep.

morning
arg-m., chin-s., grat., jac-c.[11],
lycps.[11], myric.[11], olnd., petr.

forenoon
cinnb., myric.[11]

afternoon
chin-s. gins.[11], myric.[11], ox-ac.

evening
ars., cund.[11], **graph.,** myric.[11],
nat-ar., phyt.

night[11]
phys.

alternating with frequent[8]

bell.[3], chin., cic.[14], cimic.[14], dig.,
gels., iod., **morph.**[7, 8], rhus-t.[3, 5],
stroph-h.[3]

bounding, full and[7]

visc.

chill, during[16]

mur-ac.

fever with[14]

karw-h.

lying, in[16]

dig.

slower than the beat of heart

agar., cann-s., **dig.**, dulc., hell.,
KALI-I.[3], **kali-n.**, kres.[13], laur.,
lyc.[3], **nat-m.**[3], sec., verat.

vomiting, on[16]

squil.

small

ACON., acon-s.[11], **aeth.**[2, 11],
aether[11], **agar.**, agar-pa.[11], agro.[11],
ail.[11], ald.[11], alco.[11], alum., am-c.[3],
am-caust.[11], ammc.[2], amyg.[11], ant-c.,
ant-m.[2, 11], **ant-t.**, apis, apoc.[1'], arn.,
ARS., ars-h.[2, 11], **ars-i.**, ars-s-f.[1', 2, 11],
arum-d.[2, 11], asaf., asc-t.[2, 11], aspar.[11],
aster.[2], atro.[11], **aur.**, aur-ar.[1'],
aur-m., aur-s.[1'], bar-c., bar-i.[1'],
bar-m., **bell.**, ben-n.[11], benz-ac.,
bism., bol-lu.[11], bry., caj.[11], calad.,
calc., calth.[11], **CAMPH.**, cann-i.,
cann-s., canth., carb-ac., carb-an.[3],
CARB V., carbn h.[11], catal.[11],
cham., CHEL.[2, 3], **chin., chin-ar.**[2],
chin-s.[2], **chlor.**[2, 11], cic., **cina**[2, 3, 11],
clem.[3], coca[2], **cocc.**, cod.[11], coff.[2],
colch., coloc.[2, 3, 11], **con.**, conin.[11],
cop.[11], croc.[3], **crot-h.**[2], crot-t.[11],
cub.[2, 11], cund., **CUPR.**, cupr-ar.[2],
cupr-s.[2], cyt-l.[11], delphin.[11], **DIG.,**

digin.[11], **dulc.**, euph-l.[11], ferr.,
ferr-m.[11], fl-ac.[11], frag.[11], gels.,
glon.[2, 11], graph.[3], grat., **GUAJ.**,
gymno.[11], haem.[11], **hell.**, helo.[11],
hippoz.[2], hydr-ac.[11], **hyos.**, iber.[11],
ign., **iod.**, ip., juni.[11], kali-ar.[11],
kali-bi., **kali-br.**[2], **kali-c.**, kali-chl.,
kali-cy.[11], kali-fcy.[11], kali-i.,
kali-m.[1', 2], kali-n., **kali-p.**[2], kali-s.[11],
keroso.[11], **kreos.**, lac-ac., **lach.**, led.,
LAUR., lil-t.[11], **lob.**, lyc., **lycps.**[2],
mang., meny., **merc.**, merc-br.[11],
merc-c., merc-cy., merc-d.[11],
merc-pr-r.[11], merc-n.[11], merc-sul.[2],
meth-ae-ae.[11], **mez.**[2], morph.[11],
mosch.[3], **mur-ac.**, naja[3], narcot.[11],
nat-br.[11], nat-m., nat-n.[11], nat-s.[11],
nit-ac., nit-s-d.[11], **nux-m.**, nux-v.,
oena.[11], **ol-j.**[2], olnd.[11], **op.**, ox-ac.,
past.[11], peti.[11], petr., **ph-ac., phos.**,
phys., phyt., pic-ac., **plat.**, plb.,
plumbg.[11], podo., prun.[11], prun-p.[7],
ptel.[11], puls., ran-a.[11], ran-b., ran-s.,
raph., rhod., rhus-t., ric.[11],
rumx-a.[11], russ.[11], ruta[11], sabad.,
sal-ac.[2], **samb., sang.**[2], sarr.[2, 11],
SEC., seneg., serp.[11], **SIL.**, sol-n.[11],
sol-t.[11], sol-t-ae.[11], solin.[11], spig.,
spirae.[11], spong.[2, 3], squil., **stann.**,
staph., **STRAM.**, stroph-h.[3], stry.[11],
sul-ac., sulph., tab.[3, 11], tanac.[11],
tarent.[2], tax.[11], **ter.**, thea[11], thuj.,
til.[11], upa.[11], uva[11], valer., **VERAT.**,
vesp.[2, 11], viol-o., vip.[11], visc.[7, 11],
wies.[11], zinc., **zinc-m.**[11], **zinc-p.**[1'],
zinc-s.[11]

soft

acal.[8], acet-ac., **acon.**, aesc., aeth.,
aether[11], agar., agn., ant-c.,
ant-s-aur.[11], **ANT-T.**, anth.[11], apis,
apoc., arn., **ars.**, ars-h.[2], arum-d.[11],
aspar.[11], **aster.**, atro.[11], **aur.**, bapt.,
bar-c., bar-m., bell., bism., bry.,
calc-ar.[7], calc-i.[11], camph., cann-i.,
cann-s., canth., **carb-ac., CARB-V.**,
carbn-o.[11], carbn-s.[11], cham., chin.,
chlor.[2, 11], cic., cit-l.[11], cocc.,
coffin.[8], **colch.**, con., conv., crot-h.,
cub.[2], **CUPR.**, cupr-s.[2], cyt-l.[11],

DIG., digin.[11], digox.[11], dulc., ery-a.[11], euph., ferr., ferr-m., **ferr-p.**[3, 6-8], **gels.**, glon.[11], **guaj.**, ham., hell., hep., hydr-ac., hyos., iber.[2], iod., ip., jab.[11], jal., jatr.[11], juni.[11], kali-bi., kali-br., kali-c., kali-chl., kali-cy.[11], **kali-m.**[1', 2], kali-n., **kalm.**, kreos., lac-ac., **LACH.**, lat-m.[14], laur., **lob.**, lyc., **lycps.**[2], **manc.**[2], mang., **merc.**, merc-cy., mez., morph.[11], **MUR-AC.**, **naja,** narcot.[11], nat-ar., nat-m., nat-n.[11], nitro-o.[11], nux-v., oena.[11], **ol-j.**[2], olnd., **OP.**, **ox-ac.**, ph-ac., **phos.**, phys., phyt., **plat.**, plb., polyp-p.[11], puls., ran-s., rhod.[3], rhus-t., **sang.**, santin.[11], sec., seneg., sil., sin-n.[11], sol-n.[11], **spig.**, spirae.[11], **STRAM.**, stry.[11], sul-ac., **sulph.**[2], **sumb.**[2, 11], syph.[3], **tab.**, tarax.[11], **TER.**, thuj., toxi.[11], trios.[14], uva[11], valer., **VERAT.**, **verat-v.**, vip.[11], zinc., zinc-m.[11]

spasmodic

ang.[2, 3], arn.[3], ars., bism., carbn-s.[1', 2], chin.[3], **COCC.**[2, 3], cupr., cupr-a.[11], **dig.**[2, 3], indg.[11], iod.[3], kali-bi.[3], merc., **merc-c.**[2, 3, 11], nux-m., nux-v.[11], plb.[3], sabad., **sec.**[3], sep., **stram.**[2], zinc., zinc-s.[11]

contracted

strong

achy.[14], acon., aether[11], agar.[2], agar-pa.[11], alco.[11], aloe, am-c., aml-ns.[2, 11], amyg.[2, 11], ant-t., apis, arn., ars.[11], ars-h.[2], ars-i.[2, 11], asar., aster.[14], aza.[14], **bell.**, bism.[3], **bry.**[3], caj.[11], cann-i., canth.[3], catal.[11], chel.[3], chin., chin-ar.[2], cinnb.[11], coca[11], con., crot-t., **cupr.**[2, 3], dig.[3], fago.[11], ferr-p.[1'], gast.[11], gels., gins.[11], hell.[3], hoit.[14], hydrc.[11], hyos., iber.[11], iod.[3], jatr.[11], **kali-m.**[2], kreos.[3], lach.[3], lappa[11], laur.[3],

lycps.[11], **merc.**[3], merc-c., merc-cy., merc-i-r.[11], mill., morph.[11], nat-s.[11], op., par.[11], paro-i.[14], petr.[3], **PH-AC.**[3], phys., **puls.**[2], ran-b.[3], raph., sabad., **SABIN.**[2, 3], sang., sarr.[2, 11], seneg., serp.[11], sium[11], sol-t-ae.[11], **SPIG.**[3], stram., stront-c.[3], stry.[11], tanac.[11], ter.[2], uva[11], valer.[3], **verat.**[3], **VIOL-O.**[3]

tense

acon.[3], adren.[7], agro.[11], all-c., all-s.[11], am-c., **am-m.**, ammc.[2], **ant-t.**, aphis[11], ars., atro.[11], bell., ben-n.[11], bism., **BRY.**[2, 3], cann-i., camph., canth., cham., chel.[3], chin., clem., coca[11], coff-t.[11], colch., con., corn-f.[11], **cupr.**[2, 3], dig.[3], **DULC.**[3], ferr., hyos., kali-i., merc-c.[3], **mez.**, morph.[11], nat-c., nit-ac., ox-ac., petr., plb., sabad., **SABIN.**[3], sang., sec., sol-t-ae.[11], spira.[11], squil.[3, 11], stram.[3], til.[11], **valer.**[2, 3, 11], verat.[11], verat-v., zinc.[2, 3, 11]

thready

acon., agar-pa.[11], **ail.**[3, 6], alum., aml-ns.[3, 6], amyg.[2, 11], **apis**[3, 6], arn., **ars.**, ars-s-f.[2], ars-s-r.[2], bell., camph., canth., carb-v., carbn-h.[11], chlf.[11], colch., cop.[11], crat.[6, 11], **crot-h.**[2], cupr., dig., digin.[11], hell., **hydr-ac.**[3, 6], hyos., iod., jatr.[11], kali-bi., kali-n.[11], lach.[3, 6], **LAT-M.**[7, 9, 14], merc-c.[3], merc-ns.[11], morph.[11], naja, nat-f.[9, 14], olnd., op., ox-ac., petr., phos., phys.[11], phyt., **plat.**[2], plb., ptel.[11], **pyrog.**[3, 6], raja-s.[14], rhus-t., sal-ac.[6], santin.[11], sec.[1'], sol-t-ae.[11], solin.[11], **spig.**[3, 6], stram.[2, 3], sul-ac.[11], sulph., tab.[3, 6], tax.[11], **ter.**[2, 11], **VERAT.**[2, 3, 6], verat-v.[3, 6], **verb.**[2], vip.[11], **zinc.**[2], zinc-m.[11]

tremulous

acon., ambr., **ANT-T.**, apis[2], **ars.,
bell., CALC.**, camph., cann-i.,
canth., carb-ac., **cic.**, cina,
cinnb.[11], cocc., colch.[2], crot-h.,
dig., fago.[11], gels., gins.[11], **hell.,
iber.**[2, 11], iod., kali-c., **kreos.,**
lach., merc., merc-c.,
merc-sul.[2, 11], nat-m., nux-m., op.,
ox-ac., phos., plat.[2], plb., **rhus-t.,**
ruta, **sabin., sep., SPIG., staph.,**
stram., sul-ac., valer.

night
calc., narc-po.[11]

eating, after

calc.

undulating

agar. [11, 16], amyg.[11], **ars.**, camph.,
carb-ac.[11], carbn-o.[11], chlf.[11], crot-h.,
dig., digin.[11], gins.[11], iber.[11], op.,
plb.

weak

acet-ac., acon., acon-f.[11], aesc.,
aeth., aether[11], agar.[2, 3, 16],
agar-cps.[11], agar-em.[11], **AGN.**[3],
ald.[11], aloe, alum-p.[1'],
am-caust.[11], am-m., amyg.[2, 11],
ampe-qu.[11], **ant-ar.**[6], ant-c.[3, 6],
ant-m.[2], **ANT-T.**, anth.[11], apis,
apoc.[1'], apom.[11], **arn., ARS.,**
ars-h.[2, 11], ars-s-f.[1'], arum-d.[11], asaf.,
asc-c.[2], **aspar.**, aster.[2], atro.[2, 11],
AUR., aur-ar.[1'], aur-m.[1'], **aur-s.**[1'],
aza.[14], bapt., **BAR-C.**[1', 3, 6], bar-s.[1'],
bell., benz-ac.[2], **BERB.**, bism.[3], bry.,
buth-a.[9], cact.[2], caj.[11], calad.[11],
CAMPH., cann-i., **CANN-S.**[2, 3, 6],
canth., carb-ac.[2], carb-an.,
CARB-V., carbn-chl.[11], carbn-o.[11],
cass.[11], catal.[11], cedr., cench.[11],

cham.[3], chen-a.[11], **chin., chin-ar.,**
chlol.[2], chlor.[11], **CIC.**[3], cimic.,
cimx., cinch.[11], coca[2, 11], **cocc.**[2],
cod.[11], coff.[2, 3], coff-t.[11], colch.,
coloc.[2, 3], con.[3], conin.[11], **crat.**[6],
CROT-H., crot-t., cub.[2], **cupr.,
cupr-a.**[2, 11], cupr-ar.[2, 11], cycl.,
cyt-l.[11], **dig.**, digin.[11], digox.[11],
dios.[2], dirc.[11], dor.[11], erio.[11], ery-a.[11],
eryt-j.[11], fago.[11], fagu.[11], ferr-m.,
gast.[11], **GELS., glon.**, guaj.[3], ham.,
hell., hydr-ac.[6, 7, 11], hydrc.[11], hyos.,
iber.[2, 11], **ign., iod., ip.**, iris, jasm.[11],
jatr.[11], juni.[11], kali-ar.[11], **kali-bi.,
kali-br., kali-c.**[2, 3, 6, 11], kali-n.[11],
kali-ox.[11], kali-t.[11], **kalm.**, keroso.[11],
kreos., lac-ac., **lac-c.**[2], **LACH.,**
lact.[11], lat-k.[11], **LAT-M.**[7, 14], **LAUR.,**
lil-t., lob., lyc.[3], **lycps., lyss.**[2],
manc., mang., **merc., merc-c.,**
merc-cy., merc-i-f.[2], merc-ns.[11],
merc-pr-r.[11], merc-sul.[11],
meth-ae-ae.[11], mez., mom-b.[11],
morph.[11], **mosch.**[3, 11], **mur-ac.,
NAJA**, narcot.[11], nat-f.[9, 14], nat-m.,
nit-ac.[11], nit-s-d.[11], **nux-m.**[2, 3, 6],
nux-v., oena.[2, 11], olnd., op., ox-ac.,
past.[11], peti.[11], **PH-AC., phos.,**
phys., phyt., **PLAT.**[2, 3], plb.,
plumbg.[11], podo., polyp-p.[11], prop.[11],
psor.[2], **puls.**, pyre-p.[11], raja-s.[14],
rhod., **rhus-t.**, rhus-v., ric.[11],
rumx-a.[11], sabin.[11], sacch.[11],
sal-ac.[2], sal-p.[11], **sang.**, santin.[11],
sapin.[11], **sec.**, seneg., sep., sil.[3, 6],
sol-t-ae.[11], solin.[11], **spig.**, spira.[11],
spong.[2], **staph., still.**[2, 11], **stram.**,
stront-c.[3], stry.[1], sul-ac., sul-h.[11],
sulo-ac.[11], **sulph.**[2], sumb.[11], **tab.**,
tanac.[11], **tarent.**[2], tart-ac.[11], tax.[11],
ter.[2, 11], tere-ch.[14], thea[11], **thuj.**[3, 11],
thymol.[9], trif-p.[11], upa.[11], **ust.**[2],
uva[11], **valer.**[2, 3, 11], **vario.**[2], verat.,
verat-v., verb.[11], vesp.[2, 11],
vip.[3, 6, 11], vip-a.[14], xan.[11], zinc.,
zinc-m.[11], zinc-p.[1'], zinc-s.[11],
zing.[11]

morning[16]
sep.

motion, on[1']

bar-s.

wiry

amyg.[2, 11], ars., ben-n.[11], bol-la.[11], cupr., cupr-a.[11], dig., gels., **glon.**[1', 2], ham., iber.[11], kreos., **lac-c.**[2], **lycps.**[2], oena.[11], ox-ac., phos., phys., sec., tax.[11], ter.[2], zinc.

tense

PUNISHMENT agg.[3]*

ambr., con., dig., lach., stann., staph.

PURGATIVES, abuse of[3]

hydr., **nux-v.**[3, 6], op.[3, 6], sulph.

pus see abscesses–pus

QUININE, abuse of*

am-c., **ant-t., apis, ARN., ars.,** ars-s-f.[1'], asaf., aza.[12], **bell.,** bry. **CALC.,** calc-ar.[7], caps., carb-an.[12], **CARB-V.,** cham., chelo.[12], **cina,** coloc.[8], cupr., cycl., dig., eucal.[8, 12], **FERR.** , ferr-ar., gels., hell., **hep.**[2], **IP.,** kali-ar.[1'], **lach.,** mang.[3], meny.[3, 8, 12], merc., **NAT-M.,** nat-p.[7], nat-s.[1'], nux-v., parth.[8], **ph-ac.,** phos.[1], plb., **PULS.,** ran-s.[3], samb., sel.[3, 8], **sep.,** stann., sul-ac., **sulph., verat.**

china

QUIVERING
TSSEN

agar.[3, 11], agn.[3], alum.[3], **am-c.,** am-m.[3], ambr.[3], **ang.**[3], ant-c.[3], ars.[3],

ASAF.[3], bapt.[1'], bar-c.[3], **BELL.,** berb., bism., bov.[3], bry.[3], **calc.,** calc-p.[11], camph.[3], **cann-s.**[3], canth.[3], caps., carb-v.[3], caust., chel.[3], chin.[3], cic.[3], **clem.,** cocc.[1'], colch.[3], coloc.[3], com., **CON.,** croc.[3], cupr.[3], dig., dros.[3], gels.[12], graph.[3], guaj.[3], hell.[3], hep., hyos., ign., iod., ip.[3], kali-c., kali-n., kali-s.[1'], kreos.[3], lyc., mag-c., mag-m.[3], med.[1'], meny.[3], merc.[1', 3], **MEZ.**[3], mosch., mur-ac.[3], **NAT-C.**[3], nat-m.[3], **nit-ac.,** nux-v., par.[3], petr., phos.[3], plat.[1', 3], plb.[3], puls.[3], rhod.[3], rhus-t.[3], ruta[3], sabin.[3], sars., sel.[3], seneg.[3], **sep.,** sil., **spig.**[3], stann., stram.[3], stront-c., sul-ac.[1'], **SULPH.,** tarax.[3], thuj.[3], valer.[3], verb., viol-t.[3], **zinc.**[1', 3]

all over, followed by vertigo

calc.

lying, while

clem.

glands

bell., calc., kali-c., mez., nat-c., sil.

REABSORBENT action[3]

arn., kali-i., sul-i., **sulph.**

REACTION, lack of

aeth.[3], agar., **alum., AM-C., AMBR., anac.,** ant-c., ant-t., apis[7], arn., **ars., ARS-I.**[1], ars-s-f.[1'], **asaf., bar-c.,** bar-m.[3], bar-s.[1'], bell.[7], bism., **brom., bry.**[1, 7], **CALC.,** calc-f.[3, 6], **calc-i., calc-s., camph., CAPS., carb-an., CARB-V.,** carbn-s.[8], **cast.,** caust., cham., **chin.,** cic., **cocc.,** coff., coloc.[3], **CON.**, **cupr.**, cypr.[7], dig.[3], **dulc.**, euph., **ferr.**, ferr-i., **fl-ac.**, **gaert.**[7], **GELS.**, **graph.**, **guaj.**, **HELL.**, hep.[3, 6], **HYDR-AC.**, hyos., **iod.**, **ip.**, kali-bi.[3, 6], **kali-br.**, **kali-c.**, kali-i.[3], luf-o.[14], **lyc.**, mag-c., mag-f.[10], mag-m., **MED.**, **merc.**, mez., **mosch.**, **mur-ac.**, nat-ar.[7, 8], nat-c., nat-m., nat-p., nat-s.[8], nit-ac.[3, 6], **nux-m.**, **OLND.**, <u>**OP.**</u>[1,7], ped.[7], petr., **PH-AC.**, phos., plb., prot.[7], **PSOR.**, puls.[3, 6], rhod., scut.[7], **sec.**, seneg., **sep.**, spong., **stann.**, **stram.**, **sep.**, sul-i.[1'], **SULPH.**, **syph.**, **TARENT.**, thal.[14], **thuj.**, **TUB.**[1', 3, 6-8], **valer.**, vario.[6], **verat.**, verb.[1], x-ray[7, 8], **ZINC.**[1, 7], zinc-p.[1']

irritability – lack.

weakness – reaction

acute danger[3]

ambr., ars., camph., lyc.

chill, after[3]

camph., dulc.

climacteric period, at[3]

con.

convalescence, in[3]

cast., ph-ac.

convalescence–ailments

exanthemas, in[3]

ant-t., **bry.**, cupr., dulc., psor., stram., **sulph.**, zinc.

loss of fluids, after[3]

chin.

remedies, to[3]

carb-v., laur., op.[12], teucr.[2, 12]

nervous patients, in[3]

ambr., laur., op., **VALER.**[2, 3], zinc.

old age, in[3]

con.

suppression, after[3]

lach.

eruptions, of[1']

ars-s-f.

suppressed – eruptions

suppuration, in[3]

calc-f., hep.

abscesses–chronic

REACTION, violent[3]

bell., **cupr., nux-v.,** zinc.

REBELS against poultice[15]

bor., bry., **calc.,** carb-v., **cham., lyc.,**
merc., mur-ac., nit-ac., nux-v., phos.,
puls., rhus-t., sep., spig., staph.,
sulph.

REFLEXES, diminished[3, 6]

alum., arg-n., cur.[3, 6, 8],
kali-br.[3, 6, 11], oena, op.[11], oxyt.[8],
phys., plb.[8], **sec.**[8]

increased[3, 6]

anh.[8], bar-c.[11], cann-i.[8], cic., cocc.,
lath.[3, 6, 8], mang.[8], morph.[11], nux-v.,
stry.[6]

paralysis-spastic

lost[11]

morph., nat-br., sulfon.[8, 12]

RELAXATION of connective tissue[12]

calc.[1'], calc-br., caps., ferr-i., hep.,
kali-c., mag-c., merc-i-r., nit-ac.,
sec., spong.

complexion-fair-lax

muscles, of

acet-ac.[7], aeth.[3], **agar.,** alum.[3],
ambr., amyg.[2], ang.[3], anh.[10], ant-t.,
arg-m.[1'], arn., **ars.,** asaf., atro.[11],
bar-m.[11], bar-s.[1'], bell.[2], bor., bry.,

CALC., calc-sil.[1'], camph., canth.,
CAPS., carb-ac.[3], carb-an.[11],
camph., canth., **CAPS.,** carb-an.[11],
carbn-o.[11], carbn-s.[11], caust[1', 3],
cham., chin., chin-ar., chlor.[11], cic.,
clem., coca[3], **COCC.,** colch.[1'], **con.,**
croc., crot-c., cupr., cur.[3], cycl.[1'],
dig., **dios.,** dros.[3], euph., **ferr.,**
ferr-ar., ferr-i.[12], fl-ac.[3], **GELS.,**
graph., guare.[11], **hell.,** helo.[3], hep.[12],
hydr., hydr-ac.[11], **hyos., iod., ip.,**
jug-r.[11], kali-ar.[1'], **KALI-C.,**
kali-m.[1'], kali-n.[3], kali-p.[3], kali-s.[1'],
lach., laur., **lyc., mag-c.,** mang.[1'],
merc., morph.[11], mur-ac., murx.[1'],
nat-c., nat-p.[1', 7], nit-ac.[12], nux-m.,
nux-v.[11], olnd.[3], op., oxyt., ph-ac.[3],
PHOS., phys.[11], plat., plb., puls.,
rheum, sabad., **sec., seneg., sep.,**
sil., sol-n., spig., **spong.,** stram.[3],
sul-ac., sul-h.[11], **sulph.,** tab.[3, 11],
ter.[11], thuj., **verat.**[3, 11, 12], verat-v.,
viol-o., zinc.[3]

physical[3]

acon., agar., agn., alum.,
ant-t.[3, 11], arn., ars., asar., aur.,
bell., bism., bry., camph., caust.,
cham., chel.[3, 11], chin.[3, 11], cic.,
cina, cocc., coff., colch., cupr.,
cycl., dig., dulc., euph., ferr.,
hydr-ac.[11], hyos., ign.[3, 11], ip.,
kali-c., kali-n., lach.[3, 11], linu-c.[11],
lyc., meny., merc., morph.[11],
nat-c., nat-m., nit-ac., nux-m.,
nux-v., olnd., op., par., petr.,
ph-ac., phos., plat., plb., ran-s.,
rhod., rhus-t., ruta, sabad.,
sabin., sel., sep., sil., spig.,
spong., stann., staph., stram.,
sulph., tarax., verat., viol-o.,
viol-t., zinc.

flabby
weakness

coition, after

agar.[2], sep.[11]

REST agg.[2, 3]

acon.[2, 3, 8], **aesc.**[3, 6], **agar.**[2, 3, 6],
alum.[3], **alumn.**[2], am-c., **am-m.**,
ambr., anac., ang., ant-c., **ant-t.**,
aran-ix.[14], **arg-m.**[1'-3, 6], **arn.**[2, 3, 8],
ars.[2, 3, 6, 8], **asaf.**[1'-3, 6, 8], asar.,
AUR.[2, 3, 6, 8], aur-m.[1'], bar-c., bell.,
bell-p.[14], benz-ac.[3, 6], **bism., bor.,**
bov., bry., calc., calc-f.[8],
CAPS.[2, 3, 8], carb-v., caust.,
cham., chin., cic., cimic.[14], **cina,**
cocc., **coloc.**[1'-3], com.[8], **CON.**[2, 3, 6, 8],
cortiso.[14], cupr., **CYCL.**[2, 3, 8],
dros., DULC.[1'-3, 8], **EUPH.**[2, 3, 8],
euphr., FERR.[1'-3, 6, 8], ferr-ar.[1'],
ferr-p.[1'], fl-ac.[3, 7], foll.[14], gels.[3],
glon.[3], guaj., hecla[14], hep., hyos.,
ign., indg.[8], **iod.**[3, 6], iris[8],
kali-c.[2, 3, 8, 14], kali-i.[3, 6], **kali-n.,**
kali-s.[1'], **kreos.**[2, 3, 6, 8], **lach.**[2, 3, 6],
laur., lith-lac.[8], **LYC.**[2, 3, 6, 8],
mag-c.[2, 3, 6, 8], **MAG-M.**[2, 3, 6],
mang., **meny.**[2, 3, 8], **merc.**[2, 3, 8],
merc-c.[3], merc-i-f.[1'], mez.,
mosch., mur-ac.[2, 3, 6], **nat-c.**[2, 3, 6],
nat-f.[10, 14], **nat-m.,** nat-s.[1', 3, 6],
nit-ac., **nux-m.**[2, 3, 6], olnd.[2, 3, 8],
op., par., petr., **ph-ac.,**
phenol.[13, 14], phos., **plat.,** plb.,
pneu.[14], **PULS.**[1'-3, 6, 8], pyrog.[3],
rhod.[1'-3, 6, 8], **RHUS-T.**[1'-3, 6, 8],
ruta[2, 3, 6], **SABAD.**[2, 3, 8], sabin.,
SAMB.[2, 3, 8], sars., sel.,
seneg.[1'-3, 8], **SEP.**[2, 3, 8], sil., spig.,
spong., stann., staph.,
stront-c.[2, 3, 8], sul-ac.,
sulph.[2, 3, 6, 8], **TARAX.**[2, 3, 8, 14],
tarent.[8], tell.[14], teucr., **thuj.**[1'-3, 6],
tub.[1', 7], tub-r.[14], **VALER.**[1'-3, 6, 8],
verat.[2, 3, 6], **verb., viol-t.**[3],
zinc.[2, 3, 6], zinc-val.[6]

as well as motion agg., during[3]

am-c., bov., calc., carb-an.,
carb-v., caust., mez., ph-ac.,
phos., sulph.

am.[2, 3]

achy.[14], acon.[2, 3, 7], adlu[14], aesc.[8],
agar., **agn.**[1', 3], alum.[3], alum-sil.[1'],
alumn.[2], **am-c.,** am-m., ambr.,
anac., ang., anh.[14], ant-c.[2, 3, 8],
ant-t., aq-mar.[14], arg-m., **Arn.,**
ars., asaf., **asar.,** aur., bar-c.,
bar-m.[3], **BELL.**[1'-3, 8], bism., **bor.,**
bov., **BRY.**[1'-3, 6, 8], buth-a.[10, 14],
cadm-s.[8], **calad., calc.**[2, 3, 6], calc-f.[1'],
calc-p.[1', 3], **camph.,** cann-i.[1', 8],
cann-s., canth., caps., **carb-an.,**
carb-v., caust., cham., **chel.,** chin.,
cic., cina, coc-c.[3, 6], **cocc., coff.,**
COLCH.[2, 3, 6, 8, 14], **coloc.**[2, 3, 6], con.,
crat.[8], **croc., cupr.,** cycl., des-ac.[14],
dicha.[14], **dig.,** dros., dulc., **echi.**[3, 6],
euph., ferr., fl-ac.[3], **GELS.**[2], get.[8],
gink-b.[14], **graph., guaj.**[1'-3], guat.[14],
gymno.[8], **hell., hep.,** hydr.[1'], hyos.,
ign., **iod., ip.,** kali-bi.[1'], kali-c.,
kali-i.[1'], kali-n., kali-p.[8], kalm.[1'],
kreos.[3], lac-d.[1'], lach., laur., **LED.,**
lyc., mag-c., mag-m., mag-p.[1'],
mand.[14], **mang.,** meny., **merc.**[2, 3, 8],
merc-c.[3, 8], **mez.,** mosch., mur-ac.,
nat-c., **nat-m., nit-ac., nux-m.,**
NUX-V.[2, 3, 6, 8], olnd., onop.[14], op.,
par., penic.[13], **petr.,** ph-ac.[1', 2],
penob.[13, 14], **phos.,** phyt.[8], plat.,
plb., prot.[14], pulx.[8], **ran-b., rheum,**
rhod., rhus-t., ruta, sabad., sabin..
samb., sang.[3], **sars., sec., sel.,**
seneg., sep.[2, 3, 6], sieg.[10], sil.,
spig.[1'-3], **spong., squil.**[2, 3, 8], stann.,
staph.[2, 3, 8], **stram.,** stront-c.,
stroph-s.[14], stry-p.[8], **sul-ac.,** sulph.,
teucr., ther.[1'], thuj., trios.[14], verat.,
vib.[8], viol-t.[3], zinc.

must rest[3, 6]

aesc., alum., alum-sil.[1'], **anac.**[3, 6, 14],
arn., brom., **bry.,** lach., lyc., nux-v.,
op., **ph-ac.,** sabad., **stann.**

REVELING, from night

agar.[3], ambr., ant-c., **ars.,** bry., **carb-v.,** coff., colch., ip., **laur.,** led., nat-c.[3], **NUX-V., puls.,** rhus-t., sabin.[3], staph.[3], sulph.

RICKETS[2, 3]

am-c.[3, 12], arg-m.[14], **ars.**[12], **ASAF.,** bar-c.[3], **bell.,** bufo[3], **CALC.**[2, 3, 8, 10, 12], **calc-p.**[2, 3, 6, 10-12], caust.[3], cic.[3], con.[2], **ferr., ferr-i.**[2], ferr-m.[2, 12], ferr-p.[2], **guaj.**[2], hecla[2, 12], hed.[12], **hep.,** iod., **ip.,** iris[8], **kali-i.**[3, 12], lac-c.[2], **lyc.**[2, 3, 6], **MERC.**[2, 3, 11, 12], mez., **nit-ac.**[2, 3, 12], nux-m.[2], **ol-j.**[2], op.[11], petr.[3], **ph-ac.**[3, 6, 10], **PHOS.**[2, 3, 8, 10, 12], plb.[3], **psor.**[2], **puls.,** rhod.[3], **rhus-t.**[2], ruta, sacch.[12], sanic.[12], **sep., SIL.**[2, 3, 8, 10, 12], **staph., sulph.,** tarent.[11], ther.[2, 3, 12], thuj.[2, 3, 12]

RIDING horseback agg.

arist-cl.[9], arg-n.[7], ars., **bell.,** bor.[3, 6], bry., **graph., lil-t.,** mag-m., meph., **nat-c.,** nat-m.[4, 16], psor.[3], **ruta**[2, 3, 7], **SEP.,** sil., spig., **sul-ac.,** ther.[12], valer.

ailments from[12]

ther.

am.
brom., calc., kali-c.[3, 6], lyc., tarent.[3]

cars agg., in a wagon or on the

acon.[6], alum-sil.[1'], **arg-m., arg-n., arn.,** ars., asaf.[1', 3],

aur., bell.[3], berb.[3, 8], **bor.,** bry., calc., calc-p.[3], carb-v., caust.[6, 8], coc-c.[3], **COCC.,** colch.., **con.,** croc., cycl.[2, 7], dig.[3], ferr., fl-ac.[3, 6], graph.[2, 3, 7], grat.[3], **HELON.**[2, 7], **hep.,** hyos., ign., iod., iodof.[2], kali-c., lac-d.[7], **lach.,** lyc., **lyss.,** mag-c., mag-s.[9, 10, 14], meph., nat-m., **nux-m.,** op., **PETR.,** phos., plat., **psor.,** puls., rhus-t., **rumx., sanic.**[7, 8], **sel., SEP., sil.,** spig.[1'], staph., sul-ac.[3], **sulph., TAB.**[3, 7], **ther.,** thuj., tril.[3], valer.

after r. agg.

graph., kali-n., nat-c., nat-m., **nit-ac.,** plat., **SIL.**

aversion to[7]

psor.

down hi.l agg.

BOR., psor.

ailments from[12]

lyc., petr.

am.
arg-n.[6, 7], **ars.,** bar-m.[3], brom., bry.[3], des-ac.[14], **gels.**[3, 6], glon.[3], **graph.**[2, 3], kali-n., lyc.[3], merc.[3], merc-c.[3], naja[7], nat-m.[3, 4, 16], **NIT-AC.,** nux-m.[6], phos., puls.[6], thiop.[14]

ship, ailments form r. in a[12]

ars., petr.[1', 12] ther.

RISING UP agg.

ACON., aesc.[3], agar.[3], alum.,
alum-sil.[1'], **am-m.**, ambr.[3], anac.,
ang.[3], ant-c.[3], **ant-t., apis**[3], arg-m.,
arg-n.[6, 7], **arn., ars.,** asar., aur.[3],
bar-c., bar-m., bar-s.[1'], **BELL.,**
berb.[3, 4], bov., **BRY.,** cact.,
calad., **calc.**[3], **cann-i., cann-s.,**
canth.[3], caps., carb-an.,
CARB-V.[3, 8], caust., **cham., chel.,**
chin., **cic., cina**[3], clem.[3], **COCC.,**
colch., coloc., **con.,** croc., **DIG.,**
dros., dulc.[3], **euph.**[3], **ferr., fl-ac.**[3],
graph.[3], guaj.[3], hell., hep., hyos.[3],
ign., kali-bi.[3], kali-c., kali-m.[1'],
kali-n.[3], kreos.[3], lach., laur., **led.**[3],
lept.[3], **LYC.,** mag-c.[3], mag-m.,
mang., meny., merc., merc-i-f.[3],
mosch.[3], **mur-ac., nat-c., nat-m.,**
nat.-s.[3], **nit-ac., NUX-V., olnd.**[3],
OP., osm., par.[3], **petr.**[3], ph-ac.,
phos., phyt.[6, 8], plat., plb., psor.[1'],
puls., rad-br.[8], ran-b., **rhod.**[3],
RHUS-T., rumx., **ruta**[3], sabad.,
sabin.[3], samb.[3], **sang.,** sars., **sel.**[3],
seneg., sep., **SIL., SPIG.**[3], spong.,
squil., stann., staph., stram.,
stront-c.[3], sul-ac., **SULPH.,** tarax.,
thuj.[3], valer.[3], verat., verat-v.,
viol-t., zinc.

am.

acon., **agar.**[3], agn.[3], alum., **AM-C.,**
am-m., **ambr.**[3, 8], anac.[3], **ang.**[3],
ant-c.[3], **ant-t., arg-m.**[3], ant-c.[3], **ARS.,**
asaf., asar.[3], aur., bar-c., bell.,
bism.[3], **bor.,** bov., bry., **CALC.,**
cann-s., canth., **CAPS.**[3, 6], carb-an.[3],
carb-v., caust., **cham.,** chel., chin.,
cic., **cina**[3], cocc.[3], colch.[6], coloc.,
con., cupr., **CYCL.**[3], **dig., dros.**[3],
DULC.[3], **euph.**[3], euphr.[3], ferr.,
graph.[3], guaj.[3], hell., hep., **hyos.,**
ign., iod.[3], **kali-c.,** kali-n.[3, 6], kreos.[3],
lach.[3], laur., **led.**[3, 6], lith-c.[8], **lyc.,**
mag-c., **mag-m.**[3], mang., **meny.**[3],
merc., mez.[3], mosch., **mur-ac.**[3], naja,
nat-c., nat-m., nit-ac.[3], nux-m.,
nux-v., olnd., op.[3], par.[3], parth.[8],
petr., **ph-ac.**[3, 4, 6], phos., **PLAT.**[3, 16],

plb.[3], puls., **rhod.**[3], rhus-t., **ruta**[3],
sabad.[3], sabin., **SAMB.,** sars.[3], sel.[3],
seneg.[3], **SEP., sil.,** spig., spong.[3],
squil., stann., staph.[3], sul-ac.,
sulph., **tarax.**[3], teucr., thuj.[3],
valer.[3], verat.[3], **VERB.**[3], viol-o.[3],
VIOL-T.[3], zinc.[3]

ROOM full of people agg.

ambr., **ant-c.,** apis[1', 3], **arg-n.,** ars.,
bar-c., carb-an., con., **hell.,**
iod.[1', 3, 6], kali-i.[1', 3, 6], lil-t.[1', 3],
lyc., mag-c., nat-c., nat-m., petr.,
phos., plb., **puls.,** sabin., **sep.,**
stann., stram., **sulph.**

Vol. I: *fear – narrow place – trains*

close r. agg.[5]

alum.[1'], arist-cl.[14], ars-i.[1'] bar-s.[1'],
nux-v., puls., rauw.[14], staph.,
sulph., tub.[7]

Vol. I: *fear – narrow place – trains*

RUBBING agg.

am-m., **ANAC., am., ars.,** bism.,
bor., **calad., calc.,** cann-s., canth.,
caps., carb-an., **caust.,** cham., chel.,
coff., **CON.,** cupr., dros., guaj.,
kreos., **led.,** mag-c., mang., merc.,
mez., mur-ac., nat-c., par., ph-ac.,
phos.[2, 8], **PULS.,** seneg., **SEP., sil.,**
spig., spong., squil., stann., staph.,
stram., **STRONT-C., SULPH.,**
thuj.[3]

am.

acon., agar., agn., **alum., alumn.**[2],
am-c., **am-m.**, ambr., anac.,
ang.[2, 3], ant-c., ant-t., **arn., ars.,
asaf.**, bell., bell-p.[10], benz-ac.[2],
bor., bov., bry., **CALC.**, calc-f.[7],
camph., cann-s., **CANTH.**, caps.,
CARB-AC., carb-an., cast.[3, 6],
caust., cedr., chel., chin., cic.,
cina, colch., croc.[3], **cupr.**[3], **cycl.**,
dios., **dros.**, form.[8], **guaj.**, ham.,
hed.[10, 14], hep., **ign.**, indg.[4, 8],
iod.[10], kali-c., kali-m.[1'], kali-n.,
kreos., laur., lil-t., mag-c.,
mag-m., **mag-p.**[3, 8], mang., meny.,
merc., mim-p.[14], mosch., **mur-ac.**,
NAT-C., nit-ac., **nux-v.**,
OL-AN.[1, 7], olnd., osm., pall.,
ph-ac., **PHOS.**, plat., **PLB.**,
podo.[3, 8], puls.[3, 10], ran-b.,
rhus-t., **ruta**, sabad., sabin.,
samb., sars., sec., sel., seneg.,
sep.[3], sil.[3], spig., spong., stann.,
staph., sul-ac., **sulph.**, tarax.,
tarent.[1', 3, 6-8], **thuj.**, valer.,
verat-v.[3, 6], viol-t., **zinc.**, zinc-p.[1'],

clothes am., of[3]

bufo

gently agg., stroking

teucr.

but hard r. am.[3]

rhus-t.

with hand am.[2]

arn., **asaf., CALC., caps.**, cina,
croc., **CYCL., dros.**, guaj., ign.,
mang., meny., **merc., mur-ac.,
NAT-C.**, phos., plb., puls., **ruta**,
sulph., **thuj.**, zinc.

RUNNING agg.

alum., alumn.[2], **ang.**[2, 3], arg-m., **arn.,
ARS.**, ars-i., ars-s-f.[1'], aur., aur-ar.[1'],
aur-i.[1'], aur-s.[1'], **bell.**, bor., **BRY.**,
calc., **cann-s., caust.**, chel., chin.,
cina, **cocc.**, coff., **con.**, croc.,
cupr., dros., **ferr.**, ferr-ar.[1'], hep.,
hyos., **ign.**, iod., ip., **kali-c.**, laur.,
led., lyc., merc., mez., nat-c.,
nat-m., nit-ac., nux-m. **nux-v.**,
olnd., phos., plb., **PULS.**, rheum,
rhod., rhus-t., ruta, sabin., **seneg.**,
sep., **sil., spig.**, spong., squil.,
staph., sul-ac., **SULPH.**, verat.,
zinc.

walking – fast

am.

ars.[3], brom.[3], caust., fl-ac.[3], graph.[3],
ign., nat-m., nit-ac.[3], **SEP.**, sil.,
stann., sul-ac.[3], tarent.[3], thlas.[3]

SALT abuses[12]

nit-s-d., phos.

SARCOMA

bar-c., calc-f., carb-ac.[2], **crot-h.**[2],
cupr-s.[7], graph.[2], hecla[2, 7, 12], **kali-m.**[2],
lap-a.[2, 7]

SCARLET fever, after

AM.C.[3], **AM-M.**, aur., bar-c., **BELL.,
bry., calc., carb-ac., carb-v.,
CHAM., con.**[3], dulc., euph., **hep.**,
hyos., **lach.**, lyc., **merc.**, nit-ac.,
petros.[12], phos., rhus-t., **sulph.**

exanthema repelled[4]

phos.

glands swollen[15]

am-c., **BAR-C., lac-c**[2].

SCLEROSIS, multiple[7]

alum.[8], arg-m.[14], arg-n., **aur.**, aur-m.[12], bar-c., bell.[8], calc., cann-i.[8], carbn-s.[12], caust., **con.**[8], des-ac.[14], gels., halo.[14], hyosin.[12], irid.[8], **lath.**[7, 8, 12], lyc., mand.[14], nux-v., **phos.**[7, 8], **phys.**[7, 8, 12], **pic-ac.**[8, 12], **plb.**[2, 7, 8], psil.[14], sil., sulph., tarent.[7, 12], thala.[14], thuj., wildb.[12], xan.[8]

SCURVY, scorbutus

acet-a.[8], agav-a.[8, 12], agn.[1] (non: ang.), all-s.[12], alum., alumn.[12], **am-c.,** am-m.[12], ambr., ant-c., arg-m., aran.[2, 12], **ars.**[1], ars-i., arum-m.[12], aur., bell., bor., bov., brass.[12], bry., **calc.,** canth., caps., **carb-an., CARB-V.,** cary.[12], caust., cetr.[12], chin., cic., **cist.,** c[i+]-ac.[11], cit-l.[12], cit-v., coca[12], coch.[12], con., **dulc.,** elat.[12], graph., **ham.**[12], **hep., iod.,** jug-r.[12], **kali-c.,** kali-chl.[12], **kali-m.**[2, 3, 12], kali-n., kali-p.[2], kreos., lach.[12], lyc., mag-m., **MERC., MUR-AC.,** nat-hchls.[12], **nat-m., nit-ac.,** nux-m., **NUX-V.,** petr., ph-ac., phos., plb.[11], psor.[12], rat.[12], rhus-t., ruta, sabin., sacch.[11, 12], sanic.[12], sep., **sil.,** sin-n.[12], sol-t-ae.[12], stann., **STAPH.,** sul-ac., **sulph.,** tep.[12], zinc.

seashore see air–seashore

SEASONS

autumn, agg. in

all-c.[12], **ant-t.,** aur., bani., bar-m., bry., **calc.,** calc-p.[3, 6, 7], **chin.,** cic., **colch.**[1, 7], coloc.[3],

dulc.[1', 3, 7], **graph.**[1, 7], hed.[10], hep., ign.[3, 6, 7], iris[3, 7], **KALI-BI.**[1, 7], **LACH., merc.**[1, 7], merc-c.[3, 7], nat-m.[3, 6, 7], nux-v., rhod.[7, 12], **RHUS-T., stram., verat.**

ailments since[12]

kali-bi.

am.[14]
flav.

spring, agg. in*

acon., all-c.[3, 7, 8, 12], **AMBR.**[1, 7], **ant-t., apis, ars-br.**[8], **aur.**[1, 7], bar-m., **BELL.**[1, 7], brom.[1', 7], **bry.**[1, 7], **CALC.**[1, 7], calc-p.[3, 6-8], **carb-v.**[1, 7], **cench., chel.,** cina[16], **colch.,** con.[12], **crot-h.**[1', 3, 4, 6-8], dulc., **GELS.**[2, 3, 7, 8], ham.[3], hed.[10], hep., **iris, kali-bi., LACH., LYC.**[1, 7], merc-i-f.[12], nat-c.[3, 7], **nat-m.**[1, 7], **nat-s.,** nit-s-d.[7, 8], nux-v., **puls.,** rhod.[7, 12], **rhus-t., sars.**[1, 7], sec., sel.[3], **sep.**[1, 7], **sil.**[1, 7], **sulph.**[1, 7], urt-u.[3], **verat.**

ailments since[12]

con., kali-bi., merc-i-f.

am.[14]
flav.

summer, agg. in

acon.[1', 8], **aeth.,** aloe[3, 6-8], **alum.,** alum-sil.[1'], **ANT-C.**[1, 7], apis[3, 6, 7], arg-n., ars-i., bapt.[2, 7], bar-c., **BELL.**[1, 7], bor., bov.[2, 3, 7], brom.[1', 7], **BRY.**[1, 7], calc.[3], **CAMPH.**[2, 7], **CARB-V.**[1, 7], carbn-s., cham., **chion.,** cina[3, 6, 7], cinnb., coff.[1'], croc.[8], crot-h.[3, 6, 8], crot-t.[7, 8], cupr.[3, 6, 7], dulc.[3], **FL-AC., gamb.**[2, 7], **GELS.**[2-3, 7, 8],

GLON.[1'-3, 6-8], graph., **guaj., iod.,**
iris[3, 7], **KALI-BI.,** kali-br.[7],
kali-c.[6, 7], kali-i.[3], **LACH.**[1, 7],
lyc.[1, 7], mur-ac.[3, 7], **NAT-C.**[1, 7],
nat-m., nit-ac.[8], nux-m.[3, 7],
nux-v., ph-ac.[3, 7], **phos.**[3, 7, 8],
pic-ac.[8], **PODO.**[3, 6-8, 12], **psor.,**
PULS.[1, 7], rheum[7], rhod.[3, 6, 7],
sabin.[8], **sel.,** sep.[3, 6, 7], sin-n.[12],
sul-i.[1'], syph.[1', 7, 8], thuj.,
verat.[2, 7], verat-v.[3, 7]

ailments since[12]

podo., sin-n.

am.[3]
aesc.[3, 7], alum.[8], ars-i., aur.[8],
aur-ar.[1'], calc-p.[8], calc-sil.[1'],
caust.[7], ferr.[8], kali-sil.[13], **petr.,**
psor., sil.[7, 8], stront-c.[3, 6]

children, in[7]

ip.

cool days in, after[2, 7]

BRY.

summer solstice agg.[7]

apis., **BELL.,** brom., bry., **carb-v.,**
gels, iris, **kali-bi., LACH.,** lyc.,
nat-c., **nat-m.,** nux-v., **puls.,** rhod.,
sep., **verat.**

winter, agg. in ✱

ACON.[1, 7], **aesc.,** agar., **alum.,**
AM-C.[1, 7], ammc., **arg-m.,**
ARS.[1, 7], **AUR.,** aur-ar.[1'], aur-s.[1'],
bar-c.[1, 7], **bell.,** bor.[7], bov.,
BRY.[1, 7], **calc., calc-p.,** calc-sil.[1'],
CAMPH.[1, 7], **caps.**[1, 7], carb-an.,

carb-v.[1, 7], carbn-s.[1'], **caust.,**
cham.[1', 7], cic., cina, cist.[3, 7],
coc-c., cocc.[1, 7], colch., **con.**[1, 7],
DULC.[1, 7], **ferr.,** ferr-ar., **FL-AC.,**
graph.[1', 3, 7], **HELL.**[1, 7], **HEP.**[1, 7],
hyos.[1, 7], **ign.**[1, 7], **ip.**[1, 7], **kali-bi.,**
KALI-C.[1, 7], **kali-p.,** kali-sil.[1'],
kalm.[3, 7], **LYC.**[1, 7], mag-c.,
MANG.[1, 7], **merc., mez.,**
MOSCH.[1, 7], nat-ar., nat-c.,
nat-m., **NUX-M.**[1, 7], **NUX-V.,**
PETR.[1, 7], ph-ac., **phos.,** prot.[14],
PSOR.[1, 7], **PULS.**[1, 7], rhod.[1, 7],
RHUS-T., ruta, **sabad.,**
sang-n.[7, 12], sars., sec.[3], **sep., sil.,**
spig., spong., stann.[3, 7],
STRONT-C.[1, 7], **sulph.**[1, 7],
syph.[1', 7], **VERAT.**[1, 7], viol-t.

ailments since[12]

sang-n.

am.[1']
glon., ilx-a.[8], ilx-c.[2, 7], sul-i.

winter solstice agg.[7]

aur., bry., **calc.,** calc-p., cic.,
colch., **dulc.,** graph., hep., ign.,
kali-bi., merc., nat-m., nux-v.,
rhod., RHUS-T., verat.,

SEDENTARY habits[8, 12]

acon., aloe, alum.[5, 12], am-c.[7, 8, 12],
anac.[7, 8, 12], arg-n.[8], ars.[16], asar.[12],
bry.[5, 8], **calc.**[5, 12], cocc.[12], con., **lyc.**[5],
nat-m.[12], **NUX-V.**[3, 5, 7, 8, 12], petr.[12],
rhus-t.[5], sep., sil.[12], staph.[5],
sulph.[1', 3, 12], ter.[12]

SENSITIVENESS externally

acon., aesc., agar., ail.[12], aloe,
alum., alum-p.[1'], alum-sil.[1'], am-c.,
am-m., ambr., ang.[3], ant-c., ant-t.,

APIS, arg-m., ARN., ars., asaf., aur., aur-ar.[1'], bapt., bar-c., bar-s.[1'], BELL., bor., bov., bry., calc., calc-p., calc-sil.[1'], camph., cann-s., canth., caps., carb-an., carb-v., caust., chel.[1'], CHIN., CHIN-S., cimic., cina, clem., coc-c., coff., colch., coloc., con., crot-c., cupr., dig., euph-pi.[12], ferr., ferr-p., gels., glon.[12], graph.[1'], ham.[1'], hell., hep., hist.[10], hyos., ign., ip., kali-bi., kali-c., kali-i.[12], kali-n., kali-p., kali-s., kreos., LACH., led., lyc., mag-c., mag-m., menth., meny.[3], merc., merc-c.[3], mez., mosch., mur-ac.[3], nat-ar., nat-c., nat-m., NAT-P., nat-s.[1'], nat-sil.[1'] nit-ac., nux-m., NUX-V., olnd., op., par., petr., ph-ac., PHOS., plb,, psor., PULS., RAN-B., ran-s., rhus-t., sabad., sabin., sal-ac., sars., sec., sel., seneg., sep., SIL., SPIG., spong., squil., stann., STAPH., stront-c., sul-ac., sulph., teucr., thuj., valer.[1'], verat., zinc.

internally

acon., agar., alum., alum-p.[1'], alum-sil.[1'], am-c., ant-c., ant-t., apis, arn., ars., ars-i., asaf., asar., aur., aur-ar.[1'], bapt., bar-c., bell., bism., bor., bov., bry., calad., calc., cann-s., CANTH., carb-an., carb-v., carbn-s., caust., cham., chin., cic., cimic.[1'], clem., coc-c., cocc., coff., colch., coloc., con., croc., crot-h., cub., cupr., cycl., dulc., equis., ferr., graph., hell., helon., HEP., hyos.[1], iod., ip., kali-bi., kali-i., kali-p., LACH., laur., led., lil-t., mag-c., mag-m., mang., meny., merc., merc-c., mez., mosch., nat ar., nat-c., NAT-M., nit-ac., nux-v., olnd., osm., par., PHOS., puls., ran-b., rhus-t., ruta, sars., sec., sel., seneg., sep., SIL., spong., squil., stann., stram., stront-c., sul-ac., sulph., tarax., tarent., teucr., thuj., valer., verat., zinc.

pain, to

acon., agar., alum., am-c., ambr., anac., ang.[3], ant-c., ant-t., arg-n.[3], arn., ars., ars-i., ars-s-f.[1'], asaf.[1'], asar., AUR., aur-ar.[1'], aur-m.[8], aur-s.[1'], bar-c., bar-i.[1'], bar-s.[1'], bell., bry., cact., calad., calc., calc-p., calc-sil.[1'], camph., cann-s., canth., caps., carb-an., carb-v., carbn-s.[1', 7], CHAM., chin., chin-ar., cimic.[3], cina, cocc., COFF., colch., con., cupr., dig., ferr., ferr-ar.[1'], ferr-p., graph., hell., HEP., hyos., hyper.[8], IGN., iod., ip., kali-ar., kali-c., kali-m.[1'], kali-p., lac-c.[3], LACH., lact.[10], laur., led., LYC., mag-c., mag-m., mag-p.[3, 6, 8], MED., meli.[8] merc., mez.[8], morph.[2, 8, 10] mosch.[8], mur-ac., nat-c., nat-p., nat-s.[1', 7], NIT-AC., nux-m., NUX-V., olnd., petr., ph-ac., PHOS., phyt., plat.[3] plb,, PSOR., PULS., ran-s.[8], rhus-t., sabad., sabin., sars., sel., seneg., SEP., SIL., spig., squil., STAPH., stram.[3, 6], sulph., thuj., tub., valer., verat., vesp., viol-o., zinc., zinc-p.[1'], zinc-val.[8]

Vol. I: *sensitive – pain*

bones, of

asaf., aur., bell., bry., bufo[2], calc., carb-an., chel., chin., chin-s., cupr., EUP-PER., guaj., hyper., kali-bi.[3], lach., lyc., merc., merc-c., mez., nat-c., nat-sil.[1'], PHOS., puls., rhus-t,, sil., stram., sulph., symph.[3], TELL., zinc.

pain – bones

cartilages, of

ARG-M.

pain – cartilages

glands, of

arn., **aur.**, aur-s.[1'], **BAR-C.**, bar-i.[1'],
bell., **cham.**, chin., cimic.[1'], clem.,
cocc., **CON.**, crot-h., cupr., graph.,
hep., ign., kali-c., laur., **lyc.**,
mag-c., nat-c., nat-sil.[1'], nit-ac.,
nux-v., petr., ph-ac., **PHOS.**, puls.,
sep., sil., spig., squil., sul-ac., zinc.

pain – glands

periosteum

acon.[3], ant-c., aur., bell., **bry., chin.**,
chin-s.[3], ign., **LED.**, mang.[3], merc.,
merc-c.[3], **mez.**, nit-ac.[3], **ph-ac.**,
puls., rhus-t., ruta, sil., spig.,
staph., symph.[12], tell.[3]

pain – periosteum

SEPTICAEMIA, blood-poisoning

achy.[14], **acon.**[8], agar.[12], **ail.**[1', 6],
am-c.[1', 6, 10], anthraci., ap-v.[8], **apis,**
arg-m.[14], arg-n., **arn., ARS.,**
ars-i.[6, 8], arum-t.[6], atro.[8], **bapt.,**
bell.[6, 8], bor-ac.[12], both.[8], **bry** bufo[6],
calc.[1', 2, 7], calc-ar.[6, 7], calen.[8],
carb-ac.[6, 8], **CARB-V.**, **cench.**,
chin.[10], **chin-ar.**[6, 8, 10], **chin-s.**[8, 10, 12],
chlorpr.[14], colch.[6], conch.[12],
CROT-H., dor.[6], **echi.**[3, 6-8, 10, 12],
elaps[6], **ferr.**, ferr-p.[6], gels.[6], gunp.[8],
hell.[6], **hippoz.**, hydroph.[14], hyos.[6, 8],
ip.[6, 10], irid.[8], kali-bi.[2, 6], kali-c.[6],
kali-p., kreos.[6], **LACH.**, lat-h.[8],

lob-p.[12], **lyc.**, mag-c.[10], **merc.**[8, 12],
merc-cy.[3, 6, 8], methyl.[8], mur-ac.[6, 8],
naja[6], nat-s-c.[8], **nit-ac.**[6], op.[6],
paro-i.[14], ph-ac.[6], **phos., phyt.**[6],
puls., PYROG., rad-br.[7], raja-s.[14],
rhus-t., sal-ac.[2], **sec.**[6, 8], sieg.[10], sil.[8],
stram.[1', 6], streptoc.[8], sul-ac.[6],
sulfonam.[14], **sulph.**, tarax.[6], tarent.,
tarent-c.[6, 8], **ter.**[3, 6], trach.[12],
verat.[2, 3, 6, 8, 12], **verat-v.**[3, 6, 10],
vip.[6], zinc.[6]

ailments from[12]

agar., gunp., lob-p., pyrog., tarent.

SEWER-GAS poisoning[12]

bapt., phyt., pyrog., **tub.**[7]

SEXUAL excesses, after*

acon., **AGAR.**, agn., alum.,
alum-p.[1'], anac., ant-c., arg-n.[7, 12],
arn., **ars.**, asaf., aur., aur-ar.[1'],
aven.[8, 12], bar-c., bell., bor.,
bov., bry., **calad.**[1, 7], **CALC.,**
calc-p.[12], **calc-s.**, cann-s., canth.,
caps., carb-an., **CARB-V.**[1], caust.,
cham., **chin., chin-ar.**, cina,
cocc., coff., **CON., dig.**, digin.[8],
dulc., ferr., ferr-pic.[12], **gels.**,
graph., ign., **iod.**, ip.[1], **kali-br.**,
kali-c., kali-n., **KALI-P.**, led., **lil-t.**,
LYC., lyss.[8], mag-m., **merc.**, mez.,
mosch., nat-c., NAT-M., NAT-P.,
nit-ac., NUX-V., ol-an.[6], onos.[12],
op., petr., **PH-AC., PHOS.**, plat.,
plb., **puls.**, ran-b., rhod., rhus-t.,
ruta, sabad., samb., sec., **SEL., SEP.**
SIL., spig., squil., stann., **STAPH.,**
SULPH., symph.[12], thuj.,trib.[8],
upa.[12], valer., zinc., zinc-p.[1']

excitement agg.

agar.[1'], arg-n.[12], arn.[12], **bufo.**,
calc.[2], cinch.[12], gins.[12], kali-p.[12],
LIL-T., sars., sep.[1'], staph.[12]

drunkenness, s. e. during[5]

canth., **caust.**, chin., nux-v., phos.

suppression of s. desire agg.

agn.[3, 6], **APIS**, bell.[3], berb.,
calc., **CAMPH., carb-v.**[2, 3],
carbn-o., CON., graph.[3, 6], **hell.**,
hyos.[3], **kali-br.**[2], kali-p.[12], lil-t.,
lyc.[3, 7], mosch.[2], orig.[7], **ph-ac.**,
phos.[3, 6], pic-ac., plat., **PULS.**,
staph.[3, 6], stram.[3]

ailments from[12]

con., kali-p.

am.
calad.

climacteric period, during[7]

con.

SHAVING agg.[3]

ant-c., aur., caps.[3, 6, 8], **carb-an.**[3, 6, 8],
hep., kalm., mang., ox-ac.[3, 8],
ph-ac., phos., plb.[8], **PULS.**, rad-br.[3],
stroph-s.[15]

am.[3, 6, 8]
brom.

SHINING objects, ailments from[6]

bell., canth., glon., hyos., stram.

Vol. I: *shining*

SHOCK agg.[3]

acet-ac., **acon.**[3, 12], am-c., arn.,
camph., cham., cic., coff., gels.,
hep., hyos., hyper.[3, 12], mag-c.[12],
merc., nat-m., op., ph-ac.[12], puls.,
sec., stram.[12], stront-c., sulph.,
verat.

injury see shock–injury

electric-like

acon., agar., ail., alum., alum-p.[1'],
ambr., anac., ang., apis,
aran-ix.[10], **ARG-M., arg-n.**, arn.,
ARS., ars-s-f.[1'], **art-v.**, bar-c.,
bar-m., bar-s.[1'], bell., bufo,
calad., calc., **calc-p., camph.**,
cann-s., carb-ac., carb-v., caust.,
cic., cimic., **cina, clem., cocc.**,
colch., con., croc., cupr., **dig.**,
dulc., **fl-ac.**, graph., hell., hep.,
hydr-ac.[6], kali-c., kreos., **laur.**,
lyc., mag-m., manc., mang.,
meph.[11], mez., mur-ac., nat-ar.,
nat-c., **nat-m.**, nat-p., **nit-ac.**,
nux-m., nux-v., ol-an., olnd.,
op.[3], ox-ac.[6], **phos.**, plat., plb.[6, 11],
puls., **ran-b., ruta**, sang.[6], sep.,
spig., squil., stram., **stry.**, sul-ac.,
sulph., sumb., **tab., thal.**, thuj.[3],
valer.[1', 6], **VERAT.**, verat-v.[6],
xan., zinc., zinc-p.[1']

right side of body

agar.

morning[16]
  mang.

evening in bed[16]

  sulph.

concussion of brain, from

  CIC.

  ailments–commotion of brain

convulsions, before

  bar-m., laur.

interrupted by painful shocks

  stry.

epilepsy, before

  ars.

lying, while

  clem.

motion, on beginning of

  arg-n.

during
  colch.[7], graph.

rest, during,

  graph.

return of senses, on

  cic.

sleep, during

  arg-m., ars., iod.[11], kreos., lyc., mez.[16], **nat-m., nux-m.**

  jerking – sleep.

on going to

  agar., alum., **ARG-M., ARS., bell.,** calc.[16], **ip.,** kali-c.[16], nat-ar., **nat-m., nit-ac., phos., stry.,** thuj.[16]

slow pulse, with

  dig.

touched, when[7]

  colch.

touching anything

  alum.

waking, while

  alum-p.[1'], lyc., **mag-m.,** manc.

wide awake, while

  mag-m., nat-p.

injury, from

acet-ac.[2], **ACON.,** am-c., **ARN.,**
ars.[2], bell., **calc.**[2], calen.[7],
CAMPH., caps., carb-v., cham.,
chin.[2], **chlf.**[2], **cic.,** cocc., **coff.,**
cupr., cupr-ar.[6], **DIG.**[2], **gels.,**
hell.[2], hep.[2], **hydr-ac.**[2], hyos.[6],
HYPER., ip., LACH., laur.[2], lyc.[2],
merc., **nat-m.**[2], nit-ac.[2], **nux-m.**[2],
nux-v.[2], **OP., phos.**[2], psor., **ran-b.,**
sec., sep.[2], **staph.,** stront-c.,
stry-p.[6], sulph., **tab.**[2], **VERAT.**

faintness–injury

injuries

fractures, from[7]

acon., arn.

SHORTENED muscles and tendons

abrot.[6], ambr., am-c., **am-caust.**[6],
AM-M., anac., ars., aur., **bar-c.,** calc.,
carb-an., carb-v., **CAUST.,** cic., **cimic.,**
coff.[6], **COLOC.,** con., cupr., dig., dros.,
ferr.[6], form.[6], **GRAPH., guaj.,** hell.,
hep., hyos., iod.[6], kali-c., kali-i.[6],
kreos., lach., led., **lyc.,** mag-c., **merc.,**
mez., mosch., **nat-c., NAT-M.,** nit-ac.,
nux-v., olnd.[6], ox-ac., petr., ph-ac.,
phos., plb., puls., ran-b., rheum,
rhus-t., ruta, samb., sec.[6], **sep.,** sil.,
stann., sul-ac., sulph., tell.[6]

SHOT rolling through the arteries,
sensation

nat-p.

SHRIVELLLING

abrot.[6], alum.[6], am-c.[4], am-m., ambr.[4],
ant-c.[4, 6], **arg-n.,** arn., **bar-c.**[6], bism.,
bor.[3, 6], bry.[4], **calc.**[1', 4, 6], camph.[4],
cham.[4], chin., cupr., fl-ac.[6], hell.[4],
graph.[4, 6], kali-br.[6], **lyc.**[4-6], merc.,
mur-ac.[4], nux-v.[4], op.[6], ph-ac.[4], plb.[4],
psor.[1'], rheum[4, 6], rhod., rhus-t.[4],
sabad.[4], **sars.**[1', 4], **sec.**[1', 4, 6], **sep.**[1', 4, 6],
sil.[5], spig.[4], stram.[4, 6], **sulph.**[1', 4-6],
verat., viol-o.[4, 6], vip.[4], zinc.

SHUDDERING, nervous

absin.[11], acon., acon-l.[11], aether[11],
agar.[11], aloe[11], anac., **am-m., ARN.,**
ars.[3], asar.[11, 16], aur., **bell.,** benz-ac.,
blatta-a.[11], bond.[11], bor.[11], **brom.**[11],
bry.[11], caj.[11], calc., camph., cann-s.,
caps.[11], caust., cham.[0, 11], **cimic.**[2, 3, 15],
cina, clem.[11], **cocc.,** cupr.,
cupr-s.[11], cycl.[11], dig.[11], digin.[11],
dios.[3, 11], dros.[11], dulc.[11], elae.[11],
elaps.[11], eup-per.[11], euph.[11],
gast.[11], **gels.,** gins.[11], glon.[3], graph.[11],
haem.[11], hell.[3, 11], hura[11], hydr-ac.[11],
hyos., **hyper.**[3], ign.[3, 11], ip.[11],
iris-fl.[11], junc-e.[11], kali-c.[11],
kali-chl.[11], kali-n.[11], kalm.[11], kiss.[11],
kreos., **lach.**[11], laur., **led.,** linu-c.[11].
lyc., mag-m., mag-s.[11], mang.,
merc.[11], merc-i-r.[11], merc-sul.[11],
mez., morph.[11], mosch.[3, 11], **nat-m.,**
nit-ac.[11], nux-m., **NUX-V.,** op.[11],
osm.[11], ped.[11], ph-ac., phos., phys.[3],
phyt.[11], plat.[11], plb.[11], podo.[11],
polyp-p.[11], **puls.,** ran-b.[3], raph.[11],
rheum[3, 11], **rhus-t.,** ruta[11], samb.[11],
scroph-n.[11], seneg., sep., **sil.,**
sin-n.[11], **spig.,** stann.[11], staph.,
stram.[11], tab.[11], tarent.[11], thuj.[3, 11],
til.[11], upa.[11], valer., verat., viol-t.,
vip.[11], zinc.[3, 11], zinc-s.[11]

morning from rising from bed[16]

coloc., rhus-t.

alternating with heat[11]

bol-la., mang., merc., puls., raph., stry., tab.

asleep, when falling[11]

am-c., **BELL.,** calc., ign., merc-c., mez., rhus-t.

bruised, if[3]

spig.

cold air, in[16]

cham.

dinner, before[11]

ars., cann-i., grat., sulph.

drawing pain in abdomen, with[16]

nit-ac.

drinking, when[11]

ars., calen.

after[11]
caps., carb-ac.[3'], chin., elaps, lyc., nux-v., verat.

agg.[3]: carb-ac.

eating, when[11]

cham., lyc.[11, 16], staph.

after[11]

digin., ign., lyc.[16], rhus-t.[16], sulph.[16], tab.

emotions agg.[3]

asar.

emptiness in stomach, after[16]

phos.

epileptic convulsions, before[15]

cupr.

eructations, with[16]

ip.

headache, from[16]

bor., sars.

lying down, on[11]

cit-v.

menses, before

sep.

during[11]
nux-v., sapin.

motion, during[11]

caps., caust., con., merc., nux-v.

am.[11]
dros.

nausea, with[16]

mag-c., stann.

pain, during the[11, 16]

sep., sil.[16]

umbilicus[16]

chin., ip.

part touched

spig.

rest, during[11]

dros.

rising, after[11]

lyc.

am.[11]
nat-c.

sitting, while[11]

hyper., nat-m.

starting, with[16]

sulph.

stool, before[11]

merc.

during
aesc.[11], alum., bell.[1], calad.,
calc-s.[11], cast., con.. ind., kali-c.,

mag-m., mez.[11], nat-c., nit-ac.[16],
plat., rheum[11], stann., spig.,
verat.

after[11]
acon-l., grat., mag-m., mez.[16],
plat., ptel.

supper, during[11]

bov.

thinking of disagreeable things

benz-ac., phos.

twitching of legs[16]

con.

urination, after[11]

eug., iod., plat.

vomiting, with[16]

sulph.

walking, when[11]

arn.

after[11]
meny.

waterbrash, with[16]

sil.

wine, drinking[1']

cina

yawning, when

cast.[11], **cina,** hydr.[4], ip.[16], laur.[16], mag-m.[16], nux-v.[16], olnd., sars.[16]

SIDE, symptoms on **one**

aesc., **agar.,** agn., **ALUM., ALUMN.**[2], am-c., am-m., **ambr., ANAC.,** ang.[2, 3], ant-c., ant-t., aphis, **apis**[2], **arg-m., arg-n.,** arn., ars., **ASAF.,** asar., aur., **bar-c.,** bar-m., bell., bism., bor., **bov.**[2, 3], **BRY., calc.,** camph., cann-s., **canth.,** caps., carb-ac.[11], carb-an., carb-v., caust., cham., chel., chin., **chin-s.**[6], cic., **cina,** clem., **coc-c.**[2], cocc., coff., colch., coloc., con., croc., cupr., **cycl.,** dig., dros., **dulc.,** euph., euphr., ferr., ferr-s.[11], graph., **guaj.,** hell., hep., hura[11], hyos., ign., iod., iris, **KALI-C.,** kali-m.[1'], kali-n., **KALI-P., KREOS., LACH.,** laur., led., **LYC., LYSS.,** mag-c., mag-m., mang., meny., merc., **mez.,** mosch., **mur-ac.,** nat-c., nat-m., nit-ac.[1], nux-m., nux-v., oena.[11], **olnd.,** orig.[11], **par.,** petr., **PH-AC., phos., PLAT., plb.,** puls., rad-br.[3], ran-b., ran-s., rheum, rhod., rhus-t., ruta, **sabad., sabin.,** samb., **SARS.,** sel., seneg., sep., sil., **spig.,** spong., squil., stann., **staph.,** stront-c., **SUL-AC.,** sul-i.[1'], sulph., tarax., **tarent.**[2], tell.[11], teucr., thala.[14], thuj., valer., verat., **VERB.,** viol-o., viol-t., vip.[6], xan.[11], **zinc.,** zinc-p.[1']

alternating sides

agar., ant-c., cimic., cina[3], **COCC.**[3], iris, **LAC-C.,** mang.[6], merc., onos., phos., plat., puls., rad-br.[3], sep.

crosswise, left upper and right lower

AGAR., alum., anac., ant-t.[8], **arn.,** ars., asc-t.[7], bar-c., bell., **both.**[7], brom., camph., caps., **carb-an.,** cham., chel., chin., coff., con., cycl., euphr., **fl-ac.,** hep., hyper., **kali-c.,** kali-n., lach., laur., **LED.,** mag-m., meny., merc., mill., mur-ac., nat-m., nit-ac., nux-m., nux-v., olnd., op., par., ph-ac., **puls.**[1], ran-s., rhod., **RHUS-T.,** sabad., sabin., samb., sars., sec., seneg., spong., **squil., stann.,** staph., stram., sulph., **TARAX.,** teucr., **thuj.,** valer., **verat., verb., viol-t.**

right upper and left lower

acon., **agar.**[6], agn., am-c., am-m., **AMBR., ant-c.,** ant-t., arg-m., ars-i., asar., asc-t.[7], bism., **bor., both.**[7], **bov.,** brom.[8], bry., calad., **calc.,** cann-s., carb-v., **caust.,** chel., cic., cina, colch., coloc., croc., cupr., dig., **dulc.,** euph., euphr.[1], **ferr.,** graph., hell., hyos., ign., iod., ip., kali-n.[16], **lyc.,** mag-c., mang., med.[8], **merc-i-f.,** mez., mur-ac., **nat-c.,** nux-v., **perh.**[14], **PHOS.,** plat., **plb.,** ran-b., rheum, rhus-t., ruta, sel., **sil.,** spig., **SUL-AC.,** viol-o.

left

achy.[14], acon., adon.[6], agar.[2, 3, 8], agn.[3], **all-c.,** aloe, alumn.[2], **am-br.,** am-c.[2, 3], am-m.[2, 3], **ambr.**[2, 3], **anac.,** ang.[2, 3], ange-s.[14], **ant-c., ant-t., apis, arg-m., ARG-N., arn.,** **ars.**[2, 3, 6], ars-i.[3, 6], **art-v.**[2], arum-t., **ASAF., ASAR., asc-t., aster.,** atra-r.[14], **aur.**[2, 3] aur-m-n., bapt.[2], bar-c.[2, 3], bar-m., bell.[2, 3, 11], **bell-p.**[2, 7], benz-ac.[11], **berb.,** bism., bor.[2, 3], bov.[2, 3], **brom., bry.,** buni-o.[14], **calc.,** calc-ar.[1'], calc-f.[3, 10, 14],

camph.[2, 3], cann-s., cantn.,
CAPS, carb-v.[2, 3, 6], caust.,
cean.[8], **cedr.**[3, 6], **cham., chel.,**
chin., chin-s.[3], **cic.**[2, 3], **cimic.,**
CINA, cinnb.[3, 11], **CLEM.,**
cocc., coff-t.[11], **colch., coloc.,**
con.[2, 3], cortiso.[14], **CROC.,**
crot-c.[11], crot-h.[11], **crot-t.,**
cupr., cycl.[2, 3], cyt-l.[9, 10, 14],
daph.[4, 11], dig.[2, 3], dros.[2, 3],
dulc., elat.[11], erig.[8], euon.[11],
eup-pur.[11], **EUPH., euphr.,**
ferr., ferr-p., ferr-s.[11], flav.[14],
flor-p.[14], gels., **GRAPH.,** grat.[1'],
guaj., halo.[14], hecla[14],
hed.[9, 10], hell.[2, 3], hep.,
hir.[14], hist.[14], hydroph.[14],
hyos.[2, 3], ign., ind.[11], **iod.**[2, 3],
ip., iris, kali-bi.[3], kali-c.[2, 3, 14],
kali-chl., kali-m.[1'], kali-n.[2, 3],
kalm.[11], **KREOS.,** lac-ac.[2],
LACH., lat-m.[14], laur.[2, 3],
led.[2, 3], lepi.[8, 11], **lil-t.**[3, 8, 11],
lith-c., lyc.[2, 3], lycps.[11],
mag-c.[2, 3], mag-m., mag-s.[3],
mang., meny., meph.[14],
merc., merc-c., merc-i-f.[11],
merc-i-r., MEZ., mosch.,
mur-ac., naja, nat-ar.[11],
nat-c.[2, 3], nat-f.[10, 14], nat-m.[2, 3],
nat-s., nid.[14], **nit-ac.,** nux-m.,
nux-v.[2, 3], oena.[11], ol-j.[11],
OLND., onop.[14], **onos.,** op.[11],
osm., ox-ac., **par.,** paro-i.[14],
perh.[14], **petr.**[2, 3], ph-ac.[2, 3],
PHOS., phys., pic-ac.[11], plan.[11],
plat.[2, 3, 11], plb., **podo.**[2], puls.[2, 3],
puls-n.[11], pulx.[8], ran-b., **ran-s.,**
rheum[2, 7], **rhod.,** rhus-t.[2, 3],
rumx.[8], sabad.[2, 3], **sabin.,**
sal-ac., samb.[2, 3], sapo.[8],
sars.[2, 3], **SEL.,** seneg.[2, 3], **SEP.,**
sieg.[10], **sil., spig.,** spong.[2, 3],
SQUIL., STANN., staph.,
stront-c., stroph-s.[14], sul-ac.,
sulfa.[14], sulfonam.[14], **SULPH.,**
tab., **tarax.,** tell.[14], teucr.,
thala.[14], ther., **thuj.,** ust.,
v-a-b.[14], valer.[2, 3], **verat.**[2, 3],
verb.[2, 3], vesp., **viol-o., viol-t.,**
vip-a.[14], xan., **zinc.**[2, 3, 6]

coldness of[11]

bry., carb-v.[3], caust., lyc.,
rhus-t.[3], sapin., sulph.[3]

heat of [11]

bell., lac-ac., rhus-t.

then right

acon., all-c.[1', 3, 7], aloe, arg-n.[3],
ars.[3], benz-ac.[7], brom.[3], calc.[3, 7],
calc-p., **colch.,** dulc., elaps,
ferr.[3, 7], **form.**[3, 6], form-ac.[6],
hed.[9, 10, 14], **iod.**[7], ip.[7], kali-c.,
kreos., lac-c.[8], **LACH.,** merc-i-r.[3],
naja, nit-m-ac., nux-v.[3], phyt.,
puls.[3], rhus-t., sabad.[3, 6, 7],
stann.[3], tarax.[3]

right

abies-c., **acon.,** adlu.[14], **aesc.,**
agar.[2, 3, 8], **agn., alum., alumn.**[2]
am-c., am-m.[2, 3, 4, 6], ambr.[7],
anac.[2, 3, 8], **ang.**[2, 3], ant-t.[2, 3],
APIS, ARG-M., arist-m.[11], **arn.,**
ARS., ars-i., ars-s-f.[1'], art-v.[2],
arum-t.[2], asaf.[2, 3], aster.[2],
AUR., aur-ar.[1'], **aur-i.**[1'],
aur-s.[1'], aza.[14], **BAPT.,**
bar-c.[2, 3], **bar-s.**[1'], **BELL., bism.,**
BOR., both.[3, 7, 8], **bov.**[2, 3],
brach.[11], brom., **BRY., CALC.,**
calc-i.[1'], **calc-p.,** camph.[2, 3],
cann-i., cann-s., **CANTH.,**
caps., carb-ac.[3, 6], **carb-an.**[2, 3],
carb-v.[2, 3], card-m.[3, 6], **caust.,**
cedr., cere-s.[11], cham., **CHEL.,**
chin., chloram.[14], cic.[2, 3]
cimic.[14], cina[2, 3], cinnb.[8],
clem.[2, 3], **cocc., coff.**[2, 3], **colch.,**
COLOC., CON., corn.[2], croc.[2],
CROT-C., CROT-H., culx.[1'],
cur.[7, 8], cycl.[2, 3], cyn-d.[14],
dicha.[14], dig.[2, 3], dol.[8], **dros.,**
dulc., **elaps**[3, 6], elat.[2], equis.[8],
euph.[2, 3, 6], **euphr.,** fl-ac.[11],

form., gels.³, gink-b.¹⁴, gins.⁴,
glon.¹¹, graph.²· ³, guaj., guat.¹⁴,
harp.¹⁴, hell.²· ³, **hep.,**
hip-ac.⁹· ¹⁴, hyos.²· ³, hypoth.¹⁴,
ign., indg.³, iod.²· ³· ⁸, **ip., iris,
kali-bi.**³, **kali-c.**²· ³· ⁸, kali-m.¹′,
kali-n.²· ³, kalm., kreos.,
laur.²· ³, led.²· ³, lil-t., **lith-c.,
LYC.,** lycpr.⁸, **LYSS.,** mag-c.²· ³,
mag-m., mag-p.³· ⁶· ⁸,
mand.¹⁰· ¹⁴, **mang.,** meny.,
merc., merc-i-f., methys.¹⁴,
mez., mim-p.¹⁴, moly-met.¹⁴,
mosch., mur-ac., murx.³· ⁶,
naja³, nat-ar., **nat-c.,** nat-m.²· ³,
nat-s.⁷, nit-ac., **nux-m.,
NUX-V.,** oci-s.⁹· ¹⁴, oena.¹¹,
olnd.²· ³, op., **pall.,** par.,
penic.¹³, **petr., ph-ac.**²· ³, phel.⁷,
phos.²· ³, phyt., pic-ac.¹¹,
plat.²· ³, **plb., podo., prun.,**
psil.¹⁴, **PULS., ran-b., RAN-S.,
RAT.,** rheum²· ³, **rhod.,
rhus-t.**²· ³· ⁸, rumx.³, **ruta**²· ³· ⁶,
**sabad., sabin., sang., SARS.,
SEC.,** sel.¹⁴, **seneg.**²· ³ sep.²· ³,
sil., spig., spong.²· ³, **squil.**²· ³,
stann.²· ³· ¹⁴, **staph., stront-c.,
SUL-AC., sul-i.**¹′, **sulph.,** tarax.,
tarent.³· ⁸· ¹¹, **tell., teucr.,**
thiop.¹⁴, thuj., thyr.¹⁴, tub.⁷,
valer.²· ³, ven-m.¹⁴, verb.²· ³,
viol-o., viol-t., wye.¹¹, yuc.¹¹,
zinc.

coldness of¹¹

ars., bar-c.³, par., rhus-t.,
sabin.³

heat of¹¹

op.

then left

acet-ac., acon., am-c.³· ⁷,
ambr.³· ⁷, anac.⁷, apis¹′· ³· ⁷, ars.¹¹,
ars-met. (non: ars-n.), aspar.,
bar-c.⁷, bell., benz-ac.³· ⁶, bry.³,
calc-p.³, canth.³· ⁶, **caust.**⁷, chel.³,

cupr.³, lil-t.³· ⁷, **LYC.,** merc-i-f.³· ⁷,
mez., ox-ac.³· ⁶, **phos.**³· ⁷,
ptel.¹¹, rheum⁷, rumx.³· ⁷,
SABAD.³· ⁴· ⁶· ⁷· ¹¹, sang.,
saroth.¹¹, spong., sul-ac.³· ⁷,
sulph., syph.³, thiop.¹⁴,
verat.³· ⁷

SILICA, from over use of

camph.², **FL-AC.,** hep.², merc.²,
sulph.²

SITTING agg., while

acon., **AGAR.,** agn., **aloe,** alum.,
alumn.², am-c., **AM-M., ambr.,**
anac., **ang.**²· ³· ⁶, ant-c., ant-t.,
apis³, **arg-m.,** arn., **ARS.,** ars-s-f.¹′,
asaf., asar., **aur.,** aur-i.¹′, **aur-m.,
aur-m-n., bar-c.,** bar-m., bell.,
bism., bor., bov., **bry.,** cact., calad.,
calc., camph., cann-s., canth.,
CAPS., carb-an., carb-v., caust.,
cham., chel., **chin.,** cic., cimic.¹⁴,
cina, clem., cob., **cocc.,** coff.,
colch., **coloc., CON.,** croc., cupr.,
CYCL., dicha.¹⁰, dig.²· ³· ⁸, dios.⁸,
dros., DULC., equis.⁸, **EUPH.,
euphr., ferr.,** ferr-a.⁶, ferr-ar.¹′,
fl-ac., **gamb.,** graph., grat.⁴, guaj.,
hecla¹⁴, **hell.,** hep., hydrc.⁸, hyos.,
ign., indg.⁸, iod., ip., **kali-bi.,** kali-c.,
kali-m.¹′, kali-n., kali-p., kali-s.,
kreos., **lach.,** laur., **led., LYC.,**
mag-c., **mag-m.,** mang., **meny.,**
meph.¹⁴, **merc.,** mez., **mosch.,
mur-ac., nat-c.,** nat-m., nat-p.,
nit-ac., nux-m., nux-v., olnd., op.,
par., **petr., ph-ac.,** phel.⁴, **PHOS.,**
phyt.⁸, **PLAT.,** plb., pneu.¹⁴, **prun.,**
psor.¹′, **PULS.,** pyrog.¹′, ran-b.,
ran-s.¹, rheum, **rhod.**¹, **RHUS-T.,
ruta, sabad.,** sabin., samb., sars.,
sec., sel., **seneg., SEP.,** sil., **spig.,**
spong., squil., stann., staph., stram.,
stront-c., sul-ac., sul-i.¹′, **SULPH.,
tarax.,** teucr., **thuj.,** tong.⁴, tub.¹′,
VALER., verat., **VERB.,** viol-o.,
vip-a.¹⁴, **VIOL-T., ZINC.,
ZINC-P.**¹′

am.

acon., agar., agn., alum., **alumn.²,**
am-c., am-m., **anac.,** ang.², ³, **ant-t.,**
aral.³, ⁶, arg-m.², arn., ars., asaf.,
asar.³, aur., bar-c., bell., bor., **BRY.,**
cadm-s., **calad.,** calc., camph.,
cann-s., canth., caps., carb-an.,
carb-v., caust., cham., chel., chin.,
chion., cic., cina, clem., cocc.,
coff., COLCH., coloc., con., croc.,
cupr., cycl., **DIG.², ³, dulc.²,** ferr.,
gels. **glon., graph.³, ⁷,** graph., guaj.,
hell., hep., hyos., ign., iod., ip.,
kali-c., kali-n., kreos., laur., led.,
mag-c., mag-m., mang., meny.,
merc., mez., mosch., nat-ar., nat-c.³,
nat-m., nit-ac., nux-m., **NUX-V.,**
op., par., petr., ph-ac., phos., plb.,
puls., ran-b., ran-s., **rheum, rhod.²,**
rhus-t.², ³, ⁴, sabad.³, sabin., samb.,
sars., sec., sel., **sep.², sil.,** spig.,
spong., **squil.,** stann., staph., stram.,
sul-ac., sulph., sumb., tarax., thuj.,
valer., verat., verb.², zinc.

aversion to sit[11]

iod., lach.

bent agg.², ³

acon., **agn.³,** alum.³, **alumn.²,**
am-m., ang., **ANT-T.,** arg-m.,
ars., asaf., bar-c., bor., bov., **bry.,**
caps., carb-v., caust., cham.,
chel., **chin., cic., DIG., dulc.,**
ferr., **hyos.,** ign.³, meny., nat-m.³,
nux-v., phos., plb., **puls., rhod.,**
rhus-t., sabin., samb., **sep.,** spig.,
spong., **squil.,** stann., **sulph.,**
verb., viol-t.³

am.²

anac., **ang.,** ars., bar-c., **bell.,**
bor., bry., calad., **carb-v.,** caust.,
cham., chel., chin., cina, **colch.,**
coloc., **con.,** dig., **ign., KALI-C.,**
lyc., mang., **merc., mez.,** mosch.,
nux-m., nux-v., op., puls., **rheum,**

rhus-t., **sabad.,** sars., **spig.,**
spong., stann., sulph., tarax.,
verat., verb.

cold seat agg., on a[8]

chim., dulc.³, **nux-v.**

down agg., on first

agn., alum., **AM-M., ant-t.,**
arg-m., aur., bar-c., bov., bry.,
caust., **chel.,** chin., **coff.,** croc.,
cycl., graph., **hell., ip.,** iris,
kali-c., lyc., **mag-c.,** mang.,
merc., murx., nat-s.⁶, nit-ac.,
ph-ac., phos., puls., rhus-t.³,
ruta, sabin., **samb.,** sars., **SPIG.,**
spong., squil., sulph.⁶, thuj.,
valer., verat., viol-t.

am.

acon., ambr., anac., ang.³, **ant-c.,**
ant-t., arn., ars., asar., aur.,
bar-c., bell., bov., bry., calc.,
cann-s., canth. **CAPS.,** carb-an.,
carb-v., caust., cham., chin.,
cic., cocc., **CON.,** croc., dig.,
dros., **euph., ferr.,** ferr-ar¹ʼ,
graph., kali-c., kali-n., lach.,
laur., led., lyc., mang., merc.,
mur-ac., nat-c., nat-m., nit-ac.,
nux-v., olnd., petr., ph-ac., **phos.,**
plat., puls., ran-b., rhod., **rhus-t.,**
ruta, sabad., **sep.,** sil., **spig.,**
staph., stram., stront-c., **sulph.,**
thuj., **verat.**

erect agg.², ³

anac., **ang.,** ars., aur-s.¹ʼ, bar-c.,
bar-s.¹ʼ, **bell.,** bor., bry., calad.,
carb-v., caust., **cham., chel.,** chin.,
cina, colch., **COLOC.,** con., dig.,
ign., KALI-C., kreos., **lyc.,** mang.,
merc., **mez.,** mosch., nat-m.³,
nux-m., nux-v., op., puls., rheum,
rhus-t., **sabad.,** sars., **spig.,**
spong., staph., sulph., tarax.,
verat., verb., viol-t.³

am.²

acon.², **alumn., am-m.,** ang.,
ant-t.², ³, ⁶, ⁸, apis⁸, arg-m.,
ars.², ³, ⁶, asaf., bar-c.², ⁶, bell.⁸,
bor., bov., **bry.,** caps., carb-v.,
caust., cham., chel., **chin., cic.,**
DIG.², ³, dulc., ferr., **hyos.**², ³,
kali-bi.³, ⁶, meny., nat-m.³,
nux-v., phos., plb., **puls., rhod.,**
rhus-t., sabin., samb., **sep.,** spig.,
spong., squil., stann., **sulph.,**
verb.

inability to sit erect¹¹

lyc., stram.

must sit up in bed with knees drawn
up, rests her head and arms upon
knees

ARS., glon.¹¹

impulse to sit³

acon.³, ⁴, **agar.,** alum.³, ⁴, am-c.,
am-m., ambr.⁶, anac.³, ⁴, ant-c.,
arg-m., arn.³, ¹¹, **ars.**³, ⁶, asar.,
bar-a.⁶, bar-c., **bell.,** bor., bry.³, ⁴, ⁶,
calc.³, ⁶, camph., **cann-s.,** canth.,
caps.³, **carb-v.**³, ⁶, caust.³, ⁶,
cham.⁴, ¹¹, **chel., CHIN.**³, ⁴, ⁶, ¹¹,
cocc.³, ⁶, cod.¹¹, colch.³, ⁶, **CON.**³, ⁶,
croc.³, ⁴, cupr., cycl., dulc.³, ⁴, ⁶,
euphr., GRAPH.³, ⁶, **guaj.**³, ⁶,
hell.³, ¹¹, hep., hyos., ign., **iod.,** ip.,
jac-c.¹¹, kali-c., lach., lact.⁴, laur.,
led.⁶, lil-t., lyc., m-aust.⁴, mag-c.,
mag-m., **merc.**³, ⁶, mez., mur-ac.³, ⁴,
nat-ar.¹¹, nat-c., **nat-m.**³, ⁶, nat-s.⁶,
nit-ac.³, ⁶, **NUX-V.**³, ⁴, ⁶, ¹¹,

olnd.³, ⁴, ⁶, op., petr., **ph-ac.**³, ⁶,
PHOS.³, ⁶, pic-ac.¹¹, plb.,
puls.³, ⁴, ⁶, ¹⁶, ran-b., ran-s., rheum,
rhod., rhus-t.³, ⁴, ruta, sabin.⁴, **sec.,**
sep., sil., **spong., SQUIL.,**
stann.³, ⁴, ⁶, staph.⁴, stront-c.³, ⁶,
sulph.³, ⁴, **tarax.**³, ⁴, teucr.,
verat.⁴, ⁶, verb., viol-t., **zinc.**

Vol. I: *sit*

wet ground, ailments from s. on³

ars., calc., caust., **dulc.**³, ⁶, **nux-v.**³, ⁶,
rhod., **rhus-t.**¹′, ³, ⁶, sil.

SLEEP agg., **before**

acon., agar., **agn.,** alum., am-c.,
am-m., ambr., anac., ant-c., arn.,
ARS., ars-s-f.¹′, asar., aur., aur-ar.¹′,
bar-c., **bell.,** bism., bor., **BRY.,**
calad., CALC., camph., canth.,
caps., **carb-an., CARB-V., caust.,**
cham., chel, **chin.,** clem., cocc.,
coff., coloc., con., cycl., dig., dulc.,
euph., euphr., **graph.,** guaj., **hep.,**
ign., ip., **kali-c.,** kali-n., **kreos.,**
lach., laur., led., **lyc.,** mag-c.,
mag-m., mang., **MERC.,** mez.,
mosch., mur-ac., nat-ar., nat-c.,
nat-m., nit-ac., nux-m., nux-v., par.,
petr., **ph-ac., PHOS.,** plat., plb.,
PULS., ran-b., rheum, rhod.,
RHUS-T., sabad., sabin., samb.,
sars., sel., seneg., **SEP., sil.,** spig.,
spong., stann., staph., stront-c.,
sul-ac., **SULPH.,** tarax., teucr.³,
thuj., verat., verb., viol-t., zinc.

at beginning of s. agg.

agar., agn., am-c.³, am-m., aral.,
arg-m., arg-n., arn., **ARS.,** ars-s-f.¹′,
arum-t.³, aur., bapt., bar-c., **BELL.,**
bor., **BRY.,** calad., **calc.,** camph.³,
caps., carb-an., carb-v., caust.,
cench.¹, **cham.**², chin., cocc., coff.,

con., **CROT-H.**, dulc., **graph., grin.,**
guaj., hep., ign., ip., **kali-ar.,**
KALI-C., kreos., **lac-c., LACH.,**
laur., **lyc.**, mag-c., mag-m., **merc.,**
merc-pr-r.[3], mur-ac., nat-c., nat-m.,
nit-ac.[3], nux-v., **op.,** ph-ac., **phos.,**
PULS., ran-b., **rhus-t.,** sabad.[3],
sabin., samb.[6], sars., sel., **SEP.,** sil.,
spong., stann.[3], staph., stront-c.,
sulph., tarax., teucr., thuj., **valer.,**
verat.

during s. agg.

    acon., aesc.[1'], agn., alum., am-c.,
am-m., ambr., anac., ant-c.,
ant-t., apis, arg-n., ARN., ARS.,
ars-s-f.[1'], aur., aur-ar.[1'], **bar-c.,**
bar-m., **BELL.,** bism., **BOR.,**
brom., **BRY., calad.,** calc.,
camph., **cann-i.,** cann-s., canth.,
caps., carb-ac., carb-an., carb-v.,
carbn-s., caust., **CHAM., chel.,**
chin., chin-ar., cic., cina, clem.,
cocc., coff., colch., coloc., **con.,**
croc., cupr., cycl., dig., dros.,
dulc., euph., ferr., ferr-ar.,
graph., guaj., hell., **HEP., HYOS.,**
ign., ip., **kali-ar.,** kali-br., **kali-c.,**
kali-n., kali-p., kreos., **lach.,**
laur., led., **lyc.,** mag-c., mag-m.,
mang., meny., **MERC.,** merc-c.[3],
mez., mosch., **mur-ac.,** nat-ar.,
nat-c., **nat-m., nit-ac., nux-m.,**
nux-v., **OP.,** par., petr., **ph-ac.,**
phos., plat., plb., **PULS.,** ran-b.,
ran-s., **rheum,** rhod., rhus-t.,
ruta, sabin., **samb.,** sars., sel.,
seneg., **sep., SIL.,** spig., spong.,
squil., stann., staph., **STRAM.,**
stront-c., sul-ac., **SULPH.,** syph.[7],
teucr.[3], thuj., valer., verat.,
verb., viol-t., **ZINC.,** zinc-p.[1']

am.
    am-m., calad., hell., phos., samb.

after s. agg.

    acon., aesc., ail.[2], am-c.[3, 6], am-m.,

ambr.[1], anac., **apis,** arg-m.[1', 3, 6],
arn., ars., ars-s-f.[1'], asaf.,
aur-ar.[1'], bar-m.[3], bell., bor., bov.,
bry., bufo[2, 8], cadm-s., calad.[3],
calc., calc-f.[10], **camph., carb-v.,**
carbn-s., caust., cham., **chel.,**
chin., cina, cob-n.[10], coc-c.[3, 8],
cocc., coff., **con.,** crat.[8], **CROT-C.,**
crot-h.[1'-3, 6], **crot-t.**[1], dig., **dios.**[2],
epiph.[8], **euphr., ferr.,** ferr-ar.,
graph., **hep.,** hom.[8], hyos., ign.,
kali-ar., kali-bi.[3], kali-c., kali-i.[3],
kali-n.[3, 6], kali-p., kreos., lac-c.,
LACH., lob.[3], **lyc.,** mag-c.,
mag-f.[10, 14], merc-c.[8], morph.[8],
mur-ac., myric.[2], naja, nat-ar.,
nat-sil.[1'], nux-m., nux-v., olnd.,
op., paeon., parth.[8], **ph-ac.,**
phos., phyt., pic-ac.[8], **puls.,**
rheum, rhus-t., **sabad.,** samb.,
SEL., sep., spig., **SPONG.,** squil.[3],
stann., **staph., STRAM., SULPH.,**
syph.[8], thuj., tub.[8], uran-n.[3, 6],
valer.[2, 8], **verat.,** ziz.[8]

morning on waking agg.[7]

    AM-M., AMBR., arn., **ARS.,**
bell-p.[10], cadm-met.[9, 10], **CALC.,**
carb-v., CAUST., chel., chin.,
cob-n.[10], **cocc., con., dig.,**
ferr-ar.[1'], flav.[14], **graph., HEP.,**
hyos., ign., kali-ar., kali-c.,
LACH., lyc., mag-c.[10], **NUX-V.,**
PHOS., phyt., prot.[14], **PULS.,**
RHUS-T., samb., SEP., staph.,
SULPH.

afternoon, agg

    anac., bar-c.[16], bell.[7], **bry.,**
caust.[3], chin., con.[16], **graph.**[3],
lach., mag-c.[10], mag-f.[10, 14],
nat-m.[16], phos., **puls.,** SEL.[3],
spong., **STAPH., sulph.**

am.[3]
    fl-ac., kali-bi., meph., nux-m.,
nux-v.[14], ph-ac., pneu.[14], senec.

am.
   acon., agar., am-c.[3], am-m.,
   ambr., apis, **ars.**, bry., **calad.**,
   calc., caps.[3], cham., chin., cocc.,
   colch., con., crot-t.[3, 6], **cupr.**[3],
   epiph.[3], ferr., **fl-ac.**[3], glon.[1'], hell.,
   ign., ip., iris[3, 6], kali-bi.[3], kali-p.[3],
   kreos., lach., lob.[3], **med.**[3, 6],
   meph.[3, 6], **merc.**, mygal.[8], myric.[8],
   nat-c., nid.[14], **nux-v.**, oxyt.,
   PH-AC., PHOS., puls., ran-b.[3, 6],
   ruta, sabin., samb., sang., sel.,
   sep., spig., thuj.

falling asleep am., on

   merc.

half asleep am., when

   hell.[3], **sel.**

long s. agg.

   ambr., anac., arn., ars., asaf., bell.,
   bor., bry., **calc.,** camph., carb-v.,
   caust., cham., cocc., **con.,** dig.,
   euphr., ferr., **graph., hep.,** hyos.,
   ign., kali-c., kreos., **LACH.,** lyc.,
   mag-c., **nux-v.,** ph-ac., puls.,
   rhus-t., spig., **stram., SULPH.,**
   verat.

loss of, from

   ambr., ars.[6], bry., carb-v.[2, 3], **caust.,**
   chin., **cimic., COCC.,** coff.[2, 3], **colch.,**
   cupr., ip., kreos.[3], **lac-d.**[1], laur.,
   merc.[3], nat-m., **nit-ac., NUX-V.,**
   ol-j.[2], olnd., op., pall.[3], ph-ac.,
   PHOS.[3], pic-ac.[1'], puls., ruta, sabin.,
   sang.[3], **sel.,** sep., **sulph.,** zinc.,
   zinc-a.[7, 12], zinc-o.[7]

short s. am.[3]

   carc.[9], fl-ac.[3, 7], kali-bi., med.[6],

meph.[3, 6, 14], nux-m., nux-v.,
   ph-ac.[6], senec.

slow–broken bones see injuries–bones

SLUGGISHNESS of the body

   acon.[4], agar.[4, 11], alum.[4], **alumn.**[1']
   am-m., ammc.[4], anac., **ant-t.**[4, 11],
   arn., ars., **ASAR.**[11], bar-c.[4], bell.[4],
   bor.[4], bruc.[4], bry.[1', 4], cact.[1'],
   calad.[4], calc., calc-p.[4], camph.,
   cann-s.[4], canth.[11], **caps.,** carb-an.,
   carb-v., carl.[11], casc.[4], **chel.,** chin.[4],
   cinnb., cocc., **con.,** croc.[4], cur.,
   cycl.[12], dig.[4], dirc.[11], dulc., ferr-m.[11],
   gels., graph.[4], grat.[4], guaj., hell.[4],
   hep.[4], hera.[4], hyos.[11], ign.[4], indg.[4],
   iod., ip., kali-c., kali-m.[1'], kali-p.,
   kali-s.[1'], lach.[4, 11], laur., lil-t.[11], lyc.,
   m-aust.[4], mag-c.[4], mag-m., merc.,
   mez., mur-ac., nat-c., nat-m.,
   nit-ac., nux-v., ol-an.[4], olnd., **op.,**
   petr., ph-ac., phel.[4], phos., phys.[11]
   plb., puls., rheum[4], rhod., ruta[4],
   sabin.[4], sars.[1', 4, 11], **sec.,** sel.[4], **sep.,**
   sil.[4], stann., stram., stront-c.[4],
   sul-i.[1'], **sulph.,** thea[11], thuj.[4], verb.,
   zinc.[4], zinc-p.[1']

   lassitude
   weakness

morning
      carb-an., chel., nat-c., nat-m.,
      verb.

   sitting, while

      chel.

forenoon[11]
      sars.

rising, on[11]

      ammc.

SMALLER, sensation

acon., agar., **calc.**, cact.³, croc.,
euphr., **glon.**, graph.³, kreos., naja³,
nux-m.³, nux-v.³, sabad., sulph.³,
tarent., zinc.³

Vol. I: *delusions – diminished,*
smaller

SMOKE agg., smoke inhalation

ars.³, brom.³, calc., caust., chin.³,
euphr., kali-bi.³, lyc.³, naja³, nat-m.,
nux-v., olnd., puls.³, **sep., SPIG.,**
sulph.

SNOW, ailments from bright¹²

glon.

SNOW-AIR agg.

asar.¹⁴, **calc., calc-p.,** caust., cic.,
CON., fl-ac.³, **form.**³, ⁸, lach.³, **lyc.,**
mag-m., merc., nat-c., nux-v.¹,
ph-ac., phos., puls., rhod., **rhus-t.,**
SEP., sil., sulph., urt-u., vib.³

ailments from¹²

con., sep.

SOFTENING bones

am-c., **ASAF., bell., CALC.,** calc-f.,
calc-i.⁸, calc-p., cic., con.², ferr.,
ferr-i.², ferr-m.², **ferr-p.**², guaj.⁸,
hecla², **hep.,** iod., ip., **kali-i.**², **lac-c.**²,

lyc., **MERC.,** merc-c.³, mez., **nit-ac.,**
nux-m.², **ol-j.**², parathyr.¹⁴, petr.,
ph-ac., **phos.,** plb., **psor.**², **puls.,** rhod.,
ruta, **sep., SIL.,** staph., **sulph.,** syph.¹',
ther., thuj.²

brittle bones

caries of bone

necrosis bone

x-ray, from⁹

cadm-met., cortico., cortiso.

spring see seasons

STAGNATED, sensation as if blood

acon., bar-c., bell., bry., **carb-v.,**
caust., croc., crot-t., dig., gels., hep.,
ign., **lyc.,** nat-m.⁴, nit-ac.¹⁶, nux-v.,
olnd., **pic-ac.,** puls., rhod., **sabad.,**
seneg., sep., sulph., sumb., zinc.

STANDING agg.

acon., aesc.⁸, **agar.,** agn., aloe,
alum., alum-p.¹', alum-sil.¹',
alumn.², am-c., **am-m.,** ambr.,
arg-m., arn., ars., ars-s-f.¹', asaf.,
asar., atra-r.¹⁴, **aur.,** aur-s.¹', bar-c.,
bar-m., bar-s.¹', **bell., berb.,** bism.,
bor., **bov.**², ³, **bry.,** cact., **calc.,**
calc-s., calc-sil.¹', camph.¹, cann-s.,
canth., caps., carb-an., carb-v.,
carbn-s., caust., cham., chel., **chin.,**
chin-ar., cic., cina, **COCC.,** coff.,
coloc.², ³, com.³, **CON.,** cortico.¹⁴,
croc., cupr., **CYCL.,** dicha.¹⁰, ¹⁴, **dig.,**
dros., dulc., **euph., euphr., ferr.,**
ferr-ar., ferr-p., **fl-ac.,** graph., guaj.,
hell., hep., ign., **kali-bi.,** kali-c.,
kali-n., kali-p., lach., laur., led.,
LIL-T., lyc.², ³, mag-c., mag-m.,
mand.¹⁰, mang., meny., merc., mez.,

mosch., mur-ac., **murx.**, nat-c.,
nat-m., nat-s.[3], **nit-ac.**, nux-m.,
nux-v., olnd., op., par., petr.,
ph-ac., phel.[4], phos., **plat.**, plb.,
PULS., **ran-b.**, **rheum**, rhod., **rhus-t.**,
ruta, sabad., **sabin.**, **samb.**,
sarcol-ac.[14], sars.[2, 3], sec.[3], **SEP.**,
sieg.[10], **sil.**, spig., spong., stann.,
staph., stram., stront-c., stroph-s.[14],
sul-ac., **SULPH.**, **tarax.**, teucr.,
thlas.[3], thuj., **tub.**, **VALER.**, **verat.**,
verb., viol-t., **zinc.**, **zinc-p.**[1']

weakness – standing

am.

agar., agn., am-c., anac., **ang.**[2, 3],
ant-t., arn., **ARS.**, **asar.**, bar-c.,
BELL., bor., **bov.**[2], bry., **calad.**,
calc., camph., **cann-s.**, canth.,
carb-an., carb-v., chel., chin.,
cic., cina, cocc., coff., **colch.**,
coloc.[2, 3], croc., cupr., dig., dios.,
euph., graph., guaj., hell., hep.,
ign., **iod.**, ip., kreos., **led.**, mang.,
meny., merc., merc-c.[3], mez.,
mur-ac., naja, nat-m., nit-ac.[2, 3],
nux-m., **nux-v.**, par., petr., **phos.**,
plb., **ran-b.**, rheum, rhus-t.[2, 3],
ruta, sars., sec., **sel.**, **spig.**,
spong., **squil.**, stann., staph.,
stram., sul-ac., sul-i.[1'], tarax.,
tarent., thuj., vip-a.[14]

erect[8]

ars., bell., **dios.**, kali-p.

impossible[11]

acon., acon-f., ant-t., calc-p.,
canth., cocc.[4, 6], con.[4, 6], cupr.[4, 6],
cupr-s.[4], dulc., hep.[4, 6], hydrc.,
hyos., iod., **kali-br.**[2, 11], lach.[4, 6]
merc., merc-ns., nat-m.[4, 6],
nit-ac.[4, 6], nux-v.[4, 6], op., phys.,
plb., sabad.[4], sec.[4, 8, 11], stann.[6],
staph.[4, 6], stram.[4, 6, 11], sul-ac.[4],
tarent.

till afternoon[11]

bell.

STARVING with exhaustion,
sensation of

ign.

STIFFENING OUT of body[3]

ang., camph., cham., **cina**[16], cupr.,
ign., **ip.**, just.[15], phos.[16], stram.

cough, before[15]

cina, led.

touch, from (children)[15]

apis

STONE-CUTTERS, for: silicosis

agar-t.[14], ars.[3, 6], brom.[3], **CALC.**,
ictod.[6], ip., **lyc.**, mag-m.[14], nat-c.,
nat-ar.[3], nit-ac., penic.[14], ph-ac., **puls.**,
SIL., sulph.

mining

STOOL agg., **before**[3]

acon., **ALOE**, am-c., am-m., ant-t.,
ARG-N., ars., asar., bar-c., bor.,
bry., calad., calc., canth., caps.,
carb-an., carb-v., caust., cham.,

chin., cocc., colch., dig., **DIOS.,**
dulc., ferr., **GAMB.,** kali-c., lach.,
MAG-C., mang., **MERC.,** merc-c.,
mez., nat-c., nat-s., nux-v., op.,
petr., phos., psor., puls., **RHEUM,**
rhod., rhus-t., sabad., sep., spig.,
staph., stront-c., sulph., **THUJ.,**
VERAT.

during st. agg.[3]

acon., agar., alum., am-c., am-m.,
anac., ang., ant-c., apis, **ARS.,**
bar-c., bor., bry., calad., calc.,
canth., caps., carb-an., carb-v.,
caust., **CHAM.,** chin., coloc., con.,
dulc., euph., ferr., graph., hell.,
hep., ign., ip., **IRIS, KALI-BI.,**
kali-c., lach., lyc., **MERC.,** merc-c.,
mur-ac., nat-c., nat-m., nit-ac.,
nux-m., nux-v., olnd., phos., **PULS.,**
rheum, rhus-t., sabin., sars., sel.,
sep., sil., spig., spong., staph.,
stront-c., sul-ac., **SULPH.,** verat.,
zinc.

after st. agg.[3]

aesc.[8], aeth., aloe, **ALUM.,** am-c.,
am-m., ambr., apoc., ars., bor.,
calc., calc-p., canth., caps.,
carb-an., carb-v., **CAUST.**[3, 7],
chin.[3, 7], cocc., coloc., con., fl-ac.,
GAMB., graph., hell., hep., hir.[14],
hydr., **IGN.,** iod., **IRIS,** kali-bi.,
kali-c., kali-n., lach., lept., lyc.,
mag-m., merc., **MERC-C.,** mez.,
mur-ac., nat-c., nat-m., nit-ac.,
nux-m., **NUX-V.,** petr., **PHOS.**[3, 7],
plat., podo., puls., rat., rheum[3, 7],
rhus-t., ruta, **SEL.,** seneg., sep.,
sil., stann., staph., stront-c.,
sulph., tell., teucr., verat.[3, 7]

am.[3]
acon., agar., aloe, alum., **am-m.,**
ant-c., ant-t., ars-i.[3, 6], asaf., aur.,
bar-c., bism., **bor.,** bov., **BRY.**[3, 7],
calc-p., canth., caps., caust.,

cham., cina, coff., **COLCH.,**
coloc., **con.,** croc., cycl.,
cyt-l.[10, 14], dig., dulc., ferr.,
fl-ac., GAMB., glon., guaj., hell.,
hep., ip., kali-bi.[3, 7], mag-c.,
mand.[7], mang., meny., **merc.**[7],
mur-ac., nat-c., **nat-m.**[3, 6],
NUX-V.[3, 7], op., ox-ac.[3, 6, 7], par.,
ph-ac., plb., psor., **puls.,** rauw.[14],
rheum, **RHUS-T.,** sabad., **sang.,**
seneg., sep., **SPIG.,** squil., **sulph.,**
thuj., verat.

STOOP shouldered

arg-n.[3], **calc.**[5, 7], **carb-v.**[3], cocc.[3],
coff.[7, 12], coloc.[3], **lyc.**[5, 7], **mang.**[3],
med.[7], nat-c.[7], nux-v.[7], op.[7],
PHOS.[3, 6, 7, 12], **sil.**[5, 7], **SULPH.,** ter.[6, 7],
tub., verat.[3]

STOOPING agg.[3]

am-c., bell., **BRY.,** calc., caust., lyc.,
mang., nux-v., puls., sep., sil., **spig.,**
sulph., valer.

am.[3]
colch., hyos., iris

STREAMING of blood, sensation

ox-ac.

STRENGTH, sensation of

agar., alco.[11], anh.[10], ars.[6], bell.[11],
bov.[11], bry.[11], **bufo,** calc-f.[9], carbn-o.[11],
chin-s.[11], clem.[11], cob.[11], **coca**[6, 11],
coff., corn.[11], cot.[11], elae.[11], erech.[11],
ferr.[11], **fl-ac.,** gast.[11], gels.[11], gins.[11],
helon.[11], kola[6], lach.[3, 6], lil-t.[11],
meny.[11], **nat-p.**[3, 6], nep.[10, 13, 14],
ol-j.[11], **OP.,** ped.[11], phos.[11], pic-ac.[6],

pip-m.[6, 11], plat.[11], sars.[11], stram.,
vanad.[14], wies.[11], zinc.[3, 6]

anger, after[11]

carbn-s.

coition, after[11]

merc-c.

muscular[11]

agar.[6], alco., anh.[6], ars.[6], camph.,
coca, cod., **fl-ac.**[6, 11], gels.,
keroso, kola[6], **nat-p.**[6], nitro-o.
phos., tab., thea, zinc.[6]

perspiration, during[11]

op., pilo., stach.

walking, while[11]

bapt., chin.

STRETCHING

acon., **aesc.,** agar., all-c.[8], **alum.**[3, 6, 16],
alumn.[2], **am-c.,** ambr., aml-ns.[7, 8],
ang., ant-t., apis, arn., **ARS.,** art-v.[2],
arum-t., asar.[8], bar-a.[11], bar-c.,
bell., bol-la.[11], bor.[3, 16], bov., brach.,
brom., bry.[2, 3, 4], caj., calad., **calc.,**
calc-p., calc-s.[2], camph., cann-s.,
canth., caps., **carb-ac.**[2], carb-an.,
carb-v., cast.[8], **CAUST., CHAM.,**
chel., chin., chin-s.[4], chlf., cimic.,
cimx., cina, cit-v.[2], clem.[3], cocc.[3, 4],
colch., croc.[3], cur.[2], cycl., daph.,
dig., dios., dros., dulc.[4], elat.[3, 8],
ferr., form., gins., gran., **graph.,**
guaj., haem., hell.[3, 4, 16], hep.,
hydrc.[11], hyos., ign.[3, 8], ind., ip.[3],
kali-bi., kalm., kreos., lach., lact.[4],
laur., led., lil-t., lim.[11], lob., lyc.[3],

mag-c., mang.[4, 11], **menis.**[11], meph.,
merc., merc-c., merc-i-r., **mez.,**
mur-ac.[3], nat-c., **nat-m.,** nat-s.,
nit-ac.[3], **NUX-V., olnd.**[3, 6, 16],
onis.[4, 11], op., ox-ac., petr., ph-ac..
phel., **phos.,** plan., **plat.,** plb.,
podo.[2], polyp-p.[11], prun., **PULS.,**
ran-b.[1], raph., rhod.[4], **RHUS-T.,**
rhus-v., ruta[3, 4, 6, 16], **sabad.,**
sabin.[2, 3], **sec.**[3, 4, 7, 8], sel., senec.[6],
seneg.[3], **sep.,** sil., spong., squil.,
stann., staph., stram.[3], sul-ac.[3],
sulph., tab.[4], tarent., tart-ac.[4, 11],
teucr., tong.[4, 11], tub-r.[13], valer.,
verat.[3, 4], verb., vinc.[2], viol-o.,
wildb., zinc.

daytime

mang.

morning
ars., **calc., carb-v.,** cedr.[11], ferr.,
hell.[4, 11], graph.[4], lyc., nux-v.,
phos., puls.[4], rhod.[4, 11], sep.[4, 11],
sulph.[4, 1], tab., tarent., verat.

6 h
sep.

7 h
cedr.

8–11 h[2]
nat-m.

am.[7]
sec.

bed, in

graph.[4], hell., meph.[4], merc.[4],
petr., phos.[4], puls.[4], rhod., sep.,
sulph.[4]

of arms[16]

petr.

desire to[7]

aml-ns., plb., sec.

stupefied, as if

meph.

waking, on

dulc., sep.

forenoon
aloe, ant-t., bov., mag-c., mez.,
mill., mur-ac., nat-m.

11 h
, mit.

noon
am-c., menis.[11]

afternoon
arum-t., cina[11], form.[11], jug-r.,
nux-v., plat., rhus-t.

13 h
form.

16 h
cina, plan.

17–21 h[16]: bell.

sleeping, after

verat.

evening
bell.[4], cann-s., chin.[4], graph.,
nat-c., rhus-t., sumb., tab., verat.

chill, during

tab.

night
CAUST., cocc.[11], nat-c., sulph.

bed, in

cocc.

sleep, in

nat-m.

waking, when

merc.

agg.[3]
am-c.[3, 6], calc., colch., iod., med.[7, 8],
meph.[14], merc-c., PLAT., PULS.,
rad-br., RHEUM, RAN-B.[3, 6],
rhus-t.[3, 6, 8], sep., staph.[3], sulph.,
thuj.

air am., in open

ol-an.

always[4]

puls, rhod., sabad., staph., tab.

am.[3, 6]
alet.[3], alum.[3], aml-ns.[8], ANT-T.,
arn.[3], bell., berb.[6], calc.[3, 7], carb-v.[16],
dios., graph.[3], guaj., halo.[14], hep.,
ign.[3], lyc.[3], mand.[10], nat-f.[14], nux-v.[3],
perh.[14], phos.[6], plat.[3, 6, 16], plb.[8],
podo., puls.[3, 16], pyrog.[3], rhus-t.[3, 8],
sabad., sabin., sec.[3, 7, 8], teucr.[8],
tub-r.[14], v-a-b.[14]

bending–backward am.

anguish with impending menses

carl.

anxiety, from

nat-c.

arms, the[4]

spong., squil., stann., tab.

backward

glon., hydr.

am.[16]: bor.

breakfast, after

lach.

chill, before

aesc., ant-t., aran.[2], arn., **ars.,**
bry.[1], **eup-per.,** ign., ip., **nat-m.,**
nux-v., plan., rhus-t.

during
alum., alumn.[2], ars., bry., caps.,
coff., daph., elat., **eup-per.,**
ferr-p.[3], ip., **kreos.,** laur., mur-ac.,
nat-s., nit-ac., nux-v., petr.,
rhus-t., ruta, tab., teucr.

coldness, during internal

bol-la.[2], nat-s.

continually[4]

puls., rhod., sabad., staph., tab.

violently

colic, during

haem.

convulsive, paroxysmal

ang.[4], bell., camph.[4], carbn-h.,
chin., cic.[4, 6], cimic.[6], cina, hydr-ac.,
ip.[4], lach.[4], lyc., merc.[4], nux-v.[4, 16],
op.[6], sabad.[4], sec.[4, 6], sil.[4], stram.[4, 6],
sulph.[4], thuj.[4], verat.[4]

cough, after

merc.[16], sang.

dinner, after

mag-c.

eating, after

ip.

fever, during

alum.[3], **ars.**[2], bell.[3], **bor.**[3], bry.[3],
CALC.[3, 16], **calc-p.**[2], caust.[3], cham.[3],
eup-per.[2], nat-m.[3], **nux-v.**[3],
RHUS-T.[2, 3], **SABAD.**[3], sep.[3],
spong.[3], sulph.[3], thuj.

high up to reach things[16]

rhus-t.

house, in the

ruta

impossible

acon., phos.

by pains[16]

bell.

lying down, after[2]

COCC.

menses, before

PULS.[1]

during
carb-an.

after[6]
carb-an.

out affected parts agg.[3]

alum., am-c., am-m., anac., ang.,
ant-c., arg-m., arn., aur., bar-c.,
bell., bov., **bry., CALC.,** cann-s.,
caps., carb-v., caust., **cham.,**
chin., cina, clem., **colch., coloc.,**
con., croc., dig., dros., dulc.,
ferr., fl-ac., graph., guaj., **hep.,**
ign., **IOD.,** kali-c., laur., lyc.,
mag-m., **mang.,** meny., merc.,
merc-c., mur-ac., nat-m., nux-v.,
petr., phos., **plat.,** plb., psor.,
puls., rheum, rhus-t., ruta,
sabin., sel., **SEP.,** spig., spong.,
stann., **staph., SULPH., THUJ.,**
valer., verat.

am.[3]
agar., alum., am-m., anac., **ant-t.,**
asar., bell., berb., bor., carb-an.,
carb-v., cham., chel., chin., coff.,
cupr., dig., dros., dios., dulc.,
ferr., guaj., hep., ign., kali-c.,
mag-c., mez., mur-ac., nat-m.,
nat-s., nux-m., nux-v., olnd.,
ox-ac., par., petr., phos., plat.,
puls., rheum., rhod., **RHUS-T.,**

sabad., sabin., **SEC.,** stann.,
staph., thuj., verb., zinc.

painful

sec.

perspiration, during[3]

alum., bell., **BOR.,** bry., **CALC.,**
caust., cham., **NAT-M., nux-v.,**
RHUS-T., sabad., sep., spong.,
sulph.

shuddering, during

ars., **puls.**

sitting, while[16]

alum.

sitting and reading, while

euphr.

sleep, during[11]

nat-m.

sleepiness, with[4]

ant-t., bell., chin., lach., meph.,
sabad.

sleeplessness, during[4]

dulc.

after
sulph.

slept enough, as if he had not

am-c., mill.

supper, after

nit-ac.

tossing about, with⁴

rhod.

unsatisfactory

graph.

urination, before

PULS.

violently for hours⁸

aml-ns., plb.

continually

waking, on⁴

bell.¹⁶, dulc.⁴, ¹¹, hell., **ign.²,** meph.,
nit-ac.¹⁶, merc.⁴, ¹¹, phos., sulph.

walking in open air am.

ox-ac., plan.

yawning, with³, ⁴

acon.³, ⁴, ⁸, aesc.², **agar.²⁻⁴, ⁸,**
all-c.⁸, **alum.³, am-c.³,** ambr.³,
ang., ant-t.³, ⁴, ⁸, arn.³, ⁸,
ARS.³, ⁴, ⁶, asar.⁸, bar-c., **bell.,**

bor.³, bov.³, **bry.²⁻⁴,** calc.³, ⁸,
cann-s.³, canth., caps., **carb-v.,**
cast.⁸, **caust., CHAM.³, ⁶,**
chin.³, ⁴, ⁸, chin-s.⁴, cocc., cur.²,
dig.⁴, dros., elat.³, ⁸, ferr., **form.³, ⁶,**
gran.⁴, graph.³, **guaj.²⁻⁴,** hell.,
hep.³, ⁸, **ign.³, ⁸, ip.³,** kreos.,
lach.², ⁴, lact.⁴, laur., led.³, mag-c.,
mang.⁴, meph.⁴, merc.³, merc-c.³,
mez., mur-ac.³, nat-m.⁴, nit-ac.³,
NUX-V.²⁻⁴, ⁶, ⁸, olnd.³, ⁶, onis.⁴,
petr., ph-ac., phos., plat.³,
plb.³, ⁴, ⁸, **puls.³, ⁴, ⁶,** ran-b.³,
rhod.⁴, **RHUS-T.³, ⁶, ⁸,** ruta,
sabad., sec.³, ⁴, ⁸, senec.⁶, seneg.³,
sep., sil.³, ⁸, **spong.,** squil.³, ⁴, ⁶,
stann., **staph.²⁻⁴, ⁷, sulph.³, ⁴, ⁸,**
tab.⁴, tart-ac.⁴, tong.⁴, valer.,
verat., verb.³, viol-o.², zinc.

forenoon⁴

ant-t.

without sleepiness²

viol-o.

SUDDEN manifestation⁷

ACON., BELL.

SULPHUR, abuse of

acon.², ³, ars., **calc.,** camph.², ³,
cham.², ³, chin., iod.², **merc.,** nit-ac.²
PULS., rhus-t.², ³, sep., thuj.¹²

summer see seasons

SUN, from exposure to

acon.³, ⁶, ¹², adlu.¹⁴, aeth.³, ⁶, **agar.,**

aloe³, aml-ns.³, ⁶, anh.⁹, **ANT-C.,
arg-m.,** arn.³, **ars.², ⁷, bar-c.,
BELL.¹, ⁷,** brom., **bry.,** cact.⁷, ⁸, ¹²,
cadm-s., calc., calc-f.¹⁰, ¹⁴, **camph.,
carb-v.,** cina³, ⁶, clem., cocc.⁷, ¹²,
crot-h.¹², **euphr.,** fago.⁸, **gels.¹, ⁷,
GLON.,** graph., ign., iod., ip., **kalm.,
LACH.¹, ⁷,** lappa³, **lyss.,** mag-m.,
med.⁷, merc-c.³, mur-ac.¹², **NAT-C.,
NAT-M.,** nat-n.³, **nux-v., op.,**
prot.¹⁴, prun.¹², **psor., PULS., sel.,**
stann., stram.², ³, ⁷, ¹², sul-i.¹', sulph.,
syph.¹², ther.³, ⁷, thuj.⁷, **valer.,**
verat-v.¹², zinc.

ailments from¹²

    acon., agar., ant-c., bell., cact.,
    cadm-s., cocc., crot-h., gels.,
    glon., kalm., lach., mur-ac., op.,
    prun., stram., sulph., syph.,
    verat-v.

    chronic¹²
    nat-c.

am.³, ⁷
    anac.⁶, con.³, ⁶, crot-h.³, iod.³,
    kali-c.⁷, kali-m.³, pic-ac.³, **plat.³, ⁶,**
    rhod.⁷, rhus-t.³, **stram.³, ⁶, ⁷,
    STRONT-C.³, ⁶,** tarent.³, **thuj.⁶**

exertion in

    ANT-C.

sunburn³

    acon.², ³, **agar.,** ant-c., **BELL.², ³,**
    bry., **camph.², ³,** clem.², ³, cortiso.¹⁴,
    cyl-l.¹⁴, euphr., **hyos.², ³,** lach., lyc.,
    mur-ac.⁹, nat-c., op., **PULS.,** sel.,
    sulph., **valer.**

sunstroke

    acon.², ³, ⁶⁻⁸, agar.², ⁷,
    AML-NS.², ⁷, ¹², ant-c.², ⁷, ⁸, ¹²,

apis⁶, ¹⁰, arg-m., **arn.², ⁷, ars.², ⁷,
bell.,** bry.⁸, **cact.², ⁷, ⁸, ¹²,
camph.¹, ⁷, carb-v.², ⁷,** cit-l.², ⁷, ¹²,
crot-h.¹², cyt-l.¹⁰, ¹⁴, euph-pi.¹²,
gels.², ⁶⁻⁸, ¹⁰, ¹², GLON.,
hydr-ac.⁸, ¹⁰, ¹², hyos.³, ⁶, kalm.², ⁷,
lach.⁸, ¹⁰, lyc.¹², lyss.¹²,
nat-c.¹', ², ³, ⁷, ⁸, nat-m.¹²,
nux-v.³, **op.², ⁷, ⁸, ¹⁰, ¹²,** pop-c.¹²,
rhus-t.¹², stram., syph.¹², **ther.,**
thuj.¹², usn.⁸, valer.¹², **verat.², ⁷,
verat-v.¹, ⁷**

ailments from¹²

    arg-m., camph., **LACH.², ⁷,
    NAT-C.², ⁷, ¹⁰, ¹²,** thuj.

SUPPRESSED condylomata¹'*

    merc., nit-ac., staph., **thuj.**

abscesses – pus

coryza
gonorrhoea
mucous secretions – suppressed

perspiration – suppression

Vol. III: *leucorrhoea – suppressed*

    lochia – suppressed

    menses – suppressed

eruptions*

    acon., **ail.³,** alum., am-c., ambr.,
    anac.¹², ant-c.¹², ant-t.³,
    apis³, ⁶, ⁸, ¹², ARS.¹, ⁷, ars-i.,
    ars-s-f.¹', asaf.⁸, ¹², bad.², bar-c.¹',
    bell., BRY., calad., calc.,

camph.[3, 8, 12], caps.[3], carb-an.,
carb-v., caust., cham., chin.[3],
cic.[8], clem.[6], con., **cupr.**, cupr-a.[12],
cupr-ar.[12], **DULC., gels., graph.,**
hell.[6, 8,] **hep.**, hyos.[6], iod.[3], **IP.,**
KALI-BI.[3], kali-c., **kali-s.,**
kreos.[3], lach., laur.[6], **lyc.,**
mag-c.[3], mag-s.[8], merc., **mez.,**
nat-c., nit-ac., nux-m., **NUX-V.**[3],
op., **PETR., PH-AC.,** phos., plb.[12],
PSOR., ptel.[12], **puls., rhus-t.,**
sars., sel., senec.[3], **sep.**, sil.,
staph., STRAM., sul-ac.,
SULPH., thuj., **tub.**, tub-k.[12],
verat., verat-v.[6], **viol-t.**, x-ray[9],
ZINC.

fail to break out, when

ail., am-c., ant-t., **stram., sulph.,**
zinc.

exanthemata[12]*

ail.[6], hell., verat.

mother milk *

acon.[6, 8], agar., **agn.**,, aur., aur-i.[1'],
aur-s.[1'], bell.[8], **BRY.**, calc.,
calc-sil.[1'], camph-br.[8], **carb-v.,**
CAUST., cham., chim., cimic.[1'],
cycl.[6], dulc., frag.[11], **hyos.**, ign.[11],
iod., lac-d., **lach., merc.**, mill.[12],
phyt.[8], **PULS., rhus-t., sec.,**
senec.[6], **sil.**, sul-i.[1'], **sulph., urt-u.,**
verat., zinc.[6, 8, 12]

convulsions-suppressed

anger, from

cham.

haemorrhoids

aloe[7], am-m.[7], apis[7], ars., **calc.,**

caps.[1, 7], carb-v., **coll.**[2, 6, 7], cupr.,
ign.[2], lycps.[12], **mill.**[2, 7], **NAT-M.**[2, 7],
NUX-V., OP.[2, 7], phos., puls.,
ran-b.[7], **SULPH.**

suppuration see abscess

SWELLING in **general**

acon., agar., agn., all-s.[11], aloe[3, 11],
alum., am-c., am-m., ambr., anac.,
ant-c., anthraco.[4], **APIS**, arg-m.,
arg-n.[3], **arn., ARS.**, ars-i., ars-s-f.[1'],
asaf., asar.[3, 4], aur., aur-m.[4],
bar-c., bar-m.[4], **BELL.**, bell-p.[9],
bism., bor., bov., **BRY.**, bufo,
buth-a.[9], calad., **calc.**, calc-i.[3],
calc-sil.[1'], camph., cann-s., **canth.,**
caps., carb-an., carb-v., **carbn-s.,**
caust., celt.[11], **cham.**, chel., **chin.,**
chin-s.[4], cic., cina[4], clem., cocc.,
coff., colch., coloc., com., con.,
conch.[11], cop., cortiso.[9], croc.,
crot-h. crot-t.[4], cupr., cycl., **daph.**[4],
dig., dor.[11], dros., **dulc.**, eucal.[2, 11],
euph., euphr., **ferr.**, frag.[11], graph.,
guaj., hell., **hep.**, hip-ac.[9], hydr.[3],
hyos., ign., iod., **kali-ar., KALI-BI.,**
kali-c., kali-i.[4], kali-n., kreos.,
lach., laur., led., **lyc., m-arct.**[4],
mag-c., mag-m., mang., **MERC.,**
merc-c.[4], mez., mosch., mur-ac.,
naja, narcin.[11], **nat-c.**, nat-m.,
nit-ac., nux-m., **NUX-V.**, olnd.,
op., par., ped.[11], petr., **ph-ac., phos.,**
phyt.[3], plat.[4], **plb., PULS.**, ran-b.,
ran-s.[4], raph.[11], rauw.[9], rhod.,
RHUS-T., rhus-v.[11], ruta, sabad.,
sabin., samb., sang.[3], saroth.[9], sars.,
sec., seneg., **sep., sil., spig.**, spong.,
squil., stann., staph., **stram.,**
stront-c., sul-ac., **sulph.**, tarent.[11],
ter.[4], teucr.[3], thal.[14], **thuj.**, urea[11],
urt-u.[11], valer., verat., **vip.**, zinc.,
ziz.[11]

right side, on[16]

ars.

affected parts, of

ACON., ACT-SP., agn., alum.,
alum-sil.[1'], ant-c., ant-s-aur., **apis,**
arn., **ars., ars-i.,** asaf., aur., aur-s.[1'],
bar-c., bar-i.[1'], **BELL.,** bov., **BRY.,**
calc., calc-i.[1'], calc-sil.[1'], cann-s.,
canth., carb-an., carb-v., **caust.,**
cedr., cham., chin., cic., clem., cocc.,
colch., coll., con., **CROT-H.,**
crot-t., cub., cupr., dig., dulc.,
euph., **EUPHR., ferr.,** ferr-ar.[1'],
ferr-p., **fl-ac., GELS.,** graph., guaj.,
guare.[2], hell., **hep.,** hippoz.[2], hydr.,
ign., **iod., KALI-C.[3], kali-bi.,**
kali-i., kali-m.[1'], **lach., led., lyc.,**
mag-c., mang., **MERC., MERC-C.,**
mur-ac., nat-c., nat-m., nit-ac.,
nux-v., ox-ac., **petr.,** ph-ac., **phos.,**
phyt., plb., **psor., PULS.,** ran-b.,
RHOD., RHUS-T., ruta, sabin.,
samb., sang., sars., sec., **SEP., SIL.,**
spig., **SPONG.,** stann., staph.[3],
stram., **SULPH.,** thuj., **valer.,** zinc.

inflammatory

ACON., agn., alum., am-c., ant-c.,
ant-t.[3], **apis,** arn., **ARS.,** ars-i.,
ars-s-f.[1'], asaf., **aur.[4],** bar-c.,
BELL., bor.[4], bry., **CALC.,**
calc-sil.[1'], cann-s., **CANTH.,**
carb-an., carb-v., **caust.,** chin.,
cocc., colch., **con.,** crot-h.[4], cupr.,
euph., gran.[4], graph., guaj., hep.,
hyos.[4], **iod., kali-ar., KALI-BI.,**
KALI-C., kali-i., kali-n.[4], led., **lyc.,**
mag-c., **mang.[4], MERC.,** mez.[4],
mur-ac.[4], nat-c., **nat-m., nit-ac.,**
nux-v., petr., ph-ac.[4], **phos., phyt.,**
plb., **puls., rhus-t.,** sabin., samb.,
sars., sec., seneg.[4], **SEP., sil.,**
spong., stann., stram.[4], **SULPH.,**
thuj., zinc.

painful[16]

dig.

puffy, edematous

acon., agar., am-c., **am-m., ANT-C.,**
APIS, apoc., arn., **ARS.,** ars-s-f.[1'],
asaf., aur., **aur-m.,** bar-c., **bell.,**
bry., CALC., calc-sil.[1'], **CAPS.,**
carbn-s., cedr., cham., chin.,
cina, cocc., colch., coloc., con.,
CUPR., DIG., dros., **dulc., FERR.,**
GRAPH., guaj., **HELL.,** hyos., **iod.,**
ip., kali-c., kreos., lach., laur., led.,
lith-c.[2], lyc., mag-c., merc., mez.,
mosch., nat-c., **nat-m.[2], nit-ac.,**
nux-m., nux-v.[3], **OLND.,** op., phos.,
phyt., plb., **puls.,** rheum, **rhust-t.,**
samb., sars., **seneg., sep.,** sil., **spig.,**
spong., **SQUIL.,** staph., stram.,
sulph., teucr., verat., **verb.,** zinc.,
ziz.[2]

bones, of

am-c., ambr.[4], ang.[3], ant-c.[4],
arg-m.[3], ASAF., aur., bell., bry.,
bufo[3], **CALC.,** calc-f.[3], **calc-p.,**
carb-an., clem., coloc., con.,
conch.[11], daph.[2, 4], dig., dulc., euph.,
ferr., fl-ac., guaj., hep., iod., **kali-i.,**
kreos., lac-ac.[1], lach., led.[4] **lyc.,**
mang., **merc., mez.,** nat-c., nat-m.,
nit-ac., petr., **PH-AC., PHOS.,**
phyt.[2], plb., **PULS.,** rhod., rhus-t.,
ruta, sabin., sep., **SIL.,** spig.,
STAPH., stront-c.[3], **SULPH.,** thuj.,
verat.

sensation of sw.[16]

ars.

cartilages, of

ARG-M., calc.[2], sil.[2]

glands, of

acon., acon-l.[8, 12], **aesc.,** agn.,

ail.[3, 6, 8], **aln.**[8, 12], alum.,
alum-sil.[1'], **alumn.**[2], am-c., **am-m.**,
ambr. **anthraci.**, ant-c., ant-t.,
apis[2, 3, 8], aq-mar.[6, 8], arg-m., arn.,
ars.[1], ars-br.[8], **ARS-I.**, ars-s-f.[1'],
arum-t., asaf., astac.[2, 8, 12], aur.,
aur-ar.[1'], aur-i.[1'], **aur-m.**[2, 8],
aur-s.[1'], **bad.**[2, 3, 6, 8, 10], bapt.,
BAR-C., BAR-I., BAR-M., bar-s.[1'],
BELL., berb.[1], bor., bov., **BROM.**,
bry., **bufo**, calad., **calc.**, calc-ar.[6],
calc-f.[3, 6, 8, 10], calc-hp.[6], **CALC-I.**,
calc-m.[12], calc-p., **CALC-S.**,
calc-sil.[1'], **calen.**[8, 12], camph.,
cann-s., **canth.**, caps., **CARB-AN.**,
CARB-V., carbn-s., caust., **cham.**,
chim.[12], chin., cic., cinnb.[4], **CIST.**,
CLEM., coc-c.[11], cocc., coloc.,
CON., cor-r.[3, 4, 6], cory.[6, 8], croc.,
crot-h., cupr., cycl., dig., dros.[7],
DULC., eucal.[2, 11], euph., euphr.[12],
eupi.[12], **FERR.**[1], ferr-ar., ferr-i.,
fil.[8], fl-ac.[3, 6], fuc.[6, 10], **GRAPH.**,
hall[12], ham[3, 6], **hecla**[2], hed.[10], hell.,
HEP., hippoz.[2], hydrc.[6], hyos., ign.,
IOD., iris[2, 3], **kali-ar., kali-bi.**[2],
kali-br.[2], **kali-c., kali-chl.,**
kali-bi.[2], kali-br.[2], **kali-chl.,**
kali-i., kali-m.[1', 3, 6, 12], kreos.[4],
lach., **lap-a.**[6, 8, 12], led., **lith-c.**[2, 12],
LYC., mag-c., mag-m., mang.,
med., **MERC., MER-C.**, merc-cy.[8],
merc-d., **merc-i-f., merc-i-r.**,
mez., mur-ac., **nat-c.**, nat-m.,
nat-p.[2], nat-s.[3, 6], **NIT-AC.**,
nux-v., ol-j.[6], petr., **ph-ac.**,
PHOS., phyt., plb., psor., **puls.**,
ran-b., ran-s., raph.[4], rhod.,
RHUS-T., rumx.[8], ruta, sabad.,
sabin., samb., sars., scir.[8, 12],
scroph-n.[8, 12], sec.[2, 12], **sep., SIL.**,
sil-mar.[8, 12], sol-a.[12], sol-o.[12],
spig., **SPONG.**, squil., **stann.**,
staph., stict.[12], stram., stront-c.,
sul-ac., sul-i.[1', 3, 6], **SULPH.**,
symph.[12], **syph.**[1', 2], tab.[12], tax.[8],
ter.[4], teucr., ther.[1'], thiosin.[8, 12],
THUJ., tub.[3, 6, 8], uran-n.[2], **verat.**,
viol-o., viol-t.[2], zinc.

bluish
arn., ars., aur., **carb-an.**, carb-v.,
con., ferr-i., hep., lach., mang.,

merc., merc-i-f., puls., sil., sul-ac.

cold
ars., asaf., bell., **cocc., CON.**,
cycl., dulc., lach., **merc.**[3], rhod.,
spig., **sulph.**[3], thuj.[2]

emaciation, with[2]

ars., ars-i., bar-c., calc., calc-i.,
calc-p., carb-v., caust., **cist.**, **con.**,
graph., mag-c., mag-m., nat-m.,
nit-ac., **ol-j.**, petr., ph-ac., phos.,
psor., **sil.**, staph., sul-ac., sulph.

eruption, with[16]

dulc.

hard
agn., alumn.[1'], ant-c., arn., ars.,
ars-i.[1'], asaf., **bad.**[2], bar-c.[1', 3],
bar-m.[3], bell.[3], brom.[1'], **bry.**,
calc-f.[7], calc-sil.[1'], **carb-an.**,
caust., chin., **CON.**, dig., graph.,
hep.[1', 3], **IOD., kali-i.**, lach., led.,
merc., mez., nux-v., **phos.**,
phyt.[1', 3], **puls., RHUS-T.**, sabin.,
samb., sil.[3], **spong.**, staph.[1'],
stront-c., sul-i.[1'], **sulph., tarent.**[3]

hot
acon., am-c., ant-c., ant-t.[3], arn.,
asaf., **BELL., BRY.**, bufo[3], **calc.**,
canth., **carb-an.**, carb-v., **cham.**[2],
chin., clem., cocc., euph., **hep.**,
kali-c., led., **MERC.**, nux-v.,
petr., **PHOS., phyt.**, puls.,
rhus-t., sars., sil., **sulph.**

inflammatory
acon., agn., am-c., ant-c., **arn.**,
ars., asaf., **bad., bar-c.**, bar-m.[1'],
BELL., bor., **bry.**, calc., **carb-an.,**
carb-v., caust., **cham.**[2], cinnb.,
clem., cocc., **CON.**, dros.[7], **hep.**,
hyos., **kali-i., lyc.**, mang.,
MERC., mez., mur-ac., nat-c.,
petr., ph-ac.[4], **phos., phyt.**, plb.,
puls., rhus-t., sabin., samb., sars.,
sec., seneg.[4], **SEP., sil.**, spong.,
stann., stram.[4], **SULPH.**, thuj., zinc.

knotted cords, like

BAR-M., calc., cist., con., dulc.,
hep., iod., lyc., rhus-t., sil.,
sul-i.$^{1'}$, tub.

menses, during

kali-c., lac-c.

nodes, like

bry., iod.$^{1'}$, nit-ac.

painful

acon., am-c.^{2}, anan ^{2}, ant-c.,
anthraco.^{2}, arn., ars.^{2}, aur.,
aur-i.$^{1'}$, bar-c.^{2}, BAR-M., BELL.,
calc., calc-p.^{2}, canth., caps.^{2},
carb-an., carb-v.$^{2, 6}$, caust.^{2},
cham.^{2}, chin., clem., CON.$^{2, 6}$,
cop.^{2}, cor-r., crot-t.^{2}, cupr.^{2},
graph.^{3}, hep., ign.^{2}, iod., kali-c.$^{2, 6}$,
kali-i., lyc.^{3}, merc.^{2}, mosch.^{3},
nat-m.^{2}, nit-ac., nux-v., phos.^{3},
phyt., psor.^{2}, puls., rhus-t., sil.,
spig., stann., staph., sulph.^{2}

painless

ars., asaf., CALC., cocc.^{1}, con.,
cycl., dulc., ign., lach., merc.^{3},
nit-ac., ph-ac., plb., sep., sil.,
staph., sulph., thuj., tub.^{7}

scarlet fever, after

am-c.^{15}, BAR-C., lac-c.^{2}

scarlet fever

joints, of

abrot., acon., ACT-SP., agn., anag.,

ant-c.^{3}, ant-t., apis, apoc., arn., ars.,
asc-t., aur., aur-m., BELL., berb.,
bov.^{6}, BRY., bufo, calc., calc-f.,
canth.^{6}, caust.$^{1'}$, cedr.^{6}, chin.,
chin-s.^{6}, cimic., clem., cocc.,
COLCH., coloc.^{3}, con., dulc.$^{1'}$,
ferr-p., guaj., ham., HEP., hip-ac.^{9},
iod.$^{3, 6}$, kali-ar.$^{1'}$, kali-bi.$^{1'}$, kali-chl.,
kali-i., kali-m.^{6}, kalm., kreos.^{3},
lac-ac., lac-c.$^{1'}$, lach., LED., lyc.,
mang., med., merc., nat-m., nux-v.,
puls.^{3}, ran-b.^{6}, rhod., rhus-t., sabin.,
sal-ac., samb.^{6}, sil., sol-t-ae., stict.,
SULPH., tarent., ter., thuj., verat-v.

mucous membranes, of^3

arg-n., ars-i., hydr.

periosteum, of

acon.^{3}, ant-c., ASAF., aur., bell.,
bry., chin., kali-i., mang., merc.,
mez., nit-ac., PH-AC., puls, rhod.,
rhus-t., ruta, sabin., sil., staph.,
sulph.^{3}

wounds see wounds–swelling

SWOLLEN sensation

acon., aesc.^{6}, agar., aloe, alum.,
am-c.^{4}, am-m., ambr., aml-ns.^{3},
anac., ant-c., ant-t., apis, aran.,
arg-m., arg-n., arn., ars., asaf.,
asar., aur., bapt., bar-c., bell.,
berb.^{3}, bism., bov., bry., caj.,
calad., calc., calc-p., cann-i.,
cann-s.^{3}, canth., caps., carb-ac.,
carb-an.^{4}, carb-v., carbn-s., caust.,
cedr., cench.^{7}, cham., chin., cic.^{3},
cimic., cina, coc-c., cocc., colch.,
coloc., com., con., cor-r., crot-h.,
crot-t., cupr., cycl., dig., dulc.,
euph., euphr., gels.^{3}, glon., graph.^{4},
GUAJ., ham.^{6}, hell., hep., hyos.,
ign., ip., kali-c., kali-n., kreos.,
LACH., laur., led., lyc., mag-c.,
mang., MERC., MERC-I-F., mez.,

mosch., nit-ac., nux-m., nux-v., olnd., **op., PAEON., PAR.,** petr., ph-ac., phos., plat., plb., **PULS., ran-b.**[1], ran-s., rhod., **RHUS-T.,** sabad., sabin., samb., **sang.,** sars., **seneg.,** sep., sil., **SPIG.,** spong., stann., staph., stram., sul-ac., **sulph.,** tarax., thuj., valer., verat., zinc.

bones, of

ant-c., bell., chel., guaj., **puls.,** rhus-t., spig.

glands, of

ant-c., aur., **bell.,** bry., carb-v., chin., clem., con., dulc., hep., ign., kali-n., lach., m-arct.[4], merc., nat-m.[4], nit-ac., nux-m., nux-v., **PULS., rhus-t.,** sabin., spig., **spong.,** staph., sulph.[4], zinc.

internal parts, of[3]

anac., ant-t., arn., ars., **asar.,** aur., **BELL., bism.,** bov., bry., calad., **caps.,** carb-v., cina, cocc., con., euph., guaj., hyos., **IGN.,** kali-c., laur., merc., nux-m., olnd., op., **par.,** petr., plat., ran-b., ran-s., rhod., sars., **sep., spig., stann.,** tarax., **verat.,** zinc

SYCOSIS

adlu.[14], aesc.[7], **agar.,** agn.[6], alum., alumn., am-c.[7], am-m.[7], anac., **anan.**[2, 7, 12], ang.[7], ant-c., ant-t., **anthraco.**[2, 11], **apis,** aran., **ARG-M., ARG-N.,** arn.[2], **ars.**[2, 3, 7], asaf.[2, 7], asar.[7, 14], asim.[7], aspar.[7], **aster.,** aur., **aur-m.,** aur-m-n.[12], **bar-c., benz-ac.**[1', 7, 12], berb.[2, 7], berb-a.[14], bor.[1', 7], bov.[7], bry., bufo[7], calad.[7], **calc.,** cann-i.[7], cann-s.[7], canth.[7], caps.[6, 7], carb-ac.[7], carb-an., carb-v.,

carb-n-s., cast.[12], caul.[7], **caust.,** cedr.[7], cham., chim.[7], chin.[7], cic.[7, 14], cimic.[7], cinnb., clem.[1', 6, 7], cob-n.[14], coc-c.[7], coch.[7], colch.[6, 7], coloc.[7], con., cop.[7], croc.[7], crot-h.[7], crot-t.[7], cub.[7], cupr-a.[7], cycl.[7], cyna.[14], dig.[7], dor.[7], **dulc.,** epig.[7], erech.[7], erig.[7], ery-a.[6, 7], eup-pur.[7], euph.[7], euph-pi.[7], euphr., fago.[7], **ferr., fl-ac.,** flav.[14], gamb.[7], gels.[7], gnaph.[7], **graph.,** guaj.[6], guat.[14], helon.[7], hep., hydr.[6, 7], influ.[7], **iod.,** kali-bi.[2, 6, 7, 12], kali-c., **kali-i.**[3, 6, 7], kali-m.[7, 12], kali-n.[7], **KALI-S., kalm.**[1', 3, 6, 7], kreos.[2], kres.[14], lac-c.[7], **lach.,** lil-t.[7], lith-c.[7], **lyc.,** mag-c.[2, 7], **mang., MED.,** merc., **merc-c.**[2], merc-d.[7], **merc-sul.**[2], **mez.,** mill.[12], mosch.[7], murx.[7], nat-c.[2, 7], **nat-m.**[2, 6, 7], **nat-p.**[2], **NAT-S., NIT-AC.,** nux-v.[7], ol-j.[7], orig-v.[7], pall.[7], pareir.[7], penic.[13, 14], petr., petros.[6, 7], ph-ac.[2, 3, 6, 7, 12], phos.[7], **phyt.,** pic-ac.[12], pip-n.[7], plat.[7], plb.[7], pneu.[14], prun.[7], psor.[6, 7], puls., rat.[7], rauw.[14], rhus-t.[7], sabad.[3, 6, 7], sabin., sacch-l.[7], sanic.[7], sarr.[7], **sars., sec., sel.,** senec.[7], seneg.[7], **SEI.., sil.,** spig.[7], **STAPH.,** still.[7], stram.[7], **sulph.,** tab.[7], tell.[14], ter.[7], **THUJ.**[1, 1'], thyr.[14], uran-n.[7], ven-m.[14], vib.[7], zing.[6]

SYNALGIA[3]

apis, tarent.

SYPHILIS *

aethi-a.[12], agn.[6], ail.[12], allox.[14], aln.[12], am-c.[3], anag.[2, 12], **anan.**[2, 12], **ang.**[2], ant-c.[6], **ant-t.**[2], apis[2, 12], arg-i.[12], arg-m., arg-n.[6, 12], arn.[2], **ars., ARS-I.,** ars-met.[8, 12], **ars-s-f., asaf.,** asar.[14], asc-t.[2, 12], astra-e.[14], **AUR.,** aur-ar.[1', 12], aur-i.[1', 12], **AUR-M., AUR-M-N.,** aur-s.[1'], bad., bell.[7], benz-ac.[2], berb.[2], berb-a.[12], buni-o.[14], cadm-met.[9], **calc-f.**[3, 6, 12, 14], **calc-i., calc-s.,** calo.[8, 12], **carb-an.,** carb-v., **caust.**[2, 7, 12], **cean.**[2], chim.[2, 12], chin-ar.[12], chr-o.[12], **cinnb.,** clem., cob-n.[14], **colch.**[6, 7], **con.,**

convo-s.[14], cop.[6], cor-r., cory.[6, 8, 12],
crot-h., cund.[2, 12], cupr.[6], cupr-s.[12],
echi.[12], ery-a.[6], eryth.[12], eucal.[12],
euph.[2, 6, 12], ferr.[7, 12], ferr-i.[2, 6], fl-ac.,
franc.[12], graph.[12], guaj., ham.[6],
hecla[2, 12], hep., hip-ac.[14], hippoz.[2, 12],
hir.[14], hydr.[6, 12], hydrc.[12], hyoth.[14],
iber.[14], iod., iris[2], jac.[2, 7, 12], jac-c.[12],
jatr.[3], jug-r.[12], kali-ar., kali-bi.,
kali-br.[12], kali-c.[7], kali-chl., KALI-I.,
kali-m.[2], KALI-S., kalm.[2, 3, 6, 7],
kreos.[2, 6, 12], lac-c.[2, 7, 12], lac-d.[7],
lach., LAUR.[2], led., lith-c.[12],
lyc.[1', 2, 7], maland.[12], MERC.[i, 1'],
merc-aur.[6], MERC-C., merc-d.[2, 7],
MERC-I-F., MERC-I-R., mez., mill.[7],
nep.[14], NIT-AC., nux-v.[6], ol-sant.[6],
osm.[12], penic.[14], perh.[14], petr.,
petros.[6], ph-ac., phos., PHYT.,
pilo.[12], pitu.[14], plat-m.[8], psor.[12],
reser.[14], rhod.[6], sabad.[6], sang.[2, 6, 12],
sars., sec.[7], sel.[12], sep.[2], SIL.,
spong.[6], staph., stict.[12], STILL.,
strych-g.[12], sul-i., sulph., SYPH.,
ter.[6], thala.[14], thiop.[14], thuj.,
thymol.[14], thyr.[7, 12], ulm.[12], vac.[12],
viol-t.[2, 12], xan.[6]

congenital[8]

, aethi-m., ars-i., ars-met., aur.,
calc-f., calc-i., cor-r., kali-i.,
kreos.[8, 12], merc., merc-d., nit-ac.,
pilo.[12], psor., syph.[8, 12]

serologie, with irreducible[14]

astra-e.

TALKING agg.[3]

acon., agar., alum.[3, 4], am-c.[3, 4],
am-m., ambr.[3, 4], ANAC., arg-m.[3, 14],
arg-n., arn.[3, 4], ars., arum-t., aur.,
bar-c., bell.[1', 3], bor.[3, 4], bry.,
CALC.[3, 4], CANN-S., canth., caps.,
carb-v., caust., cham., CHIN., cic.,
COCC.[3, 4], coff., con., croc., dig.,

dros., dulc., euphr., ferr., ferr-p.,
fl-ac., graph., hell., hep., hyos.,
ign., iod., ip., kali-c., led., lyc.,
mag-c., mag-m., MANG., merc.,
merc-c., merc-cy., mez., mur-ac.,
NAT-C., NAT-M., nux-m., nux-v.,
par., petr., PH-AC., phos., phyt.,
plat., plb., puls., raja-s.[14], ran-b.,
RHUS-T., sars., SEL., sep., sil.,
spig., spong., squil., STANN.[3, 4],
staph., stram., stront-c., sul-ac.,
SULPH.[3, 4], verat.

Vol. I: *conversation*

am.[3]
ferr., rhus-t., sel.

TEETH together agg., biting[3]

alum., AM-C., anac., bell., bry.,
carb-an., caust., chin., coff.,
colch., dig., graph., guaj., hell.,
hep., hyos., ip., lach., mang.,
merc., petr., puls., rhus-t., sars.,
sep., sil., spong., staph., sul-ac.,
sulph., verb.

am.[3]
ars., chin., cocc., coff., euph.,
mag-m., staph.

brushing, cleaning the, agg.[3]

carb-v., coc-c.[3, 8], lyc., ruta,
staph.[3, 8]

TENSION externally

acon., agar., agn., aloe, alum.,
alum-p.[1'], alum-sil.[1'], alumn.[2],
am-c., am-m., ambr., anac.,
ang.[3, 4], ant-c., ant-t., apis[3, 6],
arg-m., arg-n., arn., ars., asaf.,
asar., aur., aur-s.[1'], BAR-C.,
bar-i.[1'], bar-m., bar-s.[1'], bell.,
berb., bism., bor., bov., BRY.,

calc., camph., cann-s., canth.,
caps., **carb-an.**, carb-v., **CAUST.**,
cham., **chel.**, chin., chin-s.[4], cic.,
clem., cocc., colch., **COLOC.**,
CON., croc., crot-h., **cupr.**,
dig., dros., euph., euphr.,
ferr., glon., graph., guaj.,
hell., hep., hyos., ign., iod., ip.,
kali-ar., **kali-c.**, kali-n., kreos.,
lach., laur., **led.**, lyc., **m-arct.**[4],
mag-c., mag-m., mang., med.[2],
meny., **merc.**, **mez.**, **mosch.**,
mur-ac., **nat-c.**, nat-m., nat-p.,
nit-ac., nux-m., **nux-v.**, **olnd.**, op.,
par., **petr.**, ph-ac., **PHOS.**, **PLAT.**,
plb., **PULS.**, ran-b., **rheum**, rhod.,
RHUS-T., ruta, sabad., **sabin.**,
samb., sars., **sec.**, seneg., **sep.**,
sil., **spig.**, **spong.**, squil., stann.,
staph., stram., **STRONT-C.**,
sul-ac., sul-i.[1'], **SULPH.**, tarax..
teucr., **thuj.**, valer., verat.,
VERB., **viol-o.**, viol-t., x-ray[9],
zinc.

prevents motion[7]

apis

internally

acon., aesc., agar., agn., alum.,
am-m., ambr., anac., ang.[3], ant-c.,
ant-t., apis[3], arg-m., arn., **ars.**,
ASAF., asar., **aur.**, bar-c., bar-i.[1'],
bar-s.[1'], **BELL.**, **berb.**, bov., bry.,
calc., camph., cann-s., **caps.**,
carb-ac., carb-an., carb-v.,
caust., cham., chel., chin., **cic.**,
clem., coc-c., cocc., coff., colch.,
coloc., com., con., croc., crot-t.,
cupr., cycl., dig., dros., **dulc.**,
euph., euphr., ferr., gels., **glon.**,
graph., guaj.[16], hell., hep., hydr-ac.,
hyos., **hyper.**, ign., iod., ip., kali-c.,
kali-n., kreos., lach., lact.[3], laur.,
led., lob., **LYC.**, mag-c., mag-m.,
mang., meny., **merc.**, mez., **mosch.**,
mur-ac., naja, nat-c., nat-m.,
nit-ac., nux-m., **NUX-V.**, olnd., **op.**,

osm., **PAR.**, petr., ph-ac., **PHOS.**,
plat., plb., **PULS.**, **RAN-B.**, ran-s.,
rauw.[9], **rheum**, rhod., **rhus-t.**, ruta,
sabad., sabin., samb., sec., seneg.,
SEP., sil., **spig.**, spong., squil.,
stann., **staph.**, **stram.**, **STRONT-C.**,
sul-ac., sul-i.[1'], **SULPH.**, tab., tarax.,
teucr., thuj., valer., **verat.**, verb.,
zinc.

arteries, of[11]

chlor., **coff.**[7, 11], gels.

bones, of

agar., ang.[4], arg-m.[11], **asaf.**[1], bar-c.[2],
BELL., bry., **chin.**[2, 11], cimic., cocc.,
con., crot-h., dig., dulc., kali-bi.,
mang.[4], merc., nit-ac., rhod., **ruta,**
sulph., **valer.**, zinc.

glands, of

alum., am-c.[4], ambr., ang.[3, 4],
arg-m., arn., aur., **bar-c.**, bell.,
bov., **bry.**, calc., carb-an., **caust.**,
clem., coloc., **con.**, dulc., graph.,
kali-c., lyc., m-arct.[4], merc.,
mur-ac., nux-v., **PHOS.**, **puls.**,
rhus-t., sabad., sabin., sep., sil.,
spong., staph., stront-c., **sulph.**,
thuj.

joints, of[3]

am-c.[4], anac., ant-t., **ARG-M.**,
arn., ars., asaf., bell., **bov.**,
BRY.[3, 11], calc., calth.[11], caps.,
carb-an., carb-v., **carl.**[11], **CAUST.**,
cham., clem.[11], colch., coloc., con.,
croc., dig., dros., euph., euphr.,
graph., hell., hep., iod., **kali-c.**,
kali-n., kreos., lach., laur., **LED.**[2, 3],
LYC., **mag-c.**, manc.[11], **mang.**,
merc., **mez.**, mur-ac., **NAT-M.**,
nit-ac., nux-v., par., petr., phos.,
plat., **PULS.**[2, 3], rheum, **rhod.**,

rhus-t.[3, 4], ruta, samb., **seneg.**[3, 4, 11],
SEP., sil., spig., spong., **stann.**,
sul-ac., **SULPH., teucr.**, verat.,
verb., zinc.

muscles, of

ACON., am-c.[4], am-m., anac.,
ang.[3, 16], ant-c., arn., ars., bell.,
berb.[3], bufo[3], cann-i., cann-s., canth.,
caps.[3], carb-v., caust., chin., dulc.,
graph., **guaj.**, kali-ar.[1'], kali-c.,
lach., led., **mosch., nat-c., nat-m.,**
nat-p.[1'], **NIT-AC., NUX-V.**, olnd.,
ph-ac., **PHOS.**[3], **PHYS.**, phyt., **plat.,**
plb., **puls.**, rhus-t., **SEP.**, sil., stann.,
staph., sulph., verb., wies.[11], zinc.,
zinc-p.[1']

tremulous[16]

petr.

TETANUS, prophylaxis of[7]

ARN., HYPER., LED., tetox.. thuj.

THIRST for **large** quantities

acet-ac.[7], **acon., ARS.**, bad.,
BRY., calen.[2], camph., carbn-s.,
chin., coc-c., **cocc.**, cop., **eup-per.,**
ferr-p., ham., **jatr.**[2], lac-c.[3], lac-d.,
lil-t.[3], **lycps., merc-c., NAT-M.,**
PHOS., pic-ac., **podo.**[2], sol-n.,
stram., SULPH., VERAT., vip.[6]

often
acon.[2], arn.[2], ars.[10], **bell.**[2], **BRY.,**
cop., **eup-p.**[2], **lac-c., lac-d.**[2],
lil-t.[2, 3], **nat-m.**, ruta[16], samb.[2],
syph.[2], **tarent.**[2]

at long intervals

BRY., hell.[8], podo.[8], **sulph.**[8],
verat.[8]

small quantities, for

anac.[3], ant-t., apis, **ARS.,**
arum-t., bell., bry.[3], cact., calc.[3],
caps.[3], carb-v.[3], **chin.**, cimic.[7],
cupr., cupr-ar., gast.[11], **hell.,**
hep.[3], hyos., lac-c., **lach.**, laur.[3],
LYC., merc-i-r., nat-m.[3], nux-v.[3],
phos., **rhus-t.**, sanic.[7], squil.,
sulph., tab.

often
acon., ant-t., apis, **ARS.**, arum-t.,
bell., cact., **chin.**, coloc., **corn.,**
eup-per., hyos., kali-n.[6], lac-c.,
lyc., **nat-ar.**, puls., rhus-t., sanic.[7],
sulph., verat.

THIRSTLESS during heat

acet-ac.[7], aesc.[2], **aeth.**, agar., **AGN.**[3],
all-c.[3], **alum.**, alum-p.[1'], alum-sil.[1'],
am-m.[3, 6], anac.[3], ang.[3], **ant-c., ant-t.,**
APIS, arg-m., arn.[3], **ars.**[3, 16], ars-h.,
asaf., bar-c., bell.[3, 16], bov., brom.[3],
bry.[3], **calad.**[2], **calc.**, calc-p.[3], camph.,
canth.[3], carb-an., **carb-v., caust.,**
cham.[3, 6, 16], **CHEL.**[3], chin., chin-m.[2],
chin-s.[6], **cimx., CINA**, cocc., **coff.**[3, 6],
coloc.[3], **con.**[3, 16], cycl., dig., **dros.,**
DULC.[3, 6], euph.[3, 16], **ferr., GELS.,**
gran.[11], graph.[3], guaj.[3, 16], hell.,
hep.[3, 16], hydr-ac.[2], hyos.[2], **ign., ip.,**
kali-c., kali-n.[3, 16], kreos.[8], **lach.**[8],
laur.[3], lec., **led.**, lyc., mag-c.[8], mang.[3],
med., meny., **merc.**[3, 6], **mur-ac.,**
nat-c.[3], nat-m.[3], **nit-ac., nux-m.,**
olnd.[3], op., **ph-ac., phos.**[3, 16], plb.[3],
puls., rheum[3, 16], **rhod.**[3, 11], rhus-t.,
RUTA[3, 16], **SABAD.**, sabin.[3], **samb.,**
SEP., sil.[16], spig., spong.[3, 16], squil.[3, 16],
stann.[16], staph.[3, 16], stram.[2, 3, 16],
sulph., tarax.[3, 6, 16], thuj.[3], valer.[3],
verat.[3, 16], **viol-t.**[3]

THREADS, sensation of

bry., coc-c., ign., lach., **osm.**, par., **plat., VALER.**

pain–drawing–bones–thread

THROMBOSIS

acetan.[12], **ars.**[1, 7], apis[2, 7], **both.**[7, 8], calc-ar.[12], **carb-v.**[3, 16], cortico[9], **kali-m.**[2, 3, 6, 7, 12], kres.[13], lach.[8], nat-s.[7]. sec.[12], **vip.**[3, 6]

inflammation – phlebitis

albuminuria, in[7]

calc-ar.

pneumonia, in[7]

am-c.

wet agg.[7]

nat-s.

TICKLISH

KALI-C.[7], solin.[12], zinc.[11]

TOBACCO agg.*

abies-n.[3, 8, 12], acon., act-sp.[2], agar., **alum., alumn.**[2], ambr., anac.[3], ang.[2, 3], **ant-c.**, arg-m., arg-n., **ARS.**, aur-m-n.[6], bell., bor.[8], brom.[1', 3], **bry.**, cact.[3],

calad., calc., calc-caust.[6], calc-p.[8], camph., cann-i.[8], carb-an., carbn-s., caust.[3], cham.[3], chel., chin., chin-ar.[8, 12], chin-m.[12], cic., **clem.**, coca, coc-c., **cocc., coff.**[3, 6], coloc., con., conv.[3], cupr.[3], **cycl.**, dig., dor.[2], **euphr.**, ferr., **gels., hell.**, hep., hydr., **IGN.**, iod., **ip.**, kali-bi.[3, 8], kali-br.[3], kalm.[3, 6, 8, 12], lac-ac., **lach.**, lob.[8, 12], **lyc., mag-c.**, mag-m.[14], mand.[10], **meny.**, merc.[3], mur-ac.[8], naja[3], nat-c.[3], **nat-m.**, nicot.[12], **NUX-V.**, okou.[14], olnd.[3], osm., **par.**, petr., **phos., PLAN.**, plb.[8], psil.[14], **PULS.**, ran-b., rhus-t., **ruta**, sabad., sabin., sars., scut.[12], sec.[8], **sel.**, sep., sil., sol-m.[12], **SPIG., SPONG., STAPH.**, stel.[8], stront-c.[3], stroph-h.[6, 12], sul-ac., sulph., tab.[3, 8], **tarax., thuj.**, verat.

chewing agg.

ARS., carb-v., ign.[8], lyc., nux-v., **plan.**, sel.[8], tab.[2], **verat.**

nicotinism[10]*

ign., okou.[14], nux-v., tab.

smoking, when breaking off

calad.

ailments from[12]

abies-n., arg-n., ars., chin-ar., lob., lyc., phos., scut., **sep.**, spig., staph., stroph-h., thuj., **verat.**

am.

aran., aran-ix.[10], arn.[6], bor., carb-ac., coloc., **hep.**, levo.[14], merc., naja[3], nat-c., **sep.**, spig., stront-c.[3], tarent.[3, 6]. tarent-c.[3, 8]

aversion to

acon., acon-l.[11], alum.[6], ant-t.,
arg-n.[7], arn., bov., brom., bry.,
**CALC., camph., canth.,
carb-an.,** chlor., cimic., clem.[11],
cocc., con., grat.[6], **ign.,** jug-r.[11],
lach., led.[7], **lob.**[3, 4, 6, 8], **lyc.,**
mag-s., mand.[9], meph.,
nat-ar.[11], **nat-m., NUX-V.,
op., phos.,** phyt.[7], plan.[6-8],
psor., **puls.,** spig., staph.[6],
stry.[7], **sulph.,** tarax., thuj., til.,
v-a-b.[14], valer., zing.

morning
meph.

sensitive to smell of

agar.[11], ars-n.[2], **asc-t.**[2], **bell.,
casc.**[2, 8], chin., **ign., lob.**[2, 8], **lyc.**[2],
lyss., **nux-v.,** phos., **puls.,** sol-n.[11],
tab.[11]

smoking (his accustomed cigar)

alum., alum-p.[1'], ant-t.[2, 3],
arg-m., **arn.,** asar., bell.[3], bor.,
brom., bry., **calc.,** calc-p.,
camph., canth.[3], carb-an.,
casc.[2], chin.[3], clem., coc-c.,
cocc.[3], coff., con.[16], euphr.,
ferr.[1'], ferr-i.[11], grat., **IGN.,** ip.[3],
jug-r.[11], kali-bi., kali-n., lach.,
led.[3, 16], lob.[3], **lyc.,** mag-s.,
meph.[3], mez.[3], nat-ar., nat-m.,
nat-s., nicc., nux-m.[3], **nux-v.**[2, 3],
olnd., op., ox-ac., par.[3], phos.,
plat.[3, 16], psor., **puls.,** rhus-t.[3],
sars.[3, 16], sep., spig., stann.[3],
staph.[3], **sulph.,** tarax., tell.,
thuj.[3]

morning
ox-ac.

forenoon
kali-bi.

afternoon[1]

ign.

evening[2]
arg-n.

breakfast, after[11]

psor.

in spite of[14]

thiop.

• **desire** for t.

aran-ix.[9, 10, 14], **ars.**[12], **asar.**[8], bell.,
calad.[1'], **calc-p.**[3, 6, 12], **camph.**[12],
carb-ac., carb-v.[8], **chin.**[12], chlor.[11],
coca[2, 8], coff.[3], con.[11], daph.,
eug., glon.[3, 6], kreos., manc.,
med.[1', 7], narz.[11], (not [16]: nat-c.),
nicot.[7], nux-v., ox-ac., **phos.**[12],
plan.[12], plat., plb., rhus-t.[3], **spig.**[12],
staph., TAB., ther., thuj.

evening[11]
ox-ac.

dinner, after[11]

nat-c.

smoking

calad., carb-an., card-m.,
cast-eq.[2], coff.[3], daph.[3], eug.,
glon., ham., led., lyc., med.[3],
nat-c.[3, 16], nux-v.[3], staph.[3], ther.

snuff

bell.

disgust for t., remedies to [3, 5, 7]

arg-n.[7], ars.[7], calad., calc., camph.[5], caust., con.[5], ign., lach., nep.[13, 14], nicot.[7], nux-v., petr., plan.[3, 5-7], STAPH., stry.[7], sulph., tab.[7], v-a-b.[13]

TORPOR of the left side of the body

acon.

TOUCH agg.

acon., aesc., AGAR., agn., aloe, am-c., am-m., ambr., anac., ANG.[2, 3, 8], ange-s.[14], ant-c., ant-t., APIS, ARG-M., arg-n.[7], arn., ars., ASAF., asar., aur., aur-ar.[1'], aur-s.[1'], bar-c., bar-i.[1'], BELL., bor., bov., BRY., bufo[1'], cact., calad., calc., calc-f.[10, 14], calc-p., calc-sil.[1'], camph., cann-s., canth., caps., carb-an., carb-v., cast.[3], caust., CHAM., chel., CHIN., chin-ar., CHIN-S., cic., cimic.[6], cina, cinnb., clem., COCC., COFF., COLCH., coloc., com.[8], con., croc., CROT-C., crot-h., CUPR., cupr-a.[8], cycl., dig., dros., dulc., equis.[8], eup-per.[6], euph., euph-l.[8], euphr., ferr., ferr-i., ferr-p.[3, 8], fl-ac.[3], foll.[14], graph., GUAJ., HAM., hell, helon.[8], HEP., HYOS., ign., iod., ip., KALI-AR., kali-bi., KALI-C., kali-i., kali-m.[1'], kali-n., kali-p., kali-s., kali-sil.[1'], kreos., lac-c.[3], lac-d.[1'], LACH., laur., led., lil-t.[8], lob.[8], LYC., mag-c., mag-m., MAG-P., mand.[14], MANG., med., meny., meph.[4, 14], merc., merc-c., mez., mosch., mur-ac., murx.[3, 6, 8], nat-c., nat-m., nat-s.[1', 3, 7], nat-sil.[1'], NIT-AC., nux-m., NUX-V., olnd., op., osm.,

ox-ac.[8], par., petr., ph-ac., phos., plat., plb., puls., RAN-B., ran-s., RHOD., RHUS-T., ruta, sabad., SABIN., sal-ac., sang., sanic.[3], sars., sec., seneg., SEP., sieg.[10], SIL., SPIG.[1], spong., squil., stann., STAPH., stram., stront-c., stry.[8], sul-ac., sul-i.[1'], SULPH., syph.[1', 3, 7], tarax., tarent., tell., teucr.[2, 3], thal.[14], ther.[8], thuj., urt-u.[8], valer., verat., verb., viol-o., viol-t., vip-a.[14], zinc., ziz.[6]

cannot bear limbs touch each other at night[7]

psor.

children, in

ant-t.[4], apis[2], cina[2, 4]

feet, of

KALI-C.[2, 3], nux-v.[3]

slight

ACON.[3], APIS[3], ars., BELL., CHIN., coff., colch., ign., LACH., lyss.[2], mag-m., MERC., merc-c.[3], mez., nit-ac.[3], NUX-V., ph-ac., phos., stann.

throat agg., of[2, 3]

bell., LACH.

am.
agar., alum., alumn.[2], am-c., am-m., anac., ant-c., arn., ars., ASAF.[2, 3, 6, 8], bell., bell-p.[7], bism., bry., CALC., calc-a.[6], canth., cast.[3, 6], caust., chel., chin., coloc.,

con., **CYCL.**, dros., euph., euphr., **grat.**[3, 4, 6], hep.[2, 3], kali-c.[2, 3], petr., ph-ac., **phos.**, plb., sang.[3], sep., spig.[3], spong., staph.[3], sulph., tarax., **THUJ.**, viol-t., zinc.[3]

illusions of being touched

acon., **alum.**, anac., ant-t., arn., ars., **asaf.**, asar., bar-c., **bell.**, bism., bor., bov., bry., **calc.**, cann-s., canth., caps., caust., chel., coc-c., cocc., coloc., con., **croc.**, dros., dulc., glon., graph., guaj., hell., hep., hyos., **ign.**, indg., iod., kali-c., kali-n., kreos., **lach.**, laur., lyc., mag-c., mag-m., meny., merc., mosch., nat-c., nat-m., nux-v., olnd., op., **par.**, ph-ac., phos., plat., **plb.**, **puls.**, ran-b., ran-s., rheum, rhod., **RHUS-T.**, ruta, sabad., samb., seneg., sep., sil., **spig.**, spong., squil., staph., **stram.**, sul-ac., **sulph.**[1], tarax., thuj., valer., verat., verb.

pain vanishes on t. and appears elsewhere

ant-t.[2], asaf., sang., staph.[3]

TOUCHING anything agg.

acon., am-c., am-m., arg-m., arn., bell., bor., **bry.**, **calc.**, **cann-s.**, **carb-v.**, **caust.**, **CHAM.**, chin., dros., kali-c., kali-n., led., lyc., merc., nat-c., phos., plat., **puls.**, sec., **sil.**, spig., verat.

cold things agg.

calc., **HEP.**, **lac-d.**, **merc.**, **nat-m.**, **pyrog.**, **RHUS-T.**, **SIL.**, thuj., zinc.

warm things agg.

sulph.

TRAVELLING, ailments from[12]

cocc., con.

TREMBLING externally

aur., aur-ar.[1'], aur-i.[1'], aur-s.[1'], **bapt.**[1', 3, 6, 11], **bar-c.**, bar-i.[1'], bar-m., bar-s.[1'], **bell.**, ben-n.[11], benz-ac.[11], berb.[4], bism., **bor.**, both.[7], bov., brom., bruc.[4], **bry.**, bufo, buth-a.[9, 10], cadm-met.[10], cadm-s., caj.[11], **calad.**, **calc.**, calc-caust.[4, 11, 12], calc-f.[10, 14], **calc-i.**[1'], calc-m.[11], **calc-p.**, calc-sil.[1'], calth.[11], **camph.**, canch.[11], cann-i., cann-s., canth., caps., **carb-ac.**, carb-an.[4], carb-v., carbn-h.[11], carbn-o.[11], **carbn-s.**, cast.[2], **caust.**, cedr., cham., chel., chin., **chin-ar.**, **chin-s.**, chlorpr.[14], **CIC.**, cic-m.[11], **CIMIC.**, **cina**, cinch.[11], cinnm.[2], **cit-v.**[2, 11], clem., **coca**[2], **COCC.**, cod., **coff.**, coff-t.[2, 7, 11], coffin.[11], **colch.**, coloc., **CON.**, cop.[2], **cortico.**[9, 10], cortiso.[10], croc., crot-h., crot-t., **cupr.**, cupr-a.[4], cupr-ar.[6], **cupr-s.**[3], dig., digin.[11], dios., dros., dubo-h.[11], **dulc.**, echit.[11], esp-g.[13], euph.[3], euphr., fagu.[11], **ferr.**, ferr-ar.[4], ferr-ma.[4, 11], ferr-p., fl-ac.[1'], **GELS.**, gins.[6, 11], glon., gran.[3, 4, 6, 11], **graph.**, guaj., **hell.**, helo., hep., hydr-ac.[4, 11], **hyos.**, **hyper.**[2], iber.[11, 14], **ign.**, inul.[11], iod., ip., **iris**[2], jab.[6], kali-a.[11], **kali-ar.**, kali-bi.[11], **kali-br.**, **kali-c.**, kali-cy.[11], **kali-fcy.**, kali-i.[11], kali-n.[11, 16], kali-p., kali-s., kali-sil.[1'], **kalm.**, kiss.[11], kreos., lac-ac., **lach.**, lat-m.[9], lath.[3, 6], laur., **lec.**, **led.**, lil-t.[1', 2, 11], lob.[3, 4, 6, 11], lol.[3, 10-12], lon-x.[11], lyc., lycps.[2], **lyss.**, m-arct.[4], m-aust.[4], mag-c., mag-m., mag-p., mag-s., manc.[3, 11], mang., meny., meph., **MERC., merc-c.,** merc-d.[11], merc-i-f.[11], merc-ns.[11], merc-pr-r.[11], **mez.,** morph.[11], **mosch.,** mur-ac., mygal., naja[1'] **NAT-AR.,** nat-c.[1], nat-hchls.[11], **nat-m., nat-s.,** nat-sil.[1'], nicc.[4, 6, 11], nicot.[11], **nit-ac.,** nux-m., **nux-v.,** oena.[11], ol-an.[4], **olnd., OP.,** ox-ac., pall., par., ped.[11], petr., **ph-ac.,** phel.[2, 4], **phos.,** phys.[2, 3, 6, 11], **phyt., pic-ac.,** pip-n.[3], plan., **PLAT., plb.,** polyg-h., prun.[4, 11], psil.[14], **psor., PULS.,** ran-a.[11], ran-b., ran-s., rauw.[9, 14], reser.[14], rheum, rhod., **RHUS-T.,** russ.[11], ruta, **sabad.,** sabin., sal-ac.[6], sang., sars., scut.[11], **sec.,** sel., senec.[11], **seneg., sep.,** sieg.[10], **sil.,** spig., spig-m.[11], sol-n.[11], spong., squil.[3, 6], **stann.,** staph., **STRAM.,** stront-c., **stry.,** sul-ac., sul-h.[11], sul-i.[1'], **SULPH., tab.,** tanac., tarax., **tarent.,** tax.[11], teucr., thal.[11, 14], thea, **THER., thuj.,** thyreotr.[14], til.[11], valer., vanad.[7], **verat.,** verat-v.[11], verb., verin.[11], vesp.[2, 11], viol-o., vip.[3, 4, 6], **vise.,** wies.[11], **x-ray**[9], **ZINC.,** zinc-cy.[11], zinc-o.[4], **zinc-p.**[1'], zinc-s.[11]

weakness – tremulous

right side, of[11]

merc.

internally

abrot.[3, 6, 7], ambr., ang.[3], **ant-t.,** aran-ix.[10, 14], **arg-n.,** asaf., bell., bell-p.[9], **brach.,** bry., calad., **CALC.,** calc-sil.[1'], **camph.,** caps., carb-v., carbn-s., **caul., caust.,** chin-s.[11], cina, **clem.,** cocc., colch.,

con., **crot-h.,** cycl., dicha.[14], esp-g.[13], **eup-per.,** gels.[7], glon.[3], **GRAPH.,** hep.[3, 16], hura[11], **IOD., kali-c., kali-n.,** kali-sil.[1'], kreos., lach.[3, 6], **lec.,** lil-t., **lyc.,** meph., merc., mosch., nat-ar., **nat-c., nat-m.,** nep.[10, 13, 14], nit-ac., nux-m., **nux-v.,** par., petr., **phos., plat., puls., RHUS-T.,** ruta, sabad., sabin., samb., **seneg.,** sep., sil., **spig., STANN., STAPH., stront-c., SUL-AC.,** sul-i.[1'], **sulph.. teucr.,** ther.[3, 6], thuj.[3], valer., **x-ray**[9], zinc.

night[16]   :t/n~
   nat-m., plat.

climacteric period, during[7]

   caul., sul-ac.

whole body, in[2]

   alum-sil.[1'], ant-t., **arg-n.,** ars., ars-s-f.[1', 2], ars-s-r., bell., calc.[16], carbn-s., **chel., cimic.**[3], **cocc., ferr., GELS.,** inul., iod.[3], **kali-br.,** kali-sil.[1'], **nat-m., nat-s., phos.**[2, 3], sep., stram., sul-ac., sulph.[16], ther.[3], **verat.**

morning
   alumn., **arg-m., arg-n.,** ars., bar-c., calc., carb-v.[2], cimic., **con., dulc.,** gran.[11], graph., lyc., mag-c., nat-m., nicc.[6], **nit-ac.**[2], **nux-v.,** petr., phos., sil., sulph.

breakfast, before

   calc., **con.,** nat-m., nux-v., staph.

rising, on[4, 11, 16]

   bar-c.[4, 11], dulc.[11], petr.

   am.[16]: mag-c.

waking, on

   arg-m., bar-c.[4], calc.[4, 16], carb-v.[4],
   caust., **dulc.,** euphr.[4], hyper.,
   mag-c., nit-ac., phos., tarent.,
   verat.[3]

forenoon
   ars., carb-v.[11], carbn-o., lyc.,
   nat-m., ol-an.[4, 11], **plat.,** sars.,
   sulph.[4]

9.30 h[11]
   phys.

10 h
   bor.

exertion, on

   gels.

noon[4]
   sulph.

after sleep

   nat-m.

afternoon
   ant-t.[4], carb-v., **gels.,** lyc., lyss.
   pic-ac.

13 h[11]
   verat-v.

15 h[2]
   asaf., **nux-v.**

17 h[11]
   ped.

evening
   bruc.[6], caust.[6], chel., iber.[11],
   lach.[6], lyc., mez., mygal., nat-m.,
   nit-ac.[6, 16], nux-v.[6], pic-ac.[1], plb.,
   sil.[6], stront-c., sulph.

19 h[11]
   phys.

bed, in
   lιι, aι
   B
   anag.[11], eupi., lyc., nux-v., samb.

sleep, after

   carb-v.

walking, after

   sil.

night
   bell., hyos., lyc., merc.[1', 6], **op.[2],**
   phos., rat.[4]

half awake, while[16]

   sulph.

3 h
   rhus-t.

dreaming, after

   calc.[11], nicc.[11], phos., sil.

sleep, after

   sil.

affected parts, of[3]

   caust.

air, in open

   calc., **kali-c.,** laur., **plat.**

am.
   clem.

alternating with convulsions[11]

merc.

convulsive movements of limbs[11]

arn.

weakness[11]
ferr.

alone, am. when[11]

ambr.

anger, from

acon., alum.[7], ambr., arg-n., **aur.,**
cham.[3, 6], chel., cop., daph., ferr-p.[7],
lyc., m-austr.[4], merc., **nit-ac.,**
nux-v.[3, 6], pall.[1], petr.[3], phos., **plat.**[2],
ran-b., sep., **staph., zinc.**

with
acon., alum.[7], ambr., arg-n.,
aur., cham.[3, 6], chel., cop., daph.,
ferr-p., lyc., m-aust.[4], merc.,
nit-ac., nux-v.[3, 6], pall., petr.,
phos., **plat.**[2], ran-b., sep., **staph.,**
zinc.

anxiety, from

abrot.[6], aeth.[2], ambr., **ARS.,** aur.,
bell., bor., **calc.,** canth., carb-v.,
caust., **cham.,** chel., **coff., con.,** croc.,
cupr., euph.[16], ferr.[11], graph., **lach.,**
lyc., mag-c., mez., mosch., nat-c.,
nit-ac., nux-m., phos., **plat.,** psor.,
puls., rhus-t., samb., sars., sep.,
sulph.[16], valer.

with[6]
abrot., acon., agar.[16], ant-c., aur.,
bell., **cina, croc.,** petr.[16], **puls.,**
ther., verat.

ascending, on

merc.

attacks, before[3]

absin.

bed, in[11]

merc-ns.

breakfast, after

arg-n.

am.
calc., con., nat-m., nux-v., staph.

caressing, while

caps.

climacteric period, during

kali-br.[2, 7], ther.[6]

coffee, from smell of[11]

sul-ac.

coition, after[6]

calc.

cold drinks am.

phos.

coldness, during

bor.

with coldness[2]

bufo, hyos.[6], **merc., mosch., nux-m., op.**[2, 6], plat.[6]

company agg.

ambr., lyc.

conversation, from

ambr., bor.

convulsive[3]

am-c.[11], ang., ars.[11], bar-m.[2, 3], bism., canth.[11], ign., lol.[11], merc.[11], nux-v., op., plb., sabad., tab.[11]

spasmodic

coughing, from

am-c.[16], ant-t.[3], bell., **cupr., phos.,** seneg.[16]

dinner, during

mag-m.

dipsomania with[2]

ant-t., **ars.**[2, 3, 6], **crot-h., lach., mag-p., nux-v.**[2, 3, 6], sul-ac.[3, 6], **sulph.**[3, 6]

dreams, during[4]

calc., m-arct.

after[4]
ferr-ma., nicc.

drinking, after excessive

plb.

eating, after

alum., ant-c., caust.[4], lyc.[3, 4, 16], mag-m.[4], olnd.[3], phel.[4], tab.[4], zinc.[4]

emotions, after

arg-n., **COCC.,** coff.[6], cycl.[7], ferr., hep., merc., nat-c., nat-m., petr.[2], phys.[2], **plb., psor., STAPH.,** stram., thyreotr.[14], **zinc.**

exercise, from[11]

merc., plan., polyg-h.

exertion, on[6]

alco.[11], am-caust.[6, 11], anac., ant-t., **arn.,** ars., chin-s., **COCC.**[2, 6], iod., merc.[11], nat-c., **nat-m., rhus-t.,** sec.[6, 11], **sil.**[2, 6]

agg.[3]
anac., ant-t., arn., ars., chin-s., cocc., iod., nat-c., nat-m., rhus-t., sec., sil.

on slight

bor., **cocc.,** ferr., **merc.,** phos., **plat., plb.,** polyg-h., **rhus-t.,** sec., **stann., zinc.**

eyes agg., closing[11]

merc.

faintness, during[7]

asaf.[11], lach.[2], nux-v., petr.,

fatigue, after

plb.

fear, from[2]

calc.

feet, on washing[11]

merc.

fever, during

acon.[6], ars., calc., camph., cann-i.[6], caps.[6], cist., eup-per., kali-c., lach., mag-c., mygal., sep.

fright, from

acon.[2, 3, 6], arg-n., aur., calc.[3, 6], coff., glon., hura, ign., mag-c., merc., nicc., op., plat.[2], puls., ran-b.[2], rat., rhus-t., sep., stram.[2], tarent.[2], zinc.[3, 6]

headache, during[3]

arg-n.

with chill[16]

carb-v.

hungry, when

alum., crot-h., olnd., stann., sulph., zinc.

intention tremor[3]

anac., arg-n., bell., cic., cocc., gels., iod., merc., phos., phyt., rhus-t., samb., sec., zinc.

joy, from

acon., aur., cimic.[2], coff., cycl.[2], merc., valer.

looking down, on

kali-c.

lying, while

clem.

on left side agg., on back am.[2]

kalm.

meeting friends

tarent.

menses, before

alum., hyos.[2, 3], kali-c.[2, 3], lyc.[2, 3], nat-m.[2, 3], sep.[3], stann.[2, 3, 6]

during
agar.[3], arg-n., calc-p., caul.[3], caust.[3], cina[2], graph., hyos., kali-c.[3], lec., mag-c.[4], merl.,

nat-m.[2, 3], nicc.[6], **nit-ac.**, plat.[2, 3], puls.[6], **stram.**[2, 3, 6], wies.[11]

after
chin.

mental exertion, from

aur., bor.[1], **CALC.**[2], **plb.**[1], vinc.

motion, on

anac., arg-n., canth.[4], iod., kali-ar.[1'], phyt., puls.[4], sulph.[16], zinc.

hands and feet, of[11]

cann-i.

am.
merc., plat.

music, from

aloe[2, 7], **AMBR.,** thuj.[7]

nausea, with[2]

ars.[11], **calc.,** carb-v.[11], chel., cimic.[11], eup-per., plat., tab.[11], vesp.[2, 11]

noise, from

aloe[2], bar-c., caust., **cocc.,** hura, **kali-ar.,** mosch., tab.

nursing infant, after

olnd.

old age, in[3, 6]

alum.[7], ambr.[7], aur.[7], bar-c., calc., con., kali-c.[7], merc.[7], op.[7], phos.[7], plb.[3], plb-a.[6], sil., stront-c., sulph., zinc.[7]

pains, with the

bism.[7], **cocc., NAT-C.,** nit-ac.[3], **plat.,** puls., sul-ac.[3], zinc.[3]

after[11]
bry.

palpitation, with[2]

acon., benz-ac., calc-ar.

paroxysmal

anthraci.[2], arg-n.[3], crot-h.[3, 6], ferr.[3, 6], lyc.[3, 6, 16], **merc.**

periodical

ARG-N.

perspiration, with[2]

ars.[16], merc.[3, 6], mosch.[6], rhus-t.

cold[3]
merc., mosch., **puls.**[2]

after[2]
apis

playing the piano, while

nat-c.

rest, during[11]

eupi.

am.
merc.[11], nep.[10]

rising, on[3]

ambr.[7], nat-m., rhus-t.

from sitting in affected parts

CAUST.

sexual excess, t. after[2]

phos.

excitement, t. during

graph.

side lain on

clem.

sleep, before

carb-an.[4], nat-m., petr.[4], sep.[4, 16]

during
apis[2], **chlf.**[2], con., kali-c.[16], rheum[2]

starting from[16]

petr.

smoking, from

hep., nat-m., **nux-v.**[2], sil., sulph.

sneezing, on[7]

BOR.

something is to be done, when

KALI-BR.

spasmodic[3, 6]

ang., bar-m., bism., **ign., nux-v.,**
op., plb., **sabad.**

convulsive

standing, while

merc.

stitching in ear, from[16]

thuj.

stool, before

hydr., merc., sumb.

during
carbn-s.

after
ars., carb-v., caust., **CON.,** lil-t.,
merc.[2]

supper, after

alum., caust.

surprise, agg. from[11]

merc.

thunderstorm

agar., **morph.,** nat-p., **phos.**

touch, unexpected

   cocc.

urination, during[11]

   gels.

   after[16]
     ars.

vertigo with

   am-c., ars., bell., **camph.,** carb-v., crot-h., **dig., dulc., glon.,** nat-m., puls.

vexation, from

   acon., **aur.,** cham.[6], coff.[1'], lyc., nit-ac., nux-v.[6], petr.[6, 16], ran-b.

voluptuous

   calc.

vomiting, while[11]

   colch., eup-per.[2], gran.

   after[11]
     ars.

waking, on

   abrot., bar-c.[4], calc., carb-v.[2, 4], caust.[4], **cina, dulc.**[2], euphr.[4], ferr-ma.[4], **ign.**[2], lach., m-arct.[4], **merc.,** nicc.[4], nit-ac., orig.[11], **petr.**[4], phos.[3', 4], rat., samb.[4, 16], sil.[4], stront-c.[4], sulph.[4], tarent., verat.[3]

walking, while

   am-c., cupr-ar.[6], lac-ac., merc., nux-v., stry.[11]

   after
   cupr.[16], ust.

weakness, from[6]

   agar., **anac., ant-t., bapt.,** bell., bry., caust., **chin.**[3, 6], cocc., con., kali-c., mang., **nat-m.**[3, 6], **stann.**[3, 6], ther., verat., zinc.

wine, from

   con.

worm affections, in[1']

   sabad.

writing, while

   lyss.[10], **phos., sil.**

TRICKLING sensation, like drops

   agar.[3], ambr., arg-n.[3], arn., bell., berb.[3], **CANN-S.,** caust.[3], cot.[3], croc.[3], glon.[3], graph.[3], kali-bi.[3], mag-m.[3], nat-m.[3], nux-m.[3], petros.[3], phos.[3], rhus-t.[3], sep., spig., stann.[3], tarent.[3], thuj., vario.[3], verat.

hot drops[3]

   stann., sulph.

TUBERCULOSIS, prophylaxis of[7]

bac., sulph., tub.[7]

lupus vulgar

abr.[8, 12], agar., alum., alum-sil.[1'],
alumn., am-ar.[8], ant-c., apis[8],
arg-n., **ARS.**, **ars-i.**, ars-s-f.[1'],
aur-ar.[8, 12], aur-i[8], aur-m., **bar-c.**,
bell.[1], calc., calc-ar.[2], calc-i.[8],
calc-p.[2], calc-s.[8], calc-sil.[1'],
calo.[12], **carb-ac.**, **carb-v.**, **carbn-s.**,
caust., chr-o.[12], cic.[1], **cist.**,
cund.[2, 8], ferr-pic.[8, 12], form.[8],
form-ac.[8], graph., guar.[8], guare.[12],
hep., hippoz.[12], **hydr.**[2, 8, 12],
hydrc., irid.[8], kali-ar., **kali-bi.**,
kali-c., **kali-chl.**, **kali-i.**[8],
kali-m.[2], kali-s., **kreos.**, lach.,
LYC., m-arct.[1], merc-i-r.[1], **nit-ac.**,
ol-j.[1], **phyt.**, **psor.**, ran-b.[1'],
rhus-t.[1], sabin.[1], sep., **sil.**, spong.,
staph., sulph., thiosin.[8, 12],
THUJ., **tub.**[8], **tub-k.**[12], urea[8],
x-ray[8]

in rings
sep.

TUMORS, benign

polypus

**angioma, fungus haematodes,
hemangioma**

abrot.[8], ant-t., **ARS.**, bell., **calc.**,
CARB-AN., **carb-v.**, clem., **kreos.**,
LACH., lyc., manc.[8], **merc.**, **nat-m.**,
nit-ac., nux-v., **PHOS.**, **puls.**,
rhus-t., sep., **SIL.**, staph., **sulph.**,
THUJ.

atheroma, steatoma

agar., ant-c.[4], anthraci.[2], **bar-c.**,
bell.[2], benz-ac.[6, 8, 12], brom.[6], **calc.**,
caust[2], clem[2], **con.**[2, 6, 8, 12], daph[8],
GRAPH., **guare.**[2, 11], **hep.**, kali-br.[2, 6],
kali-c., kali-i.[6, 12], lac-ac.[2], lach.[7, 12],
lob., lyc., m-arct.[4], mez.[6, 8], nat-c.,
nit-ac.[2, 4, 6, 12], **ph-ac.**[2, 12], **phyt.**[2, 6, 12],
rhus-t.[2, 12], **sabin.**[4, 6], sil., spong.[4],
staph.[12], **sulph.**[2, 4, 6], thuj.[2], **vanad.**[12]

reappearing every 4 weeks

calc.

suppurating
calc., carb-v., sulph.[4]

cheloid see keloid

colloid[2]

carb-ac., hydr., phos.

cystic

agar., **apis**[1, 7], apoc.[2, 6], ars.[2, 3],
aur.[1', 3, 6], **BAR-C.**, benz-ac.[6], bov.[12],
brom., **CALC.**[1, 7], calc-f.[6], calc-p.[8],
calc-s., caust.[3], **con.**[3, 6], form-ac.[6],
GRAPH., hep.[1, 7], hydr.[3], iod.[3, 6, 8],
kali-br.[7, 8], kali-c.[3], lyc.[3, 6], med.[7],
merc-d.[6], nit-ac., **PHOS.**[3], platan.[8],
sabin.[3], sil., spong.[3], staph.[8, 12],
sulph., **thuj.**[3, 6]

bones, of

mez.

encephaloma

acet-ac., arn.², **ars.**, ars-i., art-v.²,
bell.², **calc.**, carb-ac., **carb-an.**,
caust., **croc.²**, hydr.², kali-i., **kreos.**,
lach., nit-ac., nux-v.², **PHOS.**,
plb.¹², **sil.**, sulph., **thuj.**

enchondroma⁸

calc.², calc-f., conch.¹², lap-a.
sil.¹', ², ⁶, ⁸, ¹²

erectile

lyc., nit-ac., phos., staph.

fibroid

arb.⁷, bell.², bry.², **calc., CALC-F.,**
calc-i.⁷, ⁸, **calc-s.**, chol.⁷, chr-s.⁸,
con., fl-ac.⁷, ¹⁰, frax.⁷, graph.³, ⁸,
hydr.⁷, **hydrin-m.**⁸, ¹², **kali-br.**⁷,
kali-i.⁸, ¹², **lap-a.**², ⁷, ⁸, ¹², led.²,
lil-t.¹², lyc.¹², **PHOS.**, phyt.⁷,
sec.⁸, ¹², **SIL.**, tarent.¹², ter.¹²,
teucr.¹², thiosin.⁸, thlas.¹²,
thyr.⁸, ¹², tril.³, ⁸, ust.⁷, ¹², xan.¹²

haemorrhage, with⁸, ¹²

calc.³, **hydrin-m.**, lap-a.⁸, nit-ac.³,
phos.³, sabin.⁸, sul-ac.³, thlas.,
tril., ust.

ganglion

am-c., arn., aur-m., **benz-ac.**², ³, ⁸, ¹²,
bov.¹², calc-f.⁶, **carb-v.**, ferr-ma.¹²
iod.⁶, kali-m.⁸, ph-ac., **phos.**, plb.,
rhus-t., **ruta**, sil., sulph., thuj.⁶, ¹²,
zinc.

keloid. cheloid

ars.⁷, **bad.³, bell-p.⁶, ⁷**, calc.⁷,

calc-f.⁶, ¹⁰, carb-v.⁷, caust.⁶, ⁷,
crot-h.⁷, cupre-l.¹², **FL-AC.**⁷, ⁸,
gast.⁷, **GRAPH.⁶, ⁷**, hyper.⁷, **iod.⁶, ⁷**,
junc-e.⁷, kali-bi.³, **lach.⁷**, maland.¹²,
merc.⁷, **NIT-AC.**⁶⁻⁸, ¹², nux-v.⁷,
phos.⁷, phyt.⁷, psor.⁷, rhus-t.⁷,
sabin.⁷, ⁸, **SIL.¹, ⁷**, sul-ac.⁷, sulph.⁷, ¹²,
thiosin.⁷, tub.⁷, vac.⁷, ¹², vip.⁷

lipoma², ⁸

agar.², ¹², **am-m.²**, **BAR-C.²**, ⁶, ⁸,
BELL.², **calc.**, calc-ar.⁸, croc.²,
graph.², **kali-br.⁷**, **lap-a.**², ⁷, ⁸, phos.²,
phyt., thuj.⁸, ¹², ur-ac.⁸, ¹²

naevus

abrot.³, ⁶, ¹⁰, **ACET-AC.**, arn.³,
ars.³, bell-p.¹⁰, **calc.**, calc-f.³, ⁶,
carb-an.³, **carb-v.**, con.⁸, cund.², ⁸,
ferr-p.², ³, ⁶, ¹⁰, ¹², **FL-AC., graph.³, ⁴**,
ham.³, ⁶, lach.³, **lyc.**, med.⁷,
nit-ac.³, ⁴, nux-v., **petr.³, ⁴**, **ph-ac.³, ⁴**,
PHOS., rad.³, rad-br.⁶, ⁸,
rumx.³, ⁶, **sep.³**, **sil.³, ⁴**, sul-ac.³, ⁴,
sulph.³, ⁴, **thuj.**, ust.³, vac.

neuroma

all-c.⁸, calc., calen.⁸, staph.

noma

alum., alumn., **ars.**, bapt.⁸, calc.,
carb-v., **con.**, elat., **guare.²**, hydr.⁸,
kali-chl.⁸, **kali-p.⁸**, **kreos.⁸**, **lach.⁸**,
merc., **merc-c.⁸**, **mur-ac.⁸**, sec.⁸,
sil., sol-t-ae.¹², sul-ac.⁸, sulph.,
tarent-c.³

osteoma², ¹²

mez.

papillomata⁸

ant-c., **calc.**¹', ², nit-ac., **staph.**,
thuj.

TURNING around agg.

agar., aloe, calc., cham., **ip.**, kali-c., merc., nat-m., par., **phos.**, sil.

bed, in

acon., agar., am-m., anac., ars., asar., **bor.**, **brom.**[3], **bry.**, calc., **cann-s.**, **caps.**, **carb-v.**, caust., chin., cina, cocc., **con.**, cupr., dros., **euph.**, ferr., graph., **hep.**, kali-c., kreos., lach., led., **lyc.**, mag-c., merc., **nat-m.**, nit-ac., **nux-v.**, petr., phos., plat., plb., **PULS.**, ran-b., rhod., rhus-t., ruta, sabad., sabin., samb., sars., **sil.**, **staph.**, **sulph.**, thuj., valer.

head

am-m., anac., **arn.**, ant-c., ars.[3], asar., bar-c., **bell.**, bov., **bry.**, **CALC.**, camph., cann-s., canth., carb-an., carb-v., caust., cham., chin., **CIC.**, cocc., coff., coloc., con.[3], cupr., dros., dulc., glon., **HEP.**, hyos., **ign.**, ip., kali-c., lach., lil-t.[3], **lyc.**, mag-c., mez., **nat-c.**, **nat-m.**, nit-ac., **nux-v.**, par., petr., ph-ac., **phos.**, plat., **puls.**, **rhus-t.**, sabad., sabin., samb., **sang.**, sars., **sel.**, **sep.**, spig., **SPONG.**, stann., staph., sulph., thuj., verat., viol-t., zinc.

left agg., right to[3]

sulph.

right am., left to[3]

lach., phos.,

---

twisting involuntarily, t. and[16]

lyc.

TWITCHING

abies-c.[11], acon., acon-c.[11], **AGAR.**, agn., alum., alum-p.[1'], alum-sil.[1'], alumn.[2, 11], am-c., am-m., **ambr.**, ant-c., **ant-t.**, apis, aran.[2], **arg-m.**, **arg-n.**, arn.[2, 3, 11], **ars.**, **ars-i.**, ars-s-f.[1', 11], ars-s-r.[11], arund.[2, 11], **ASAF.**, asc-t.[2], aster., atro., **bar-c.**, bar-i.[1'], bar-m., **bell.**, bism.[3], bor., brom., bruc.[11], **bry.**, bufo, **CACT.**, cadm-s.[2, 11], **calc.**, **calc-i.**[1'] calc-p.[11], **calc-s.**, calc-sil.[1'], **camph.**, cann-i., cann-s.[3, 11], **canth.**, caps., carb-ac., carb-v., **carbn-s.**, carc.[9], **caust.**, cedr.[2], cerv.[11], cham., **chel.**, **chin.**, **chin-s.**, chlf.[2], chlor., **cic.**, cic-m.[11], **cimic.**, cina, **clem.**, cocc., **cod.**, coff.[1', 2], coff-t.[11], colch., coloc., **con.**, croc., crot-h., **cupr.**, cupr-s.[2, 11], cypr.[2], cyt-l.[11], dig., dol.[2, 11], dor.[2], dros., dulc.[3, 11], ferr.[1'], form.[3], **gels.**[2], **glon.**[2, 3, 6], graph., guaj., hedeo.[11], **hell.**, hep.[5], hydr-ac.[3, 11], **HYOS.**, **IGN.**, **IOD.**, ip., juni.[11], **kali-ar.**, kali-br., **KALI-C.**, **kali-i.**[2], kali-m.[1'], kali-n.[11, 16], kali-p., **kali-s.**, kali-sil.[1'], kreos., **lach.**, lact.[11], laur., lipp.[11], lon-x.[11], **lyc.**, **lyss.**, mag-c.[3], mag-m., mag-p., meny., **merc.**, **merc-c.**, **MEZ.**, morph.[11], **mosch.**[2], **mur-ac.**, mygal., **nat-ar.**, **NAT-C.**, nat-f.[9], **nat-m.**, **nat-p.**, nat-s.[1'], nat-sil.[1'], **nit-ac.**, nitro-o.[11], **nux-m.**[2, 6, 11], **nux-v.**, oena.[2, 11], ol-an.[3], olnd., **op.**, ox-ac., **par.**, petr., **ph-ac.**, **phos.**, phys.[2, 3, 11], phyt.[1'] pic-ac.[11], plat., **plb.**, **podo.**[6], psor., puls., **ran-b.**[2, 3], rat.[3, 11], rhod., **rhus-t.**, **rhus-v.**[11], ruta, sabad.[2, 3], sabin., salin.[11], sarcol-ac.[9], scut.[11], **sec.**, sel., senec-j.[11], seneg., **sep.**, **sil.**, sol-n.[11], **spig.**, spong., squil.[3], **stann.**, staph.[3, 11], **STRAM.**,

stront-c., **stry.**, sul-ac., sul-i.[1'],
sulph., tab.[11], tanac., tarax.,
tarent.[3], ter.[2], thuj., valer.,
verat.[2, 3], **verat-v.**[2, 3], viol-t.,
vip.[3, 11], **visc.**, x-ray[9], ZINC.,
zinc-m.[11]- **zinc-p.**[1']

daytime[2]

bar-c., lyss

morning[11, 16]
rheum

waking, on

chel.[2], menth-pu.[11]

noon[11]
petr., ZINC.

evening[11]
aether

bed, in[11]

ped., petr., ran-b., sil.

night[11]
ambr., cupr.-a., op., staph., tab.

sleep, during[11]

graph., nat-c., petr., sel., ZINC.

chill, during[2, 11]

stram.

dentition, during[2]

cham., ter., **zinc.**

dipsomania, in[2]

crot-h., phos.

electricity, as from[11]

acon., arn., clem., **daph.,** dulc.,
plb., sec.

fever with[2]

bell., nit-s-d., rhus-t.[11], **spong.**

typhoid[2]

CALC., cham., **colch.,** crot-h.,
cypr., gels., HYOS., lyc., ter.,
zinc.

fright, after

op., stram.

haemorrhage with[2]

chin.

here and there

alum.[16], agar., ant-c.[3], chel.[3], **cocc.,**
colch., **kali-c.,** kali-n., lyc., mez.,
nat-c.[16], nat-m., ph-ac., phos., rhod.,
sep., **stry.,** sulph., ZINC.

internally

atro., bov., **cann-s.,** cic.[11], seneg.

leucorrhoea with[3]

alum.

menses, during[3]

bell., calc-s.[2], chin., cocc., coff.,
kali-c., plat., sec., sulph.

after[3]

    chin., cupr., kreos., **nat-m.**[2, 3],
    puls.

one-sided[15]

    apis

paralysed part, of

    apis, **arg-n.**, merc., nux-v., phos.,
    sec., stram., stry.

parturition, during[2]

    cinnm.

    labor ceases, t. beginns when[2]

    sec.

rest, during[1']

    valer.

right side

    caust., tarent.[3]

single parts, of[3]

    agar., alum., chin., **cocc.**, nux-v.,
    puls., zinc.

sleep, during

    alum.[1], **ant-t.**[2], anac., **ars., bar-c.**[2],
    bell., brom.[11], caust., **cham.**[2, 6],
    chlf.[2], cina[6], cinnb., **colch.**[2], con.,
    cupr., dulc., graph.[16], **hell.**[2],
    HYOS.[2], hyper.[2], ign.[6], **kali-c.**,
    kiss.[11], **lyc.**[2, 6, 16], mag-c., merc.[16],

mez., nat-c., nat-m., op.[11], petr.[16],
ph-ac., phos., puls.[11], rheum[2],
seneg., **sep.**[2], sil., stann., **stram.**[2],
stront-c., sul-ac., **sulph.**, tep.[11],
thuj., **ZINC.**

on going to

    acon., **agar.**, all-s.[2], **aloe**[2], **alum.**,
    arg-m., **ARS., BELL.**[3], calc.[3],
    carb-v.[1'], cham.[3], cob., hyper.,
    ign., iodof.[2], **KALI-C.**, mag-m.[11],
    phys., puls.[3], **sel.**, sep.[3], stront-c.,
    stry., sul-ac., sulph., zinc.

subsultus tendinum

    agar., am-c., ambr., **ars., asaf.**,
    bell., **calc., camph., canth., chel.**,
    chlor., cupr.[6], **HYOS., IOD.**, kali-c.[6],
    kali-i., lyc., mez., mur-ac., ph-ac.,
    phos., rhus-t., **sec.**, squil.[6], **stry.**,
    sul-ac.[16], **ZINC.**

touch, on[11]

    morph., phos., stry.

    agg.
      stry.

upper part of body on lying down[16]

    nat-m.

waking, on[4]

    ars., bell., camph.[2], carc.[9], cham.[6],
    chel.[2], **cod.**[2], **hyos.**[6], laur.[2], lyc.,
    mag-m., op.[11], sang.[11], stront-c.

worm affections, in

    cina, sabad.[1', 2]

ULCERS, glands

ambr., ant-c., arn., **ARS.**, asaf., aur., aur-ar.[1'], **bell.**, calc., **canth.**, carb-an., carb-v., caust., clem., coloc., **con.**, cupr., dulc., **hep.**, hyos., ign., kali-c., kali-p., kreos., **lach.**, lyc., merc., nit-ac., **ol-j.**[2], ph-ac., **PHOS.**, **phyt.**, rhus-t., **rhus-v.**[2], sars., sep., **SIL.**, spong., squil., sul-ac., **sulph.**, thuj., zinc.

cancerous see cancerous–ulcers

UNCLEANLINESS agg.

CAPS., chin., psor., puls., **sulph.**
all-c.[3], **CAPS.**, **chin.**, **psor.**, **puls.**, **sulph.**

UNCOVERING agg.

acon., acon-f., **agar.**, am-c., ant-c., arg-m., **arg-n.**, arn., **ARS.**, asar., **atro.**, **aur.**, aur-ar.[1'], **bell.**, **benz-ac.**, bor., **bry.**, calc-sil.[1'], camph., cann-s.[3], canth., **caps.**, **carb-an.**, caust.[3, 6], **cham.**, **chin.**, **cic.**, **clem.**, **cocc.**, **coff.**, **colch.**, **con.**, dios., dros.[8], **dulc.**, **graph.**, hell., **HEP.**, hyos., **ign.**, **KALI-AR.**, kali-bi., **KALI-C.**, kali-i., **kali-sil.**[1'], kalm.[12], kreos., **lach.**, led.[2, 3], **LYC.**, lycps., **mag-c.**, **mag-m.**, **MAG-P.**, mang.[16], meny., **merc.**, mur-ac., **nat-c.**, **nat-m.**, **NUX-M.**, **NUX-V.**, ph-ac., **phos.**, psor.[3, 6], puls., rheum, **RHOD.**, **RHUS-T.**, **rumx.**, sabad., **SAMB.**, sang-n.[12], sep., **SIL.**, **SQUIL.**, staph., stram., **STRONT-C.**, sulph.[3], thuj., **ZINC.**, zinc-p.[1']

least[3]

hep., nux-v., rhus-t., **sil.**

single part agg.

bry., **HEP.**, ip.[2], **nat-m.**, **RHUS-T.**, **SIL.**, squil., stront-c., **thuj.**

cold becoming

feet, of[8]

calc., cupr., nux-m., sil.

ailments from[12]

kalm.. sanq-n.

am.[3]

acon., alum., apis[1', 3, 8], ars., asar.[3, 6], aur., **bor.**[3, 6], bry., **calc.**[3, 6], camph.[3, 8], cann-s., carb-v., cham., chin., coff., **ferr.**, ign., **IOD.**[3, 6], kali-i., kali-s., lach., led.[3, 6], **LYC.**[3, 8], merc., mosch., mur-ac., nit-ac., nux-v., onos.[8], op., phos., plat., **PULS.**[3, 6], rhus-t., **sec.**[1', 3, 8], seneg., sep., **spig.**[3, 6], staph., sulph.[3, 6], **tab.**[8], **verat.**[3, 6]

aversion to[6]

arg-n.[7], **ars.**[3, 6], aur.[1', 6], **bell.**[3, 6], calc-s.[1'], clem., colch., hep., mag-c., nat-m., nux-m., **nux-v.**[3, 6], samb., sil., **squil.**[3, 6], **stront-c.**[3, 6]

desire for[6]

acon.[3, 7], **aloe[1', 6]**, **apis**, ars-i.[1'], asar., calc.[6, 7], calc-s.[1'], **camph.**[1', 3, 6], ferr., **iod.**[3, 6], kali-i.[1'], led.[1'], manc.[11], merc.[1']

mosch.$^{1'}$, op.$^{1', 6}$, **puls.**$^{3, 6}$,
sec.$^{1', 3, 6, 7}$, spig., stram.,
sulph.$^{3, 6}$

morning^{11}
fl-ac.

sleep, on going to^{11}

op.

waking, on^{11}

plat.

kicks the covers off^{6}

BRY.^{7}, camph., **cham.**, iod.

in coldest weather^{7}

hep., sanic., sulph.

UNDRESSING agg., after

am-m., **ARS.**, calc., carc.^{9}, **cocc.**,
crot-t.^{3}, **DROS., dulc.**^{3}, hep., mag-c.,
merc.^{3}, mez., mur-ac., nat-s.,
NUX-V., olnd., plat., **puls.,
RHUS-T.**, rumx.^{3}, sep., **sil., spong.**,
stann.,sul-ac.^{3}, tub.^{3}

air, in open

phos.

URAEMIA^{3}

apis, ars., bapt., bell., **canth., hyos.,
op.**, sulfa.^{14}, **stram., verat-v.**

URIC ACID diathese, lithaemia^{3}

berb., chin-s., coc-c., **lyc.**, nat-s., sep.,
urt-u.

URINATION, am. after$^{3, 7, 8}$

benz-ac.$^{1'}$, bor.^{3}, bry.^{7}, chin-s.^{3}, cyt-l.^{9}
eug.^{7}, **GELS.**, ign., **LYC.**^{3}, ph-ac.,
sang.^{3}, sil.$^{3, 7, 8}$, **tab.**^{7}, ter.^{3}, verat.^{3}

VACCINATION, after *

acon.$^{8, 12}$, **ant-t.**$^{3, 6-8}$, apis$^{1, 7}$, ars.,
bell.$^{6, 8, 12}$, bufo^{7}, crot-h.$^{8, 12}$, echi.,
graph.^{12}, hep., kali-chl.,
kali-m.$^{2, 3, 6-8, 12}$, lac-v.^{12}, **MALAND.**,
merc.$^{3, 6, 8, 10, 12}$, **MEZ.**$^{7, 8, 12}$, **ped.**^{7},
phos.^{12}, **psor.**^{7}, rhus-t.^{3}, sabin.$^{2, 7}$,
SARS.$^{7, 8}$, sep.^{8}, <u>**SIL.**</u>$^{1, 7}$, skook.^{12},
<u>**SULPH.**</u>$^{1, 7}$, <u>**THUJ.**</u>$^{1, 7}$, tub.$^{2, 7}$,
VAC.$^{6, 7, 12}$, **vario.**$^{3, 6, 7, 10, 12}$

prophylactic$^{3, 7}$

sulph., thuj., vario.^{3}

VARICOSE veins

alum.^{4}, alum-sil.$^{1'}$, **alumn., am-c.**^{4},
ambr., ang.^{4}, **ant-t.**, apis^{12},
arist-cl.^{10}, **ARN., arg-n., ars.**,
ars-s-f.$^{1'}$, **asaf.**, bar-c.^{4}, **bell.**,
bell-p.$^{6, 12}$, **berb.**^{1}, brom.$^{1'}$, **bry.**^{4},
CALC., calc-f., calc-p., calc-s.$^{1'}$,
calen.^{12}, camph.^{4}, **carb-an.**,
CARB-V., carbn-s.$^{1'}$, card-b.^{12},
card-m.$^{6, 10, 12}$, **caust.**, chel.^{4},
chin.$^{4, 12}$, chin-s.^{12}, cic.^{4}, clem.,
coll.^{10}, coloc., con.^{4}, **croc.**^{4}, **crot-h.**,
cycl.^{4}, **ferr.**, ferr-ar., **ferr-p.**^{6}, **FL-AC.**,
form-ac.^{6}, **graph., HAM.**, hecla^{14},
hep., hyos.^{4}, kali-ar.^{12}, kali-n.^{4},
kreos., lac-c.^{12}, **lach., lyc., LYCPS.**,

m-aust.[4, 12], mag-c., mag-f.[10], mand.[10], meli.[10], meny.[4], merc-cy.[12], mez.[6], mill., mosch.[4], **mur-ac.**[4, 12], **nat-m., nux-v.,** olnd.[4], op.[4], **paeon.,** petr.[12], ph-ac.[4, 12], **phos.**[4, 6], **plb., PULS.,** pyrog.[12], **ran-s.**[2, 12], rhod.[4], **rhus-t.**[4], ruta[10], sabin., sars.[4], scir.[12], sec.[3], **sep.,** sil., sol-n.[12], **spig.,** spong.[4, 12], staph.[4], stront-br.[12], stront-c.[4, 12], sul-ac., **sulph.,** thuj., **vip., zinc.**

*inflammation – blood vessels –
    phlebitis*

blue

carb-v., lycps., mur-ac.[4], PULS.[2]

burning

apis, ARS., calc.

night
ARS.

bursting, as if[7]

vip.

constricting sensation[2]

ang.

dipsomania, from[2]

crot-h.

*inflamed see inflammation–blood
    vessels–phlebitis*

itching

ant-t.[4], berb.[4], bruc.[4], **caps.**[4], carb-v.[4], caust.[4], **graph.,** lach.[4], m-aust.[4], nux-v.[4], plb.[4], puls.[4], **sep.**[4], sil.[4], sul-ac.[4], **sulph.**[4]

net work in skin

berb., **calc., carb-v., caust.,** clem., **crot-h., lach.,** lyc., nat-m., ox-ac., plat., sabad., thuj.

painful

brom., caust., ham., lyc., mill., petr.[2], PULS., sang., thuj.[3], vip.[7], zinc.[3]

pimples, covered with

graph.

pregnancy, during

FERR., lyc., lycps., mill., nux-v.[2], PULS., zinc.

soreness

am-c.[4], ang.[4], bar-c.[4], **caust.**[4], graph., grat.[4], HAM.[1], hep.[4], ign.[4], **kali-c.**[4], kali-n.[4], m-arct.[4], merc.[4], mur-ac.[4], nat-m.[4], **nux-v.**[4], **phos.**[4], puls., rhus-t.[4], sil.[4], sul-ac.[4], **sulph.**[4], vip.[7]

stinging

apis, graph., **ham., PULS.**

stitching

alum.[4], **ant-t.**[2, 4], **ars.**[4], bar-c.[4],

caust.[4], grat.[4], kali-c., **kali-n.**[4], lyc.,
merc.[4], nat-m.[4], nux-v.[4], phos.[4],
sil.[4], sul-ac[4], sulph.[4]

ulceration

aesc., alumn.[1'], anac., ant-t.,
arist-cl.[14], arn.[14], ars., calc., calc-f.[14],
carb-v., card-m., CAUST., cecr.[14],
cham.[4], cinnb., crot-h., crot-t.[6],
des-ac.[14], **fl-ac., graph.,** grin., **ham.,**
hydr., hydr-ac., kali-s., kreos.,
LACH., LYC., merc., mez., **nat-m.,**
parath.[14], **PULS.,** pyrog., raja-s.[14],
rhus-t., rib-ac.[14], sars., sec., **sil.,**
sul-ac., **sulph.,** syph., thuj., **zinc.**

swollen

apis, berb.[1], puls.

young persons, in[7]

ferr-p.

VALUTS, cellars agg.

aran.[3], **ARS., bry.,** calc., **carb-an.,**
caust., dulc.[3], **kali-c.**[3], lyc., merc-i-f.[3],
NAT-S.[3], **PULS., sep., stram.**

VEINS swollen evening[16]

carb-v.

VENESECTION, ailments from[12]

senec., squil.

*inflammation – blood vessels –
    phlebitis*

VENOUS pulsations[1]

asaf.

VIGOR, decreased[3, 6]

ars-i.[1'], carb-an.[1', 3, 6], carb-v., cocc.,
ferr-p.[1'], laur., mag-m., op., ph-ac.[7],
phos.[1'], sulph., tub.[1', 7], verat.[3],
vinc

VIOLENT EFFECTS[3]

acon., alum., anac., **ars., BELL.,** bry.,
canth., carb-v., **CHAM.,** cupr., glon.,
hep., **hyos.,** ign., iod., **lach.,** merc.,
NUX-V., STRAM., sulph., **tarent.,**
verat.

VOMITING agg.

acon., **AETH.**[3, 8], **ant-t.,** arn., **ARS.,**
asar., bell. bry., **calc.,** caps., cham.,
chin., cina, cocc., **colch.,** coloc.,
con., **CUPR.,** dig., **dros.,** ferr.,
graph., **hyos.,** iod., **IP.,** lach., **lyc.,**
mez., mosch., nat-m., **nux-v.,** op.,
phos., plb., PULS., ran-s., ruta,
sabin., **sars.,** sec., **sep.,** sil., stann.,
SULPH., verat.

am.
acon., agar., anac.[15], ant-t.[3], ars.,
asar.[14], carbn-s., **coc-c.,** colch., **dig.,**
eup-per.[3], helia.[8], hell.[3], hyos.,
kali-bi.[3], lat-m.[9], nux-v., op., plb.[3],
puls., **sang., sec., tab.**[3]

WAKING, on

acon., agar., agn., alum., alum-sil.[1]
alumn.[2], **am-c., AM-M., AMBR.,**
anac., **ant-c.,** ant-t., apis[3], arg-n.[7],
arn., ARS., aur., bapt.[6], bar-c., bell.,
benz-ac., bism., bor., bov., bry.,
bufo., cact., cadm-s., calad., **CALC.,**

calc-p., calc-s., cann-s., canth.,
caps., carb-an., carb-v., CAUST.,
cench., cham., **chel., chin.,** cic.,
cina, clem., coc-c., **cocc.,** coff.,
colch., **con.,** corn., croc., **crot-h.,**
crot-t., cupr., cycl., **dig.,** dros.,
dulc., euph., euphr.[3], ferr., ferr-ar.[1'],
fl-ac.[3], form., **graph.,** guaj., **HEP.,**
hydr., **HYOS., ign., ip., kali-ar.,**
KALI-BI., kali-c., kali-i., kali-n.,
kali-s., kreos., **LACH.,** laur., led.,
lyc., lycps.[3], mag-c., mag-m., mang.,
meny., **merc.,** merc-c.[3], **merc-i-f.,**
mez., mosch., mur-ac., naja, nat-c.,
nat-m., NIT-AC., nux-m., **NUX-V.,**
op., **ONOS.,** palo.[14], par.[3], petr.,
ph-ac., **PHOS., phyt.,** plat., psor.,
PULS., ran-b., ran-s., rauw.[14],
rheum, rhod., **rhus-t.,** ruta, sabad.,
sabin., **samb., sang.,** sars., sel.,
seneg., **SEP., sil.,** spig., spong.,
squil., stann.[3], **staph.,** stram.,
stront-c., sul-ac., **SULPH.,** tarax.,
teucr.[3], thuj., trios.[14], tub.[3],
VALER., ven-m.[14], verat., viol-o.,
viol-t., **zinc.**

sleep–after–morning

agg. on w. at night[3]

ambr., bry.[3, 4], carb-v., chin.,
COCC., colch., ip., lach.[4], nat-c.,
nat-m., **NUX-V.,** ph-ac., **puls.,**
ruta sabin., **sel.,** sep.

siesta, from[3]

caust.

am.
am-m., ambr., **ars.,** bry., **calad.,**
calc., cham., chin., cocc., **colch.,**
hell., ign., ip., kreos., lach., meph.[4],
nat-c., **nux-v., onos.,** ph-ac., **PHOS.,**
puls., ruta, sabin., samb., sel., **SEP.,**
spig., thuj., vip.[1]

WALK, late learning to

agar., **bar-c.,** bell., **CALC.,**
CALC-P., CAUST., lyc.[6], merc.[6],
NAT-M., nux-v., **ph-ac.[6], phos.[6],**
pin-s.[6], **sanic., sil.,** sulph.

tardy development of bones[8]

calc.[1', 8], calc-f., **calc-p.,** sil.

WALKING agg.

acon., **AESC., agar., agn.,** aloe,
alum., alum-p.[1'], am-c., am-m.,
ambr., anac., ang.[3], ant-c., **ant-t.,**
apis, arg-m., arg-n.[3], **arn., ars.,**
ars-i., asaf., **asar.,** atra-r.[14], **atro.,**
aur., aur-ar.[1'], aur-m.[1'], **bapt.,**
bar-c., bar-i.[1'], bar-s.[1'], **BELL., berb.,**
bor.[3], **bov., BRY., cact.,**
cadm-met.[14], cadm-s., **calad.,**
CALC., CALC-S., camph., cann-s.,
canth., caps., **carb-ac., carb-an.,**
carb-v., **carbn-s., CAUST.,** cham.,
chel., CHIN., chion., cic., cina,
clem., **COCC., coff., COLCH.,**
coloc., **CON.,** conv., cortico.[14],
croc., cupr., cycl., dicha.[14], **dig.,**
dros., dulc., euph., euphr.[3], **ferr.,**
ferr-ar.[1'], ferr-i., ferr-p.[1'], **FL-AC.[3],**
form., gels., **glon., gran., graph.,**
guaj., **hell., hep.,** hyos., ign., **iod.,**
ip., kali-c., kali-n., kali-p., kali-sil.[1'],
kreos., **lach.,** laur., **LED., lil-t.,** lyc.,
mag-c., mag-m., **mag-p.,** mang.,
meny., **merc.,** merc-c.[3], methys.[14],
mez., mosch., mur-ac., **murx.,** nat-c.,
nat-m., nat-p., nat-s., nat-sil.[1'],
NIT-AC., nux-m., **NUX-V.,** olnd.,
op., paeon., par., **petr., ph-ac.,**
PHOS., phyt., plat., plb., **psor.,**
puls., **ran-b.,** ran-s., **rheum,** rhod.,
RHUS-T., ruta, sabad., **sabin.,**
samb., **sars.,** sec., **sel.,** seneg., **SEP.,**
sil., SPIG., spong., squil., **STANN.,**
staph., stram., stront-c., sul-ac.,
sul-i.[1'], **SULPH.,** tab.[3], **tarax.,**

tarent., teucr., thiop.[14], thuj., tub., valer., verat., **verat-v.**, verb., viol-o., viol-t., **zinc.**

am.

    acon., agar., agn., alum., alumn., am-c., **am-m.**, ambr., anac., ang.[3], ant-c., ant-t., apis, apoc., aran-ix.[14], arg-m., arg-n.[3], arn., **ars.**, ars-s-f.[1]′, asaf., asar., **AUR.**, aur-m.[3], aur-s.[1]′, bar-c., **bell.**, bism., bov., **brom.**, **bry.**, buni-o.[14], calc.[3], calen.[4], canth., **caps.**, carb-v., caust., cham., chin., cic., cina, cocc., coloc., **CON.**[3], cortiso.[14], crot-h., cupr., **CYCL.**, dios., **dros.**, **DULC.**, **EUPH.**, euphr., **FERR.**, ferr-ar., **fl-ac.**, glon., graph., guaj., halo.[14], hep., hyos., ign., indg., iod., kali-bi., kali-c., **KALI-I.**, kali-n., kali-p., **kali-s.**, kreos., lach., laur., **lyc.**, lycps.[3], **mag-c.**, **mag-m.**, mag-p.[3], mang., **meli.**, **meny.**, meph.[14], **merc.**, mez., **mosch.**, mur-ac., nat-c., **nat-m.**, nat-s.[1]′, nid.[14], nit-ac., nux-m.[1], olnd., op., palo.[14], par., petr., **ph-ac.**, phos.[3], **plat.**, plb., **PULS.**, pyrog., **ran-b.**, raph., **rhod.**, **RHUS-T.**, **ruta**, **SABAD.**, sabin., **SAMB.**, sars., sel., seneg., **sep.**, sil., spig., spong.[3], stann., staph., stront-c., sul-ac., **SULPH.**, **TARAX.**, tere-ch.[14], teucr., thal.[14], thuj., tub.[1, 7], **VALER.**, verat., verb., **viol-t.**, vip-a.[14], **zinc.**

after w. agg.[3]

kali-bi., **kali-c.**, lyc., ruta, stann. stram., sulph.,

ailments from[12]

sel.

air agg., in open

    acon., **agar.**, agn., alum., alum-p.[1]′, **am-c.**, am-m., ambr.,

anac., ang.[3], ant-c., arg-m., arn., **ARS.**, ars-s-f.[1]′, asar., aur., aur-ar.[1]′, aur-s.[1]′, bar-c., **bell.**, bor., bov., **bry.**, calad., **calc.**, calc-sil.[1]′, **camph.**, cann-s., canth., caps., **carb-ac.**, **carb-an.**, **carb-v.**, carbn-s.[1]′, **CAUST.**, cham., **chel.**, chin., chin-ar., cic., **cina**, clem., **COCC.**, coff., **colch.**, coloc., **con.**, croc., dig., dros., dulc., euph., **euphr.**, ferr., ferr-ar.[1]′, **FL-AC.**[3], graph., **guaj.**, hell., **hep.**, hyos., ign., iod., ip., **kali-c.**, kali-n., **kali-p.**, kreos., lach., laur., **led.**, lyc., mag-c., mag-m., **MAG-P.**, mag-s.[4], mang., meny., **merc.**, merc-c., mez., mosch., mur-ac., nat-ar., nat-c., nat-m., nit-ac., **nux-m.**, **NUX-V.**, olnd., op., par., petr., ph-ac., **phos.**, **plan.**, plat., plb., **psor.**, **puls.**, ran-b., **ran-s.**, rheum, rhod., **rhus-t.**, ruta, sabad., sabin., sars., **SEL.**, **seneg.**, **sep.**, **sil.**, **SPIG.**, **spong.**, **stann.**, staph., **stram.**, stront-c., sul-ac., **SULPH.**, tarax., teucr., thuj., valer., verat., **verb.**, viol-t.[1], zinc.

am.

    acon., aesc.[6], agar., aloe, **ALUM.**, am-c.[3], am-m., ambr., anac., ang.[3], ant-c., ant-t.[4], aran.[6, 14], arg-m., **ARG-N.**, arn., ars.[3], asaf., **asar.**, **aur.**, bapt., bar-c., bar-s.[1]′, bell., bism., bor., bov., **brom.**, **bry.**, calc., calc-s., caps., carb-ac., carb-v., carbn-s., caust., cic., cimic.[14], cina, **con.**, croc.[4], dios.[6], **dulc.**, **FL-AC.**, gamb., **graph.**, hed.[10], hep.[3], hyos., ign., iod.[6, 10], ip.[4], kali-c., **KALI-I.**, kali-n., **KALI-S.**, lach.[6], laur., **lil-t.**, **LYC.**, **mag-c.**, mag-f.[10, 14], **mag-m.**, mag-s.[4, 10, 14], mand.[10], mang., meny., merc., **merc-i-r.**, mez., mosch., mur-ac., **naja**, nat-ar., nat-c., nat-m., nat-s.[1, 7], nicc.[4], nit-ac., op., ox-ac., par., petr., **ph-ac.**, phel.[4], phos., pip-n.[3], plat., plb., **PULS.**, rauw.[14], rhod., **RHUS-T.**, ruta[3],

sabin., **sang.**, sars., sel., **seneg.,
sep.,** spig., spong.[3], **stann.**, staph.,
stront-c., sul-ac., **sulph., tarax.,**
tarent.[1,7], **teucr., thuj.,** verat.,
verb., vinc.[4], viol-t., zinc.

aversion to[11]

agar., aza.[14], cham., clem., fago.,
kali-bi., nit-ac.

backward impossible[3]

cocc., mang.

beginning of w. agg

acon., **agar.,** am-c., ambr., anac.,
ang.[3,6], ant-c., ant-t., arn., ars.,
asar., aur., bar-c., bell., bov., **bry.,
cact., calc.,** cann-s., canth., **CAPS.,**
carb-an., **carb-v., caust.,** cham.,
chin., cic., cina, cocc., **CON.,** croc.,
cupr., cycl., dig., dros., **EUPH.,
FERR.,** graph., kali-c., kali-n., lach.,
laur., led., **LYC.,** mag-c., mang.,
merc., mur-ac., nat-c., nat-m.,
nit-ac., nux-v., olnd., petr., ph-ac.,
phos., phyt.[6], plat., plb., **PULS.,**
ran-b., rhod., **RHUS-T., ruta,
sabad.,** sabin., **samb.,** sars., sep.,
sil., spig., staph., stram., stront-c.,
sulph., **thuj.,** valer., verat., **zinc.**

bent, agg.[3]

bry.

am.[3]
arn., **CON., hyos., lyc.,** nux-v.,
phos., rhus-t., sabin., sulph.,
viol-t.

bridge agg., on a narrow[3]

bar-c., ferr., sulph.

circle. in a[16]

bell.

desire for[3,6]

acon.[3], arg-m.[1,6], arg-n., **ars.**[3,11],
aur., bism.[6], caj.[11], calc.[3,16],
chlor.[11], cod.[11], fl-ac.[3], gins.[11],
iod., lepi.[11], lil-t.[3], lyc.[3], mag-c.[3],
merc., mosch.[6], naja[3,11], **op.,**
paeon.[3], paull.[11], phos.[3], ruta[3],
sep., spirae.[11], **stront-c.,** tarent.[3],
thlasp.[3], thuj.[3], valer.[8], zinc-a.[11]

night[6]
iod., merc.[11], **op.**

air, in open[4]

asaf.[11], clem., crot-t., fla-ac.[7],
lach., lact., lyc., mez.[11], phos.[4,11],
puls., teucr.

down stairs agg.[1']

bor.

descending

easily

thuj.[16], zinc.[6]

fast agg.

alum., alum-sil.[1'], **ang.**[3], arg-m.,
apis, arn., ARS., ars-i., ars-s-f.[1'],
aur., aur-ar.[1'], aur-i.[1'], **aur-m.,**
aur-s.[1'], **BELL.,** bor.[3], **BRY., cact.,**
calc., calc-s., calc-sil.[1'], **cann-s.,
caust.,** chel., chin., cina, cocc.,
coff., **CON.,** croc., **cupr.,** dros.,
ferr., ferr-ar., hep., hyos., **ign.,
iod.,** ip., **kali-ar., kali-c.,** kali-p.,

kali-sil.[1'], laur., **led.**, **lyc.**, **merc.**, mez., nat-ar., nat-c., **nat-m.**, nit-ac., nux-m., **nux-v.**, olnd., **PHOS.**, **plb.**, **PULS.**, rheum, **rhod.**, **rhus-t.**, ruta, sabin., **seneg.**, sep., **SIL.**, **spig.**, spong., squil., staph., sul-ac., **SULPH.**, verat., zinc.

running

am.

ant-t.[3], **arg-n.**, ars.[1'], aur-m.[3], brom.[1'], canth., carb-ac., **ign.**, **mag-c.**[3], **mag-m.**[3], nat-m., petr. **rhus-t.**[3, 7], **sabin.**[3], **SEP.**, sil., **stann.**, sul-ac., **TUB.**

level agg., on a[3]

ran-b., verat.

rough ground agg., over[3]

clem., lil-t., phos., podo.

running water agg., over[3]

ang., bar-c., brom., **ferr.**, hyos., **sulph.**

slowly am.

agar., **AUR.**, aur-i.[1'], **AUR-M.**, cact., calc-s., **FERR.**, ferr-ar., iris, **kali-p.**, lyc.[7], **PULS.**, sep., **tarent.**

stone pavement agg., on[3]

aloe, ant-c., ars., **con.**, **hep.**, nux-v., sep.

wind agg., in the

acon., **agar.**, **ars.**, asar., aur., aur-ar.[1'], **BELL.**, **calc.**, carb-v.,

cham., chin., con., euphr., **graph.**, lach., **lyc.**, mur-ac., nat-c., nux-m., **NUX-V.**, **phos.**, plat., **puls.**, rhus-t., **SEP.**, spig., **stann.**, thuj.

WARM agg.

acon., adlu.[14], **aesc.**[7], aeth.[8], **agar.**, agn., **all-c.**, aloe[1', 7], **ALUM.**, alumn.[2], ambr., **anac.**[2, 3, 8], **ant-c.**, **ant-t.**, **APIS**, aq-mar.[14], **ARG-N.**[1, 7], arn., **ARS-I.**, asaf.[6-8], asar.[2, 3], aster.[14], aur., **auri.**[1', 7], **aur-m.**, bar-c., bar-i.[1'], bell., beryl.[14], **bism.**, **bor.**, brom.[1'], **bry.**, **calad.**[1, 7], **calc.**[2, 3, 5, 8], **calc-i.**[1', 7], **calc-s.**[7], **camph.**, cann-s., canth., carb-v., **carbn-s.**, caust., cench.[1'], cham., chin.[2, 3, 8], cimic.[14], cina, clem.[8], **coc-c.**[1], cocc., coff.[1'], colch., coloc., **com.**[8], conv.[8], cortico.[9], cortiso.[9, 14], **croc.**[1, 7], **crot-h.**[3], dig., **dros.**, **dulc.**, euph., euphr., ferr.[2, 3, 8], ferr-i., **FL-AC.**[1', 3, 6-8], flav.[14], foll.[14], gels., **glon.**, **graph.**, **grat.**[7], **guaj.**, **ham.**[7], hed.['0], helio.[8], hell., hep.[3], hip-ac.[14], hist.[14], hydroph.[14], **hyos.**[3, 8], iber.[8, 14], ign., **ind.**, **IOD.**, **ip.**, jug-c.[8], just.[8], kali-br., kali-c.[2, 3, 14], **KALI-I.**[3, 7, 8], **kali-m.**[8], **KALI-S.**[1, 7], **lac-c.**, **lach.**, laur., **LED.**, lil-t.[3, 6, 7], **lyc.**, mag-c.[10], med.[7, 8], **merc.**, **mez.**, mur-ac., nat-c., **NAT-M.**[1, 7], **NAT-S.**[1, 7], nit-ac.[2, 3, 8], nux-m.[2, 3, 8], nux-v.[2, 3], **op.**, ph-ac., phenob.[13, 14], **phos.**, phyt.[1'], pic-ac.[1'], pitu.[14], **PLAT.**[1, 7], prot.[14], **PULS.**, rauw.[9, 14], rhus-t.[2, 3, 4], sabad., **sabin.**[1, 7], **SEC.**, sel., **seneg.**, sep.[2, 3], sil.[2, 3], spig., **spong.**[1, 7], staph., stel.[8], sul-ac.[8], **sul-i.**[1', 7], **SULPH.**[1, 7], tab., teucr., **thuj.**[1, 7], trios.[14], **tub.**[7], **verat.**, vesp.[7], visc.[14], **zinc.**

heat, sensation – vital, lack

ailments from[12]

acon., gels., nat-c.

am.[2]

acon., agar.[1, 2], alum-sil.[1], alumn.,
am-c.[2], anac., ant-c.[1, 2, 6, 7],
arg-m.[2, 6], arist-cl.[9, 10], **arn.**[2],
ARS.[1, 2, 4, 6-8], asar., **aur.**[2, 8], bad.[8],
bar-c.[2, 6], **bell.**[1, 2, 8], bell-p.[10, 14],
bor., bov., bry.[1, 2, 8], calc.,
calc-f.[1, 7, 8, 10, 14], calc-p.[1], calc-s.[1],
CAMPH.[2, 8], **canth., caps.**[2, 6, 8],
carb-an., carb-v., cast.[6],
CAUST[1, 2, 4, 8], cench.[1],
cham.[1, 2, 4, 6, 7], chel.[1], **chin.**[2, 6],
cic.[2, 14], cimic.[8], **clem., cocc.,**
coff.[2, 7, 8], colch.[1, 2, 6, 14], coll.[8],
coloc.[1, 2, 6, 8, 10], **con.**[2, 6], cor-r.[8],
cupr-a.[8], cycl.[6, 8], cyn-d.[14], **dig.,**
DULC.[2, 6, 8], **ferr.**[1, 2], flor-p.[14], form.[8],
gink-b[14], **graph.,** gymno [2, 9] **hell.,**
HEP.[2, 3, 6, 8], **hyos.**[2], **ign.**[2, 9, 8], ip.,
kali-ar.[1], kali-bi.[1, 8], **KALI-C.**[2, 6, 14],
kali-p.[8], **kreos.**[2, 6, 8], lac-d.[1],
lach.[2, 8], laur., led., levo.[14], lob.[8],
lyc.[1, 2, 4, 8], lycpr.[8], **mag-c.**[2, 3, 10],
mag-m.[2, 14], **mag-p.**[1, 8], mand.[9, 10],
mang., med.[1], **meny., merc., mez.,**
moly-met.[14], **MOSCH., mur-ac.,**
nat-c., nat-m.[2], nid.[14], nit-ac.,
nux-m.[2, 6, 8], **NUX-V.**[2, 6, 8], onop.[14],
ph-ac.[2, 6, 8], **petr., phos.**[1, 2], phyt.[8],
psor.[8], puls., pyrog.[1, 6], **ran-b.,**
rheum[2], **rhod.**[2, 8], **RHUS-T.**[1, 2, 3, 6, 8],
rumx.[8], **ruta, SABAD.**[1, 2, 4, 8],
samb., sars.[1, 2], seneg., **sep.**[2, 4, 8],
sil.[2, 3, 6, 8], **spig.**[1, 2], **spong.**[2, 6],
squil., staph.[2, 8], **stram.**[2, 3, 8],
STRONT-C.[2, 4], **sul-ac.**[2, 8], **sulph.**[2, 4],
syph.[1], thea[8], ther.[1], **thuj.**[2, 6],
tub.[1, 7], **verat.**[2, 8], **verb., viol-t.,**
xero.[8], **zinc.**

air agg.

agn., **aloe,** ambr., anac.[2, 3], **ant-c.,**
ant-t., arg-n., arsi-i., asar.[2, 3, 6],
aur., aur-i.[1], **aur-m., bry.,** calad.,

calc., calc-i.[1], **calc-s.,** cann-s.,
carb-v., cham., cina, **coc-c.**[2], cocc.,
colch., croc., dros., **euph., fl-ac.,**
GLON., ign., **ind., IOD., ip.,**
kali-bi., **KALI-S., LACH.,** led.,
lyc., MERC., mez., nat-m., nat-s.,
nit-ac.[2, 3], nux-m., nux-v., **op.,**
ph-ac.[3], phenob.[13, 14], **phos.,**
pic-ac., plat., podo., **PULS.,**
rhus-t.[2, 3], sabin., sars., **sec.,** sel.,
seneg., sep.[2, 3], **sul-i.**[1], **sulph.,**
teucr., thuj., xan.

am.[2]

acon., agar., alumn., **am-c.,** anac.,
ant-c., arn., **ARS.**[2, 6], asar.,
AUR.[2, 8], **bar-c.**[2, 6], **bell.,** bor.,
bov., bry., calc.[2, 8], **CAMPH.,**
canth., **caps.**[2, 6], **carb-an., carb-v.,**
CAUST.[2, 6, 8], **cham.,** chin., **cic.,**
cina, coc-c., coff., **colch.**[2, 6],
coloc.[2, 6], **con.,** dig., **DULC.**[2, 6],
ferr., graph., **HELL., HEP.**[2, 6],
hyos., ign., ip., **KALI-C.**[2, 6],
kreos., lach., laur., led.[8], **lyc.,**
mag-c.[2, 8], mag-m., mag-p.[6],
mang., meny., **merc.**[2, 8], **mez.,**
MOSCH., mur-ac., nat-ar.[1],
nat-c., nat-m., nat-s.[6], **nit-ac.,**
NUX-M., NUX-V., par., petr.[2, 8],
ph-ac.[2, 6], **phos.,** psor., ran-b.,
rhod.[2, 6], **RHUS-T.**[2, 6, 8], **ruta,**
SABAD., samb., **sars., sel.,**
seneg., **sep., sil.**[2, 6], **spig.,**
spong.[2, 6], squil., staph., stram.,
STRONT-C.[2, 6], sul-ac., **sulph.,**
thuj.[2, 6], **verat.,** verb., viol-t.,
zinc.

becoming warm agg.[2, 3]

acon.[2, 3, 8], am-c., **ANT-C.**[2, 3, 8],
bar-i.[1], **bell.**[2, 3, 8], bor.[2],
brom.[3, 7, 8], **BRY.**[2, 3, 8], calc.[3, 8],
caps., carb-v.[2, 3, 8], coff., **dig.,**
gels.[2], **glon., hep., ign., ip.,**
KALI-C., lach.[1], lyc.[3, 8], mez.,
nat-m., nux-m.[2, 3, 8],
nux-v.[2, 3, 8], olnd., **op., sep.,**
sil., staph., **thuj,** zinc.

air agg., in open

acon., agn., alum., alumn.[2], ambr., anac.[2], **ant-c.**, asar.[2], aur., aur-i.[1'], **aur-m.**, bar-c., **bell.**, bor., bov., **BRY.**, calad., calc., cann-s., **carb-v.**, caust., cham., chin., cina, cocc., coff., colch., coloc., croc., dros., **dulc.**, euph., **GELS.**[2], **glon.**, graph., ign., **IOD.**, ip., kali-c., lach., led., **LYC.**, mang., **merc.**, mez., nat-c., nat-m., **nat-s.**, nit-ac., nux-m.[2], nux-v.[2], olnd., **op.**, petr., ph-ac., **phos.**, plat., **PULS.**, rhus-t.[2], **sabad.**, sabin., **sec.**, sel., **seneg.**, sep., **sil.**, **spig.**, spong., staph., **sulph.**, teucr., thuj., **verat.**

am.[2]

acon., **agar.**, am-c., ant-c., **arn.**, **ARS.**, asar., **aur.**, **bar-c.**, **bell.**, **bor.**, bov., **bry.**, **calc.**, **camph.**, canth., **caps.**, carb-an., carb-v., **caust.**, **cham.**, **chin.**, **cic.**, clem., **coc-c.**, colch.[1'], **con.**, dig., **dulc.**, ferr., **GRAPH.**, **hell.**, **hep.**, **hyos.**, **ign.**, **KALI-C.**, kreos., lach., **lyc.**, **mag-c.**, mag-m., **mang.**, meny., **merc.**, mez., **MOSCH.**, mur-ac., **nat-c.**, nat-m., **nit-ac.**, **nux-m.**, **NUX-V.**, petr., **ph-ac.**[1', 2], **phos.**, ran-b., rhod., **RHUS-T.**, ruta, **SABAD.**, samb., **sars.**, sel., **sep.**, **sil.**, spig., **spong.**, staph., stram., **stront-c.**, sul-ac., **sulph.**, thuj., **verat.**, **verb.**, viol-t., zinc.

bed agg.

aeth., agn., **alum.**, alumn.[2], ambr., anac.[2, 3]. **ant-c.**, **ant-t.**, **APIS**, arg-n., arn., ars-i., **asaf.**, asar.[2, 3], aur., aur-i.[1'], **aur-m.**, aur-s.[1'], bar-c., bell-p.[8], bov., **bry.**, calad., calc., calc-f.[10], calc-i.[1'], **calc-s.**, **camph.**, cann-s., **carb-v.**, carbn-s.[1', 7], **caust.**[2, 3], cedr., **CHAM.**, chin.,

cina, cinnb.[1'], **clem.**, **coc-c.**, **cocc.**, colch., coloc.[3], croc., daph., **DROS.**, dulc., **euph.**, **fl-ac.**, **glon.**, goss., **graph.**, hell., hyos., ign., **iod.**, **ip.**, **kali-c.**[2, 3], **kali-chl.**, kali-m.[1'], **kali-s.**, **lac-c.**, **lach.**, **LED.**, **lyc.**, **mag-c.**, med.[7], **MERC.**, **mez.**, mur-ac., **nat-c.**, **nat-m.**, nit-ac., **nux-m.**[2, 3], **nux-v.**[2, 3], **OP.**, **ph-ac.**, phenob.[13, 14], phos., phyt., **plat.**, psor., **PULS.**, **rhod.**[3, 4, 6], **rhus-t.**[2, 3, 4, 6], sabad., **SABIN.**, sars., **SEC.**, sel., **seneg.**, sep.[2, 3], **sil.**[3, 6], spig., **spong.**, staph., stram., stront-c.[3], **sul-i.**[1'], **SULPH.**, teucr., **thuj.**, **verat.**, visc.[8], x-ray[9]

cold extremities, with

CAMPH., LED., mag-c., med., SEC.

am.

agar., **am-c.**, arn., **ARS.**, ars-s-f.[1'], **aur.**, bapt.[3], bar-c., bell., **BRY.**, **calc-p.**, camph., canth., **caust.**, cic., cocc., **coloc.**, con., **dulc.**, **graph.**, **HEP.**, hyos., **kali-bi.**, **KALI-C.**, **kali-i.**, kali-p., lach., **LYC.**, **mag-p.**, mosch., nit-ac., **NUX-M.**, **NUX-V.**, petr., ph-ac., **phos.**, **RHUS-T.**, **rumx.**, sabad., sep., **SIL.**, spong., squil., **stann.**, staph., stram., stront-c., sul-ac.[3, 6], sulph., **tarent.**, thuj.[6], **TUB.**, verat.[2, 3]

room agg.

acon., aeth.[6], **agn.**, **all-c.**[1', 8], **alum.**, alum-sil.[1'], **alumn.**[2], am-c.[3], ambr., **anac.**[2, 3, 6], **ant-c.**, ant-t., **APIS**, aran-ix.[10], aran-sc.[8], **arg-n.**, ars-i., arn., **asaf.**, **asar.**[2, 3, 6], aur., aur-i.[1'], **aur-m.**, aur-s.[1'], bapt.[3, 8], bar-c., bar-i.[1'], bell., bor., **brom.**, **bry.**, bufo,

calad., calc., calc-i.[1'], calc-p.,
CALC-S., cann-s., **carb-ac.,
carb-v., CARBN-S.**, caust., cina,
coc-c., cocc., colch., crat.[8],
CROC., culx.[1'], **dros.**, dulc.,
euphr.[8], **fl-ac., glon.**, **GRAPH.**,
hell., hep.[2, 3], hip-ac.[9, 14], hyos.,
hyper.[8], ign., **ind., IOD., ip.**,
kali-c., **KALI-I., KALI-S.**, lach.[1'],
laur., **led.**, lil-t., luf-op.[14], **LYC.**,
mag-m.[1], med.[7], **merc., merc-i-f.,**
mez., mosch., mur-ac., nat-ar.,
nat-c., nat-m., **nat-s.**, nit-ac.,
nux-v.[2, 3, 8], **op.**, oxyt., ph-ac.,
phos., **pic-ac.**, plat., pneu.[14], **ptel.,
PULS.**, ran-b., rhus-t.[2, 3, 8],
SABIN., sanic., SEC., sel.,
SENEG., sep.[2, 3, 6, 8], spig.,
spong., staph., **sul-i.**[1'], **SULPH.,
tab., thuj., til., tub., verat.**, vib.[8]

am.[6]

aur-ar.[1'], carb-v., **caust.**, cham.,
chel., chin., chin-ar.[1'], cocc.,
cycl.[1'], guaj., **hep.**[1, 6], mag-p.[1'],
mang., merc., nux-m., nux-v.,
plat., rhus-t.[1'], **rumx., sil.**

stove agg.

ant-c., apis, arg-n., ars.[3], **bry.**,
bufo, **cimic.**[3], **cocc., con.**,
cupr.[3], **euph., iod., GLON.,
kali-i., laur.**, mag-m., **merc.**,
nat-m., nux-v.[3], op., psor.[3],
puls., SEC., thiop.[14], **zinc.**[2, 3]

he is cold and stiff on approaching

laur.

ailments from[12]

glon.

am.

acon., agar., am-c., **ARS.**, aur.,
bar-c., bell., bor., bov.[3], camph.,
canth., caps., caust., cic., cocc.,
con., conv., **dulc.**, graph.[3], hell.,
HEP., hyos., **IGN.**, kali-c., lach.[3],
mag-c., **MAG-P.**, mang., **meny.**[2, 3],
mosch., **nux-m., NUX-V.**, petr.,
ran-b., rhod., **RHUS-T.**, sabad.,
SIL., stront-c., sulph., tub.[1']

wraps agg.

acon., ant-c.[1'], ant-t.[1', 6], **APIS,
arg-m., arg-n.**, arn.[3], **ars-i.,
asar.**[2, 3], aur., aur-i.[1'], **aur-m.**,
aur-s.[1'], **bor.**, brom.[1'], **bry., calc.**,
calc-i.[1'], calc-s., **camph.**, carb-v.,
carbn-s., **cham.**, chin., **coc-c.**,
coff., **crot-h.**[3], cupr.[3], **ferr.**, ferr-i.,
fl-ac., glon., ign., **IOD., ip.**[3],
kali-bi.[3], kali-i.[3], **KALI-S.,
lac-c.**, lach., **LED., LYC.**,
MAG-P.[3], merc., mosch., mur-ac.,
nit-ac., nux-v., op., phos., plat.,
PULS., rhus-t., sabin.[1', 3], **SEC.**,
seneg., sep., **spig.**, staph., **sul-i.**[1'],
SULPH., tab., thuj., **verat.**

am.[2]

ars.[1'], colch.[1'], **HEP.**, psor.[2, 3],
rhod.[1'], rhus-t.[15], sabad.[3], **SIL.**

desire for warm bed[11]

spig.

clothing[1']

alum., ars., **bar-c.**[6], bell., calc.[1'],
caul., graph., hep., kali-c.,
nat-c., nat-s., plb., psor.[6],
sabad.[6], sil.

Vol. I: *fur*

afternoon[11]

nux-v.

in spite of sensation of heat[14]

achy.

stove[11]

bar-c.[6], cic., ptel., **sil.**[6], tub.[1']

warmth[3, 6]

alum., am-br.[6], arg-m., **ars.,**
bar-c.[3], calc.[1'], caps., **caust.,**
colch., con., **hep., kali-c.**[3, 6, 14],
moly-met.[14], ph-ac., psor., **sabad.,**
sil., thuj.[3], tub.

WASHING clothes, laundry, ailments
from[12]

phos., sep., ther.

WATER, dashing against inner parts,
sensation of

ars.[3], bell., carb-ac.[3], carb-an.[3],
chin.[3], cina, **crot-h.**[3], **CROT-T.,** dig.,
ferr., glon.[3], hell., **hep.**[3], **hyos.**[3],
jatr.[3], kali-c.[3], kali-m.[1'], laur.,
nat-m.[3], ph-ac., **rhod., rhus-t.**[3],
spig.

heat—warm water—dashed

seeing or hearing of running w. agg.[3]

ang., apis, arg-m., bell.[3, 6], brom.,

---

canth., **LYSS.**[3, 6, 8, 10], nit-ac.,
stram.[3, 6], sulph.[3, 6], ter.

Vol. I: *hydrophobia*

pouring out of w. agg.[10]

lyss.

wading in, ailments from

ars., dulc., mag-p.

working in w. agg.[3, 6, 8]

calc., calc-p.[3, 6], mag-c.

ailments from[12]

calc.

hands in cold w. agg., with[3]

lac-d., mag-p., phos.

am.[3]
jatr.

WAVELIKE sensations

acon.[o], am-c.. aml-ns.[3], anac.[3], ant-t.[3],
arn.[3], asaf.[3], **BELL.,** bism., caps.,
caust., chin.[3], clem., cocc.[3], coff.[3, 6],
con., dig., dulc.[3] ferr-p.[3], fl-ac.[3],
glon.[3], hyos.[3, 6], iod.. kali-c., kali-n.,
lach.[3], lyc., mag-c., mez.[3], **nit-ac.,**
nux-v., olnd.[3], par.[3, 6], petr., plat.[3],
rhod.[3], sars., senec.[3], **sep.,** sil., spig.[3],
stann., stict.[3, 6], stront-c., **SULPH.,**
teucr.[3], verb., viol-t.[3]

WEAKNESS, enervation

abies-c., abies-n., abrot., absin.,
acet-ac., achy.[14] **acon.,** acon-c.[11]
acon-f.[11] adlu.[14] adox.[11]
adren.[7, 8, 12] aesc., aesc-g.[2, 11]
aeth., aether[11] agar., agar-cpn.[11]
agar-em.[11] agar-pa.[11] **agar-ph.**[11]
agar-pr.[11] agar-st.[11] agav-t.[14] **agn.,**
ail., alco.[11] **alet.**[1', 2, 6, 8, 12] alf.[7, 8]
all-c., all-s., **aloe,** alst.[8, 12] alst-s.[11]
alum., alum-p.[1'] alum-sil.[1'] alumn.,
AM-C., am-caust.[11] am-m., **ambr.,**
aml-ns.[2, 11] ammc.[4, 11] amor-r.[14]
amph.[11] amyg.[11] **ANAC., anag.**[2]
anan.[2] **ang.**[2, 3, 4, 7, 11, 16] anil.[11]
ant-ar.[2, 6, 11] **ant-c.,** ant-m.[2, 11]
ant-o.[11] **ANT-T.,** anth.[11] anthraci.,
anthraco.[2, 11] **antip.**[8] aphis[4, 11]
APIS, apoc., apoc-a.[11] apom.[11]
aq-m.[14] aq-pet.[11] aral.[11] **aran.,**
aran-sc.[11, 12] arg-cy.[11] **ARG-M.,**
arg-n., arist-cl.[10] **ARN., ARS.,** ars-h.,
ARS-I., ars-m., ars-s-f., ars-s-r.[2]
arum-d.[2, 11] arum-i.[11] arum-m.,
arum-t., asaf., asar., asc-t., asim.[11]
aspar.[2] astac.[11] aster., atha.[4, 11]
atra-r.[14] atro.[11] **aur.,** aur-ar.[1']
aur-fu.[4, 11] **aur-m.**[2, 8, 11] aur-m-n.[11]
aur-s.[1'] **aven.**[7, 8, 12] bals-p.[8] **BAPT.,**
bar-a.[6, 11] **BAR-C.,** bar-i.[1'] **bar-m.,**
bart.[11] bell., bell-p.[8, 9, 14] ben.,
ben-n.[11] **benz-ac.,** berb., berbin.[11]
beryl.[10] **bism., bol-la.,** bol-s.[11] bor.,
both.[11] bov., brach., **BROM.,**
bruc.[4] brucin.[11] **bry.,** bufo,
buth-a.[9, 10, 14] buni-o.[14] **cact.,**
cadm-met.[10, 14] cadm-s.[6, 7] cain.,
caj.[11] calad., **CALC.,** calc-ar.[1']
calc-caust.[6, 11] calc-hp.[8] **CALC-I.**[1, 1']
calc-m.[11] **calc-p.,** calc-s., calc-sil.[1']
camph., cann-i., cann-s., **canth.,**
caps., **CARB-AC., carb-an., carb-v.,**
carbn-chl.[11] carbn-h., carbn-o.[11]
carbn-s., card-m., **carl.**[11, 12] casc.[4]
cass.[11] cast.[6, 11] cast-v., **caul.,**
caust., cedr., cench.[1', 11] cent.[11]
cere-b.[11] cerv.[11] **cham., CHEL.,**
chelo.[12] **chim., CHIN.,** chin-ar.,
CHIN-S., chion., chlf., chlol.,

chloram.[14] chlorpr.[14] chr-ac.[2, 11]
cic., cich.[11] cimic., cimx., **cina,**
chinch.[11] cinnb., cinnm.[2] cist.[12]
cit-l.[2, 11] cit-v.[11] **clem.,** cob.,
cob-n.[9, 10, 14] coc-c.,
COCA[2, 6, 8, 11, 12] **cocc.,** coch.[2]
cod.[11] **coff., COLCH.,** colchin.[11, 12]
coll.[11] coloc., colocin.[11, 12] com.,
CON., conin.[11] conin-br.[12] conv.[7]
cop., cor-r.[6] corn.[2, 11] cortico.[9]
cot.[11] crat.[6, 8] croc., **crot-c., crot-h.,**
crot-t., cub., culx.[1'] **cupr.,**
cupr-a.[4, 11] **cupr-ar.,** cupr-s., cur.,
cycl., cyn-d.[14] cyt-l.[10, 11] **daph.**[4, 11]
der.[11] dicha.[10, 14] **DIG., digin.**[11]
digox.[11] dios., dip.[8] diph.[8] dirc.[11, 12]
dor., **dros.,** dubo-m.[11] **dulc.,**
echi.[3, 6, 8] elat., equis.[11] erig.[11]
ery-a.[11] ery-m.[12] eryt-j.[11] eucal.[2, 11]
eug., eup-per., eup-pur., **euph.,**
euph-a.[12] euph-c.[11] euph-hy.[11]
euph-ip.[11] euphr., eupi.[11] fago.,
fagu.[11] **FERR.,** ferr-ar., ferr-cit.[8]
FERR-I., FERR-M., ferr-ma.[4, 11]
ferr-p., fic.[10] fil.[12] **fl-ac.,** flor-p.[14]
form., frag.[11] franz.[11, 12] **gad.**[11]
gal-ac.[11, 12] galeg.[12] galin.[14]
gamb.[2] gast.[11, 12] **GELS.,** gent-l.,
gent-q.[12] get.[11] gink-b.[14]
gins.[4, 6, 11, 12] glon., goss., gran.,
GRAPH., grat., guaj., guan.[11]
guar.[2] guare., haem.[6] hall[11] **ham.,**
hed.[14] hedeo.[11] **hell.,** hell-o.[11]
helon., **HEP.,** hera.[11, 12] hip-ac.[14]
hipp., hir.[14] hist.[9, 14] home.[11]
hydr., hydr-ac., hydrc.[11] **HYOS.,**
hyosin.[11] **hyper.,** hura, iber.[2, 11, 14]
ign., ind., indg., **IOD., ip., irid.**[8, 12]
iris, jab., jal.[11] jasm.[11] jatr.,
jug-c.[11] jug-r., juni.[11] **KALI-AR.,**
kali-bi., kali-br., **KALI-C.,** kali-chl.,
kali-cy.[11] **KALI-FCY., kali-i.,**
kali-m.[1'] kali-n., kali-ox.[11]
KALI-P., kali-perm.[11] kali-s.,
kali-sil.[1'] kali-t.[11] **KALM.,** kino[11]
kiss.[11] kou.[11] kreos., kres.[10, 13, 14]
lac-ac., **lac-c., lac-d.**[1', 2, 7] **LACH.,**
lachn., lact.[4, 11] lam.[4] lapa.[11]
lat-k.[11] lat-m.[9, 14] **LAUR., LEC.,**
led., lepi., lept., lil-s.[11] lil-t., lim.[11]
lina.[11] linu-c.[11] lipp.[11] lith-c.[8]

lith-m.[8], lob., lob-c.[11, 12], lob-p.[8],
lob-s., **lol.**[11], luf-op.[10, 14], **lyc.**,
lycps., lyss., m-arct.[4], m-aust.[4],
marco.[11], mag-c., mag-f.[10, 14],
mag-m., **mag-p.**[2, 8], mag-s., manc.,
mand.[10, 11, 14], mang.[1', 3, 4, 6],
mang-o.[11], **MED.**, mela.[11], meli.,
menis.[11], meny., meph., **MERC.**,
merc-br.[11], **MERC-C.**, **MERC-CY.**,
merc-d.[11], merc-i-f., merc-i-r.,
merc-meth.[11], merc-ns.[11],
merc-sul.[2, 11], merl.[2, 11], methys.[14],
mez., mill., mit.[11], moly-met.[14],
mom-b.[11], morph., mosch., murx.,
MUR-AC., mygal., **myric.**[2, 11],
nabal.[11], naja, napht.[11], narcin.[11],
narz.[11], nat-ar., **nat-c.**, nat-f.[9],
NAT-HCHLS., nat-lac.[11], **NAT-M.**,
nat-n., **NAT-P.**, **NAT-S.**, **nat-sal.**[8, 12],
nat-sil.[1'], nat-sula.[11], nep.[10, 13, 14],
nicc., nicot.[11], nid.[14], **NIT-AC.**,
nit-m-ac.[11], nit-s-d.[4, 11], nitro-o.[11],
nuph., **nux-m.**, **nux-v.**, oena.,
okou.[14], ol-an., **ol-j.**, **OLND.**,
onos.[12], **op.**, opun-v.[11], orch.[12],
orig.[11], orni.[11], osm., ost.[11],
ox-ac., oxyg.[11], paeon., pall.,
palo.[14], pana.[11], par., parathyr.[14],
parth.[12], paull.[11], ped., penic.[13, 14],
perh.[14], **petr.**, **PH-AC.**, phal.[11],
phel., **PHOS.**, **phys.**, **phyt.**, **PIC-AC.**,
pilo.[11], pimp.[11], pip-m.[11], pitu.[9],
pix.[11], plan., **plat.**, **PLB.**, plb-chr.[11],
plect.[11], plumbg.[11], podo., polyg-h.,
polyp-p.[11], prun-p.[11], **PSOR.**, ptel.[1],
(non: petl.), **puls.**, puls-n.[11],
pyrog.[3, 6], pyrus[11], ran-a.[4], **RAN-B.**,
ran-s., **raph.**, rat., rham-f.[11], rheum.,
rhod., rhus-g.[11, 12], **RHUS-T.**,
rhus-v.[2, 11], ric.[11], **rob.**[2, 11], **rumx.**,
rumx-a.[11], ruta, **sabad.**, sabin.,
salin.[11], samb., samb-c.[11], **sang.**,
sanic., santin.[11], sapin.[11],
sarcol-ac.[8, 9, 14], saroth.[14], sarr.,
sars., scor.[11], scorph-n.[11], scut.[11, 12],
SEC., **SEL.**, senec., **seneg.**,
senn.[11, 12], **SEP.**, sieg.[10], **SIL.**,
silphu.[12], sin-n., sium[11], sol-m.[11],
sol-n., sol-t.[11], sol-t-ae., solid.[3, 8],
solin.[11], sphing.[11], spig., spira.[11],
spirae.[11], **spong.**, **SQUIL.**, **STANN.**,

STAPH., **sfict.**, still., **stram.**,
stront-c., stroph-h.[8], stry., stry-p.[7],
SUL-AC., sul-h.[11], sul-i., sulfa.[9, 14],
sulfon.[8], sulfonam.[14], **SULPH.**,
sumb., syph., **TAB.**, tanac.[8, 11],
tang.[11], tann-ac.[11], tarax.,
TARENT., tarent-c.[6], tart-ac.[11],
tax.[4, 11], **tell.**, **TER.**, tere-ch.[14],
teucr., thal.[11], thea[8, 11], **ther.**,
thiop.[14], **thuj.**, thymol.[9, 14], thyr.[3],
til., tox-th.[11], trach.[11], tril., trom.,
TUB., tub-r.[13, 14], tus-p.[11], upa.[11],
uran.[6], uran-n.[6-8, 11], urea[10], ust.,
uva[2], v-a-b.[13, 14], vac.[11], valer.,
ven-m.[14], **VERAT.**, verat-v., verb.,
verin.[11], vesp., vib.[3, 6], vip-a.[14],
vichy[11], vinc., viol-o.[2], viol-t., vip.,
visc.[9], voes.[11], wies.[11], wildb.[11],
wye.[11, 12], x-ray[14], xan., **zinc.**,
zinc-ar.[8], zinc-m.[11], zinc-o.[4, 12],
zinc-p.[1'], **zinc-pic.**[8, 12], zinc-s.[11],
zing., ziz.[11]

convalescence
flabby feeling

heaviness
lassitude
lie down
relaxation

weariness

daytime

agar., **am-c.**, cench.[1'], cob-n.[9],
corn., graph., iod., indg., lyc.,
lyss.[2], mag-c., mosch., nat-ar.,
nat-c., **nat-m.**, nit-ac., op., ph-ac.,
phos., phys., pip-m., plan., **stann.**,
sulph., tarent., ter., uran-n.[2]

heat of day, during

sel.

w.-heat

walking am.

ph-ac.

w.-walking

morning
acon-l.[11], agar., alum.[4], am-c.,
am-m., **ambr.**, amph.[11], ant-c.,
ant-s-aur., apoc., aran.[6], **arg-m.**,
ARS., ars-i., ars-s-f.[1'], asc-t.,
atra-r.[14], atro., aur., aur-ar.[1'],
aur-i.[1'], bell., bism.[6], bor., bruc.[4]
bry., bufo, caj.[11], **calc.**, calc-i.[1'],
calc-s., canth.[4], caps., carb-an.,
carb-v., carbn-s., celt.[11], cham.,
chel., chin-s., cimic., cinnb.,
clem., coc-c., colch., **con.**, corn.[11],
croc., crot-h., cycl., dig., digin.[11],
dios., dros., erig., euphr., eupi.,
fago., flor-p.[14], form., **gels.**,
gnaph., **graph.**, ham., hyper.,
hom.[7], **iod.**, jal., kali-bi., kali-c.,
kali-m.[1'], kali-n., kali-p., lac-c.,
lac-ac., **LACH.**, lact.[4], levo.[14],
LYC., mag-c., mag-m., meli.,
merc., merc-c., merl.[11], morph.,
mur-ac., naja, **nat-ar., nat-c.,
nat-m., nat-p., nat-s.**, nat-sil.[1'],
nit-ac., nux-v., op., osm., ox-ac.,
ped., perh.[14], **petr., PH-AC.,
phos.**, pic-ac., plat., prun.,
pulm-a.[13], **puls.**, ran-b., **rhus-v.**,
rob., ruta, sabad., sang., **SEP.,
sil., spig.**, stach.[11], **stann., staph.,
stront-c.**, stry.[11], sul-ac.[16], **sulph.**,
sumb., syph., tab., ther., thuj.,
til., valer., **verat.**, viol-t.. zinc.,
zinc-p.[1']

bed, in

ambr., arn., **carb-v.**, caust.,
chin., cinch.[11], **con.**, ham.[12],
hell., hep., hom.[7], lach., mag-c.,
nat-m., phos., **PULS., sil.,
staph.**, stront-c.

while sitting up in

nat-m.

fasting

con.

ideas at night, after copious
flow of

tab.

lying

PULS.

w.-lying

rising, on

alum., asc-t., aur-m-n., bov.,
BRY., calc-caust.[11], carbn.[11],
caust., chin., cina, colch.,
corn., crot-t., dig., dios.,
dulc., eupi., **ferr.**, ham., hep.,
ign., iris, lac-ac., **LACH.,
lyc.**, mez., nat-m.[4, 16], nux-v.,
op., petr., **PH-AC.**, phos.,
plb., puls.[4], puls-n., rhus-v.,
scut.[11], **sep., sil., stann.**,
sulph., thuj., ust.

am.
acon., carb-v., caust., con.,
kali-c., mag-c., nat-c.,
nat-m., phos., **puls.**

after

alumn., **arg-m., arg-n.**, bry.,
carb-an., hep., kali-n., **lach.,
nit-ac., nux-v.**, peti.[11],
PH-AC., rhod., til.

waking, on

acon., agar., alum., alum-p.[1]',
am-c.[6], ambr., ant-c., **arg-m.,**
arn.[4], aur., bell.[4], berb., **bry.,**
calc., calc-sil.[1]', cann-s.,
carb-an., carb-v., cast.,
cast-v.[11], cham., chel., chin.,
clem., coca, colch., coloc., con.,
corn., crot-t., cycl., dros. **dulc.,**
euph.[4], fago., gels., gnaph.,
graph., grat., hep., hyper., ign.,
iod.[4], jab., kali-c., kali-sil.[1]',
lach., lyc., mag-c., mag-s.[4],
mang.[16], nat-m., **nux-v.[1], phos.,**
pic-ac., plb.[4], podo., rhus-t.,
sabad., **sang., sep., sil., spig.,**
staph., stram., **syph.**[1', 7], tab.,
ter., thuj.[4], verat., xan., zinc.

5 h[11]
napht.

6 h
pic-ac.

6.30 h
ham.

7 h
cham., elat., graph.

8 h
dios., phys.

8.30
fago.

10 h, until
nit-ac.

forenoon

abrot.[11], acon., alum., am-c.,
ambr., ang., ant-t., bart.[11], bruc.[4],
BRY., calc.[16], carb-an., carb-v.,
corn., fago., fl-ac., graph., grat.,
hell., indg., kali-cy., kali-n., lach.,

lyc., mag-m., mang., nat-m.,
nux-m., ox-ac., **ph-ac.,** phel.,
phys., **plat.,** ptel., ran-b., sabad.,
sars., scroph-n.[11], sep., staph.[3],
tab., tarent.

agg.[8]
acal., bar-m., bry., calc., con.,
corn., lac-c., lach., lyc., **nat-m.,**
nit-ac., phos., psor., sep., stann.,
sulph., tub.

9 h
chin-s., cocc., merl., nat-s.,
ox-ac., ped., perh.[14], peti.,
phys., ptel., sep.

am.
tarent.

9–11 h
tarent.

10 h
aq-mar.[14], bor.[6], cast., cench.[1]',
equis., gels., lycps., merc-d.,
phys.

am.
gels.

10–12 h
calc-s.

11 h
arg-m., **lach.[2]**, nat-c.[6], phos.[3, 11],
ptel., sep.[3], **sulph.,** thuj., zinc.

noon

bov., carb-v., caust., clem., con.,
cycl., fago., helon., hyper.,
nat-m., nit-ac., ox-ac.[11], ph-ac.[4],
phos., phys.[11], phyt., ptel., sil.,
sulph., teucr., thuj., zinc.[4]

12.30 h
gels., sol-t-ae.

15 h, until
hyos.

18 h, until
    phyt.[11], ptel.

am.
    hyper.

sleep, after[11]

    bor., con., cycl., nat-m.

    w.-afternoon-sleep

afternoon

    acon., aeth., **alet.**, am-c., amyg.,
    anac., apis, aq-pet.[11], arg-n., aur.,
    bar-c.[16], bell., bor.[16], brom., **bry.**,
    cast., carb-an.[16], carbn.[11], cinch.,
    coc-c., coca, colch.[14], con.[16],
    coloc., com., digin.[11], erig., fago.,
    ferr., **gels.**, glon., ham., helon.,
    hydr-ac., hyos., ign., iod.[16], iris,
    kali-c.[2, 4], kali-n.[4, 16], lyc., lycps.,
    mag-c., merl., mez., mur-ac.,
    nat-c.[4], nat-m., nat-p., nat-s.,
    nit-ac., nux-v., ol-an.[4], phys.,
    phyt., plb.[4], ptel., ran-b.[4], rhus-t.,
    ruta, sang., sep.[16], **sil., spirae.[11]**,
    staph., stram., stry., **SULPH.**,
    thuj., zinc., zing.

13 h
    astac.[11], ferr-p., phys., pic-ac.,
    verat-v.

13.30 h
    lyc.

14 h
    chel., gels., nux-v., sulph.

14–15 h
    guan.[11], plb-chr.[11], sulph.

14–16 h
    ign.

15 h
    ham., lyss.[2], mag-c., nat-s.,
    nep.[13, 14]

15–16 h[14]: reser.

16 h
    caust., **gad.[11]**, hydr., iris, lyc.,
    mang., merc-i-f., phys.

17 h
    coff., coloc., **lac-d.[2]**, lyc., merc.[16]

17 h, until
    tarent.

17–23 h[14]: perh.

17.30 h
    stram.

18 h[16]: merc.

18 h, until
    merc.

sleep, after

    bor.[16], chin-s., ferr., gels.,
    kali-c.[16], nat-m.[16]

    w.-noon-sleep

walking, while

    caust.[16], lyc., mag-c., pic-ac.,
    ran-b.

am.[11]
    nat-s.

after
    ery-a., euph., hyper.

evening

    acon., aloe, alum.[4], **am-c.**,
    am-m.[16], aphis[4, 11], apis, apoc.,

ars., asaf., asar.[4, 16], bapt.,
bell.[4, 16], berb., bor., bov.,
brom., bruc.[4], bry., calc.,
calc-p., **calc-s.**, carb-v., carl.,
caust., chin.[4], clem., cob., coc-c.,
coca, coloc., colocin.[11], con.,
croc., cycl., dios., dirc., erig.[11],
ery-m.[11], euphr., eupi., fago.,
ferr., ferr-ar.[1'], form., **graph.**,
grat., haem., helon., hep., hydr.,
hydr-ac., **ign.**, indg., iris, itu[11],
jac., jac-c.[11], **kali-bi.**, kali-c.,
kali-m.[1'], kali-n.[16], kali-sil.[1'],
kalm., **lach.**, laur.[4], lim.[11], lob.,
lyc., lycps., mag-c., merc.,
merl., mez., mur-ac., murx.,
naja, **NAT-M.**, nat-n., nicc.[2],
nit-ac., nux-v., ox-ac., pall.,
petr., phos., plat., plb., psor.,
puls-n., rat.[4], rhus-g., rhus-t.,
rumx., ruta, senec., **sep.**, sil.,
spig.[4], stront-c., sulfonam.[14],
sulph., sumb., tab., **tart-ac.**[11],
thuj., tub.[1'], upa., valer., zinc.,
zinc-p.[1']

18 h
helon., lyc.

19 h
gins., mag-c., nat-m., phys.,
pic-ac., sep., verat-v.

20 h
astac.[11], bar-c., mang., pana.[11],
phys., sep.

20.30 h
pip-m.

21 h
  dirc., mag-s., op., phys., pic-ac.

am.
  phos.

21.30 h
lyc., sep.

am.
  asc-t., calc-s., colch., nit-ac.

in open air[11]

  chel., **CON.**, grat., naja
  nat-m., pic-ac., sabad.

bed, in

  lyc.

eating, after

  bov.[11], **croc.**

  w.-supper

night

  acon-l.[11], am-c.[4], ambr., ant-c.,
  anthraci., anthroco.[11], calc.,
  canth., carb-an., carb-v., chel.,
  coca, crot-t.[4], ferr-i., gnaph.,
  hell., hyper., kreos., mur-ac.[11, 16],
  naja, nat-m., nux-v., rhus-t.,
  sep.[16], **sil.**, sulph., tab., thuj.

22 h
elat., fago., phys.

23 h
nat-m.

midnight

  ambr., op., **rhus-t.**

after
  nat-m., rhus-t.

2 h[16]: sep.

3 h
nat-m., **sec.**[2], zing.[11]

4 h
sulph.

abortion, after[11]

ruta

from w.[8]

alet., caul., chin., chin-s., **helon.,**
sec., **sep.**[6], sil.[6]

acute diseases, with[3]

aeth., ail.[3, 7], ant-t., apis, ars.,
calc-p.[7], gels., guar.[7], kali-m.[1'],
merc-cy., mur-ac., psor.[7], verat.

w.–sudden

Addison's disease, in[2]

calc., iod.

air, in open

am-c., am-m., ambr., **atro.**[11],
bry., calc., chin., clem., coff.,
coloc., con., ferr., grat., kali-c.,
mag-c., merc., merc-c.[11], mur-ac.,
nux-v., **plat.,** sang., **spig.,** verat.

am.
chel., colch., **CON.,** croc., gels.,
grat., hed.[10, 14], naja, nat-m.,
pic-ac., sabad.

w.-evening-am.

for want of

meli.

fresh air am.

calc.

albuminuria, in[2]

ars., calc-ar., dig., iod., merc-c.,
nat-c., **ter.**

alcoholic drinks am.

canth., nit-s-d.[11], thea[11]

alternating with sensation of
strength[4.]

ars., chin., colch.[14]

trembling
ferr., plb.[7]

anaemia, in[2]

chin., **FERR.**[2, 3, 6], **KALI-C.,** nat-c.,
nat-m.[2, 6], **PHOS.**

anaemia

anger, after

mur-ac.[6], zinc.

anxiety, with[16]

am-c., aur., calc., caust., rhus-t.

appetite, w. increases with[3]

ail.

apoplexy, from[7]

bar-c.

apoplexy

ascending stairs, from

alum-sil.[1'], **anac.**, ars., ars-i.,
ars-s-f.[1'], bar-m.[1'], blatta-a.[11],
CALC., **calc-p.**, calc-sil.[1'],
carbn-s.[1'], coff., colch., croc.[7],
fago., **IOD.**, kali-ar.[1'], **lyc.**, m-arct.[4],
mag-c.[16], nat-m., nat-n.[11], nux-v.[4],
ox-ac., ph-ac., phys., pic-ac., puls.,
sarcol-ac.[8], spig., **stann.**, sulph.,
zinc-a.[11]

ascites, from[15]

LYC.

bed, on going to

arn., cinnb., lycps., mur-ac., rumx.,
ter.

beer, after

coc-c.

am.
thea

breakfast time, about

sep.

after
arg-n., brom., carb-v., cham.[16],
con.[16], dig., lach., nux-v.,
ph-ac., sil., still.[11], thea, verat.

am.
calc., **con.**, nat-m., nux-v.,
staph.

businessman, worn out[11]

clem., lyc.

Vol. I: *business–man*

children, in

bar-c., bell., calc., carb-v.[12], cham.[4],
cina[4], kali-c.[4], lach., **lyc.**, nux-v.,
sil., **sulph.**

chill, before

ars., **chin.**, nat-m., thuj.

during
agar.[2], aran., ars., asar.[16], astac.[2],
chin., coc-c., ip., lach., **nat-m.**,
petr.[16], **phos.**, psor.

after[2]
apis, sulph.[16]

chilliness, with[16]

sep.

climacteric period, during[7]

CHIN.[2, 3, 6, 7], chin-ar.[6], **cocc.**,
con.[6, 7], **crot-h.**[2, 7], dig.[8], helon.[2, 3, 6, 8],
kali-p.[2, 7], **lach.**[3, 6, 8], magn-gl.,
phos.[3, 6], sabin.[1'], **sep.**[3, 6, 8], sul-ac.,
tab.[3, 6]

cloudy, damp weather, in

sang.

coffee am.[11]

eug.

from odor of

sul-ac.

coition, after

agar., ambr.[6], berb., **CALC.,**
carb-an.[4], chin., clem., **con., dig.,**
graph., kali-c., kali-p., lil-t., lyc.,
mosch., nat-c.[8], **nat-m.,** nit-ac.,
nuph.[2], petr., **ph-ac., phos.,** plat.[6],
SEL., sep., sil., staph., tarent.,
tax.[11], vichy[11], **ziz.[2]**

cold, after exposure to[11]

ars.

cold weather, in

apis, lach.

coldness, during

aeth., apis, atha.[11], con., guare.,
nat-m., thuj.

from[2]
ars., CARB-V., VERAT.

colic with[3]

cast., tab.

company, in[16]

sep.

conversation, from[16]

sil.

convulsions, after

acon., agar.[16], **alm-ns.[2],** ars.,
art-v.[2], carbn.[11], **cupr.[2], ip.[2],**
merc-c., **oena.[2],** sec., stram.[16],
stry., sulph.[16], tab.

epileptic

aster.[2], camph., **plb.[2], sulph.[2]**

hysterical

ars.

coryza, during[16]

calc., graph.

cough, after[3]

cor-r., verat.

from[16]
ars.

dampness, from exposure to

ars.

death, as of approaching

ars., con.[4], dig.[4], mag-m[4]., nat-c.[4]
olnd., op.[4], sec.[4], spig.[4], **vinc.[4, 7]**

dentition, in[2]

calc., calc-p., **ip.**

descending steps

stann.

diabetes mellitus, in[2]

arg-m., ars., lac-ac.

diarrhoea, from

acet-ac.[7],**alum.,** alum-p.[1'],**alumn.[2],**

ambr., ant-c.², ant-t.²˒⁶, **apis,
ARS.,** bar-m.², **bor.,** both., bry.,
carb-v., **CHIN.,** chin-ar.¹', coloc.,
con., **corn.²,** crot-t.², **dulc.,**
euph-a.², **ferr.,** gast.¹¹, gnaph.,
graph., hura, hydr., hyos.¹⁶,
iod., ip., iris, kali-c., kali-chl.,
kali-m.², kali-p.², lil-t., mag-c.,
merc., merc-cy., **NAT-S.,
NIT-AC.,** nuph.², **NUX-M.²,**
nux-v., **OLND.,** op., ox-ac., petr.,
PHOS., phyt., **PIC-AC., PODO.,**
ric.¹¹, **rhus-t.¹⁴,** sec., senec., sep.,
SIL., sul-ac., tab., **tarent.,**
tart-ac.², **VERAT., zinc.**

does not weaken³'

ph-ac.

dinner, before

nat-m., sabin.¹¹, sil.¹⁶, thuj.

during
am-c.¹⁶, bov., nat-ar.¹¹, nat-s.,
teucr.

after
alum.¹⁶, am-c., am-m., ant-c., ars.,
ars-h.², asar., bapt., bov., cain.,
calc., carb-v., cast., chel., **chin.,**
cob., cycl., dig., euph-a.¹¹, graph.,
grat., ign., indg., iod., **lach.²,** lyc.,
mag-c., mur-ac.¹⁶, nat-m., nat-p.,
nit-ac.¹⁶, ol-an., ox-ac., perh.¹⁴,
phel., **ph-ac.,** phos., plat., plect.,
sars., sep.¹⁶, **sil.,** squil., **sulph.,
thuj.,** zinc.

am.
ambr., sars.¹⁶

diphtheria, in²

ail., alum-sil., apis, brom., canth.,
chin-ar., crot-h., diph.⁸, ign.,
kali-bi., kali-perm., lac-c., **LACH.,
MERC-CY., merc-i-f., mur-ac.,**

nat-ar., nux-v., **PHYT.,** sal-ac., sec.,
sulph.

dipsomania, in²

ars., **carbn.-s.**¹'˒⁷, **kali-br., nat-s.²˒¹²,**
phos., ran-b.⁷, sel.

drawing and jerking in limbs, after

sulph.

dream, after a

calc-s., op., teucr.

drinking, after¹⁶

nat-m.

dropsy, in²

APIS, ars., **eup-pur, hell.,** seneg.

eating, before

cinnb.

while
am-c.², bufo, mag-c., ptel., sulph.⁴

after
act-sp., alum.³, **anac., ant-c.³˒¹⁶,
ARS.,** ars-s-f.¹', asar.³, bar-a.¹¹,
BAR-C., bar-s.¹', brom., calc.³˒⁶,
calc-p., cann-s., carb-an., **chin.,**
cina³, clem., **con., croc.,** crot-c.,
cycl., dig., ferr.⁶, ferr-ma., hep.,
hyper., kali-c., kali-sil.¹', lach.³˒⁴,
lyc.¹, mag-c., mag-m.³, meph.,
merc-c., mur-ac., **nat-c.³˒⁶,**
nat-m., **nit-ac.³,** nux-m.³, nux-v.,
ox-ac.², **PH-AC.,** phos., rhod.,

rhus-t., ruta, sang., sars.², sel.,
sep.⁶' ¹⁶, **sil., staph.,** sul-ac.,
sulph., tell., teucr., thea, thuj.,
uran-n.³

am.
aster., **hep.²**, **IOD.²**, nat-c.¹⁶, petr.,
sapin.¹¹, sil.

emissions, after

acet-ac., agar., aur., **bar-c., calad.²,**
calc., calc-p.⁸, canth., carb-an.,
carl., **chin.,** chin-b.², **cob.³' ⁶' ⁸,**
coff.², con., cupr., **cypr.²,** dam.⁸,
dig., **dios.³' ⁶' ⁸,** ery-a.⁸, ferr.³,
form.⁸, **gels.,** ham.², **hydr.,** iod.,
KALI-BR.², kali-c., lach.³' ⁴, **LYC.,**
med.²' ⁸, naja, **nat-m.,** nat-p., **nuph.²,**
NUX-V., op.², PH-AC., PHOS.,
pic-ac., plb., puls., **sabad.³, sars.,**
sel., sep., **SIL., stann., STAPH.,**
sul-ac.³, **sulph.²' ⁸,** ust., zinc.⁸

erections, from

aur., aur-m.¹¹, carbn-s.

excess, after any

agar.ˣ, **anac.⁸, calc-p.⁸, carb-v.⁸,**
caust.ˣ, **chin.⁸,** chin-ar.⁸, corn-f.⁸,
cur.ˣ, gins.⁸, kali-c.⁸, nat-m.⁸,
ph-ac.ˣ, phos.⁸, plb., sel.⁸, stroph-h.⁸

excessive³

ars., bapt., chin., ferr., **ferr-pic.⁷,**
gels., ph-ac., tab.

excitement, after

con., phos.⁶, stry., thea

exertion, from⁷

acon., **alum-p.¹',** ambr., **arn.,**

ars-s-f.¹', aur-ar.¹', aur-m.¹', bry.,
calc., chin., cocc., coff.,
ferr-ar.¹', ferr-i.¹', kali-ar.¹',
kalm.¹¹, macro.¹¹, mag-c., merc.,
nit-m-ac.¹¹, nit-s-d.¹¹, rhod.¹',
rhus-t.¹'' ⁷, sil., sul-i.¹', verat.

from slight

acon., **agar.,** ail., apis, **ARS.,**
ars-i., ars-s-f.¹', alum., **am-c.,**
anac., bapt., berb., **BRY.,**
CALC., calc-sil.¹', **carb-v.,**
carbn-s.¹', cham., clem., **cocc.,**
colch., CON., CROT-H., dor.,
ferr., ferr-i., **gels.,** ham.⁷, ign.,
jatr., kali-c., kali-n., kalm.,
lac-d.¹', **LACH., lyc., mag-m.,**
merc., merc-c., nat-ar., NAT-C.,
nat-m., nat-p., nux-m., petr.,
PH-AC., PHOS., PIC-AC., plb.,
psor., ptel., **RHUS-T., SEL.,**
sep., sol-n., **spig., SPONG.,**
stann., staph., stram., sul-i.¹'
sulph., sumb., ther., thuj.,
TUB.¹⁵, verat., ziz.

w.-motion – least

am.
ferr., kali-n.

exhilaration, as after

cinnb.

faintlike⁴

ant-t., **ars.²,** bar-c., berb.⁴' ¹¹,
carb-v.²' ⁴' ¹¹, CAUST.²' ³' ⁴' ¹¹,
cham.³, **coca², cocc.³,** croc.³,
cupr-c., **dig.²,** digin.¹¹, dulc.,
EUP-PER.², ferr., **goss.²,** ign.,
kali-c., kali-i.¹¹, lyc.¹¹, mez.¹¹,
mosch., **NUX-V.²' ³,** olnd., **petr.²' ⁴,**
sep., sil., spong.³, sulph., upa.¹¹,
verat.²' ³, zing.²' ¹¹

febrile[11]

ang., cham., kali-n., nit-ac.

feet, while washing the

merc.

fever, during

acon., alum.[16], am-m.[11], ant-t.,
anthraci.[2], **apis**[2, 11], aran., **ARS.,
bapt., bry.,** calc.[11, 16], carb-v.,
crot-h.[11], **eup-per.**[2], eup-pur.,
ferr., **ign.,** lyc., morph.[11], **mur-ac.,**
nat-c., **nat-m.,** nicc.[11], nit-ac.,
petr.[16], **ph-ac., PHOS., puls., rob.,
rhus-t.,** sarr., sep.[11, 16], sul-ac.[11].
sulph., thuj.[11]

after
apis[11], **aran., gent-l.**[11], **morph.**[11],
sal-ac.[2], sulph.[11], syph.[2]

following prolonged fever

colch.[7], **psor.**[7], **SEL.**

convalescence

food, from sour

aloe

fright, from

coff., merc., op.

grief, from

caust., ign., ph-ac., pic-ac.[2]

growing fast, after[7]

hipp., ph-ac.

haemorrhage, in[2]

**carb-v., CHIN., chin-s., ferr.,
hyper., ign., rat.**

headache, from

ars-h., bufo, calc.[16], cob., fago.,
glon., kali-c.[16], lac-d.[7], naja, sil.[16]

during[2]
ANT-C., aran., ars-h.[11], bism.,
bufo[11], calc-ar., carb-v., chin.,
chin-s., cob.[11], fago.[11], glon.[11],
lil-s.[11], naja[11], **sil., thuj.,** thymol.[9],
verat.

heartburn, from[16]

lyc.

heat, from

aster., **carbn-s.,** coc-c., **lach.,
nat-c.,** nat-p., **puls., puls-n.**[11],
rhod., **SEL., sulph.,** tab., vesp.

bed, of

aster.

room, in hot

cinnb., **puls.**

entering, from bed

aloe

summer, of

alum., **ant-c.**[8], **ars.**[2], **carbn-s.**[1', 7], **corn., GELS.**[2, 8], **IOD., lach., NAT-C.,** nat-m., **SEL.**

sun, of the

ars.[2], **GELS.**[2], **NAT-C., SEL.**

w.-walking – heat

thrills of heat, from

cocc.

walk and rapid cooling, after heated

bry.[11], **rhus-t.**

heat, after flushes of

dig.[12], nat-c.[16], **SEP.**[2, 7], **SULPH.**[2], **xan.**[7]

hunger, from

alum., crot-h.[2], **IOD.,** nat-c.[16], **phos., spig.**[1, 16], sul-i.[1'], **SULPH.,** ter.[2], **zinc.**

hysteric[16]

phos.

injuries, from[8]

acet-ac.[2, 7, 8], arn.[6, 8], calen., camph.[2], carb-v., dig.[2], **sul-ac.**[7, 8]

intermittent

apis, nat-ar.[1] (non: nat-c., nat-s.)

jaundice, from[8]

ferr-pic., pic-ac., tarax.

joints, of

acon., aesc., agar.[3], agn.[3], **aloe,** alum.[3], am-c.[3], anac.[3], ang.[3], **ant-t.**[3], **arg-m., ARN.,** ars., asar.[3], aur., bar-c.[3], bell.[3], bor., bov., **bry., CALC.,** calc-p.[3, 6], cann-s.[3], canth.[3], **carb-an.,** carb-v., carbn-s., **caust.,** cham., chel., **chin.,** chin-ar., cimic., clem., cocc.[3], colch.[3], coloc., **CON.,** cupr.[3], cycl.[3], dig.[3], dros.[3], dulc.[3], euph., **ferr.,** ferr-ar., ferr-p., graph., hep.[3], hyos.[3], ign.[3], **KALI-C.,** kali-n.[3], **kali-s.,** kreos.[3], **lach., led., LYC.,** mang., **MERC.,** merc-c., mez., morph., mosch.[3], murx., **nat-c.**[3], **nat-m., nit-ac.,** nux-m.[3], **nux-v.,** olnd.[3], par.[3], **petr., ph-ac.**[3], **phos.,** plat.[3], plb., podo., **PSOR., puls.,** ran-b.[3], raph., rheum[3], rhod., **RHUS-T., ruta**[3], sabad.[3], sars.[3], **SEP., sil.,** spong.[3], stann.[3], **staph.,** stront-c.[3], sul-ac.[3], **SULPH.,** tarax.[3], thuj., valer.[3], **verat.,** viol-o.[3], zinc.[3], zing.

leaning towards left during menses am.

phel.

leucorrhoea with[2]

aesc., alet.[2, 8], alum.[3, 8], **arg-n.,** bar-c.[3, 4], berb.[2, 6], **CALC.**[2, 8], calc-p., **calen.,** carb-an.[8], **caul.**[2, 8], **caust.**[2, 8], **CHIN.**[3, 6, 8], **cocc.**[6, 8], coll.[6], con.[2, 6, 8],

frax.[6], **GRAPH.**, gua.[8], **ham.**, helin.[8],
helon.[2, 8], hydr.[2, 8], **iod.**, **kali-bi.**[3],
kali-c.[6], **KREOS.**[2, 3, 4, 8, 11], **lyc.**, lyss.,
nabal.[1], **NAT-M.**, nicc.[6], onos.[8],
petr., **ph-ac.**, phos.[8], **phys.**, **psor.**[8],
puls.[8], rob., **senec.**[6], sep.[8],
STANN.[2, 8], sul-ac., tarent.[2, 11], tril.,
vinc.[6], zinc.

from[16]
   con.

lifting, from

CARB-AN., kali-sil.[1'], nat-c.[16]

looking down, on

kali-c.

loss of fluids, from[2]

calc., **CHIN.**[2, 6], **cur.**, ferr.[1'],
ferr-ar.[1'], ham.[7], hydr.[7], lachn.,
nat-m., **nuph.**, **PH-AC.**[1', 2], **phos.**,
psor., sec., **sep.**

loss of sleep, from

COCC., colch.[8], cupr., glon.[2],
hydr.[2], ip.[2], **nat-m.**[2, 11], nux-v.[8],
osm.[11], **puls.**[11]

love, from unfortunate

ph-ac.

Vol. I: *ailments–love*

lying agg.

agar., alum., bar-c., bry., carb-v.,
carl., coca, cycl., gels., nat-c.,
nat-m., nit-ac., nux-v., petr.,
phys., pip-m., **puls.**, rhus-g.[11],
spig., zinc-m.

am.

acon-f., ars., bry.[4], hedeo.[7],
lach., mag-c., nat-m.[4], nit-ac.[4],
ph-ac.[16], **psor.**, sabad.[4], **sep.**

on back

cast.

shower, before

gels.

masturbation, from[6]
aven., bell-p.[9], **nat-m.**, **phos.**[2, 6]

meeting am., in interesting

pip-m.

menses, before

alum.[3, 8, 16], **am-c.**[8], aur-s., **bell.**,
brom., calc.[3, 3'], carb-ac.,
carb-an[8], carb-v.[3], **chin.**[8], cimic.,
cinnb.[2, 3], **cocc.**, ferr., glyc.[8],
graph.[8], **haem.**[8], **helon.**[8], ign.[3, 8],
iod., kali-p.[3], **mag-c.**, merc.[3],
nat-m., nicc.[8], nux-m., phel.,
phos.[3], puls.[8], sec.[3], **verat.**[8], zinc.

at beginning

brom.[3], cocc.[3], ferr.[3], mag-m.[3],
phel.

appearance of m. am.

cycl., mag-m.

during
   agar., **aloe**, **alum.**, alum-p.[1'],
   am-c., am-m., **ars.**, ars-i.,
   ars-s-f.[1'], bar-c., bar-i.[1'], bar-s.[1'],
   bell., berb., bor., bov., brom.[7],
   bufo, cact., calc., calc-i.[1'],

calc-p., **calc-s., cann-s.³,**
CARB-AN., carb-v., carbn-s.,
caul., **caust.,** cimic., **cinnb.,**
cocc., eupi., ferr., ferr-i.,
graph., helon., ign., **iod.,** ip.,
kali-c., kali-n.¹⁶, **kali-s., lach.,**
lil-t., lyc., **mag-c., mag-m.,**
mag-s.⁹, mosch., **murx.,** nat-ar.,
nat-c., nat-m., **nicc., nit-ac.,**
nux-m., **nux-v.,** ol-an.³, **petr.,**
phel., **phos., sabin., sec.,**
senec., **SEP.,** stann., **sulph.,**
tarent., thuj., tril., **tub.¹,** uran.,
verat., vinc., wies.¹¹, zinc.³,
zinc-p.¹'

am.
  sep.¹

can scarcely breathe, must lie
  down

nit-ac.

desire to lie down, with

bell., ip., **nit-ac.**

end of
  bov., iod.

going up stairs, when

iod.

  w.-*ascending*

painful

bell., bufo

stool, after

nux-v.

w.-*stool*

talk, can scarcely

carb-an., cocc.², stann.

after.
  agar.³, **alum., alumn.²,** am-c.⁸,
  am-m.⁸, aran.³, **ars.³, ⁶, ⁸,**
  bell.³, ³', benz-ac., berb., cact.³,
  calc.³, ⁸, calc-p., carb-ac.³,
  carb-an., carb-v.⁶, ⁸, cast.³,
  chin., chin-s.², cimic.,
  cocc.³, ⁶, ⁸, ferr.³, ⁶, ⁸, ferr-pic.⁶,
  glyc.⁶, graph.³, ⁸, **helon.², ³, ⁶,**
  iod., **IP.,** kali-c.³, ⁸, kali-p.³, ⁶,
  mag-c.⁸, nat-m., nit-ac.³,
  nux-v.³, **phos.,** pic-ac.⁶, plat.,
  sapin.¹¹, sec., sep.³, stann.³,
  sulph., thlas.⁸, thuj., **tril.⁸,**
  verat.⁸, vinc.⁸

disproportionate to loss of blood

ham.², **ip.**

mental exertion, from

aloe, anag.², apis, arn., ars., aur.,
aur-ar.¹', bar-a.⁶, **bell., CALC.,**
calc-sil.¹', cham., **chin.²,** cocc.,
CUPR., FERR-PIC., ign., **kali-c.,**
kali-n., kali-p.⁷, **LACH., LEC.,**
lil-s.¹¹, **lyc.,** mag-c.⁷, **NAT-C.,**
nat-m., **nux-v.⁷,** okou.¹⁴, **par.²,**
ph-ac., pic-ac.², **PSOR., PULS.,**
sabad., **SEL.,** sep., sil., spong.,
sulfonam.¹⁴, **sulph.,** thuj.

occupation am.

croc.

milk, after¹⁶

sul-ac.

mortification, after

ign.

motion, from

agar., ammc., apoc., **arg-m.,**
ARS., asaf., bry., cann-s., cocc.,
hydr-ac., kali-bi., kali-n., lach.,
mang-o.[11], merc., merl., mur-ac.[4],
narcin.[11], nat-m.[4], nit-ac.[16],
nux-v., phel., **phos.,** plb., sep.[4],
spig.[4, 16], **SPONG.,** stann.[16],
staph., sulph., tab.

am.

cham.[16], colch., coloc., cycl., gels.,
kreos., **lyc.,** mosch., pip-m., **plat.,**
plb., **rhod.,** stann.[4]

gentle m. am.

kali-n.

least m., on[3']

anac., lyc., nux-m., spig., verat.

w.-exertion

when moved from horizontal
position

rob.

moving arms, on

nat-m.

muscular[3]

acon., agar., alum.[3, 8], alumn.[1'],

am-c., am-m., anac., ant-c., arn.,
ars.[3, 8], asaf., aur., **BAR-C.,**
bar-m.[2, 3], bell., berb., bry.[3, 8],
calc.[2, 3, 8], cann-s., canth., **carb-ac.,**
carb-v.[3, 8], caust.[3, 8], cham.,
chin., chlol.[2], cimic.[3], cocc.[1', 3],
colch.[3, 8], **con.**[3, 8], cortico.[9], **croc.,**
dig., dros., **dulc.,** euphr., **ferr.,**
ferr-m.[2], ferr-p., **GELS.**[2, 3, 8], graph.,
hyos., iod., kali-bi., kali-c.[3, 8],
kali-n., **kali-p.**[3, 8], laur., **lyc.,**
macro.[11, 12], mag-c., mag-m.,
mag-p.[3, 8], mang., meny., merc.[3, 8],
mez., mur-ac.[1'], **nat-c., NAT-M.**[3, 6],
NIT-AC., nux-v.[3, 8], olnd., **op.**[2],
petr., ph-ac.[1', 3], phos., phys.[3, 12],
PIC-AC.[1', 2], **plat., plb.**[2, 3, 6], puls.,
rad-br.[3], rheum, **rhod.,**
sabad.[3, 8, 11, 12], sarcol-ac.[9], sec.,
sep., sil.[3, 8], sin-n.[2], spig., stann.,
stram., stront-c., sul-ac.[3], **sulph.,**
ter.[2], thuj., **verat.**[2, 3], verat-v.[3],
zinc.[3, 8]

paralytic[1']

alumn.

music, from[7]

lyc.

nausea, with[11]

aeth., **agar.**[2], alumn.[2], ang.[2],
calc.[2, 11], **camph.**[2], cimic., cob.,
crot-t., gran., hell., sabad., sang.,
sep., stront-c.[11], **verat.**

nervous

acon., aesc.[2], **agar.**[2], **agn.**[2, 3, 11],
alet.[2], **alum.,** alum-p.[1'], alumn.[2],
am-c., am-m.[2], ambr., **anac.**[2, 8],
ang.[3], **aran.**[2], **arg-n.**[2, 3, 6], arn.,
ars., asaf.[2, 3, 6], **asar.,** aur.,
aven.[6, 10], **bar-c.,** bar-i.[1'], **bell.,**
bry., **calc.,** calc-p., calc-sil.[1'],

calen.[11], camph., carb-an.,
carb-v., carbn-s., cast.[3, 6, 10],
caust.[3, 6], cham., **CHIN.**, chin-ar.[6],
chin-s.[2], cic.[1], **cimic.[2, 3], COCA[2],**
COCC., coff., colch., **con.,** croc.,
cupr., cur., cycl.[2], cypr.[12],
dig., dios.[2], **fl-ac.[3, 6], form.[3],**
GELS.[2, 8], graph., **guaj.,** hedeo.[11],
helon.[2], hell., hep., hydr-ac.[4],
hydrc.[2], hyos., **ign., iod.,** kali-br.[8],
kali-n., **KALI-P.,** lac-c.[2], lach.,
lact., laur., **LEC.,** led., **lil-t.[3],**
lyc., mag-m.[3], meph.[6], **merc.,**
mosch., mur-ac., **NAT-C.,** nat-m.,
NAT-P., nat-s.[2], **NAT-SIL.[1'],**
NIT-AC., nux-m., **NUX-V.,** op.,
petr., **PH-AC.[1], PHOS.,** phys.[2],
PIC-AC., pip-m.[6], **plat., plb.,**
PULS., rhus-t., sabin., sars.,
scroph-n.[11], sec., **SEL.[1], SEP., SIL.,**
spig., spong., squil., **STANN.,**
STAPH., stram., stry-n.[10], stry-p.[6],
sul-ac., **sulph.,** sumb.[2], tab.[6],
tarent.[2, 3, 11], teucr., **ther.[2, 3],**
valer., verat., vib.[3], **viol-o.,** zinc.,
zinc-m., **ZINC-P.[1', 10],**
zinc-pic.[3, 6, 10]

afternoon
  cimic.

walk, after a

  petr.

nursing the sick, from

  cimic., **COCC., nit-ac.,** olnd.,
  zinc., **zinc-a.[7]**

sit up with sick person[7]

  carb-v., cocc., **nux-v.,** puls.

nursing women, in

  calc.[2], calc-p.[2], carb-an., **CARB-V.[2],**

CHIN., lyc.[2], olnd., **PH-AC., phos.[2],**
phyt.[2], sil.[2], sulph.[2]

nursing agg

old people, of

  ambr., aur., **BAR-C.,** carb-v.[8], **con.,**
  cur., eup-per.[8], glyc.[8], nit-ac.[8, 12],
  nux-m., op., **phos.,** sec., **sel., sul-ac.**

w.-sudden – eruption

operation, from

  acet-ac.[7, 8], carb-v.[1'], hyper.[8]

injuries – operation

pain, from

  arg-m., **ARS.,** carb-v., cham.[16],
  hep.[1'], hura, kali-p., kalm.[1'],
  pic-ac.[3], plb., **rhus-t.**

sacrum, in

  sep.

palpitation, with[16]

  aur., caust., sang., sul-i.[1']

paralytic

  agar.[1'], **alum.,** alum-p.[1'],
  alumn.[1', 7], am-m., ambr.[1'], anac.[1'],
  ang.[3, 4], **arg-m., ARS.,** art-v.[2],
  bapt.[1'], **bar-c., bar-m.,** bell., **bism.,**
  bry., **calc.,** calc-ar.[1'], camph.,
  cann-i.[1'], canth., caps.[4], carb-v..

caust., cham., chel., chin.,
cimic.¹', cina, COCC., colch.,
con., crot-h., cupr.⁷, dig., dros.,
euph., ferr., ferr-ar., ferr-ma.⁴,
GELS., HELL., hyos., ign.¹', ind.,
kali-n., lach., laur., merc., mez.,
mosch., MUR-AC., nat-c., nat-m.⁴,
nat-p., nit-ac., nux-m.¹', nux-v.,
olnd., PH-AC., PHOS., plat.¹',
plb., psor.¹', puls., rhod., rhus-t.,
sabad., sarcol-ac.¹⁴, sil., stann.,
stront-c., sulph.³, valer., VERAT.,
zinc.¹', ⁴

morning after rising¹⁶

phos.

motion, on

aeth., arg-m.

pain, with

arg-m., verat.

painful parts, in

cham., verat.

sliding down in bed

ant-t.², apis, arn.⁶, ars., arum-t.,
bapt.², ³, ⁶, bell.², carb-v., chin.², ³,
colch.¹', ³, croth-h.¹', hell., hyos.¹', ⁶,
lyc.², mosch., MUR-AC., nux-m.,
nit-ac., PH-AC., PHOS., rhus-t.,
zinc.², ³, ¹⁶

parturition, in³

arn., asaf., BELL., bor., bry., calc.,
camph., carb-an., carb-v., caul.², ³,
caust., cham., chin., cimic., cocc.,
coff., con.², gels., graph., hyos.,
ign., KALI-C.³, ¹⁶, KALI-P., kreos.,

lyc., mag-c., mag-m., merc., mosch.,
nat-c., nat-m., nux-m., nux-v., OP.,
phos., plat., PULS., rhus-t., ruta,
sabad., SEC., sep., stann., sul-ac.,
sulph., thuj., zinc.

periodica'

ARG-N., hep.²

every other morning

nit-ac.

perspiration, from

acon., agar., am-c., ambr.,
aml-ns., ant-c., ant-t.³, ant-o.¹¹,
anthraci., apis, ARN.³, ars.,
ars-i.⁶, ars-s-f.¹', bar-c., ben.,
BRY., bov., caj.¹¹, calad., calc.,
CAMPH., canth.³, ⁶, CARB-AN.,
carb-v., carl.¹¹, cast.⁶, CAUST.³,
CHIN., chin-ar., CHIN-S., coca¹¹,
cocc., croc., dig., FERR., ferr-ar.,
ferr-i., ferr-p., gels.¹¹, graph.,
hep.⁶, hist.⁹, hura¹¹, hyos., ign.,
IOD., jatr.¹¹, kali-bi., kali-n.,
lac-c., lyc., mag-c.⁷, MERC.,
morph.¹¹, nat-c.¹¹, nat-m.¹, nit-ac.,
nux-v.³, op., ph-ac., PHOS.,
PSOR., puls., pyrog., ran-s.¹¹,
rhod., SAMB., sec., senec.⁶, SEP.,
sil., stann., sulph., tarax.,
tarent.¹¹, TUB., verat., verat-v.

night
ars., bar-c., bry., carb-an., chin.,
eupi., ferr., hall¹¹, merc., nat-c.¹¹,
ph-ac.¹¹, phos.², samb., stann.,
tarax., TUB.

parturition. after⁷

samb.

suppressed foot sweat, from[2]

sil.

while awake; dry, burning heat
while sleeping

SAMB.

with perspiration, w.[2]

ALOE, calc., chin., chin-m.,
dig., **jab., lyc., ph-ac.,** sal-ac.,
sul-ac., **tarent.**

with cold[2]

camph., carb-v., cupr., **merc.,
ph-ac.,** ter., **VERAT.**

playing piano, from[1']

anac.

pleasant[11]

cann-s., morph.

pleasure, from

crot-c.

pregnancy, in[2]

alet.[1'], alum., alumn., calc-p.,
helon., murx., **sulph., verat.**

progressive[2]

acon., ars.[3], caust.[3], cupr-ar., **dig.,**
kreos.[3], **ol-j., phos., plb.,** verat.[3]

quinine, from abuse of[1']

ars-s-f.

rapid

ARS., laur., **sep., VERAT.**

w.-*sudden*

reaction, with lack of[2]

am-c., laur., **OP., sulph., valer.**

reaction, lack

fat people, in[2]

CAPS.

reading, from

anac., **aur.,** ph-ac., plb., **sumb.**

aloud

stann.

rest, during[11]

coloc., con., kreos., lyc.[2, 11, 16],
rhod.[1']

w.-*lying*
w.-*sitting*

am.[11]
bry.

resting head on something and clothing eyes am.

anac.

restlessness, with[2]

ARS.[2, 3], bism., colch., lycps., lyss., ph-ac., RHUS-T.[2, 3], zinc.[3]

riding, from

cere-b.[11], cocc., petr., psor.[1], sep., sulph., tet.[1] (non: ter.)

in open air am.

cinnb.

rising, on

acon-c., ammc., arn., ARS., atro., BRY., clem., coca, fago., ham., hydr., hyper., jab., lyc., mag-c., nat-ar., nat-m., olnd., osm., phyt., pic-ac., ptel., rhus-g.[11], rhus-t., sol-t-ae., teucr., thuj., uran.

w.-morning – rising

after
am-c., coc-c., hydr., mag-c.

seat, from a

chin.

room, in[14]

asar.

agg. from closed[14]

asar.

sea-bath, after

mag-m.

sedentary habit, from[7]

nux-v., sulph.

sexual excesses, after[2]

ars., aven.[6], chin.[6], coca, con.[6], dig., gins.[6], kali-c.[6], nat-m.[2, 6], ph-ac.[6], phos., ust.

side, of left[2]

arg-n., lach.

sit down, desire to[6]

alum.[4], ambr., anac.[4], ars., bry.[4, 6], calc., caust., cham.[4], chin., cocc.[4, 6], colch., croc.[4], dulc., kali-n., led., lil-t., m-aust.[4], merc., mur-ac.[4], nat-m., nat-s., nux-v.[4, 6], ol-an.[4], olnd., ph-ac., rhus-t.[4], sabin.[4], stann., staph.[4], stront-c., sulph.[4], tarax.[4], verat.

sitting

agar., anac., arg-m.[4], ars., aur., bry., carl., caust.[4], chel., chin., cocc., colch., fago., graph., kali-n., led.[4], lyc., m-aust.[4], mag-c., mang., merc.[4, 6], merc-i-f., mur-ac.[4], nat-m., nit-ac., nux-v.[4], phos.[4], plat., plb., ptel., ran-b.[4], RHUS-T., ruta, sabad., staph., stront-c.[4], sulph., thuj.[4]

w.-rest

am.
  bry., euph-a.[11], glon., nux-v.,
  sapin.[11]

walk, after a

RUTA

sleep, during

  bufo

after,
  agar., ambr.[2], bor., bor-ac.,
  camph., carl., chel., chin-s., coca,
  colch., con., cycl., dor., ferr.,
  gels., gent-l., **kali-n.[6], lach.,** lyc.,
  mez., nat-n., sec., sep., sil.,
  sin-n.[2], zinc.

am.
  alum.[16], mez., **ph-ac., phos.**

loss of, from

  COCC., colch.[8], cupr.[1], glon.[2],
  hydr.[2], ip.[2], nat-m.[2, 11], nux-v.[8],
  osm.[11], **puls.[11]**

as from[16]

  plat.

sleepiness, from

  coff., chlol.[2], gran., hep.[11], nit-ac.,
  rhus-t.[11]

as from
  aeth.[2], chen-v.[2], cimic., dig.,
  kali-n., merc-sul.[2], peti.[11], petr.,
  phel., plat., **rhus-t.,** thuj.

  morning
    verat.

afternoon, walking am.

  ruta

sleeplessness, from

  cypr.[2, 11], kreos.[2]

smoking, from

  asc-t., clem.[3], **hep.**

  w.-*walking – smoking*

somnambulism, after

  sulph.

sporting[7]

  arn., ars., coca, fl-ac., rhus-t.

spring, in

  apis, **BRY.[2]**

standing, on

  acon.[2], acon-c.[11], agn., **apis**[2], asaf.,
  aster.[2], berb., **cic., cocc.[4],** crot-h.,
  cupr.[4], cur., ham.[11], hep.[4], **kali-c.[2],**
  kali-n.[4], lach.[4], led.[4], merc.,
  MERC-CY.[2, 11], mur-ac., nat-m.,
  nit-ac.[4], nux-v.[4], ol-an.[4], ped.[11],
  plat.[4], ran-b., spig., staph.[4],
  sul-ac.[1', 4, 6], **sulph.,** ther.[4], zing.

stimulants am.

  phos.

  w.-*coffee*
  w.-*tea*

stomach, in[2]

calc-p., calc-s., crot-t., HYDR., podo.

as from[16]

mag-c.

pain in, from

nux-v.[2], podo.

and back

sep.

stool, before

hydr., mez., nat-hchls., **rhus-t., verat.**

during
aesc., apis, atro., bell., **bor.,** carbn-s., cob., colch., crot-h., crot-t.[2], **cupr-a.[2],** kali-i., lact., **nit-ac.[2],** pic-ac., plan., **PLAT.,** sec., **verat.**

after
aeth., **aloe,** ant-t., apis, apoc., arn., **ARS., ARS-MET.,** ars-s-f.[1'], bapt.[2], bism., bov., **calc.,** carb-an.[16], **carb-v., carbn-s.,** cast-v.[11], caust., chin., **chin-s.,** clem., cocc.[3], coch.[3], colch., coloc., com., **CON.,** cop., crot-h., crot-t., dios., **dulc.,** eupi., ferr-ma., **graph.,** ign., **iod.,** ip., **jatr.[2], lach.,** lil-t., lipp.[11], **lyc.,** mag-c., **med., MERC.,** mez., nat-m., **NAT-S., NIT-AC., nux-m.[2],** nux-v., petr., **phos.,** phys., **PIC-AC.,** plan., **PODO.,** pyre-p.[11], rham-f.[11], sabad., sacch., **SEC., sep., sil.[2], sulph., ter.,** thuj., trio.[1] (not : tril.), trom., tub.[3], **VERAT.,** vinc.

stooping, on

grapn.

storm, before and during a

sil.

thunderstorm, during

caust., nat-c., nat-p., nit-ac., petr., rhod., sil.

sudden

acon., act-sp., **aeth.[6],** ail.[3], **am-c.[3, 6],** am-m.[4], ambr.[3, 4], **ant-ar.[6],** ant-c.[1', 6], **ant-t.[3, 6], apis,** apoc.[6], **arg-m.,** arg-n.[3], arn.[3, 6], **ARS.,** ars-h., **ars-i.[6], bapt.[3, 6],** bell.[2, 3, 16], bry.[3, 6], calc., camph., cann-s.[4], carb-ac.[6], **carb-v., caust.[3, 6, 16],** cham., colch., con., **CROT-H., cupr.[3],** cupr-ar., dig.[3, 6, 16], dulc.[4], fl-ac.[3], **gels.[3, 6],** glon.[3], **GRAPH., hell.[3, 6], hep., hydr-ac.[3, 6], ip.,** jatr.[6], kali-br.[6], kali-c.[16], kali-cy.[7], kalm.[3], lach., laur., lith-c.[3, 6], lyc., mag-c.[3], merc-c.[3], merc-cy.[3], naja[3], nit-ac.[3], **nux-v.,** petr.[4, 16], **phos.,** ran-b., rhus-t.[3, 6], sabad.[3, 6], sec., **sel., SEP.,** sil.[3], spong., stann., stram., **sulph.[3, 6], tab.[3, 6],** tarent., tax., thuj.[3], **verat., verat-v.[3, 6],** vip.[4], zinc.[3, 6, 16]

collapse

daily
hep.

afternoon
lyc., ran-b.

13.30 h
iodof.

walking, after

graph.

evening
fl-ac.

chilliness, during

sep.

diarrhoea, with[2]

crot-t.

dressing after rising, while

stann.

eruption comes out, after the

ars.

old people, in[7]

kali-cy.

sitting, while

cham., lyc., ran-b.

w.-sitting.

vanish, as if senses would

ran-b.

walking, from

carb-v.[16], con.[16], sabad., wildb.

w.-walking

sunstroke, from[2]

glon., verat-v.

supper, after

alum., bov., chin., lach., mag-c., sil.

w.-evening – eating

suppressed eruptions, from[1']

ars-s-f.

syphilis, in[2].

kali-i., lyc., staph.

talking, from

act-sp., **ALUM.,** am-c.,
am-caust.[11], ambr., arn.[7], **calc.,**
cocc., dor., **ferr.,** hydrc.[11], **hyos.,**
iod., jac-c.[11], **nat-m., ph-ac.,**
psor., sep., sil., **STANN., SULPH.,**
ust.[2], wies[11]

of peoples, from the

alum., am-c., ars., verat.

Vol. I: *talk – others*

tea am.[11]

dig.

tobacco, from[4]

clem., hep.

w.-smoking
w.-walking – smoking

toothache, after[16]

nat-c.

with[16]
mang.

tremulous

agar., **alum., anac.,** anag.[2],
ant-t.[3, 6], **apis, ARG-N., ars.,**
bapt., bell.[3, 6], berb.[3, 6], bor.[4],
bry.[3, 6], calc-ar.[1'], caps.[4], carb-v.,
caul., caust.[3, 4, 6, 16], **chin.**[2, 3, 4, 6],
chin-s.[4], clem., **cocc., CON.,**
crot-h., cupr.[16], **gels.,** graph.[4],
hep., hyos.[4], kali-c.[3, 4, 6, 16],
kali-n., **kalm., LACH.**[2], lyc.,
lycps.[2], mang.[3, 6], med.[1'],
nat-m.[3, 16], **nit-ac.,** ol-an.[4], olnd.[4],
ox-ac., petr.[7, 16], **phos., plat.,**
plb.[4], **puls.,** rhus-t.[16], **sep.,** spig.[4],
STANN., ther., thuj.[3], verat.[3, 6],
vip.[3], zinc.[6]

night, on waking

brom.

dinner, after

ant-c.

w.-dinner

stool, after

ARS., carb-v., caust., **CON.**

w.-stool

urination, after

cimic., **lyss., phos., pic-ac.**[2]

after copious

caust., gels., med.

vertigo, with[2]

acet-ac., crot-t.[11], cupr-s., dulc.[7],
graph.[11], hell.[11], **sil.,** uran-n.

vexation, after

ars., calc-p., lyc., **nat-m.,** nux-v.,
petr., sep.[16], verat.

vomiting, with[11]

aeth., ars., bol-s., **calc.**[2], crot-t.,
gran., kali-c.[11, 16], phos.[16],
SANG.[2, 11], sulph.[16], tab.

after[11]
aloe, ant-c.[2], ant-t., apom.,
ars.[11, 16], bar-c.[2, 11], cadm-s.[2, 11],
colch.[2], der., gran., mag-c.[11, 16],
nat-s., op., phyt., sel.,
verat.[2, 11, 16], zinc.[16]

waking, on

aeth., alco.[11], aloe, ambr.,
aq-pet.[11], arg-m., ars-h., bell.,
bism., bry., carbn-s., card-m.,
cham., chel., chin., clem., **cycl.,**
dig., dios., **dulc.**[2], **echi.**[3, 6], equis.,
erig., erio.[11], euphr.[4], ferr.,
ferr-p., form., hipp., hura, ign.[6],
lac-ac.[1] (not : lac-c.), lyc., mang.,
myrig., nabal.[11], nat-ar., nat-m.,
nat-p., nux-m., nux-v.[6], op.,
ph-ac., podo., ptel., **PULS.,**
puls-n.[11], rhod., rhus-t., sang.,
sec.[6], sel.[6], **sep.,** sulph., sumb.,

syph.[3], tab., teucr., thuj., upa., xan.

w.-*dream*

morning[16]
mag-c.

dream, from a

calc-s.[1], op., teucr.

after
arg-m., calc-s., cedr., cycl., iod., wildb.

walking, from

acon., acon-f.[11], aesc., agar., ALUM., ALUM-P.[1'], alum-sil.[1'], am-c.[4], ambr.[4], **anac.,** ang.[11], arg-m.[1', 4], arn., ARS., ars-i., aur-ar.[1'], aur-m.[1'], aur-s.[1'], bar-c., bar-i.[1'], bar-m., bar-s.[1'], **berb.,** bov., brom., BRY., CALC., CANN-I., carb-an., **carb-v., carbn-s.,** caust.[8, 16], cench.[1'], cham., chel., **chin.,** chin-ar., clem.[16], coca, cocc., **coloc., CON.,** cupr., **cupr-ar.,** cycl.[8], digin.[11], ery-a.[11], ery-m.[11], euph., euph-a.[11], fago.[11], FERR., ferr-ar., ferr-i., ferr-ma., **fl-ac.,** franz.[11], gins., graph.[4], ham., helon., hep., hyper., ind., indg., **iod.,** kali-ar.[1'], **kali-c.,** kali-m.[1'], kali-p., kali-sil.[1'], **lac-d., LACH.,** led.[4], **lyc.,** lyss.[11], mag-c., mag-m., mag-s.[4], **med.,** meny., merc., merl., mez., morph.[11], **MUR-AC.,** narcin.[11], **nat-ar., nat-c.,** nat-hchls., **nat-m.,** nat-n.[11], **nat-s.,** nat-sil.[1'], nicot.[11], NIT-AC., nux-m., nux-v.[4], pall., petr., **PH-AC., PHOS.,** phys., phyt., **PIC-AC., plb.,** polyg-h., **PSOR., puls.,** puls-n., ran-b.[4, 11], rheum, rhod., rhus-d.[8], RHUS-T., ruta, sabin., sarcol-ac.[8], SEP., sil., spig.[1], SQUIL., stann., **staph.,**

stram., stront-c.[4], sul-i.[1'], SULPH., sumb., tarent., tell., thea[4], thuj., til., tril., tub.[1'], **verat.,** wies.[11], wildb.[11], **zinc.,** zinc-p.[1']

w.-*afternoon – walking*

am.
ambr.[16], anac., bry.[16], calc.[11, 16], coloc., merc., nat-m., RHUS-T., **ruta, SULPH.**

w.-*daytime – walking*

air, in open

act-sp., agar., ALUM., alumn.[2], **am-c.,** ambr., ang.[16], arg-m., ars-s-f.[1'], berb.[4], bry., calc., calc-sil.[1'], carb-v., caust., chin.[4], coff., chel., **cocc.**[1], **coll.,** coloc.[4, 16], **con.,** euph.[4, 16], ferr., graph., grat.[4], hep., hyos., kali-bi., kali-c., lact., lyc.[4, 16], m-arct.[4], m-aust.[4], mag-c., mag-m.[4], merc., nat-m., **nux-v.,** ph-ac.[4], puls., rhod., RHUS-T., sang., sep., **sil., spig.,** sulph., **zinc.**

am.
agar., am-c., asar.[14], caust., chin-s.[4], croc.[4], **fl-ac.,** grat.[4], **kali-i.,** ox-ac., sapin.[11], **sulph.**

after w. in open air[16]

graph., sil.

breakfast am., after

coca

commencing to walk, on

carb-v.

cough and expectoration, from

nux-v.

dinner, before[11]

hyper.

w.-dinner

eating, after[11]

hep.

w.-eating

heat of the sun, in

lach., nat-c.

w.-heat – sun

house, in the

agar., ferr-ma., sapin.[11], sec., sumb.

menses, during

murx.[2], phel.

rapidly

agar., coc-c., olnd.

am.
stann.

riding, after

petr.

w.-riding

short walk, from[2]

calc., cann-i., **con.**

after a[2]
nat-c., ruta, **sulph., ter.**, tub.[1, 7]

slowly am.

ferr.

smoking, after

sulph.

w.-smoking

w.-tobacco

storm, before and during a

sil.

warm room, in

aloe, ambr., croc., **iod.**, merl., **PULS.**

w.-heat – room

weather agg.

ANT-C., camph.[3], **iod.**, lach.[3], **nat-ar.**, nat-c.[3], nat-m., nat-p., podo.[3], **sel., SULPH.**[1], vip.[11]

wine agg.[1] (non: am.)

ars., lyc., phos., **thuj.**

am.[11]
ars., **thuj.**, visc.[14]

worms, with[2]

cic., cina, merc.

writing, from

cann-s., ran-b., sil.

yawning, after

eug., **nux-v.**

WEARINESS

acon., adlu.[14], aesc., agar., **ALUM.,**
alum-p.[1'], **am-c.,** ambr., **anac.,**
ang.[3, 4], **anh.**[9, 10], **ant-c., ant-t.,**
aphis[4], aran.[4], aran-ix.[10], arg-m.,
arg-n., arist-cl.[9, 10], **arn., ars., ars-i.,**
asaf., asar., aur., aur-ar.[1'], aur-m.,
aur-s.[1'], **bapt.,** bar-c., bar-m., bell.,
bell-p.[9, 10], **BENZ-AC.,** berb.,
beryl.[9], bism., bor.[3, 4], bov., bruc.[4],
bry., cadm-met.[9, 10], calad.[4], **calc.**[1'],
calc-f.[9], **CALC-P., calc-sil.**[1'], camph.,
CANN-S., canth., caps., **carb-ac.,**
carb-an., **carb-v., CARBN-S.,** carc.[9],
caust.[1], cecr.[14], cench.[1'], cham.,
CHEL., chin., cic., cimic., cimx.,
cina, cist.[4], clem., cob-n.[9, 10],
coc-c., cocc., coff., colch., coloc.,
con., cortico.[9], cortiso.[9], **CROC.,**
crot-c., cupr., cycl., dicha.[10], dig.,
dros., dulc., erig.[10], esp-g.[10, 13],
euph., euphr., **FERR.,** ferr-ma.[4],
ferr-p., **GELS.,** gran.[4], **GRAPH.,**
grat.[4], guaj.[4], guat.[9], **ham.,** harp.[14],
hecla[14], hed.[9, 10], hell., helon., **hep.,**
hist.[9, 10], **hyos.,** ign., iod.[4], **ip.,**

kali-bi.[1', 3], kali-c., kali-chl.[4],
kali-m.[1'], kali-n., **KALI-P.,** kali-s.,
kali-sil.[1'], kalm.[1'], **kreos.,** lac-ac.,
LACH., lact.[4], **laur., LEC.**[1], led.,
luf-op.[10], **LYC.,** m-arct.[3], m-aust.[4],
mag-c., mag-f.[10], mag-m., mand.[9, 10],
mang., med.[7], meny., meph.[4, 14],
MERC., mez., mosch., **mur-ac.,**
murx.[4], naja[14], **nat-c., NAT-M.,**
nat-s., nat-sil.[1'], nep.[10], nit-ac.,
nux-m., NUX-V., ol-an.[4], olnd., op.,
par., petr., PH-AC., phenob.[13],
PHOS., phyt.[3], **PIC-AC., plat.,** plb.,
prun.[4], psil.[14], **psor., PULS.,** ran-b.,
rauw.[9], **rheum, rhod., rhus-t.,**
rib-ac.[14], **RUTA,** sabad., sabin.,
samb., saroth.[9], sars., sec., senec.,
seneg., **SEP.,** sieg.[10], **SIL.,** spig.,
spong., squil., **stann., STAPH.,**
stram., stront-c., **sul-ac.,** sulfa.[9],
SULPH., sumb., **tab.,** teucr., ther.[4],
thiop.[14], thuj., **TUB.,** v-a-b.[13], valer.,
verat., verb., viol-o., visc.[9], x-ray[9],
ZINC., zinc-p.[1']

flabby feeling

heaviness
lassitude
lie down.
relaxation

weakness

morning
alum.[4], am-c., ambr., ant-c.[4], **ars.,**
aur.[4], bar-c.[4], bell.[4], bov.[4], **bry.**[1],
calad., carb-an.[4], **carb-v.,**
carbn-s., cast.[6], caust.[4], **cham.,**
chel.[4], chin.[4], cob-n.[9, 10], con.[4],
cortiso.[9], croc.[4], dros.[4], erig.[10],
ferr.[4], hep.[4], kali-c.[4], **kali-chl.,**
lac-ac., **LACH.,** lact.[4], lyc.[4],
m-aust.[4], **mag-c.**[1], mag-m.,
meph.[14], mur-ac.[4], **nat-m.,**
NUX-V., petr., phos.[4], prun.[4],
puls.[4], rhus-t.[4], sabad.[4], **SEP.,**
sil.[4], spig.[4], stann.[4], staph.,
stront-c.[4], sul-i.[1'], **sulph.,** teucr.[4],
ther.[4], thuj.[4], valer.[4], zinc.

rising, on[4]

bov., ferr., hep., puls., stann.,
teucr.

waking, on[4]

alum., am-c., ambr., ant-c., aur.,
bar-c., bell., bism., **bry., calc.,**
cann-s., **carb-an., caust.,** chel.,
chin., cob-n.[9], **con.,** cycl., dros.,
dulc., hep., kali-c., lact., **lyc.,**
m-aust., **mag-m., nat-m., nux-v.,**
phos., prun., rhus-t., sabad., sep.,
spig., staph., stront-c., teucr.,
ther., **thuj.,** valer., **zinc.**

forenoon[4]
am-c., erig.[10], esp-g.[13, 14], hell.,
mag-m., nat-s., phel., seneg.

noon[13, 14]
esp-g.

afternoon[4]
adlu,[14] am-c., iod., kali-c., mag-c.,
mag-m., nat-c., ol-an., phos., staph.,
thuj.

am.[14]: kali-c.

evening
berb., carb-v., ign., meph.[14],
methys.[14], **mur-ac.,** pall., **sulph.**

air, in open

carb-v.

night[4]
dulc., kreos., merc., sabad., sabin.

agg.[7]
arn., ars., cann-s., chin., **coff.,**
RHUS-T., verat.

air am., in open[9, 10]

hed.

ascending stairs, from[1']

sul-i.

climacteric period, during[8]

bell-p., calc.

coition, after[3]

agar., calc., kali-c., lyc., nit-ac., sel.

conversation, from

ambr.

diarrhoea, after[1']

sul-i.

eating, while

kali-c.

after
ant-c., **ARS.,** bar-c., **carb-an.,**
card-m., chin., kali-c., **lach.,**
mur-ac., **nat-m., nux-m., rhus-t.,**
ruta, sang.

emissions, after[3]

chin., led., plb., puls., sabad., staph.

exertion, from mental

alum., **aur., lach., LEC., PIC-AC.,**
puls., thuj.

Vol. I: *work–fatigues*

physical e. am.[9]

hed.

leucorrhoea with[4]

prun.

after[4]
con.

menses, before

alum., **bell., nat-m.**

during
am-c., bor., calc-p., **caust., ign.,**
iod., kali-c., mag-c., **nit-ac.,**
nux-m., petr., sul-i.[1'], thuj.

am.[9]
hed.

after
alumn.[2], bell.[2, 6], carb-an.[2, 6]
cub.[2], nat-m.[2], nux-v.[6], phos.[6],
plat.[2, 6], thuj.

playing piano

anac.

reading, from

aur.

sexual excitement, from[6]

sars.

sit down, desire to[4]

dulc., stann., sulph.

sitting, while

bry.[4], chin.[4], led.[4], mag-c.[4], **merc.,**
ol-an.[4], plat.[4], plb.[4], rhus-t.[4]

standing, when

led.[4], **mur-ac.,** nat-m.[4], plat.[4]

talking, after

ALUM., calc-p., sulph.

much t.[16]

calc.

waking, on[4]

alum., am-c., ambr., ange-s.[14],
ant-c., aur., bar-c., bell., bism.,
bov., **bry., calc.,** cann-s., **carb-an.,**
caust., chel., **con.,** cycl., dros., dulc.,
ferr., lact., **lyc.,** m-aust., **mag-m.,**
nat-m., prun., rib-ac.[14], sep., spig.,
teucr., **thuj.,** valer., **zinc.**

am.[14]: thiop.

walking, on[4]

bry., chin., con., ferr., lach., led.,
mag-c., mag-m., plb., stram.

air, in open[4]

alum., coff., ferr., m-arct.,
mag-c., nat-m., rhod., sep.,
sulph.

am.[4]
caust., croc., ruta, sul-ac.

after

agar.[4], alum.[4], anac.[14],
carb-an.[4], caust.[4], clem.[4], coff.[4],
con.[4], graph.[4], iod.[4], **lac-d.**[1', 7],
mur-ac., nux-v.[4], ph-ac.[4], plat.[4],
sabad.[4], sabin.[4], sul-i.[1'], valer.[4]

pregnancy, in[7]

calen.

WEATHER

change of w. agg.

abrot., achy.[14], acon.[1'], alum.[1, 3, 6],
alumn., **am-c.**[1, 7], anh.[14], ant-c.,
ant-t., apis, aran.[3, 6, 7], ars.,
asar.[14], bar-c.[1', 3, 6, 7], **bell.,**
benz-ac., bor., brom., **BRY.**[1, 7],
calc., calc-f.[1', 7, 8, 10], **calc-p.,**
carb-v.[7, 12], carbn-s., **caust.,**
cham.[2, 7, 11], **chel.,** chin.[7, 8], cinnb.[1'],
colch., crot-c.[7], crot-h.[3, 6], cupr.[3, 11],
cur.[7], **dig., DULC.**[1, 7], euph.,
galph.[14], **gels., graph.**[1, 7], harp.[14],
hep.[1, 7], hyper., **ip.**[1', 7], kali-bi.,
kali-c., kali-i.[3, 6, 7], **kalm.**[2, 7], lach.,
lept.[12], mag-c.[3, 6-8], mand.[14],
mang., meli., **merc.**[1, 7], merc-i-r.[12],
mez., mosch.[7], **nat-c.,** nat-m.[7],
nat-p.[1'], nat-sil.[1'], nit-ac.,
NUX-M., nux-v., **petr., ph-ac.,**
PHOS., phys.[3], phyt.[7], **PSOR.,**
puls., RAN-B., rheum[1, 7], **RHOD.,**
RHUS-T.[1, 7], **rumx.,** ruta[7, 8],
sang.[3, 6, 7], sep., **SIL.,** spig.[1', 3, 6, 7],
stann.[1', 14], stict.[7, 8], stront-c.,
sulph., tarent.[7, 8], **teucr.**[3],
thuj.[3, 6, 7], **TUB., verat.**[1, 7],
vip.[3, 6, 7, 11]

ailments from[12]

carb-v., merc-i-f., ra.ı-b.

am.[14]: onop.

spring, in[8]

all-c., ant-t., gels., kali-s., nat-s.

cold to warm agg.

ant-c.[3, 6], brom.[1'], **BRY.,** carb-v.,
chel., crot-h.[3, 6], **ferr.,** gels.,
KALI-S., lach., lyc., nat-c.[3, 6],
nat-m., nat-s., nux-v.[3, 6], **PSOR.,**
puls., sep.[3, 6], **SULPH., TUB.**

warm to cold agg.[3, 6]

acon.[3], **ars.,** calc.[1'], calc-p.[1'],
calc-sil.[1'], carb-v., **caust.,**
DULC.[1', 3, 6, 15], hep.[1'], **MERC.**[15],
nat-s¡l.[1'], nit-ac.[1'], **nux-v.,** puls.,
ran-b.[1', 3, 6], **rhus-t.**[15], sabad., **sil.,**
stront-c., tub.[1'], **VERAT.**[15]

clear w. agg.

acon., aloe[7], asar., **bry., caust.,**
hep., nux-v., plb., sabad., spong.

cloudy w. agg.

aloe[3], am-c., ammc.[3], aran.[3],
arn.[3], ars.[3], aur.[3], bar-c.[3], ben-n.[3],
bry., calc., calen.[3, 7], **cham., chin.,**
dulc., hyper.[3], gels.[3], lach.[1'],
mang., merc., naja[3], nat-c.[3],
nat-m.[3], nat-s.[3], **nux-m.,** phys.[3],
plb., **puls.,** rhod., **RHUS-T.,**
sabin.[3], sang.[3], **sep.,** stram.[3],
sulph., verat., viol-o.[3]

am.[3]
caust.

cold dry w. agg.

abrot.[8], **ACON.**, aesc.[8], agar.[8], alum.[1, 3, 8], alumn.[2], am-c.[4], apoc.[8], **ars.**, ars-i.[3], **ASAR.**, aur.[8], bac.[8], **bar-c.**[8], bell., bor., **bry.**, calc.[1, 4, 8], calc-i.[1'], calc-p.[1'], **camph.**[4, 8], caps.[4, 8], carb-an., carb-v., **CAUST.**, cham., **chin.**[8], **cist.**[8], coc-c.[1'], cocc.[4], coff.[1'], **crot-h.**, cupr.[8], cur.[8], daph.[4], dulc.[1, 4, 8], euph.[8], ferr-ar.[1'], fl-ac.[3], **HEP.**, ign.[8], **ip.**, **KALI-C.**, kali-sil.[1'], kreos.[8], lach.[4], lappa[3], laur., lyc.[4], mag-c., mag-p.[8], med.[3], mez., mur-ac., nat-c.[8], nat-s.[3], nit-ac.[1, 3, 4], nit-s-d.[8], nux-m.[1, 4], **NUX-V.**, **petr.**[8], ph-ac.[4], phos.[1, 4], phys.[3], physal.[3], phyt.[1'], plat.[3], plb.[3, 8], **psor.**[1, 8], **puls.**[3], rhod., rhus-t.[4, 8], **rumx.**[8], **sabad.**, sel.[8], sep., **sil.**, spig., **spong.**, staph., sulph , tub.[8]. urt-u.[8], **verat.**[2], viol-o.[8], visc.[8], zinc.

am.
led.[3, 6], sil.[1']

cold wet w.

abrot.[1'], aesc.[1'], **agar.**, all-c.[3, 6, 12], all-s., **AM-C.**, **ant-c.**, **ant-t.**[1, 3, 8], **apis**, **aran.**, **arg-m.**, **arg-n.**, arn.[8], **ARS.**, ars-i., ars-s-f.[1'], asc-t., **aster.**, aur., aur-ar.[1'], **aur-m-n.**, **BAD.**, **bar-c.**, bar-i.[1'], bar-s.[1'], bell., bell-p.[10], bor.[1], bov., bry., **CALC.**, **CALC-P.**, calc-s., calc-sil.[1'], **calen.**[7], canth., **caps.**[3, 6], carb-an., **carb-v.**, **carbn-s.**, cham., chin., **cimic.**[1], clem., **COLCH.**, coloc.[3], con., cupr., **DULC.**, elaps[3, 6], erig.[6], eucal.[3, 6], **ferr.**, fl-ac., **form.**, **gels.**, glon.[3], **graph.**, **guaj.**[8], hep., **hyper.**, **iod.**, ip., **kali-bi.**, kali-c., kali-i., kali-m.[1'], kali-n.,

kali-p., kali-sil.[1'], **lach.**, **lath.**, laur., lept.[3, 6], **lyc.**, mag-c., mag-p.[1'], **mang.**, **MED.**, **merc.**, merc-c.[3], merc-i-f., **mez.**, mur-ac., naja[14], **nat-ar.**, **nat-c.**, nat-m.[3, 6], **NAT-S.**, **nit-ac.**, **NUX-M.**, nux-v., onop.[14], paeon., penic.[13, 14], **petr.**, phos., physal.[8], **phyt.**, polyg-h.[7], psor.[1'], **puls.**, **PYROG.**, ran-b., **RHOD.**, **RHUS-T.**, rumx.[3, 6], **ruta**, sars., seneg., sep., **SIL.**, **spig.**, stann., staph., **still.**[3, 6], **stront-c.**, **sul-ac.**, **sulph.**, **tarent.**, teucr.[3], **thuj.**, **TUB.**, urt-u.[8], **verat.**, zinc., zinc-p.[1'], **zing.**[3, 6]

night and warm days in autumn agg.[8]

merc.

old people, in[12]

ammc.

ailments from[12]

all-c., dulc., gels., lath., merc-i-t., phyt.

am.[1']
aur-m.

dry w. agg.

acon.[2], alum., alumn.[2], ars., **ASAR.**, bell.[2], bor.[2], **bry.**, carb-an., carb-v., **CAUST.**, **cham.**[2], **HEP.**, ip.[2], **kali-c.**, laur.[2], mag-c.[2], mez.[2], mur-ac.[2], **NUX-V.**, phos., rhod.[2], sabad., **sep.**, sil., spig.[2], spong., staph., sulph., zinc.

am.[2]

agar., **am-c.**[2, 8], **ant-c., aur.,** bar-c.,
bell., **bor.,** bov., bry., **CALC.**[2, 8],
canth., **carb-an., carb-v.,** cham.,
chin., clem., con., **cupr., DULC.,**
ferr., hep., ip., kali-c.[2, 8], **kali-n.,**
lach., laur., lyc., mag-c.,
magn-gr.[8], **mang., merc.,** merc-c.,
mez., moly-met.[14], **mur-ac.,**
nat-c., nit-ac., NUX-M., nux-v.,
petr.[2, 8], **phos., puls., rhod.,**
RHUS-T., ruta, sars., seneg.,
sep., sil., **spig.,** stann., **staph.,**
still.[8], **stront-c., sul-ac., sulph.,**
verat., zinc.

dry warm w. agg.[6]

ant-c., carb-v., cocc., lach.

ailments from[12]

ant-c., kali-bi., lach.

am.[8]

alum., **calc-p.,** nat-s., nux-m.[3, 6, 8],
penic.[13, 14], rhus-t., **sulph.**[3, 6, 8]

foggy w. agg.

abrot.[6], aloe[3], **aran.**[3, 6], ars.[3], bapt.[8],
bar-c.[6], bry., calc.[3], calen.[3], cham.,
chin., dulc.[3, 6], **gels.**[3, 8], **HYPER.,**
mang., merc.[3], mosch., nat-m.[3],
nat-s.[3, 6], nux-m., plb., **rhod.,**
RHUS-T., sep., **sil.,** sulph., **thuj.**[3, 6],
verat.

frosty w., hoarfrost agg.[3]

agar., calc., carb-v., caust., **CON.,**
lyc., mag-m., merc., nat-c., nux-v.,
ph-ac., phos., **puls.,** rhus-t., **SEP.,**
sil., sulph., syph.

hot w. agg.[8]

acon.[1', 8], aeth.[1', 8], aloe[6, 8],
ant-c.[3, 6, 8], ant-t.[6], apis[6], bapt.[6],

bell., bor., brom.[1'], **bry.**[3, 6, 8],
carb-v.[3], cocc.[3], croc., **crot-h.**[6, 8],
crot-t., **cupr.**[6], **gels., glon.,** hep.[3],
kali-bi.[1', 8], **lach.**[3, 6, 8], **nat-c.,**
nat-m., nat-s.[1'], nit-ac., **op.**[6],
phos.[3, 6, 8], pic-ac., **podo., puls.**[3, 8],
sabin., sel.[3, 6, 8], syph.

and cold night[3]

acon.

ailments from[12]

ant-c., kali-bi., lach.

rain, aqq. during[3]

aran., elaps, erig., glon., ham.,
lac-c., lach.[1'], mag-c., mang.,
merc.[8], nat-s.[1'], oci-s.[14], phyt.,
ran-b.[1', 3], **rhus-t.**[15], sabin., senn.,
tub.[1']

storm, approach of a

agar., arg-m.[3], aur., **bell-p.**[8],
berb.[3], bry., calc.[1'], calc-f.[3],
caust., **cedr.,** dulc.[3], **gels.,**
hep.[3, 6], hyper., **kali-bi., lach.,**
lyc., mag-p.[3], mand.[10], mang.[1', 3],
med., meli., **nat-c.,** nat-m., nat-p.,
nat-s.[8], nit-ac., petr., **phos.,**
phyt.[8], **PSOR.,** puls., **ran-b.,**
RHOD., rhus-t., sep., sil., sul-ac.[3],
sulph., syph., thuj., **tub.,** zinc.[3, 6]

during.*

agar., aran.[3'], arg-m.[6], aur.,
bry., calc.[7], carb-v., caust.,
conv.[3'], elaps[1'], erig.[3'], **gels.,**
glon.[3'], ham.[3'], **lach.,** mag-c.[3'],
mand.[14], mang.[3'], **med.,**
morph.[2, 12], **NAT-C.,** nat-m.,
nat-p., nit-ac., nit-s-d.[12], petr.,
phos., phyt.[3', 8], prot.[14], psor.,

puls.[2, 12], ran-b.[3'], **rhod.**,
sabin.[3'], **sep., sil.**, syph., thuj.,
tub.[1']

am.[7]
   carc., **sep.**

Vol. I: *cheerful – thunders*

after
   asar.[14], calc-p.[3], carc.[7], rhus-r.[3, 6],
   sep.[3, 7], tub.[1']

ailments from[12]

   crot-h., gels., morph., nat-c.,
   nat-p., nit-s-d., phos., psor.,
   puls., rhod., syph.

lightning-stroke[12]

   morph., phos.

warm and **wet** w. agg.

   aloe[3, 6], aran-ix.[10], bapt.[8], bell.[6],
   brom.[1', 3, 6, 8], bry.[3], calc-f.[10],
   CARB-V., carbn-s.[1', 3, 7, 8], caust.[1'],
   erig.[10], **gels.**, ham.[3, 6-8], **iod., ip.**[3],
   kali-bi., LACH., lath.[12], lyc.[3],
   mand.[10], mang.[3, 6], merc-i-f.[12],
   nat-m.[3, 6, 7], **NAT-S.**, phos.[8],
   puls.[3], rhus-t.[3], sabad.[3],
   SEP.[3, 6, 8, 15], **sil., SYPH.**[7, 12],
   tub.[1'], **verat.**[3], vip-a.[14]

ailments from[12]

   carb-v., gels.

am.[6]
   aloe, bell., brom., **carb-v.**, cham.[8],
   gels., ham., hep., **ip.**, kali-c.[8],
   nat-m., sep., sil.[8]

wet w. agg.

   achy.[14], agar., alum-sil.[1'], **AM-C.**,
   amph.[8], anac.[7], ant-c., **ant-t.,**
   ARAN.[1, 7], arg-m., **arg-n., ARS.,**
   ars-i., ars-s-f.[1'], aster.[8], aur.,
   BAD., bar-c., bar-m., bell.,
   blatta[12], bor., bov., brom., bry.,
   CALC., calc-f.[1', 7], **calc-p., calc-s.,**
   calc-sil.[1'], calen.[7, 8], canth.,
   carb-an.[1], **carb-v.**, caust.[1'], cham.,
   chim.[8], chin., chin-s.[8], **cist.**, clem.,
   colch., con., crot-h.[8], cupr.,
   cur.[7, 8], **DULC.**, elaps, elat.[8],
   erig.[3, 3'], euphr.[8], **ferr.**, form.[8],
   gels.[2, 8, 12], **glon.**[2, 3], **graph.**[2, 3],
   ham., hep., hyper., **iod.**, ip.,
   kali-c., **kali-i.**, kali-m.[1'], kali-n.,
   lac-ac.[2, 7], lac-c.[3], lac-d.[1'], **lach.**,
   lath.[8, 12], laur., **lem-m., lyc.**, lyss.[2],
   mag-c., **mag-p.**, magn-gr.[8], **mang.**,
   meli., **merc.**, mez., mur-ac., **naja,**
   nat-ar., nat-c., NAT-HCHLS.,
   NAT-S., nit-ac., **NUX-M.**, nux-v.,
   oci-s.[9], onop.[14], paeon., petr.,
   phos., **phyt., PULS.**, rad-br.[8],
   ran-b., rauw.[9], **RHOD., RHUS-T.,**
   ruta, sabin.[3], sang., sars., seneg.,
   senn.[3], **sep., sil.**, sin-n.[12], spig.,
   stann., staph., stict.[12], still.[8],
   stront-c., sul-ac., sul-i.[1'], **sulph.**,
   sumb., syph.[12], teucr., **thuj., tub.**,
   verat., zinc., zinc-p.[1'], zing.[2]

am.[2, 7]
   acon.[2], alum.[1', 3, 6-8], alumn.[2],
   ars., **ASAR.**[2, 3, 7, 8], aur-m.[3], **bell.,**
   bor.[2], bov.[7], **BRY., carb-an.,**
   carb-v., **CAUST.**[2, 3, 6-8], **cham.,**
   fl-ac., **HEP.**[2, 3, 6-8], ip., laur., mang.,
   MED.[7, 8], mez., mur-ac.[2, 7, 8],
   nit-ac., NUX-V.[2, 3, 7, 8], oci-s.[9, 14],
   plat., rhod., **sabad., sep., sil.,**
   spig., **spong.**, staph., sulph., zinc.

wind

   acon., anac.[4], **ars.**, ars-i., arum-t.[8],
   asar., **aur.**[1, 7], aur-ar.[1'], **bell.**, bry.,
   bufo, calc., **calc-p.**, canth.[3],

caps.³, carb-an.³, carb-v., caust.,
CHAM., chin., coff.¹′ ⁷, colch.³,
coloc.³, con., cupr., elaps, **euphr.,**
graph., **HEP.**³′ ⁸, hyos.³, ip.³′ ⁷,
kali-c.³, **lach.,** LYC., mag-c.³′ ⁸,
mag-p.¹′, med.³, mur-ac., nat-c.,
nit-ac.³′ ¹⁶, **nux-m.**¹′ ⁷, **NUX-V.,**
ph-ac.³, **PHOS.,** plat., **psor.,**
PULS., rheum³, **RHOD., rhus-t.**³,
sabad.³, samb.³, sel.³, sep.³′ ⁴′ ⁶,
sil.³, spig., **SPONG.**³, squil.³,
stram.³, stront-c.³, sul-ac., sulph.,
tab.³, thuj., tub.³, verb.³, zinc.

ailments from¹²

kalm.

am.³′ ⁶

arg-n., ferr.³, iod.³, nux-m.,
sec.³, tub.³

cold

acon., all-c.², apis³, arn.³, **ars.,**
ars-i., **asar., BELL.,** bell-p.⁹,
bry., cadm-s.⁷′ ¹², calc-p.,
carb-an., carb-v., **caust.,**
cham.¹, cupr., ferr-ar., **HEP.,**
ip., **kali-bi.,** lach.³′ ⁶,
mag-p.¹′′ ³′ ¹², nit-ac.⁴′ ⁷′ ¹¹′ ¹⁶,
NUX-V., psor., **rhod.**¹′ ⁸,
RHUS-T.²′ ³, rumx.³, sabad.,
sep., sil., SPONG., thlas.³,
tub.⁷, verat.², zinc.³

ailments from¹²

acon., bry., cadm-s., hep.,
mag-p.

riding in, am.

arg-n., tub.¹′′ ⁷′ ¹⁵

ailments from¹²

sang-n.

cold and wet, ailments from

all-c.¹′ ¹², calc.¹²

desire to be in⁷

tub.

sensation of

agar.¹′, **camph.**³, canth., **chel.,**
chin.³, **cist.**⁶, cor-r., croc.³,
graph., lach.⁶, **LYSS.,** med.³,
mez.³′ ⁶, **mosch.,** naja³, nat-m.³,
nux-v., olnd., petr.³, puls.,
rhus-t., sabin., sep.³, spig.,
squil., stram., syph.³, ther.³,
thuj.⁶, thyr.³

blowing on covered parts

camph.

cold

camph., croc., **lac-d., laur.,**
LYSS., mosch., rhus-t., samb.

warm, south

ars-i., asar.¹⁴, bry.³′ ⁶,
carb-v.³′ ⁶, euphr.³′ ⁶, **gels.**²′ ⁷,
ip., lach.¹′, nat-c.³, rhod.³′ ⁶,
sil.³′ ⁶

warm and wet w. agg.²

acon., HEP.

windy and **stormy** weather*

acon., **all-c.**[2], **am-c.**[2], arg-m.[1'],
ars., asar., aur., aur-ar.[1'], **BAD.**,
bell., bry., carb-v., caust.[3], **cham.**,
chel.[3], **chin.**, chin-ar., con.,
erig.[10], euphr., gels.[3], graph.,
hep., hyper.[2], ip.[2], **KALM.**[2], **lach.**,
lyc., mag-c., **mag-p.**, mez.[1'],
mur-ac., nat-c., nat-m.[3], nit-s-d.[12],
NUX-M., **nux-v.**, petr., **phos.**,
plat., **psor.**, **puls.**, ran-b.[1', 8],
RHOD., rhus-t., ruta, **sep.**, spig.,
sul-ac., sulph., tab.[3], thuj.

ailments from[12]

nit-s-d., psor., rhod.

WET

applications

AM-C., am-m., **ANT-C.**, bar-c.,
bell., bor., bov., bry., **CALC.**,
cann-s.[3], **canth.**, carb-v., **CHAM.**,
CLEM., con., crot-h.[8], dulc.,
kali-c., **kali-n.**, **lach.**[3, 6, 8], laur.,
lyc., mag-c., **merc.**, mez., mur-ac.,
nat-c., nit-ac., nux-m., nux-v.,
phos., puls., **RHUS-T.**, sars., **sep.**,
sil., **spig.**, stann., staph., **stront-c.**,
sul-ac., **SULPH.**, zinc.

am.[2]

alumn., am-m., ant-t., **ars.**,
ASAR.[2, 3, 6, 8], bor., bry.,
caust.[2, 3, 6], cham., **chel.**[2, 3, 6],
euphr.[2, 3, 6], laur., **mag-c.**, mez.,
mur-ac., **nux-v.**, **PULS.**[2, 3, 6],
rhod., sabad., sep., **spig.**[2, 3, 6],
staph., zinc.

cold, wet a. agg.[2]

AM-C., am-m., **ANT-C.**, apoc.[1'],
ars.[6], bar-c., **bell.**, **bor.**, bov.,
bry., cadm-met.[14], **CALC.**,
canth., carb-v., **cham.**, **CLEM.**,
con., dulc., graph.[6], **hep.**[6],
kali-c., **kali-n.**, lach.[6], **laur.**,
lyc., mag-c., **merc.**, **mez.**,
mur-ac., nat-c., **nit-ac.**[2, 6],
nux-m., nux-v., **petr.**[2, 6], ph-ac.[6],
phos.[1', 2], puls.[1', 2], **RHUS-T.**,
ruta[6], **sars.**, sep., sil.[2, 6], **spig.**,
stann., **staph.**, **stront-c.**, sul-ac.,
SULPH., syph.[1'], **zinc.**

am.[7]

aloe[7], alum.[8], aml-ns., anac.[14],
apis[7, 8], argn-n.[7, 8], arn., aur.,
asar.[8], bell.[8], bry.[1', 6, 7], ferr-p.[8],
fl-ac.[6, 7], glon., iod.[6, 7], kali-m.[8],
kali-p., **led.**[1', 6, 7], lyc.[8], merc.[8],
nat-hchls.[14], phos.[8], pic-ac.,
puls.[6-8], sabin.[8], sec.[1', 7], spig.[6]

warm, wet a. agg.[6]

apis, bry., **fl-ac.**, lach.[1', 6, 10],
led., phyt.[1'], **puls.**, **sec.**

am.[6]

alum-sil.[1'], anac.[3], ant-c.[3, 6],
ars.[1', 3, 6-8], ars-i.[3], bry.[8],
calc-f.[1', 7, 8], coloc., fl-ac.[7],
hep.[3, 6], kali-bi.[3, 6], kali-c.[3],
lach.[8], **mag-p.**[3, 7, 8], nux-m.[8],
paraph.[14], ph-ac., phos.[1'],
pyrog.[3], rad-br.[3, 8], **rhus-t.**[3, 8],
ruta, sep.[8], **sil.**[6, 7], sulfa.[14],
thiop.[14], thuj., x-ray[14]

getting *

acon.[3], **ALUM.**[3], am-c., ant-c.,
ant-t.[2, 3], **apis**, arn.[3], ars.,
bell., bor., **bry.**, **CALC.**,
calc-p., **calc-s.**, camph., carb-v.,
CAUST., cham.[6], **chin.**, colch.,
dulc., euph., fl-ac.[3], **hep.**, hyos

ip., kali-bi.³, **kali-c.³**, lach., **lyc.**, malar.¹², merc-i-r.¹², nat-m.³, **NAT-S.³, ⁶**, nit-ac., **nux-m.**, nux-v.³, phos., phyt.³, **PULS.**, ran-b.⁶, rhod.¹², **RHUS-T., sars.**, sec., **SEP., sil.³**, sulph., thuj.⁶, urt-u.³, verat., visc.¹², xan.¹², zinc.

feet, from wet

agn., **all-c., bar-c.³**, bry.³, **calc.², ³, ⁸, ¹⁶, camph.³**, caps.³, cham., **colch.³**, cupr.³, **dulc.**, fl-ac.³, graph.³, ⁶, guaj.³, **lach.³**, lob.¹², lem-m.³, **lyc.³**, merc., nat-c., nat-m., nit-ac.³, **nux-m., NUX-V.³, phos., PULS., rhus-t.**, sep., **SIL.**, stram.³, **sulph.⁶**, tub.³, xan.

am.³

calad., led., puls.

head, from wet

bar-c., **BELL.**, hep.³, hyos.³, led., phos.³, **puls.**, rhus-t.¹², **sep.³**

heated, when

bell-p.⁹, ¹², rhus-t.¹²

perspiration, during

acon., ant-c.³, ars.³, **bell-p.³, ¹²**, bry.³, calc., **clem.³**, colch., con.³, **dulc.**, nat-c.³, **nux-m., RHUS-T., sep., verat-v.²**

rooms, in wet²

aloe, ant-t.⁸, **aran.³, ⁶⁻⁸, ARS.², ⁸**, ars-i.⁸, atro., **bry., calc.², ³, ⁶, ⁸**, calc-p.⁶, calc-sil.⁸, **carb-an., carb-v.³**, caust., **DULC.¹'⁻³, ⁶, ⁸**, form., lyc., nat-n.⁶, **NAT-S.¹', ³, ⁶, ⁸**,

nit-ac.⁶, nux-m.⁸, **PULS.², ³**, rhod.³, **rhus-t.¹', ³, ⁸, sel., sep.**, sil.³, **stram.**, ter.⁸, ¹², **thuj.³, ⁶**, verat.³

sheets, ailments from wet¹²

rhus-t.

WHITENESS of parts usually red

ambr., **ars.**, anac.³, ang.³, **BOR.**, calc., canth., caust., coloc.³, **ferr., HELL., kali-c.**, lac-d.³, lyc., **MERC., merc-c.**, nat-c.³, **nit-ac.**, nux-v., olnd., op., petr., phos., **plb.**, puls.³, sabin.³, **sec.**, sep., **staph., sul-ac.**, sulph., valer., verat., viol-t.³, **zinc.**

WHOOPING-COUGH, ailments after⁷

sang.

wine see food–wine

winter see seasons–winter

WORMS, ailments from¹²

cina, sabad.

under the skin, sensation

COCAIN.

WOUNDS

anag.¹², **apis**, arist-cl.⁹, ¹⁰, **arn.**, ars.⁶, ¹², bell-p.⁶, ⁹, ¹⁰, bor., bor-ac.¹², bov.¹², bry.¹², bufo⁶, calc-p.⁶,

calen.[1', 6, 7, 10, 12], carb-ac.[7], carb-v.,
cham.[10], cic., cist.[6], con., croc.,
echi.[6, 10], erig.[12], ery-a.[·2], eup-per.[12],
ferr-p.[12], ham.[6, 10, 12], helia.[7, 12],
hell.[12], hep., **hyper.**[6, 12], iod.,
kali-p.[12], kreos., **lach.**, lappa[10],
LED., merc., mez., mill.[6, 10],
nat-c., **nat-m.**, nit-ac., ph-ac., **phos.**,
phys.[12], plan.[12], plb., **puls.**, rhus-t.,
ruta, sec.[6, 8], senec.[12], seneg., sil.,
staph., stront-c.[6], **sul-ac.**, sulph.,
symph.[6, 12], zinc., zinc-m.[12]

ailments from[12]

arn., bry., calen., ferr-p., hyper.,
kali-p., led., phos., plan., senec.

bites[2, 4]

acet-ac.[1'], all-s.[2], **arn.**, grind.[12],
hyper.[2, 12], **led.**[1', 2, 12], **plan.**[2],
sul-ac.

ailments from[12]

hyper., led.

dogs, of

hyper.[1'], **lach.**[2, 12], led.[12]
LYSS.[2, 10, 12], ter.[2]

ailments from[12]

lyss.

rabid[7]

arist-cl.[9], ars., bell., canth.,
chr-ac.[2], echi.[12], hyos., **lyss.**[7, 10]

poisonous animals, of

am-c.[1', 2, 4], **apis,** arn., **ars.,**

aur., bell., calad., **caust.**[2, 4],
cedr., echi., hyper., **lach.,**
LED., lob-p.[7], **lyss.**[2], nat-m.[2, 4],
puls.[2, 4], **seneg.**[1, 7], stram.,
sul-ac.

ailments from[12]

seneg.

snakes, of[7]

anag.[2, 12], **apis.,** arist-cl.[9], arn.,
ars.[2, 7], aur., **bell.**[2, 7], calad.,
camph.[2, 12], **cedr.**[2, 7, 12], **echi.**[7, 12],
gua., gymne.[12], hyper., **LACH.,**
LED., lob-p.[12], lycps.[12],
plan.[7, 12], seneg.[2, 7, 12], stram.,
sul-ac., **thuj.**[1', 7], **vip.**

ailments from[12]

lob-p., plan.

chronic sequel[2]

merc., ph-ac.

tarentula, of[12]

lycps.

black[2]

chin., lach., trach.[11], vip.[11]

bleeding freely

acon.[3, 4], am-c.[3', 7], ant-t.[4], aran.,
arn., ars.[4], asaf.[4], bell-p.[10],
bor.[4], both.[11], **carb-v.,** caust.[4],
cench., **chin.**[3, 4], clem.[4], con.[4],
cop.[2, 4], croc., crot-h., **dor.**[7],
eug.[4], **euphr.**[4], ferr., ferr-p.[3],
ham.[3, 7, 8], hep., **HIR.**[7], hydr.[1', 2],

kreos., **LACH.**, **LAT-M.**[7], led.[1'],
merc., mez.[4], mill., **nat-c.**[4],
nat-m., **NIT-AC.**[3', 4, 7], **nux-m.**[4],
nux-v.[4], **ph-ac.**[1, 7], **PHOS.**, plb.[4],
puls., rhus-t., ruta[4], sec.[2, 3'], sep.[4],
sil.[4], **staph.**[4], sul-ac., **sulph.**, vip.[4],
zinc.

black blood[11]

vip.

small w.

am-c., carb-v.[6], hydr.[1'],
kreos.[1', 6, 7], lach.[1'], ph-ac.[6].
phos.[1', 16], sul-ac.[6], **zinc.**[6]

bluish[2, 8]

apis[2], lach., lyss., **vip.**[11]

burning[4]

acon., arn., **ars.**, bry., **carb-v.**,
caust., hyper.[1'], merc., mez., nat-m.,
rhus-t., **sul-ac.**, **sulph.**, zinc.[7]

cold, become

led.

constitutional effects of

arn., carb-v., con., hep., **iod.**, **lach.**,
LED., nat-m., **nit-ac.**, **phos.**, puls.,
rhus-t., **staph.**, **sul-ac.**, zinc.

corrosive, gnawing[16]

mez.

crushed and lacerated finger-ends

arist-cl.[9], **carb-ac.**[7], **HYPER.**, led.,
ruta[3, 7]

cuts

arn., **calen.**[1', 2, 7, 8], **carb-v.**[2],
cic.[2], con.[2], dig.[2], **ham.**[2, 7, 8], hep.[2],
hyper.[7, 8], kali-m.[12], **lach.**[2], **led.**[1],
merc., nat-c., **nit-ac.**[2], ph-ac.,
plan.[12], plb.[2, 3, 4], sil., **STAPH.**,
sul-ac., sulph.

ailments from[12]

kali-m., plan., staph.

dissecting

anthraci., apis, ars., crot-h.[7, 8],
echi.[7, 8], ham.[2], kreos.[8], **lach.**, led.
pyrog., **ter.**[2]

ptomaine poisoning

ailments from[12]

pyrog.

foreign bodies, from*

arn.[7], **hep.**[1', 2], **lob.**[7, 12], **SIL.**[2, 7, 12]

ailments from[12]

lob., sil.

gangrenous[2, 4]

acon., am-c., **anthraci.**[2], **ARS., bell.,
brom.**[2], calen.[7, 8], **carb-v., chin.,
eucal.**[2], euph., **LACH.**[1', 2, 4],
sal-ac.[7, 8], sec.[2], **sil.**, sul-ac.[7, 8],
trach.[11], vip.[11], **vip-a.**[14]

granulations, proud flesh[2]

alum.[3], **alumn., anac., ant-t., ARS.,
calc., calen.**[1', 2, 8], carb-v.[3], cund.,
hep.[3], **hydr.**[1'], **kali-m.,** kreos.[3],
lach., merc.[1'], nit-ac.[3, 8], **sabin.**[7, 8],
SIL.[3, 7, 8], sulph.[4], thuj.[8]

greenish[7]

senec.

gunshot[2, 3, 4]

ARN.[2, 3, 4, 7, 8], calen.[7, 8], **euphr.,
hyper.**[2, 12], **nit-ac.**[2, 3], **plb.,** puls.,
ruta, **sul-ac.,** sulph., symph.[12]

heal, quick tendency to[2, 10, 12]

lyss.

slow
all-c.[2, 7], alum., alum-p.[1'],
alum-sil.[1'], am-c., ars.[1'], **bar-c.,
bor.,** both.[11], **calc., carb-v.,** caust.,
cham., chel., clem.[4], con.,
cortiso.[14], croc.[4], crot-h., **graph.,**
hell.[4], **HEP.,** hyper.[1'], kali-c.,
LACH., lyc., lyss.[10], mag-c.,
mang., **merc., merc-c.,** mur-ac.,
nat-c.[4], **NIT-AC.,** nux-v.[4], **PETR.,**
ph-ac., phos., plb., puls., **rhus-t.,**
sars.[1'], sep., **SIL.,** squil.[4], **staph.,
SULPH., tub.**[7]

*inflammation see inflammation–
wound*

injection, from painful[7]

crot-h., led.

lacerations[7, 8]

arist-cl.[10], arn., **CALEN.**[1'-3, 6-8, 12],
CARB-AC., ham.[2, 7, 8],
hyper.[1', 2, 3, 7, 8], led.,
staph.[1', 2, 3, 7, 8], sul-ac.,
symph.

ailments from[12]

calen.

lead colored

lach.[2], vip.[11]

painful

all-c.[7], am-c.[4], **apis,** arist-cl.[9], bell.[4],
calc.[2], calc-f.[2], calen.[2], cham.[2],
con.[4], croc.[4], crot-h.[11], eug.[2, 4, 11],
hep.[4], **HYPER.,** led., nat-c.[2, 8],
nat-m., **nit-ac.,** nux-v., **ph-ac.**[2, 4],
STAPH., sulph.

w.-pulsating

w.-stinging

penetrating, punctured

APIS, aran.[12], arn.[3], **carb-v.,** cic.,
hep., **hyper.,** lach.[12], **LED.,
NIT-AC.,** phase.[7, 8, 12], plan.[3, 12],
plb., sil., sul-ac.[3], sulph.

stab

ailments from[12]

   lach., led., plan.

palms and soles, of

HYPER., LED.[1, 7]

poisonous plants, from[7]

   echi.

pulsating[4]

bell., cham., clem., **hep., merc.,**
mez.[16], **puls., sulph.**

reactionless[3]

ars., camph., carb-v., con., laur.,
op., ph-ac., sulph.

reopening of old[3, 4, 6]

asaf.[1'], **carb-v., caust.**[2, 3, 4, 8], con.,
croc.[2, 3, 4], **crot-h.**[3, 4], eug.[4],
fl-ac.[8], **glon.**[3, 4], **graph.**[8], kreos.[3],
lach., nat-c., **nat-m., nit-ac.**[4],
nux-v.[4], **PHOS.**[2, 3, 4, 6],
sil.[1', 3, 4, 6, 8], **sulph., vip.**[3, 6]

abscesses–recurrent

   cicatrices

asaf., **bor.,** calc-p., **carb-an.,**
carb-v.[16], **caust.,** con., croc.,
crot-h., fl-ac.[3], glon.[7], **iod., lach.,**
nat-c., **nat-m., PHOS., SIL.,**
sulph., **vip.**[6]

scurfiness, with[2]

   calen., carb-ac., hyper.

septic[3, 6]

   ars.

splinters, from

acon., **anag.**[2], **apis, arn., carb-v.,**
CIC., colch., **hep., HYPER.,** lach.,
led., lob.[12], **nit-ac.,** petr., plat.,
ran-b., **sil., staph.,** sulph.

w.-foreign bodies

ailments from[12]

   sil.

stab wounds

acet-ac.[7], **all-c.**[2], **apis,** arn., carb-v.,
cic., con.[3, 4], eug.[4], hep.[3, 4],
HYPER.[3, 6, 8], lach., **LED.**[1'-3, 6-8],
nat-m.[4], nit-ac., phase.[8], **phos.**[3],
plb.[3, 4], puls.[3], **rhus-t.**[2], sep.[2, 4], sil.,
staph., sul-ac.[3], sulph.[3, 4, 6]

penetrating

stinging, in

acon., **apis,** arn., bar-c., bell.[4],
bry., caust., chin.[4], clem.[4], **led.,**
merc., mez.[4], nat-c., **nit-ac.,** sep.[4],
sil.[4], **staph.,** sulph.

w.-painful

suppurating[2]

arn.[7], asaf.[2, 4], **bell.[4]**, bor.[11], **bufo,
calc.**, calc-f., calc-s., **calen.[2, 7]**,
caust.[4], **cham., chin.[4], croc.[2, 4]**,
echi.[7], **hep.**, lach.[4], led.[7], **merc.[4]**,
nat-m., plb.[2, 4], **puls.[2, 4], sil., sulph.[4]**,
vip-a.[14]

abscesses

swelling of[2, 3, 4]

acon.[2], **arn., bell., bry.**, kali-m.[2],
nux-v., **puls., rhus-t.**, sul-ac.,
sulph., vip.[11]

YAWNING agg.[3]

acon., agar., am-c., am-m., anac.,
ant-t., arg-m., **arn.**, ars., aur., bar-c.,
bell., bor., bry., calad., calc., canth.,
caps., carb-an., **caust., chel.**, chin.,
CINA, cocc., croc., cycl., dig., ferr.,
graph., hep., **IGN.**, ip., kali-c.,
KREOS., laur., lyc., mag-c., mag-m.,
mang., **meny.**, mez., **mur-ac.**, nat-c.,
nat-m., **NUX-V., olnd.**, op., par.,
petr., ph-ac., **phos.**, plat., puls.,
RHUS-T., ruta, sabad., **SARS.**, sep.,
sil., stann., **staph.**, sul-ac., **sulph.**,
teucr., thuj., verat., viol-o., zinc.

after, agg.[3]

am-m., croc., **nux-v.**

am.[3]
chin-s., croc., plat.[4], **staph.**

INDEX — ENGLISH

(Black type for the column numbers of the headings with additional references and alternating symptoms. **agg.** = ⟨. **am.** = ⟩)

abortion (+ Vol. I index, Vol. III):
  convulsions after 134
  faintness 183
  weakness after 705
adenitis → inflammation 320
alcohol 216–7
  convulsions in drunkards 111
  dropsy from 159
  paralysis after abuse 477
  trembling, dipsomania 649
  twitching, dipsomania 665
  varicose veins, dipsomania 673
  Voal. I: dipsomania **398–400**
  weakness ⟩ + dipsomania 706, 712
alternating states **31**
  change of symptoms **62**
  contradictory, altern. states **95**
  metastasis 369
apoplexy **35–6**
  convulsions after 103
  paralysis after 481
  threatening 36
  weakness 706
arteritis → inflammation 316
arthritis → inflammation 321
asphyxia → death, apparent 152–3
atheroma → tumors, atheroma 660
autumn → seasons 569–570

band → constriction, band 94–5
bandaging → binding up 47
belt → constriction, belt 95
biting nails → children 64
blood → haemorrhage 288–293
  → loss of 352
  → stagnated 602
bones:
  brittle 53
  cancerous affections of 55
  caries of **58**
  constriction of, sensation 93–4
  fistulae of 214
  formication in 284
  inflammation of 317–8
  injuries of 329–330, 581
  necrosis **307–0**
  osteoma 662
  pulsation in 527
  softening **601–2**
  swelling of 622

swollen sensation of 627
tardy development 678
tension of 632
bursitis → inflammation 318

cars → riding 563–4
cartilages, affections **59**
  enchondroma 621
  inflammation of 318
  swelling of 622
  ulcers of 59
cellulitis → inflammation 318
change-weather → weather 751–2
childbed (+ Vol. I index, Vol. III) 63
  convulsions, puerperal 138–9
  faintness, puerperal 201
children, affections **63–4**
  biting nails 64
  chorea, grown too fast **68**
  convulsions in 105–6
  delicate, sickly 64
  dentition, difficult, slow **154–5**
  development, arrested 156
  emaciation in + appetite, ravenous **173**
  growing too fast **64–5, 288**
  obesity in 394
  weakness in 708
clear weather → weather 752
climacteric period, during (+ Vol. I index, Vol. III):
  chorea 68
  convulsions 106
  faintness 186
  flushes of heat 300
  obesity 394
  reaction, lack of 557
  trembling 648
  weakness 708
  weariness 748
climbing → mountain sickness 377
cloudy weather → weather 752
coition, during, after + ⟨ (+ Vol. I index, Vol. III) 76–7
  chorea after (woman) 68
  convulsions during, after 107
  faintness during, after 186
  flushes of heat after 300
  interruptus 77
  lassitude after 342
  orgasm of blood after 398
  paralysis after 478

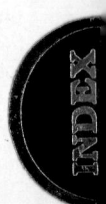

1

iodine 331
iron 332
lead **345**, 487
meat, bad 253
medicaments **364–5**
mercury 134, **368**, 487
mushrooms 386
narcotics 387
nicotinism 480, 636
ptomaine, dissecting wounds 521, **768**
purgatives 555
quinine **555**
radiotoxemie 53
sausages 267
sewer-gas 577
silica 592
smoke 601
sulphur 616
vegetable medicaments 365
vegetables, decayed 277

joints:
abscesses of 19
constriction of, sensation 94
dry sensation in 165
fistulae of 214
inflammation of 321–2
jerking in 336
pulsation in 527
swelling of 625–6
tension of 632–3
weakness of 718

loss of blood 351
ailments 289
anaemia after 33
congestion of blood after 91
convulsions with, after 130
faintness from 193, 195
loss of fluids **352**
ailments 352
chorea from 70
emaciation from 174
faintness from 195
nursing **393**
reaction after, lack of 558
weakness from 719
luxation → injuries 325–6
lymphangitis → inflammation 322

marasmus → emaciation 171–4
masturbation, from 363–4
chorea 70
convulsions 133
paralysis 479
weakness 720

mental exertion (+ Vol. I index e.):
convulsions after 134
faintness from meditating 195
flushes of heat from 302
lassitude from 343
trembling from 653
weakness from + ⟩ 722
weariness from 748
mercury, abuse of **368**
convulsions from 134
paralysis from 487
mother milk → suppressed 619
multiple sclerosis → sclerosis 569
muscles:
abscesses of 20
cramps of 150
induration of 315
inflammation of 322
injuries, rupture of 327, 330
jerking of 336–8
myatrophy, progresse spinal 386
relaxion of 559–560
tension of 633
weakness, muscular· 723–4
music (+ Vol. I index):
chorea, m. ⟩ 71
faintness on hearing 197
trembling from 653
weakness from 724
myositis → inflammation 322

nerves:
encephaloma 661
ganglion 661
inflammation of 322
injuries of 330
neuroma 662
new moon **370**
chorea during 71
nicotinism 480, 636
nodosites → indurations 313–5
non-union of bones → injuries-bones
329–330
nursing ⟨ **393**
trembling after 653
weakness 725

old people 395–6 (+ Vol. I index)
arteriosclerosis **37**
blackness 48
convulsions 136
emaciation 174
obesity 395
paralysis 480
pulse, hard 540
reaction, lack of 558
weakness 726, 737–8

tendons:
  inflammation of 323
  injuries of 331
  subsultus tendinum 668
tobacco 636–9
  nicotinism 480, 636
  smoking (index)
turning → bending 43–6, 663–4

vaccination, after 672
  convulsions after 146
vital heat, lack of → heat 307–9

washing → bathing 40–3
wet, getting 762–4
  chorea after 74

convulsions from 147
faintness after 210
paralysis after 487
weakness from dampness 710
whisky → food, brandy 222–3
wind → weather 758–760
windy, stormy → weather 761
wine 280–2
  chorea, w. ⟨ 74
  faintness, w. ⟨ 210
  trembling from 658
  weakness, w. ⟨ , ⟩ 745
winter → seasons 571–2
  chlorose in 66

x-ray → burns, from 53

ALPHABETICAL REPERTORY OF CHARACTERISTICS
OF HOMOEOPATHIC MATERIA MEDICA
By Dr. G.D. Srivastava & Dr. J. Chandra

Pages : 1612   Size : 26cm x 18cm. in 2 columns

FOREWORD

" . . . . . his monumental work represents a life time of homoeopathic practice and prescribing and incorporates many Valuable therapeutic hints from his own wealth of experience.

"The book is unique in that the author has adopted the original concept of classifying the symptoms alphabetically rather than under the different body symptoms as in Kent, Clarke, et al. He uses modern terminology eliminating the obsolete words and obscure lessen rubrics which tend to make Kent difficult to use and unwieldly. In places he recaptures the patient's own words and their descriptions of symptoms that the remedy has cured . . . . "As far as I am aware this is the first successful attempt at publishing a repertory as comprehensive as Kent in the last half century . . . . ".

DR. R.A.F. JACK
M.B.Ch.B., M.R.C.G.P., M.F. Hom., Lecturer at the Royal London Homoeopathic Hospital &Member of the Council of the Faculty of Homoeopathy, U.K.

PREFACE

"The only available Repertory is that of Dr. Kent, ... For purposes of prescribing, he is required to re-assemble the scattered fragments to form an image similar to the case in hand which being an uphill task is generally given up for want of a direct approach.

"My Repertory is in the form of a dictionary without any division or sub-divisions, direct in approach and easy to handle even by a lay man. The moment a symptom is conceived by its clue, it is reached together with its concomitants, its emphasis and its contextual significance in the form of a completed symptom . . . To be more concise, **it is a ready-reckoner-cum-analytical Repertory** not aiming to supersede but to serve only as a supplement to Kent . . . . "

· "The rubrics consist of carefully selected clues from the essential components of a symptom, viz, the locality, sensation and modality . . . . When a symptom is approachable by more than one clue, it appears under all the various clues even at the cost of repetition . . . . . ."

Published by
B. JAIN PUBLISHERS OVERSEAS
NEW DELHI - 110 055 (INDIA)

WORD INDEX OF EXPANDED REPERTORY OF MIND SYMPTOMS

(Based on Barthel's Synthetic Repertory Vol. I and Phatak's Repertory)
By Dr. H.L. Chitkara

The importance of Mind symptoms in homoeopathy is being underlined more and more. A Word Index listing all nouns, adjectives, verbs and adverbs occuring in all the rubrics of the **Synthetic Repertory** Vol. I, as also of all those rubrics of **Phatak's Repertory** which are not represented in the Synthetic Repertory has been prepared (on the lines of Dr. R.P. Patel's monumental work Word Index with Rubrics of Kent's Repertory). It is a comprehensive Index comprising more than 15,000 entries.

If one remembers even one word of the rubric, one can come upon the complete rubric by referring to that one word in the Index.

Other Advantages

In many of the Mind symptoms, there are two components, the mind component and the body component. In the Index, these body components have been highlighted and therefore many Mind symptoms which otherwise would have been overlooked have come to the fore.

Edition 1990, Pp. 256, Hard Bound *US $* 20.

B. Jain Publishers Overseas,
1920, Street 10th, Chuna Mandi, Paharganj,
New Delhi - 110 055 (INDIA)

V